Laboratory Testing for Ambulatory Settings: A Guide for Health Care Professionals

SECOND EDITION

evolve
learning system

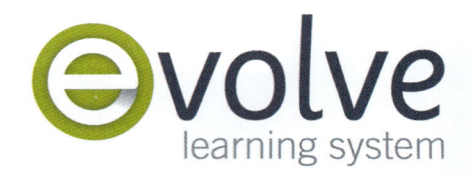

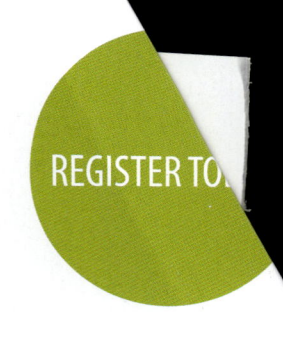

To access your Student Resources, visit:

http://evolve.elsevier.com/Garrels/laboratory

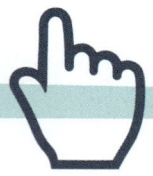

REGISTER TO

- **Structured Notes**
  These comprehensive chapter outlines provide an excellent review tool for students.

- **Clinical Skills Videos**
  These videos provide students with the opportunity to visualize concepts taught in the textbook chapters.

- **Drag and Drop Terminology**
  These activities give students a chance to interactively practice their knowledge of key terms.

- **PowerPoints**
  PowerPoint slides with images from the textbook are available on the Evolve site so that students can access them electronically.

- **Log Sheets**
  These log sheets, taken from the appendices of the Workbook, allow students to interactively engage in their laboratory experience.

- **Labeling Exercises**
  Students can use these activities to practice key concepts and important terms learned in the textbook.

- **Animations, Videos, and Lessons**
  Additional chapter resources are provided so that students can study using a variety of stimulating learning methods.

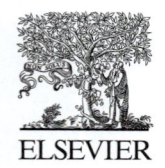

ELSEVIER

Laboratory Testing for Ambulatory Settings: A Guide for Health Care Professionals

SECOND EDITION

Marti Garrels, MSA, MT (ASCP), CMA (AAMA)
Medical Assisting Program Director
Lake Washington Technical College
Kirkland, Washington

Carol S. Oatis, MSEd, MT SM (ASCP), CMA (AAMA)
Microbiology Adjunct Instructor
Lake Sumter Community College
Leesburg, Florida

ELSEVIER
SAUNDERS

ELSEVIER
SAUNDERS

3251 Riverport Lane
St. Louis, Missouri 63043

ISBN: 978-1-4377-1906-2

Copyright © 2011, 2006 by Saunders, an imprint of Elsevier Inc.

No part of this publication may be reproduced or transmitted in any form or by any means, electronic or mechanical, including photocopying, recording, or any information storage and retrieval system, without permission in writing from the publisher. Details on how to seek permission, further information about the Publisher's permissions policies and our arrangements with organizations such as the Copyright Clearance Center and the Copyright Licensing Agency, can be found at our website: www.elsevier.com/permissions.

This book and the individual contributions contained in it are protected under copyright by the Publisher (other than as may be noted herein)

Notice

Knowledge and best practice in this field are constantly changing. As new research and experience broaden our understanding, changes in research methods, professional practices, or medical treatment may become necessary.

Practitioners and researchers must always rely on their own experience and knowledge in evaluating and using any information, methods, compounds, or experiments described herein. In using such information or methods they should be mindful of their own safety and the safety of others, including parties for whom they have a professional responsibility.

With respect to any drug or pharmaceutical products identified, readers are advised to check the most current information provided (i) on procedures featured or (ii) by the manufacturer of each product to be administered, to verify the recommended dose or formula, the method and duration of administration, and contraindications. It is the responsibility of practitioners, relying on their own experience and knowledge of their patients, to make diagnoses, to determine dosages and the best treatment for each individual patient, and to take all appropriate safety precautions.

To the fullest extent of the law, neither the Publisher nor the authors, contributors, or editors, assume any liability for any injury and/or damage to persons or property as a matter of products liability, negligence or otherwise, or from any use or operation of any methods, products, instructions, or ideas contained in the material herein.

Library of Congress Cataloging-in-Publication Data

Garrels, Marti.
  Laboratory testing for ambulatory settings : a guide for health care professionals / Marti Garrels, Carol Oatis. — 2nd ed.
      p. ; cm.
  Includes bibliographical references and index.
  ISBN 978-1-4377-1906-2 (pbk. : alk. paper) 1. Diagnosis, Laboratory. 2. Physicians' assistants 3. Medical technologists. 4. Ambulatory medical care. I. Oatis, Carol. II. Title.
    [DNLM: 1. Clinical Laboratory Techniques—methods. 2. Ambulatory Care—methods. 3. Laboratory Techniques and Procedures. QY 25]
  RB37.G37 2011
  616.07′56—dc22

2010030279

Executive Editor: Susan Cole
Developmental Editor: Jennifer Bertucci
Publishing Services Manager: Catherine Jackson
Senior Project Manager: David Stein
Design Direction: Teresa McBryan

Printed in China

Last digit is the print number: 9 8 7 6 5 4 3

Working together to grow
libraries in developing countries

www.elsevier.com | www.bookaid.org | www.sabre.org

ELSEVIER   BOOK AID International   Sabre Foundation

Reviewers for the Second Edition

MICHALEY GILGER, MLT (ASCP)
Medical Laboratory Technician
Saint Francis Hospital
Tulsa, OK

DIANA LEE-GREENE, RMA (AMT), MT (ASCP), MBA
Program Coordinator, Medical Assisting
Columbia Gorge Community College
The Dalles, OR

LISA MILLER, BBA, RMA (AMT), CPC (AAPC), MLT (ASCP), EMT-B
Medical Assistant Program Director
Coffeyville Community College
Coffeyville, KS

KAREN NELSON, RN, BA
Associate Professor
Medical Assistant Program Chair/Instructor
Iowa Western Community College
Council Bluffs, IA

DIANA REEDER, CMA (AAMA), AAS
Program Coordinator, Medical Assisting
Maysville Community Technical College
Maysville, KY

Reviewers for the First Edition

RHONDA ASHER, MT (ASCP), CMA (AAMA)
Instructor
Pitt Community College
Greenville, NC

LYNN AUGENSTERN, CMA (AAMA), BS, MA
Medical Assisting Program Director
Ridley-Lowell Business and Technical Institute
Binghamton, NY

JEANNE K. BARNETT, PHD
Professor of Biology
University of Southern Indiana
Evansville, IN

JULIE A. BENSON, RMA, EKG-PHBT TECHNICIAN
Program Director
Oklahoma Health Academy
Tulsa, OK

CYNTHIA BOLES, MBA, MT (ASCP), CMA (AAMA)
Medical Assisting Program Director
Bradford School
Pittsburgh, PA

PAMELA CARLTON, AB, MS, ABD
Director of Medical Assisting and Physician Assistant
    Program (retired)
The City University of New York/College of Staten Island
Staten Island, NY

PATRICIA A. CASTALDI, RN, BSN, MSN
Director
Union County College
Plainfield, NJ

DOLORES COTTON, RN, BSN, MS
Practical Nursing Coordinator
Meridian Technology Center
Stillwater, OK

PHYLLIS COX, MA ED, MT (ASCP)
Assistant Professor of Allied Health Sciences
Program Director of Medical Assistant and Medical
    Technology Programs
Arkansas Tech University
Russellville, AR

LORRAINE FLEMING-MCPHILLIPS, MS, MT (ASCP), CMA (AAMA)
Allied Health Education Specialist
Medical Assisting Program Coordinator (retired)
Quinebaug Valley Community College
Danielson, CT

RAUL GARZA, MD
Director of Education
Caliber Training Institute
New York, NY

J. KEITH HIATT, RRT, CPHT
Medical Assisting Program Director
Clarian Health Education Center
Indianapolis, IN

CONSTANCE L. LIESEKE, MLT, ASCP
Coordinator of Medical Assistant Program
Olympic College
Bremerton, WA

SUSAN MALEKPOUR, EDD, MS, MT (ASCP)
Curriculum Chair
Robert Morris College
Chicago, IL

WILLIAM S. SOTTILE, PHD, ABMM
Laboratory Director, Upper Peninsula Regional
    Laboratory
Michigan Department of Community Health
Houghton, MI

DICK Y. TESHIMA, MPH, MT (ASCP)
Associate Professor
University of Hawaii at Manoa
Honolulu, HI

SUSAN ANN WEITH, RN, MSN
Public Health Nurse
Marathon County Health Department
Wausau, WI

STACEY F. WILSON, MT/PBT (ASCP), CMA (AAMA)
Medical Assisting Program Coordinator
Cabarrus College of Health Sciences
Concord, NC

Reviewers for the First Edition

RHONDA ASHER, MT (ASCP), CMA (AAMA)
Instructor
Pitt Community College
Greenville, NC

LYNN AUGENSTEIN, CMA (AAMA), BS, MA
Medical Assistant Program Director
Ridley-Lowell Business and Technical Institute
Binghamton, NY

JEANNIE K. BARNETT, PHD
Professor of Biology
University of Southern Indiana
Evansville, IN

JULIE A. BENSON, RMA, SPD, PHLEBOTOMY TECHNICIAN
Program Director
Community Care College
Tulsa, OK

CYNTHIA BOLES, MBA, MT (ASCP), CMA (AAMA)
Medical Assistant Program Director
Bradford School
Pittsburgh, PA

PAMELA CARLTON, AS, MS, AuD
Director of Audiology/Assistant Clinical Assistant Professor
Truman University Speech and Language Clinic
Kirksville, MO

PATRICIA A. CASTALDI, RN, BSN, MSN
Director
Union County College
Plainfield, NJ

DOLORES COTTON, RN, BSN, MS
Practical Nursing Coordinator
Meridian Technology Center
Stillwater, OK

PHYLLIS COX, MBA, CO, MT (ASCP)
Assistant Professor, Allied Health Division
Program Coordinator of Surgical Technology and Medical Technology Programs
Arkansas State University
Russellville, AR

LORRAINE FLEMING-MCPHILLIPS, MS, MT (ASCP), CMA (AAMA)
Allied Health Education Specialist
Medical Assisting Program Coordinator
Gateway Community Colleges
Derwood, CT

RAUL GARZA, MD
Director of Education
College Training Institute
New York, NY

J. KEITH HIATT, RRT, CPFT
Medical Assisting Program Director
United Health Education Center
Indianapolis, IN

CONSTANCE D. LIESEKE, MLT, ASCP
Coordinator of Medical Assistant Program
Olympic College
Bremerton, WA

SUSAN MALEHORN, EDD, MS, MT (ASCP)
Coordinator Ithaca
Robert Morris College
Chicago, IL

WILLIAM E. SOTTILE, PHD, ABMM
Education Director (Lyon Hospital and Keweenaw Laboratories)
Michigan Technological Community College
Houghton, MI

DICK Y. TESHIMA, MPH, MT (ASCP)
Associate Professor
University of Hawaii at Manoa
Honolulu, HI

SUSAN ANN WEITH, RN, MSN
Public Health Nurse
Mendocino County Health Department
Ukiah, CA

STACEY F. WILSON, MT/PBT (ASCP), CMA (AAMA)
Medical Assisting Program Coordinator
Cabarrus College of Health Sciences
Concord, NC

Preface

This text is designed to provide students with a thorough understanding of the most common procedures and techniques of the current CLIA-waived tests, point-of-care tests, and some moderately complex tests as they apply to the ambulatory care setting. Each chapter presents a consistent "triad" organization by first focusing on the fundamental concepts, followed by the application of these concepts to the CLIA-waived procedures, and then concluding with advanced concepts to stimulate thinking. Procedure boxes are integrated throughout with step-by-step instructions and reinforced with numerous full-color photographs or illustrations. Throughout the text there is also a strong emphasis placed on proper specimen collection, safety, and government compliance. Measurable outcome-based written tests and evaluation forms are provided for each of the objective-based cognitive and procedural skills.

When writing the workbook and instructor materials, our intention was to provide instructors with many customizable tools that will help them produce well-trained, qualified allied health professionals who are able to effectively work in the CLIA-waived laboratory setting.

OUTSTANDING FEATURES

Over 450 full-color photographs, illustrations, and tables provide powerful visual learning tools that are reinforced in the PowerPoint lectures and in the workbook. Each chapter is organized into three sections to bring the reader through progressive levels of learning:
- Fundamental concepts
- Procedures
- Advanced concepts

This organization allows students and instructors to move from "seeing and understanding" the basic concepts to "performing the procedures" to "problem solving and more difficult concepts."

NOTE: In general, the first two sections of each chapter consist of material students must know and be able to perform, whereas the last section, "Advanced Concepts," allows instructors to determine the level of information the students will need to learn.

Laboratory terms are presented at the beginning of each chapter and are bolded throughout the chapter. The terms are also reinforced via the workbook and Evolve glossary exercises. Laboratory medicine has an abundance of terms that must be mastered to understand and communicate laboratory concepts and procedures effectively.

The text also includes comprehensive appendices containing:
- Common laboratory test reference values in conventional units and international units
- List of herbs and their effect on laboratory test results
- Summary of common laboratory tests
- Most common diagnoses and their related laboratory tests

These appendices provide an excellent reference tool for students and clinicians when dealing with questions regarding laboratory results and their significance to the diagnosis and treatment of the patient.

Included with the purchase of this book is access to interactive web resources, located at http://evolve.elsevier.com/Garrels/laboratory, which provides a variety of exercises and activities to reinforce learning, including:
- Comprehensive printable "structured notes" outlines for each chapter. Students are able to print out chapter outlines with fill-in-the-blanks that can be found in their text or during the instructor's PowerPoint lecture. The filled-out "structured notes" outline provides an excellent source of review for each chapter.
- PowerPoint lectures that are enhanced with corresponding text images and that provide the answers to the fill-in-the-blanks structured notes.
- Clinical Skills Videos that show various skills essential to students' success. Topics of the videos range from asepsis, infection control, and sterilization to assisting with diagnostic testing, to collecting and testing urine and microbiological specimens, to phlebotomy and hematologic, blood chemistry, and immunology. The videos provide students with a great tool to visualize concepts learned in the textbook chapters.
- Drag-and-Drop Terminology, which quizzes students on essential key terms and topics learned in the chapters.

- Log sheets, which are taken from the appendix in the workbook. On the Evolve site, they are available so that students can print them out as needed.
- Labeling exercises that give students a chance to practice key concepts learned in the textbook, like labeling the parts of a microscope.
- Animations, videos, and lessons that complement the content in the textbook and give students a chance to interactively engage in learning the material.

New to This Edition

In this new and exciting second edition, the text has been updated and expanded to provide better coverage on a multitude of topics. This additional material will help students and instructors to work together as a team in order to discover and learn about the most up-to-date procedures and concepts. The reader will find that every chapter has been updated for this new edition, and each chapter incorporates new information to assist in the learning process. Important additions include the following:
- Over 60 new pictures and drawings
- Chapter 1 has been split into two chapters and contains updated quality assurance and quality control concepts
- Updates on proper collection and processing of urine specimens, microbiology specimens, blood capillary and venipuncture specimens, which include new urine culture using a vacutainer system, new drawings for urine and influenza specimen collections, and the latest order of blood draw including the plasma separator tube
- Six new procedures with corresponding skill check sheets—Clinitek Analyzer, Standard Hematocrit (in addition to the Hemostat method), INRatio (replaces the previous Protime 3), New A1c+ Kit (replaces the DCA2000 analyzer), the new iFOB method for fecal occult blood, and new i-STAT chemistry tests
- New complete chapter on toxicology (Chapter 9)

Workbook for *Laboratory Testing for Ambulatory Settings,* ISBN 978-1-4377-1908-6

This valuable learning tool for the student contains measurable outcomes for all the conceptual and competency-based objectives in each chapter in order to fulfill CAAHEP accreditation standards. Accreditation agencies now require measurable outcomes along with competency-based objectives.

It contains *Skill Competency Check Sheets and Analytical Testing Competency Check Sheets.* The testing procedures are organized into preanalytical, analytical, and postanalytical testing phases. These sheets can be used in the classroom and clinical laboratory settings to verify individual competency that meets the "Good Laboratory Practice" criteria for quality assurance. In this new edition, five new procedure sheets have been added (to correspond with the five new procedures in the text).

The appendix includes useful quality control log sheets, lab maintenance log sheets, report forms, and a sample health screening assessment form. These forms provide the necessary documentation needed to prove laboratory quality assurance, safety compliance, and proper charting of test results. For this new edition, quality control Levy-Jennings charts have also been added.

Instructor's Resource Manual for *Laboratory Testing for Ambulatory Settings,* located on the Evolve site at: http://evolve.elsevier.com/Garrels/laboratory

The *Instructor's Resource Manual* was created to provide instructors or CLIA-waived lab supervisors with a wealth of material needed to run a successful class or clinical laboratory. All the material has been "field-tested" to help ensure the accuracy and quality of material. For the second edition, this valuable tool has been made available online in Word document format, so that instructors can have the ability to edit and update the files to suit their own needs. The *Instructor's Resource Manual* on Evolve contains:
- Information on how to set up course schedules, grading, record keeping, and so forth.
- Field-tested tips and supplies needed for each chapter.
- Chapter outlines with fill-in-the-blank answers to the students' structured notes.
- Answer keys to student workbook exercises.
- Interactive skill check-off sheets.
- Test questions and answer keys for each chapter.
- Appendices with additional laboratory forms, record-keeping logs, generic procedure sheets (if the program uses a method other than what is presented in the book).
- Comprehensive PowerPoint lecture slides that follow the chapter outlines and provide the answers to the students' structured notes.
- PowerPoint lectures with pictures from each chapter.
- Test Bank in ExamView format.
- All the forms from the workbook to allow for customization to fit individual needs.
- Complete Image Collection from the textbook with figure legends.

Evolve Course Management System for *Laboratory Testing for Ambulatory Settings:* http://evolve.elsevier.com/Garrels/laboratory

Evolve is an interactive learning environment that works in conjunction with *Laboratory Testing for Ambulatory Settings: A Guide for Health Care Professionals,* providing Internet-based course content that reinforces and expands on the concepts that instructors deliver in class. In addition to the resources available to students, instructors are able to access all of the components of the *Instructor's Resource Manual* listed above.

Instructors can also use Evolve to:
- Publish class syllabi, outlines, and lecture notes.
- Set up "virtual office hours" and email communication.
- Share important dates and information through the online class *Calendar.*
- Encourage student participation through *Chat Rooms* and *Discussions Boards.*

Acknowledgments

I would like to acknowledge the valuable input of all the reviewers, medical assisting educators, and students that have helped to make this second edition even better than the first.

I am grateful to all the Elsevier publishers, editors, reviewers, and staff who have personally supported and guided us through this exciting adventure, especially the following: Adrianne Rippinger, Rae Robertson, Katherine Judge, and Elizabeth Tinsley on the first edition, and Michael Ledbetter, Susan Cole, Jennifer Bertucci, Jennifer Hermes, and David Stein on the second edition. I am blessed by the wonderful talents of my son-in-law and daughter, Zack and Gala Bent, who have graciously provided us with all of the high-quality, up-to-date procedure photos and drawings. I have also been blessed by my husband, Mike, who has provided unwavering support through this process. Finally, I am so thankful to have had the opportunity to work with a terrific co-author during the first edition, Carol Oatis.

Marti Garrels, MSA, MT (ASCP), CMA (AAMA)

I would like to thank my family for all of their support during the time that I was involved in the writing of the first edition of this textbook. Also, it has been a great pleasure to work with my co-author, Marti Garrels, who is a tremendous asset to the medical assisting profession.

Carol Oatis, MSEd, MT SM (ASCP), CMA (AAMA)

Contents

List of Procedures, *xvii*

1 Introduction to the Laboratory and Safety Training, *1*
    Fundamental Concepts, *3*
    Overview of the Laboratory, *3*
    Safety Training in the Laboratory, *14*

2 Regulations, Microscope Setup, and Quality Assurance, *32*
    CLIA: Government Regulations, *33*
    CLIA Levels of Complexity and Their Certification Requirements, *33*
    Microscope Procedure, *36*
    Preparation: Identifying the Parts and Functions of a Microscope, *36*
    Good Laboratory Practices, *41*
    Quality Assurance, *41*
    Quality Control, *44*
    HIPAA Privacy Rule, *48*
    Risk Management, *48*
    Electronic Medical Records and Bar Coding, *48*

3 Urinalysis, *51*
    Fundamental Concepts and Collection Procedures, *52*
    Anatomy of the Urinary System, *52*
    Urine Specimen Collection, *55*
    CLIA-Waived Tests, *60*
    Urinalysis, *60*
    Advanced Concepts, *72*
    Microscopic Urinalysis, *72*
    Calculating a Microscopic Urinalysis, *75*

4 Blood Collection, *86*
    Fundamental Concepts, *87*
    Function and Structures of Blood Vessels, *87*
    Federal Law Concerning Safety Equipment, *89*
    Procedure Preparation, *90*
    Blood Collection Procedures, *91*
    Capillary Puncture, *91*
    Venipuncture, *95*
    Preparing Blood Specimens for Laboratory Pickup, *104*
    Advanced Concepts, *123*
    Complications, *123*
    Risk Management, *126*

5 Hematology, *128*
    Fundamental Concepts, *129*
    Overview of Hematology and Blood, *129*
    Preparing a Blood Smear for Observation by Physician or Laboratory Technician, *135*
    Theory of Hemostasis, *139*
    Summary of Fundamental Concepts, *144*
    CLIA-Waived Hematology Tests, *146*
    Hemoglobin, *146*
    Hematocrit, *147*
    Erythrocyte Sedimentation Rate, *148*
    Prothrombin Time, *149*
    Becoming Proficient at CLIA-Waived Hematology Tests, *149*
    Advanced Concepts, *159*
    Complete Blood Count, *159*
    Abnormal Complete Blood Count Findings, *162*
    CLIA-Nonwaived (Moderately Complex) Automated Hematology Systems, *165*

6 Chemistry, *171*
    Fundamental Concepts, *172*
    Blood Plasma, *172*
    Blood Chemistry Specimens, *173*
    Glucose Metabolism and Testing, *176*
    Lipid Metabolism and Testing, *179*
    CLIA-Waived Chemistry Tests, *181*
    Principle of Photometers and Spectrophotometers, *181*
    CLIA-Waived Glucose Tests, *183*
    Cholesterol and Lipid Profiles with the Cholestech LDX, *183*
    Fecal Occult Blood Testing with the Guaiac Method, *184*
    Summary of CLIA-Waived Tests, *184*
    Becoming Proficient at CLIA-Waived Chemistry Testing, *184*
    Advanced Concepts, *198*
    i-STAT, *198*
    Piccolo, *199*
    Metabolic Panels: Basic and Comprehensive, *199*
    Individual Analytes and Their Disease Associations, *201*
    Summary, *201*

7 Immunology, 209
Fundamental Concepts, 210
Overview of Immunology, 210
Two Types of Allergy Testing, 215
CLIA-Waived Immunology Tests, 215
CLIA-Waived Enzyme-Linked Immunoassays, 215
Pregnancy Testing, 216
Mononucleosis Testing, 217
Helicobacter pylori Testing, 217
Human Immunodeficiency Virus, 218
Fecal Occult Blood Testing Using iFOB Kits, 218
Advanced Concepts, 225
Agglutination Reactions (Non–CLIA-Waived Tests), 225
Enzyme-Linked Immunosorbent Assay: Quantitative Analysis, 226
Summary of Immunological Tests, 227

8 Microbiology, 236
Fundamental Concepts, 237
Overview of Microbiology, 237
Collecting, Transporting, and Processing Microbiology Specimens, 239
Microbiology Smears, Stains, and Wet Mounts, 243
Pinworm Specimen Collection and Microscopic Results, 246
CLIA-Waived Microbiology Tests, 251
Streptococcus Group A Testing, 251
Influenza, 252
Advanced Concepts, 257
Growth Requirements of Bacteria, 257
Media Used for Growing Bacteria, 258
Microbiology Equipment, 259
Culturing Methods, 259
Biochemical Testing, 261
Sensitivity Testing, 261
Pathogenic Organisms Seen Frequently in Physician Office Laboratories, 262
Emerging Infectious Diseases, 264
Bioterrorism, 264

9 Toxicology, 274
Fundamental Concepts, 275
Overview of Toxicology, 275
Drugs of Abuse, 275
CLIA-Waived Drug Screening Tests, 281
Advanced Concepts, 283
Therapeutic Drug Monitoring, 283
Pharmacokinetics, 283
Drug Half-Life and Specimen Collection, 285
Other Toxicology Tests, 285
Summary, 285

Appendices
A Reference Values, 289
B Herb/Laboratory Test Interactions, 293
C Common Laboratory Tests, 296
D Frequent Medical Diagnoses and Laboratory Tests, 304

Glossary, 315

Index, 321

Procedures

CHAPTER 1: Introduction to the Laboratory and Safety Training
Procedure 1-1: Proper Use of Personal Protective Equipment, 27

CHAPTER 2: Regulations, Microscope Setup, and Quality Assurance
Procedure 2-1: Using a Microscope, 38

CHAPTER 3: Urinalysis
Procedure 3-1: Instructing Patients How to Collect a Clean-Catch Urine Specimen, 57
Procedure 3-2: Instructing Patients How to Collect a 24-Hour Urine Specimen, 60
Procedure 3-3: Manual Chemical Reagent Strip Procedure, 68
Procedure 3-4: Clinitek Analyzer Method for Chemical Reagent Strip, 70
Procedure 3-5: Clinitest Procedure for Reducing Substances Such as Sugars in the Urine, 72
Procedure 3-6: Procedure for the Preparation and the Microscopic Examination of Urine, 82

CHAPTER 4: Blood Collection
Procedure 4-1: Capillary Puncture Procedure, 106
Procedure 4-2: Heel Stick for Neonatal Screening Test Procedure, 109
Procedure 4-3: Vacutainer Method, 112
Procedure 4-4: Syringe Method, 116
Procedure 4-5: Two Butterfly Methods from a Hand and Training Model, 118

CHAPTER 5: Hematology
Procedure 5-1: Diff Staining Procedure, 145
Procedure 5-2: Hemoglobin: HemoCue Method, 149
Procedure 5-3: Hematocrit: General Procedure, 151
Procedure 5-4: Hematocrit: HemataSTAT Method, 153
Procedure 5-5: ESR: SEDIPLAST System Procedure, 155
Procedure 5-6: Prothrombin Time INRatio (HemoSense) Method, 157

CHAPTER 6: Chemistry
Procedure 6-1: Glucometer Procedure, 185
Procedure 6-2: A1c NOW+ Glycosylated Hemoglobin Procedure, 187
Procedure 6-3: Cholestech Method of Measuring Lipids and Glucose, 190
Procedure 6-4: Occult Blood: ColoScreen III Method and ColoCARE Method, 194
Procedure 6-5: i-STAT Chemistry Analyzer Procedure, 205

CHAPTER 7: Immunology
Procedure 7-1: SureStep Pregnancy Test Procedure, 219
Procedure 7-2: QuickVue+ Mononucleosis Test Procedure, 221
Procedure 7-3: QuickVue *Helicobacter pylori* gII Test (CLIA-Waived) Procedure, 224
Procedure 7-4: Agglutination Slide Testing Procedure for ABO Blood Typing, 229
Procedure 7-5: Rh Blood Typing Procedure by the Slide Method, 232

CHAPTER 8: Microbiology
Procedure 8-1: Procedure for Collecting a Throat Specimen, 247
Procedure 8-2: Gram Stain Procedure, 248
Procedure 8-3: Wet Mount Procedure, 251
Procedure 8-4: KOH Preparation Procedure, 251
Procedure 8-5: Acceava Strep A Test Procedure, 253
Procedure 8-6: OSOM Influenza A and B Test Procedure, 255

CHAPTER 9: Toxicology
Procedure 9-1: Assisting with Urine Collection for Drug Screening, 279
Procedure 9-2: Assisting with Blood Collection for Alcohol Testing, 280
Procedure 9-3: Urine Drug Panel Testing Procedure, 282

CHAPTER 1
Introduction to the Laboratory and Safety Training

Objectives
After completing this chapter you should be able to:

Introduction to the Clinical Laboratory
1. List the reasons why laboratory tests are ordered, and describe how specimens are analyzed.
2. Describe the organization and function of medical laboratories.
3. Compare the advantages and disadvantages of performing laboratory tests in a physician's office laboratory versus an outside reference laboratory.
4. Identify the educational credentials of various personnel who work in laboratories.
5. Describe the necessary attributes required of the laboratory professional.
6. Identify and use laboratory requisitions and reports with proper documentation and confidentiality.
7. Interpret common metric system values used in laboratory test reporting.

Safety Training
1. Identify and apply the CDC's latest Standard Precautions for infection control and its recommendations regarding proper hand hygiene.
2. Explain the latest OSHA regulations regarding the Bloodborne Pathogens Standard and the Hazard Communication Program.
3. Identify waste classified as biohazardous, and select appropriate containers for disposal.
4. Describe the proper actions to take after exposure to bloodborne pathogens.
5. List and explain the safety rules that must be observed in the laboratory.
6. Successfully complete a posttest on safety training.
7. Locate Internet sources for updates on OSHA regulations and CDC recommendations regarding laboratory safety.
8. Identify and note the location of safety equipment, apparel, and safety manuals in the classroom laboratory.
9. Perform a medical hand wash followed by application of PPE and proper removal of PPE.
10. Complete a mock exposure incident report in the workbook appendix.

Key Terms

ambulatory setting outpatient facility versus hospital or bedridden setting

analyte the substance being tested, such as glucose or cholesterol in a blood specimen

biohazard danger related to exposure to infectious and bloodborne pathogens

bloodborne pathogens infectious microorganisms that are transmitted by the blood or bloody body fluid from an infected host into the blood of a susceptible host

Bloodborne Pathogens Standard (BBPS) rigorous standard of policies and procedures developed by OSHA to protect employees who work in occupations where they are at risk of exposure to blood or other potentially infectious materials (i.e., other body fluids that may contain blood)

chemical hazard danger related to exposure to toxic, unstable, explosive, or flammable substances

chronic disorders long-lasting, debilitating conditions

CLIA-waived tests tests that provide simple, unvarying results and require a minimum amount of judgment and interpretation

clinical laboratory a facility or an area within a medical setting in which materials or specimens from the human body are examined or analyzed

coagulation clotting ability of blood

contaminated an area that has been in contact with infectious materials or surfaces where infectious organisms may reside

C-reactive protein (CRP) protein associated with myocardial infarctions (heart attacks)

critical value a test result far from the reference range indicating a threat to a patient's health (also referred to as "panic value")

cross-contamination transmitting a pathogen from one individual to another

diabetes mellitus disease caused by the lack of insulin or the inability to regulate blood sugar levels

Key Terms—cont'd

don to put on

engineering controls efforts and research toward isolating or removing bloodborne pathogens from the workplace (i.e., biohazard disposal containers, safety devices on needles, and sharps containers)

ergonomic practices proper movements and conditions that make a worker less prone to work-related injuries

exposure control plan documented plan provided by a facility to eliminate or minimize occupational exposure to bloodborne pathogens

glucose sugar

Hazard Communication Standard federal law protecting employees' "right to know" about the dangers of all the hazardous chemicals they may be exposed to under normal working conditions

hepatitis A virus (HAV) highly contagious virus that enters the body through the gastrointestinal tract and attacks the liver

hepatitis B virus (HBV) most prevalent bloodborne virus that attacks the liver: an individual can build a protective resistance against this virus by prior immunization or vaccination

hepatitis C virus (HCV) bloodborne virus that attacks the liver and is very likely to reach the chronic stage later in life

homeostasis steady state of internal chemical and physical balance

human immunodeficiency virus (HIV) retrovirus that attacks the immune system by destroying the white blood cells known as CD4+ T lymphocytes

laboratory reports results of laboratory tests that have been ordered

laboratory requisitions laboratory orders indicating what tests are to be performed

medical assistants multiskilled professionals dedicated to assisting in patient care management in medical offices, clinics, and ambulatory care centers

nosocomial infection disease spread within a health care facility (also referred to as HCAIs [health care associated infections])

occupational exposure occurs when blood or other potentially infectious material comes in contact with open skin, eye, or mucous membrane or parenterally in the workplace

opportunistic infections infections that occur because of the body's inability to fight off pathogens normally found in the environment

panels/profiles a series of tests associated with a particular organ or disease

parenteral contact when blood enters the body through the skin or mucous membrane by means of a needle stick, bite, cut, or abrasion

pathogen disease-causing microorganism

patient compliance a patient's willingness to follow a treatment plan and take an active role in his or her health care

percutaneous through the skin

physical hazards dangers related to electricity, fire, weather emergencies, bomb threats, and accidental injuries

polydipsia excessive thirst

polyphagia excessive hunger

polyuria excessive urination

portal of entry a body opening or break in the skin through which an infectious agent enters the body

portal of exit the route by which an infectious agent leaves the host's body, such as through the mouth, broken skin, rectum, or body fluids

reagent substance or ingredient used in a laboratory test to detect, measure, examine, or produce a reaction

reference range the range of analyte values with which the general population will consistently show similar results 95% of the time

reservoir host an infected person who is carrying an infectious agent (pathogen)

Standard Precautions CDC recommendations for infection control within health care facilities

susceptible host an individual who is unable to defend herself or himself against a pathogen

transient microorganisms organisms from contaminated objects or infectious patients that adhere to the skin and can be transmitted to others

transmission the means by which an infectious agent or pathogen is transported from an infected individual to another person by indirect or direct contact

Universal Precautions assumption that blood or other potentially infectious material from any patient or test kit could be infectious

venipuncture removal of blood from a vein

Abbreviations

CDC	Centers for Disease Control and Prevention
HCAIs	health care associated infections
HHS	Department of Health and Human Services
HMIS	hazardous materials information system
MSDS	material safety data sheets
NFPA	National Fire Protective Association
OPIM	other potentially infectious material, such as bloody body fluids
OSHA	Occupational Safety and Health Administration
PEP	postexposure prophylaxis; preventive treatment after exposure to blood or OPIM
POCT	point-of-care testing
POL	physician's office laboratory
PPE	personal protective equipment

FUNDAMENTAL CONCEPTS

To enter the investigative world of medical laboratories, a general understanding of the various laboratories that perform medical tests on specimens is needed. Before laboratory procedures can be performed in the **ambulatory setting** (outpatient facility versus hospital or bedridden setting), a solid foundation is required in laboratory safety issues and government regulations regarding which tests can be performed and how to perform them.

Overview of the Laboratory

The medical laboratory plays a critical role in patient care. This section provides information on the following:
- Why and how laboratory tests are performed
- Where the tests are performed
- How various medical laboratories are organized
- The people involved in the testing process
- The basic terminology and paperwork used in the laboratory

Purpose of Medical Laboratories

A medical or **clinical laboratory** is defined as a facility or an area within a medical setting in which materials, or specimens, from the human body are examined or analyzed. The results of the various laboratory tests performed on the specimens give the physician a wealth of information regarding the status of the patient or client. Physicians and health care providers use medical laboratories to collect and test specimens for three basic reasons and in three ways.

Why Laboratory Tests Are Ordered

Physicians order laboratory tests for one or more of the following reasons:

1. *To screen patients for possible disorders.* Screening test results are used to determine if a disease or medical condition exists in patients who may not have signs or symptoms of an underlying disease process. These tests are becoming increasingly popular because they can detect potential **chronic disorders** (long-lasting, debilitating conditions) such as coronary heart disease and diabetes well before irreversible damage sets in. Primary care physician offices and community health centers are encouraged by the latest Medicare policies to participate in screening programs. The workbook has a health screening report form that includes the various screening tests that will be presented throughout the text and in the laboratory sessions.
2. *To establish a diagnosis.* Diagnostic test results help identify or confirm a disease or medical condition. These results can significantly affect the medical care and treatment of the patient. Diagnostic tests should be run by well-trained individuals and must correlate with other clinical findings (e.g., the patient's medical history and physical examination).
3. *To monitor the patient's condition or treatment.* Monitoring test results helps the physician keep track of the patient's specific medical condition or response to treatment on a periodic basis. The following three medical conditions commonly require routine testing to monitor the effects of medication treatments:
    - Patients at risk of heart disease who are taking cholesterol-lowering medications are checked periodically for cholesterol levels and liver enzymes. The medication goal is to bring cholesterol levels below 200 and to determine whether the medication is harming the liver, which would raise the blood enzymes ALT and AST (this will be covered in Chapter 6). They may also be tested for **C reactive protein (CRP)**, which is associated with myocardial infarction (heart attack) and indicates the health status of the patient's cardiovascular system.
    - Patients at risk of forming internal clots **(thrombosis)** who are taking anticoagulant medications are checked to see if their blood **coagulation** (clotting) time is too fast or too slow.
    - Patients with diabetes have their blood sugar levels checked periodically at the office. They also may have their self-monitored blood sugar results interpreted by the physician. In both cases the physician needs to determine if these patients are maintaining blood sugar levels within the recommended **reference range** (the range of analyte values with which the general population will consistently show similar results).

Advances in medical instrumentation have allowed the monitoring of all these patients to take place in an ambulatory setting rather than in a hospital or reference laboratory. This allows the physician to see the results immediately, while the patient waits, and then advise the patient accordingly.

Three General Ways to Analyze Specimens

Medical laboratories analyze specimens in the following three basic ways:

1. *Measuring the levels of analytes compared with reference values.* The human body is a remarkable organism, capable of maintaining **homeostasis** (a steady state of internal chemical and physical balance). This universal ability is seen when a healthy population is tested for the presence of a particular **analyte** (a substance being tested, such as the level of glucose or cholesterol in a blood specimen). Most of the population will test within a range of similar results. This is referred to as the *reference*

range for that analyte. When disease strikes, a person's homeostatic balance is disrupted, causing the analyte results to fall outside the reference range.

The following is an example of the information that can be obtained by monitoring the level of a patient's **glucose** (sugar) analyte and comparing it to its established population's reference range. A physician obtained a variety of abnormal clinical signs and symptoms when examining a female patient—rapid weight loss, lack of energy, **polyphagia** (excessive hunger), **polydipsia** (excessive thirst), and **polyuria** (excessive urination). These symptoms caused the physician to suspect the disease **diabetes mellitus** (a disease caused by the lack of insulin or the inability to regulate blood sugar levels). The physician then ordered a blood glucose test and received a result of 300 mg/dL (milligrams per deciliter). The population's reference range for blood glucose levels was 70 to 110 mg/dL. The patient's extremely high glucose result, along with all the other signs and symptoms, indicated that her pancreas was unable to produce the insulin necessary to regulate glucose in a homeostatic way. A repeat fasting blood glucose test showed the same high result that confirmed the diagnosis of diabetes. The physician then prescribed a course of treatment and continued to monitor the blood glucose levels until the patient's test results returned to the proper reference range.

Fig. 1-1 is an example of a reference laboratory's comprehensive report for blood tests. Note that the reference range for each analyte tested is listed above the patient's test value. If a test result is far from the reference range, it may be referred to as a **critical value or panic value** (indicating a threat to a patient's health). The laboratory report must mark or highlight the critical result requiring immediate attention. In the figure, Judith Johnson does not have any critical values. A variety of **laboratory reports** (results of laboratory tests that have been ordered) are shown and discussed throughout this text.

2. *Observing and detecting abnormal cells under the microscope.* Another way to analyze a specimen is to search for abnormal cells or **pathogens** (disease-causing microorganisms) under the microscope. In the ambulatory setting this form of testing is generally limited to basic identification of abnormal cells and microorganisms found in urine, blood, or samples taken from infected tissues. Fig. 1-2 shows the abnormal presence of red blood cells and yeast cells in a urine specimen.

This book discusses some of the normal and abnormal microscopic findings in urine, blood, and microbiology specimens to highlight their significance. Additional training beyond this text is required to identify and report microscopic findings.

3. *Detecting the presence or absence of an infection.* The third way to analyze specimens is to test for the presence of pathogens causing an infection. In the ambulatory setting increasing numbers of rapid screening tests are available to help the physician identify the presence of common pathogens. For example, test **kits** (all components of a test packaged together) are available that can detect the presence of bacteria that cause strep throat, peptic ulcers, and Lyme disease as well as the viruses that cause influenza, mononucleosis, and AIDS. Note the Rapid Strep test results from two throat-swabbed specimens in Fig. 1-3. The left test result is negative for streptococcus A, and the right test is positive for streptococcus A. Further microscopic, chemical, and growth analysis of the pathogen, along with analysis of the pathogen's sensitivity to antibiotics, is performed by sending the infected swabbed specimen to a microbiology laboratory.

Types of Medical Laboratories and Personnel

The types of medical laboratories range from large, departmentalized institutions to small designated laboratory counters within an ambulatory setting. Personnel in the ambulatory setting interact with staff from all the other types of laboratories and need a basic understanding of how the various laboratories are organized and what types of health care professionals work in each setting.

Reference (or Referral) Laboratories

Reference, or referral, laboratories tend to be the largest laboratories, with specialized departments and extensive state-of-the-art equipment. Fig. 1-4 is a sample organizational chart showing the departments typically found in a reference laboratory facility: Specimen Collection and Processing, Hematology, Chemistry, Immunology/Immunohematology, Microbiology, Pathology, and Toxicology.

The reference laboratory is typically staffed with the following trained laboratory professionals:

- **Pathologists** are physicians with doctorate degrees who have specialized in test methodology and the diagnosis of diseases.
- **Clinical laboratory scientists** and **medical technologists** have master's and bachelor's degrees, are specialists in laboratory testing, and have received one of the following nationally recognized credentials: MT (ASCP), MT (AMT), CLS (NCA), RMT (ISCLT), or CLT.
- **Medical technicians** have 2-year associate degrees in laboratory training and have received one of the following nationally recognized credentials: MLT (ASCP), MLT (AMT), CLT (NCA), or RLT (ISCLT).

These teams of laboratory professionals process and evaluate volumes of tests daily and are heavily regulated by the government to ensure that they produce accurate and reliable test results. It is interesting to note that 80% of final definitive diagnoses come from the results of laboratory tests. The testing methods in each department require extensive training in instrument maintenance, problem-solving, test interpretation, and statistical monitoring of test reliability.

Medical offices, health clinics, and hospitals send either their clients or their clients' specimens along with **laboratory requisitions** (laboratory orders indicating what tests are to be performed) to the reference lab. Some insurance companies require a specific

LABORATORY REPORT
Biomedical Laboratories, Inc
100 Main Street
Athens, Georgia 30601

DATE REPORTED	DATE RECEIVED	PATIENT NAME—I.D.		PHONE	AGE	SEX
4/12/10	4/11/10	Judith Johnson	08575	(614) 592-1100	26	F
DATE COLLECTED	**TIME COLLECTED**	**HOSPITAL I.D.**	**REQUISITION NO.**		**ACCESSION NO.**	
4/11/10	8:30 AM		91449		1235-G8	

CLIENT NAME/ADDRESS	TEST REQUIRED
Woodside Medical Clinic 400 Main Street Athens, Ohio 45701	Comprehensive Metabolic Profile Lipid Profile CBC with Differential

PHYSICIAN	VOLUME	FASTING	PATIENT SS #	COMMENTS
J. Camerson, M.D.		X	248-71-2669	

CHEMISTRY — RENAL / ELECTROLYTES

GLUCOSE 70–110 mg/dL	B.U.N. 7–25 mg/dL	CREATININE 0.6–1.5 mg/dL	BUN/CREAT RATIO 6–20	CALCIUM 8.5–10.8 mg/dL	MAGNESIUM 0.6–1.0 mmol/L	PHOSPHORUS 2.5–4.5 mg/dL	SODIUM 135–147 mmol/L	POTASSIUM 3.5–5.3 mmol/L	CHLORIDE 96–109 mmol/L	CARBON DIOXIDE 21–28 mmol/L	FERRITIN M 20–450 F 8–350 ng/mL
91	24	1.3	18.5	9.8		3.3	140.6	4.45	105	24	

PROTEIN / LIVER

URIC ACID M 3.9–9.0 F 2.7–7.7 mg/dL	TOTAL PROTEIN 6.0–8.5 g/dL	ALBUMIN 3.5–5.5 g/dL	GLOBULIN 2.0–3.5 g/dL	ALB/GLB RATIO 1.0–2.4	TOTAL BILIRUBIN 0.2–1.3 mg/dL	DIRECT BILIRUBIN 0–0.4 mg/dL	ALK. PHOS 25–140 U/L	LD £ 240 U/L	AST (SGOT) £ 40 U/L	ALT (SGPT) £ 45 U/L	GGT M 0–65 F 0–45 U/L
	6.8	4.1	2.8	1.5	0.3		82		29	38	

THYROID / LIPIDS

T_3 UPTAKE 25–35 %	T_4 TOTAL 4.5–12 mg/dL	FTI (T_3U×T_4) 1.2–4.2	TSH 0.4–6.0 mIU/mL	T_4 FREE 0.70–1.53 ng/dL	T_3 TOTAL 85–205 ng/mL	TOTAL CHOL < 200 mg/dL	HDL CHOL > 40 mg/dL	LDL CHOL < 130 mg/dL	VLDL CHOL 5–40 mg/dL	TRIGLYCERIDES < 150 mg/dL	TOTAL CHOL/ HDL RATIO < 4.5
						158	43	83	32	*160	3.7

HEMATOLOGY

WBC 4.5–11 ×10³/mL	RBC M 4.5–6.2 F 4–5.5 ×10⁶/mL	HGB M 14–18 F 12–16 g/dL	HCT M 40–54 F 37–47 %	MCV 80–100 fL	MCH 27–34 pg	MCHC 31–36 %	RDW 11.5–14.5 %	PLATELET COUNT 150–400 ×10³/mL	RETICULOCYTE COUNT 0.5–2.5 %	ESR M 0–15 F 0–20 mm/Hr	PROTHROMBIN TIME 9–12 seconds
*12.3	4.27	13.4	39	91	31.3	34.5	13.7	258			

DIFFERENTIAL / SEROLOGY

NEUT 50–70 %	LYMPH 20–35 %	MONO 3–8 %	EOSIN 1–4 %	BASO 0–1 %	SYPHILLIS SCREEN NON-REACTIVE	MONO TEST NEG	RHEUMATOID FACTOR < 1:10	CRP < 0.8 mg/dL	ANTINUCLEAR ANTIBODY < 1:140	BLOOD GROUP	$RH_o(D)$
*83	*12	3	2	0							

URINALYSIS

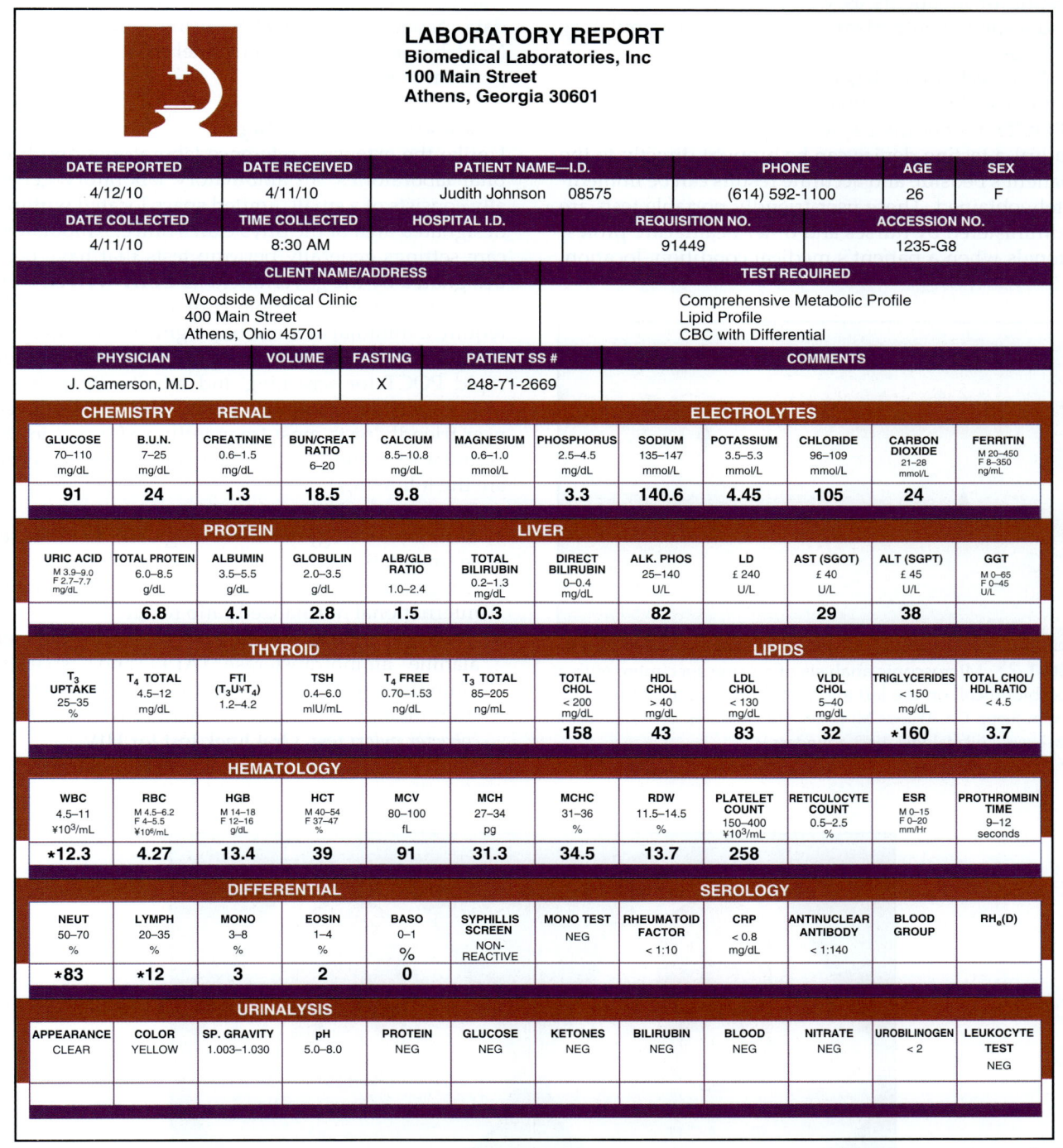

APPEARANCE	COLOR	SP. GRAVITY 1.003–1.030	pH 5.0–8.0	PROTEIN NEG	GLUCOSE NEG	KETONES NEG	BILIRUBIN NEG	BLOOD NEG	NITRATE NEG	UROBILINOGEN < 2	LEUKOCYTE TEST NEG
CLEAR	YELLOW										

Fig. 1-1. Blood test report showing the levels of a comprehensive panel of analytes. Compare the patient's results with the reference range above each one. Note the four results that fall outside of their reference ranges. In this report the TRIGLYCERIDES, WBC (white blood cells), and NEUT (neutrophils) are high, and the LYMPH (lymphocytes) are low. (From Bonewit-West K: *Clinical procedures for medical assistants,* ed 7, St Louis, 2008, Saunders.)

reference laboratory for their clients. The client's specimen and requisition must go to the correct reference laboratory for proper insurance reimbursement.

Hospital Laboratories

Hospital laboratories are organized into departments and staffed similarly to reference laboratories. They are involved in diagnostic testing and monitoring the testing of inpatients as well as specimen collection and testing of outpatient specimens from ambulatory settings.

New technology has provided a new approach to patient testing in hospitals called point-of-care testing **(POCT)**. Rather than sending specimens to the laboratory, a testing device can be brought directly to the patient's bedside and accurate results can be immediately obtained. These user-friendly portable tests are administered by nurses and other health care professionals when a patient's medical condition, location, or treatment requires immediate results to determine proper medical care. Fig. 1-5 shows a patient's blood glucose readout of 71 mg/dL on a point-of-care glucometer. Another popular point-of-care instrument is the I-STAT Portable Clinical Analyzer (PCA). It uses disposable cartridges to determine a variety of analytes in whole blood. The analyzer stores up to 50 patient records and permits on-screen viewing of test results. It is capable of transmitting the results to a data management system by using infrared signals. Nonlaboratory hospital personnel must be trained to perform POCT properly.

Ambulatory Care Settings

Unlike the extensive reference laboratories and hospital laboratories, an ambulatory laboratory generally consists of a small, limited space located within a designated area of the physician's office. Ambulatory care settings generally perform tests that have been designated by the government as **CLIA-waived tests** (tests that provide simple, unvarying results and require a minimal amount of judgment and interpretation). These government-approved tests provide rapid POCT for screening and monitoring patients in a variety of laboratory areas. The CLIA-waived user-friendly tests most frequently performed in the ambulatory setting that will be presented in this text are the following:

- Routine urinalysis and pregnancy testing
- Basic hematology tests—hemoglobin, hematocrit, sedimentation rate
- Coagulation—prothrombin time and its computed international normalized ratio result
- Chemistry—glucose, hemoglobin A1c, lipid panel, alanine aminotransferase (ALT) and aspartate aminotransferase (AST), electrolytes, and BUN
- Immunology/serology—mononucleosis test, *Helicobacter pylori* test, OraQuick test for HIV

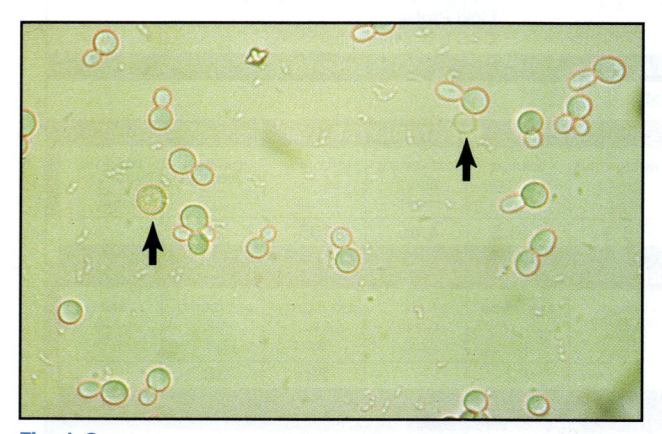

Fig. 1-2. Microscopic analysis of a urine specimen, with a red blood cell on the left and a budding yeast on the right. (From Stepp CA, Woods M: *Laboratory procedures for medical office personnel*, Philadelphia, 1998, Saunders.)

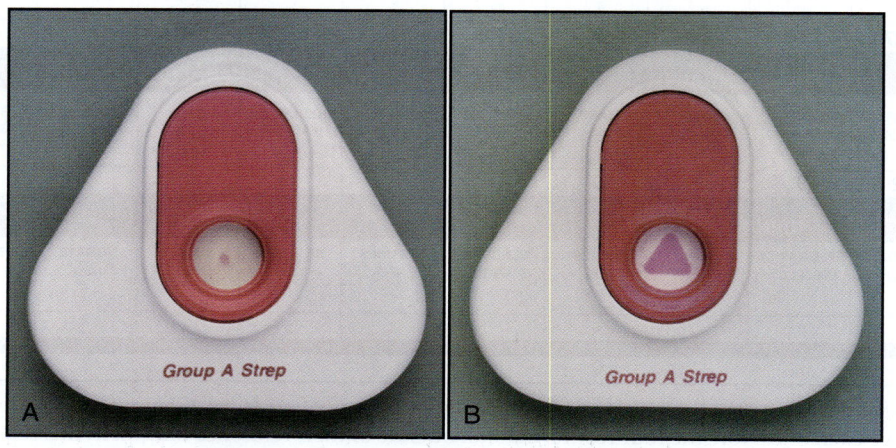

Fig. 1-3. Analyzing the presence of group A strep. **A** is negative and **B** is positive for strep throat infection. (From Mahon CR, Manuselis G: *Textbook of diagnostic microbiology*, ed 3, St Louis, 2006, Saunders. Courtesy Becton Dickinson.)

Fundamental Concepts

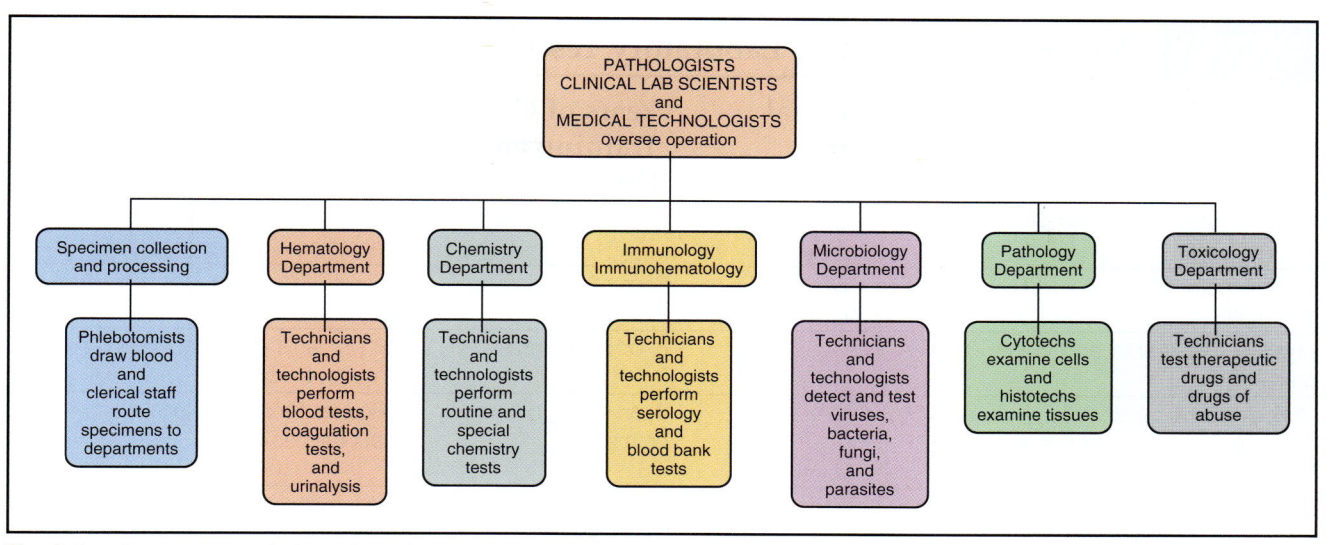

Fig. 1-4. Organizational chart for reference and hospital laboratories showing the departments and individuals involved in testing.

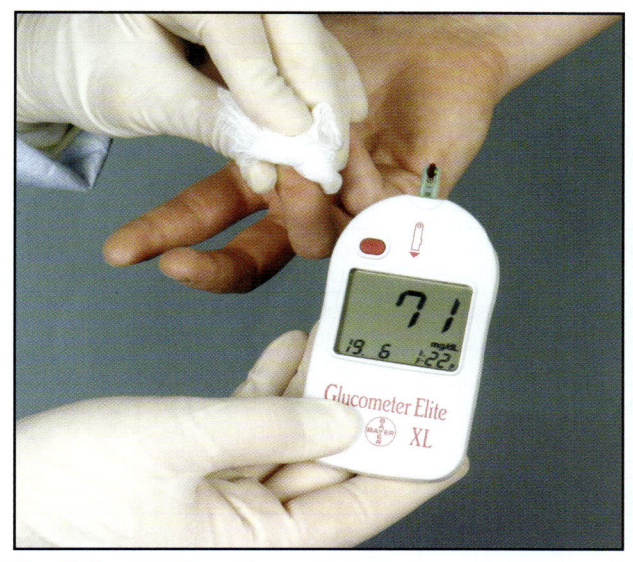

Fig. 1-5. POCT with a glucometer to determine the patient's blood glucose level. The specimen, taken from the patient's finger, registers 71, normal for a fasting glucose.

- Microbiology—rapid tests for streptococcus A, influenza A/B
- Fecal occult blood

The physician's office laboratory (**POL**) has greatly benefited and will continue to benefit from the technical advancements that have improved and simplified so many medical testing methods. A major benefit of POL testing is that ambulatory patients can now obtain their screening and monitoring test results immediately rather than needing to drive to an external laboratory. Also, the physician's interpretation and therapeutic recommendations can now be given during the same office visit. This has led to better patient care and **patient compliance** (a patient's willingness to follow a treatment plan and take an active role in his or her own health care). Many physicians may also perform basic microscopic procedures that have been CLIA approved. NOTE: The CLIA-waived approval process and basic microscopy will be presented in Chapter 2.

Reference and hospital laboratories will continue to provide physicians with the results of the more complex tests. Patient specimens must be sent to these laboratories for the critical test results that provide the doctor with sufficient information to make definitive diagnoses. Because of the complexity of these diagnostic tests, they must be performed by individuals with extensive laboratory training, education, and credentialing. A complete description of such knowledge and training is beyond the scope of this book.

Physician office laboratories are generally staffed by physicians, physician assistants, nurse practitioners, and medical assistants. **Medical assistants** are multiskilled professionals who assist in the patient-care management in medical offices, clinics, and ambulatory care centers. They perform administrative duties and clinical procedures, including the basic CLIA-waived laboratory tests. Medical assistants attend a 1- or 2-year program and are nationally credentialed as CMA (AAMA) or RMA (AMT). There may also be trained laboratory technicians working in the larger POLs that service multiple physicians.

Table 1-1 lists all the health care professionals involved in medical laboratory testing. They are organized by educational credentials, from doctorates to associate degrees and to technical certification. (Nurses are not listed because laboratory training is not part of their education. They are often trained on the job in physicians' offices.)

TABLE 1-1 Personnel Involved in Laboratory Testing

Title	Credential	Years of College Training and Degree	Laboratory Setting
Board-certified pathologists	MD or DO	8 or more: doctorate	Reference and hospital laboratories
Primary care physicians and specialists	MD or DO or ND (naturopathic doctor)	6 or more: doctorate	Physician's office laboratory and health clinics
Physician assistants and nurse practitioners	PA, NP	6 or more: master's	Physician's office laboratory and health clinics
Clinical laboratory scientist, National Certification Agency for Medical Laboratory Personnel	CLS (NCA)	4 or more: bachelor's or master's	Reference and hospital laboratories
Medical technologist, American Society of Clinical Pathologists	MT (ASCP)	4 or more: bachelor's	Reference and hospital laboratories
Medical technologist, American Medical Technologists	MT (AMT)	4 or more: bachelor's	Reference and hospital laboratories
Registered medical technologist, International Society for Clinical Laboratory Technology	RMT (ISCLT)	4 or more: bachelor's	Reference and hospital laboratories
Clinical laboratory technologist, Department of Health and Human Services	CLT (HHS)	4 or more: bachelor's	Reference and hospital laboratories
Medical laboratory technician, American Society of Clinical Pathologists	MLT (ASCP)*	2: associate degree	Reference and hospital laboratories and physician's office laboratories
Medical laboratory technician, American Medical Technologists	MLT (AMT)*	2: associate degree	Reference and hospital laboratories and physician's office laboratories
Clinical laboratory technician, National Certification Agency for Medical Laboratory Personnel	CLT (NCA)*	2: associate degree	Reference and hospital laboratories and physician's office laboratories
Registered laboratory technician, International Society for Clinical Laboratory Technology	RLT (ISCLT)*	2: associate degree	Reference and hospital laboratories and physician's office laboratories
Registered phlebotomist	National certification*	1: technical certificate	All laboratories
Certified medical assistant, American Association of Medical Assistants and CAAHEP	CMA (AAMA)*	1: associate degree or 2: technical certificate	Physician's office laboratory and ambulatory settings
Registered medical assistant, American Medical Technologists	RMA (AMT)*	1: associate degree or 2: technical certificate	Physician's office laboratory and ambulatory settings

*This book is designed to provide these professionals with the necessary information to perform CLIA-waived tests in ambulatory settings with confidence, accuracy, and precision.

Attributes of a Laboratory Professional

Everyone performing laboratory tests, regardless of educational background and credentials or place of work, must possess the following personal characteristics to guarantee proper patient care:
- Professional attitude—discreet, respectful, proper attire and personal hygiene
- Strong interpersonal communication skills with patients, co-workers, and supervisors
- Motivation, efficiency, commitment, and dedication to serving others in need
- Good organizational skills when setting up a series of tests—ability to manage time and multitask
- Focus, good power of observation, ability to pay attention to details during entire process
- Ability to solve problems if test results are not working as expected

Fundamental Concepts

- Honesty, integrity, ability to admit when unsure of procedure or results
- Manual dexterity, using both hands to accomplish the task
- Ability to perform precise calculations and measurements and neatly document all findings
- Good eyesight and normal color vision for reading color changes on test strips

Laboratory Documentation

Everyone involved in medical laboratory testing and specimen processing must understand and complete the paperwork and the electronic data accurately and completely. The documentation begins with the physician's laboratory test order being entered onto a requisition form and ends with the laboratory report being evaluated and filed in the patient's chart.

Laboratory Requisitions

When ordering tests from outside reference and hospital labs, the laboratory professionals must understand all forms of written and electronic communication between their office and the laboratory. Communication begins when the physician orders a particular test or series of tests. The laboratory order is recorded on a requisition that must be completely filled out. Different laboratories have different requisition forms, but most will cover the following areas (Fig. 1-6):

1. Where and how the final laboratory report is to be sent back to the physician and any consulting physicians (fax, call, or mail)
2. Information on the patient and the proper specimen collection
3. Numerical identification of the physician and the patient (for electronic and confidential reporting)
4. Insurance and billing information for the patient (The diagnosis/signs/symptoms section requires a proper ICD-9 coding format. This is a numerical diagnostic code required for insurance reimbursement.)
5. A listing of laboratory tests to be ordered that are organized into the following categories:
   - **Panels/profiles**—a series of tests associated with a particular organ or disease
   - Hematology/coagulation tests—focus on the numbers and quality of blood cells and coagulation
   - Chemistry tests—measure the levels of various chemicals, enzymes, and hormones
   - Serology/immunology tests—analyze blood serum for evidence of infection or disease by evaluating antigen–antibody reactions in the laboratory
   - Microbiology tests—determine what pathogen is causing the disease
   - Toxicology tests—measure the therapeutic levels and abuse of toxic drugs
   - Urinalysis tests—indicate the health status of the urinary tract and the liver and the presence of diabetes

Each test has a five-digit procedure code that is also used for insurance billing (see Fig. 1-6). Each test also has a collection container abbreviation that tells the office which color-coded blood collection tube to use or which type of microbiology or urine specimen container to use. The codes are explained at the bottom of the requisition.

When the requisition is completely filled out, it goes to the laboratory with the patient or with the patient's specimen (e.g., blood, urine).

Electronic bar codes on requisitions are becoming more common, along with stick-on labels for the specimens, in an effort to eliminate specimen identification errors and maintain confidentiality (Fig. 1-7). When these convenient labels are used, confirmation of the patient's identity with at least two identifiers is crucial (e.g., driver's license, birth date, Social Security number, phone number). As an additional safeguard, the patient should write his or her name on the bar code label placed on the requisition and on the specimen labels.

Laboratory Reports

After the specimen has been tested, the laboratory calls in or sends the results on a **laboratory report** (results of laboratory tests that have been ordered; see Fig. 1-1). Another type of report is a computer printout, which shows the results of a chemistry panel of tests (Fig. 1-8).

All laboratory reports must be reviewed by the physician as soon as possible. The physician must sign and date the report. Depending on the results of the test, the physician may need to see or otherwise get in touch with the patient. Each office has a specific protocol regarding how the patient is notified. Be sure to follow the protocol, and then file the report in the patient's file folder after charting any additional information. Understanding the process and making sure all parties are informed in a timely manner are crucial.

Fig. 1-9 is a basic flow chart of the laboratory process. The details of each step are discussed later in Chapter 2.

Laboratory Measurements

Medical laboratories must communicate their test results in a universal way. Therefore all laboratories do their reporting with international metric units for weight, volume, and length. Tables 1-2, 1-3, and 1-4 show the most common metric units used in medical laboratory reports.

Analytes measured in a liquid such as blood or urine are frequently expressed on laboratory reports

LABORATORY REQUISITION
Biomedical Laboratories, Inc.
100 Main Street
Athens, Georgia 45760

☐ Fax — Send additional copy of report to: ( )
☐ Call — Client Number/Physician's Name — Phone/Fax number
☐ Mail — Physician's Address — City, State, Zip

Patient's Name (Last) (First) (MI) | Sex | Date of Birth MO | DAY | YEAR | Collection Time : AM PM | Fasting YES NO | Collection Date MO | DAY | YEAR

NPI/UPIN | Physician's ID # | Patient's SS # | Patient's ID # | Urine hrs/vol hrs_____ vol_____

Physician's Name (Last, First) | Physician's Signature

Medicare # (Include prefix/suffix) ☐ Primary ☐ Secondary

Medicaid # | State | Physician's Provider #

Diagnosis/Signs/Symptoms in ICD-9 Format (Highest Specificity)

REQUIRED

PATIENT: Patient's Address | Phone
City | State | ZIP

RESP. PARTY: Name of Responsible Party (if different from patient)
Address of Responsible Party (if different from patient) | APT #
City | State | ZIP

INSURANCE: Patient's Relationship to Responsible Party ■ 1–Self ■ 2–Spouse ■ 3–Child ■ 4–Other

Insurance Company Name | Plan | Carrier Code
Subscriber/Member # | Location | Group #
Insurance Address | Physician's Provider #
City | State | ZIP
Employer's Name or Number | Insured SS # (If not patient) | Worker's Comp ☐ Yes ☐ No

Performance Lab ☐ | Carrier | Group # | Employee # | Mem

I hereby authorize the release of medical information related to the service subscribed herein and authorize payment directed to LabCorp.
X _____ Patient's Signature _____ Date

MEDICARE ADVANCE BENEFICIARY NOTICE

I have read the ABN on the reverse. If Medicare denies payment, I agree to pay for the identified test(s).
X _____ Patient's Signature _____ Date

NOTE: WHEN ORDERING TESTS FOR WHICH MEDICARE OR MEDICAID REIMBURSEMENT WILL BE SOUGHT, PHYSICIANS SHOULD ONLY ORDER TESTS THAT ARE MEDICALLY NECESSARY FOR THE DIAGNOSIS OR TREATMENT OF THE PATIENT. COMPONENTS OF THE ORGAN OR DISEASE PANELS/COMBINATIONS PRINTED BELOW ARE SHOWN ON THE REVERSE SIDE AND MAY ALSO BE ORDERED INDIVIDUALLY BELOW. COMPONENTS MAY BE BILLED SEPARATELY PER CARRIER POLICY.

PROFILES (See reverse for components)

80049	Basic Metabolic Profile	SST
80054	Comp Metabolic Profile	SST
80051	Electrolyte Profile	SST
80058	Hepatic Profile	SST
80059	Hepatitis Profile	SST
80061	Lipid Profile	SST
80091	Thyroid Profile	SST
80055	Prenatal Profile	RED LAV
80072	Rheumatoid Profile	SST

HEMATOLOGY/COAGULATION

85025	CBC w Diff	LAV
85027	CBC w/o Diff	LAV
85014	Hematocrit	LAV
85018	Hemoglobin	LAV
85595	Platelet Count	LAV
85041	RBC Count	LAV
85048	WBC Count	LAV
85007	WBC Differential	LAV
89190	Nasal Smear, Eosin	Nasal Smear
85060	Pathologist Consult–Peripheral Smear	LAV
85651	Sed Rate	LAV
85610	Prothrombin Time (PT)	BLU
86900 86901	PT and PTT Activated	BLU
85730	PTT Activated	BLU

CHEMISTRY

82040	Albumin	SST
84075	Alkaline Phosphatase	SST
84460	ALT (SGPT)	SST
82150	Amylase, Serum	SST
84450	AST (SGOT)	SST

ALPHABETICAL TESTS CON'T

82607 82746	B_{12} and Folate	SST
82250	Bilirubin, Total	SST
84520	BUN	SST
82310	Calcium	SST
82378	CEA	SST
82465	Cholesterol, Total	SST
82565	Creatinine	SST
82670	Estradiol	SST
82728	Ferritin, Serum	SST
82985	Fructosamine	SST
83001	FSH	SST
83001 83002	FSH and LH	SST
82977	GGT	SST
82947	Glucose, Plasma	GRY
82947	Glucose, Serum	SST
82950	Glucose, 2-hr. PP	SST
83036	Glycohemoglobin, Total	LAV
84703	hCG, Beta Subunit, Qual	SST
84702	hCG, Beta Subunit, Quant	SST
83718	HDL Cholesterol	SST
83036	Hemoglobin A_{1C}	LAV

SEROLOGY/IMMUNOLOGY

85610 85730	ABO and Rh	LAV
86038	Antinuclear Antibodies	SST
86677	*Helicobacter pylori*, IgG	SST
86706	Hep B Surface Antibody	SST
87340	Hep B Surface Antigen	SST
86803	Hep C Antibody	SST
86701	HIV Antibodies Serology	SST

ALPHABETICAL TESTS CON'T

83540	Iron, Total	SST
83540 83550	Iron and IBC	SST
83615	LDH	SST
83002	LH	SST
83690	Lipase	SER
83735	Magnesium, Serum	SST
84132	Potassium	SST
84146	Prolactin, Serum	SST
84153	Prostate-Specific Antigen	SST
84066	Prostatic Acid Phos	SST
84155	Protein, Total	SST
86431	Rheumatoid Arthritis Factor	SST
86592	RPR	SST
86762	Rubella Antibodies, IgG	SST
84295	Sodium	SST
84403	Testosterone	SST
84436	Thyroxine (T_4)	SST
84478	Triglycerides	SST
84480	Triiodothyronine (T_3)	SST
84443	TSH, High Sensitivity	SST
84550	Uric Acid	SST

TOXICOLOGY

80156	Carbamazepine (Tegretol®)	SER
80162	Digoxin	SER
80178	Lithium (Eskalith®)	SER
80184	Phenobarbital (Luminal®)	SER
80185	Phenytoin (Dilantin®)	SER
80198	Theophylline Toxicology	SER
80164	Valproic Acid (Depakene®)	SER

URINALYSIS

81003	Urinalysis — Microscopic on Positives	URN
81001	Urinalysis — with Microscopic	URN

MICROBIOLOGY See Reverse Side
■ ENDOCERVICAL ■ THROAT ■ URINE
■ STOOL ■ URETHRAL INDICATE SOURCE

87070	Aerobic Bacterial Culture	Bact Trnspt
87490 87590	*Chlamydia*/GC DNA Probe w/ Confirmation on Positives	Probe Trnspt
87490 87590	*Chlamydia*/GC DNA Probe Without Confirmation	Probe Trnspt
87490	*Chlamydia* DNA Probe	Probe Trnspt
87081	Genital, *Beta-Hemolytic Strep Cult, Group B*	Bact Trnspt
87070	Genital Culture, Routine	Bact Trnspt
87070	Lower Respiratory Culture	Steril Trnspt
87590	*N. gonorrhoeae* DNA Probe	Probe Trnspt
87015 87211	Ova and Parasites	O & P Kit
87081 X2 87045	Stool Culture	Fecal Trnspt
87081	Throat, *Beta-Hemolytic Strep Cult, Group A*	Bact Trnspt
87060	Upper Respiratory Culture, Routine	Bact Trnspt
87086	Urine Culture, Routine	Urn Cul Trnspt

Clinical Information/Comments

OTHER TESTS/INDIVIDUAL COMPONENTS
TEST # | TEST NAMES

LAB USE ONLY

STAT	VENIPUNCTURE	TRAVEL	NON LABCORP	VERBAL ORDER	CHART ORDER	HANDWRITTEN	24 HR TUV	PST/PSC #
☐ 998074	☐ 998085	☐ 998096	☐ 998239	☐ 998250	☐ 998261	☐ 998272	☐ 998283	

CONTAINERS RECEIVED →

SST	USST	SER	FRZ	RED	LAV	SLD	BLU	GRY	GRN	RYB	YEL	PLS	URN	24U	TA-U	FL	OT	BACT TRNSP	O & P KIT	PROBE TRNSP	URN CULT TRNSP	STERIL TRNSP	FECAL TRNSP	VIRAL TRNSP
SPUN	UNSPUN	SERUM TRNSPT	FRZ TRNS	RED	LAVENDER	SLIDE	LT. BLUE	GREY	GREEN	RYL BLU	ACD	PLASMA	URINE	24 HR URINE	TART. ACID	FLUID	OTHER							

300-0384

Fig. 1-6. Laboratory requisition. (From Bonewit-West K: *Clinical procedures for medical assistants,* ed 7, St Louis, 2008, Saunders.)

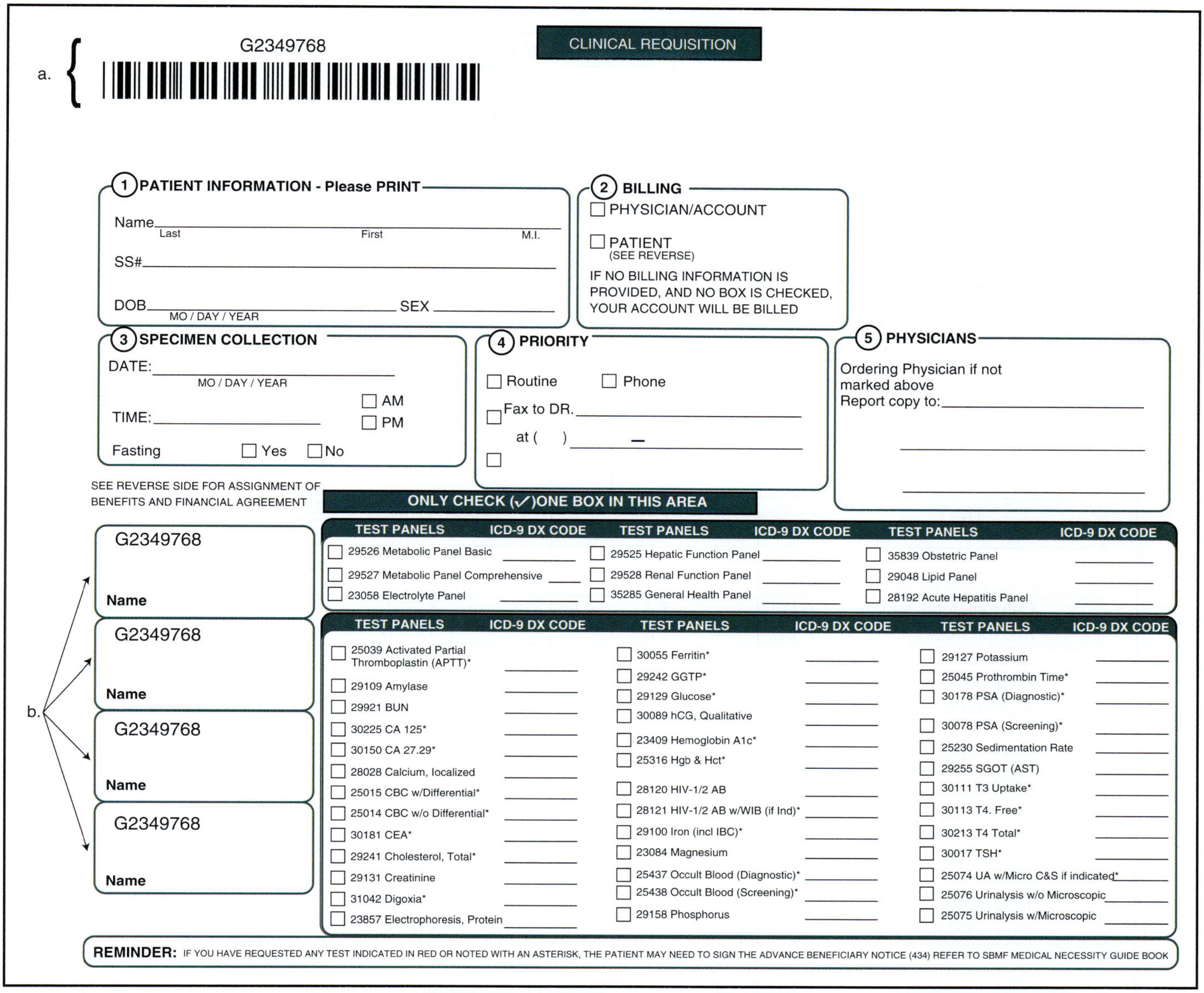

a. G2349768

CLINICAL REQUISITION

(1) PATIENT INFORMATION - Please PRINT

Name ______ Last ______ First ______ M.I.

SS# ______

DOB ______ MO / DAY / YEAR SEX ______

(2) BILLING

☐ PHYSICIAN/ACCOUNT

☐ PATIENT (SEE REVERSE)

IF NO BILLING INFORMATION IS PROVIDED, AND NO BOX IS CHECKED, YOUR ACCOUNT WILL BE BILLED

(3) SPECIMEN COLLECTION

DATE: ______ MO / DAY / YEAR

TIME: ______ ☐ AM ☐ PM

Fasting ☐ Yes ☐ No

(4) PRIORITY

☐ Routine ☐ Phone

☐ Fax to DR. ______

at ( ) ______ –

☐

(5) PHYSICIANS

Ordering Physician if not marked above

Report copy to: ______

SEE REVERSE SIDE FOR ASSIGNMENT OF BENEFITS AND FINANCIAL AGREEMENT

ONLY CHECK (✓) ONE BOX IN THIS AREA

b.

G2349768 Name

G2349768 Name

G2349768 Name

G2349768 Name

TEST PANELS	ICD-9 DX CODE	TEST PANELS	ICD-9 DX CODE	TEST PANELS	ICD-9 DX CODE
☐ 29526 Metabolic Panel Basic		☐ 29525 Hepatic Function Panel		☐ 35839 Obstetric Panel	
☐ 29527 Metabolic Panel Comprehensive		☐ 29528 Renal Function Panel		☐ 29048 Lipid Panel	
☐ 23058 Electrolyte Panel		☐ 35285 General Health Panel		☐ 28192 Acute Hepatitis Panel	

TEST PANELS	ICD-9 DX CODE	TEST PANELS	ICD-9 DX CODE	TEST PANELS	ICD-9 DX CODE
☐ 25039 Activated Partial Thromboplastin (APTT)*		☐ 30055 Ferritin*		☐ 29127 Potassium	
☐ 29109 Amylase		☐ 29242 GGTP*		☐ 25045 Prothrombin Time*	
☐ 29921 BUN		☐ 29129 Glucose*		☐ 30178 PSA (Diagnostic)*	
☐ 30225 CA 125*		☐ 30089 hCG, Qualitative		☐ 30078 PSA (Screening)*	
☐ 30150 CA 27.29*		☐ 23409 Hemoglobin A1c*		☐ 25230 Sedimentation Rate	
☐ 28028 Calcium, localized		☐ 25316 Hgb & Hct*		☐ 29255 SGOT (AST)	
☐ 25015 CBC w/Differential*		☐ 28120 HIV-1/2 AB		☐ 30111 T3 Uptake*	
☐ 25014 CBC w/o Differential*		☐ 28121 HIV-1/2 AB w/WIB (if Ind)*		☐ 30113 T4. Free*	
☐ 30181 CEA*		☐ 29100 Iron (incl IBC)*		☐ 30213 T4 Total*	
☐ 29241 Cholesterol, Total*		☐ 23084 Magnesium		☐ 30017 TSH*	
☐ 29131 Creatinine		☐ 25437 Occult Blood (Diagnostic)*		☐ 25074 UA w/Micro C&S if indicated*	
☐ 31042 Digoxia*		☐ 25438 Occult Blood (Screening)*		☐ 25076 Urinalysis w/o Microscopic	
☐ 23857 Electrophoresis, Protein		☐ 29158 Phosphorus		☐ 25075 Urinalysis w/Microscopic	

REMINDER: IF YOU HAVE REQUESTED ANY TEST INDICATED IN RED OR NOTED WITH AN ASTERISK, THE PATIENT MAY NEED TO SIGN THE ADVANCE BENEFICIARY NOTICE (434) REFER TO SBMF MEDICAL NECESSITY GUIDE BOOK

Fig. 1-7. Bar code requisition and labels for matching specimens with their laboratory order. Note the bar code and its number at the top *(a)* as well as its corresponding peel-off labels with the same requisition number and space for the patient's name *(b)*. The reference laboratory may also have the patient sign the requisition and initial the labels to confirm identity.

in milligrams per deciliter (mg/dL). This is an expression of concentration, which is the *weight* of the analyte per the *volume* of the specimen. If the analyte is very small, it is expressed in micrograms (μg or mcg), which are 1/1,000,000 of a gram.

When a *liquid* is measured in the laboratory, the most common volume is milliliter (mL or ml), which may also be referred to as a cubic centimeter (cc).

When the *length* of a test tube or a specimen within a capillary tube is measured, millimeters (mm) are used. There are approximately 25 mm in 1 inch, so 100 mm is approximately 4 inches.

Many tests are temperature sensitive and must be stored at either room temperature or refrigerated. The Centigrade temperature for refrigeration is usually 4° to 8° C (Fig. 1-10), and room temperature is 15° to 30° C. (The workbook contains a daily temperature monitoring chart that must be filled out daily if test kits or supplies are refrigerated.)

NOTE: When recording whole numbers, *do not place a zero after the decimal* (e.g., the whole number 2 should be written 2, *not* 2.0). When recording a fraction, *a zero must be placed in front of the decimal* (e.g., one half should be written as 0.5, *not* .5).

DATE AND TIME RECEIVED	ACCESSION NUMBER
10/20/2010 20:45	
LOCATION	**DATE REPORTED**
	10/21/2010

PHYSICIAN	PATIENT'S INFORMATION

TEST		RESULTS	REFERENCE RANGE	UNITS
Chemistry 23 - panel B				
Calcium, total, serum	LO	7.4	8.5-10.5	MG/DL
Phosphorus	LO	2.8	3.0-4.6	MG/DL
Uric acid	LO	3.2	3.5-7.2	MG/DL
Cholesterol	LO	123	151-240	MG/DL
Triglyceride		121	58-258	MG/DL
LDH		217	118-242	IU/L
SGOT (AST)	HI	41	10-37	IU/L
SGPT (ALT)	HI	45	10-40	IU/L
GGTP	LO	8	11-51	IU/L
Alkaline phosphatase		63	39-117	IU/L
Bilirubin, total		0.3	0.1-1.5	MG/DL
Albumin	LO	2.4	3.7-5.2	G/DL
Total protein	LO	3.6	6.0-8.5	G/DL
Albumin/globulin ratio		2.0	1.0-2.2	RATIO

Final report   (Summary)   Page 2 of 2

Fig. 1-8. Blood chemistry laboratory report. Note the patient's results compared with the reference range and the additional column indicating if the result is "HI" or "LO" compared with the reference range. (From Zakus SM: *Clinical skills for medical assistants,* ed 4, St Louis, 2001, Mosby.)

Fundamental Concepts

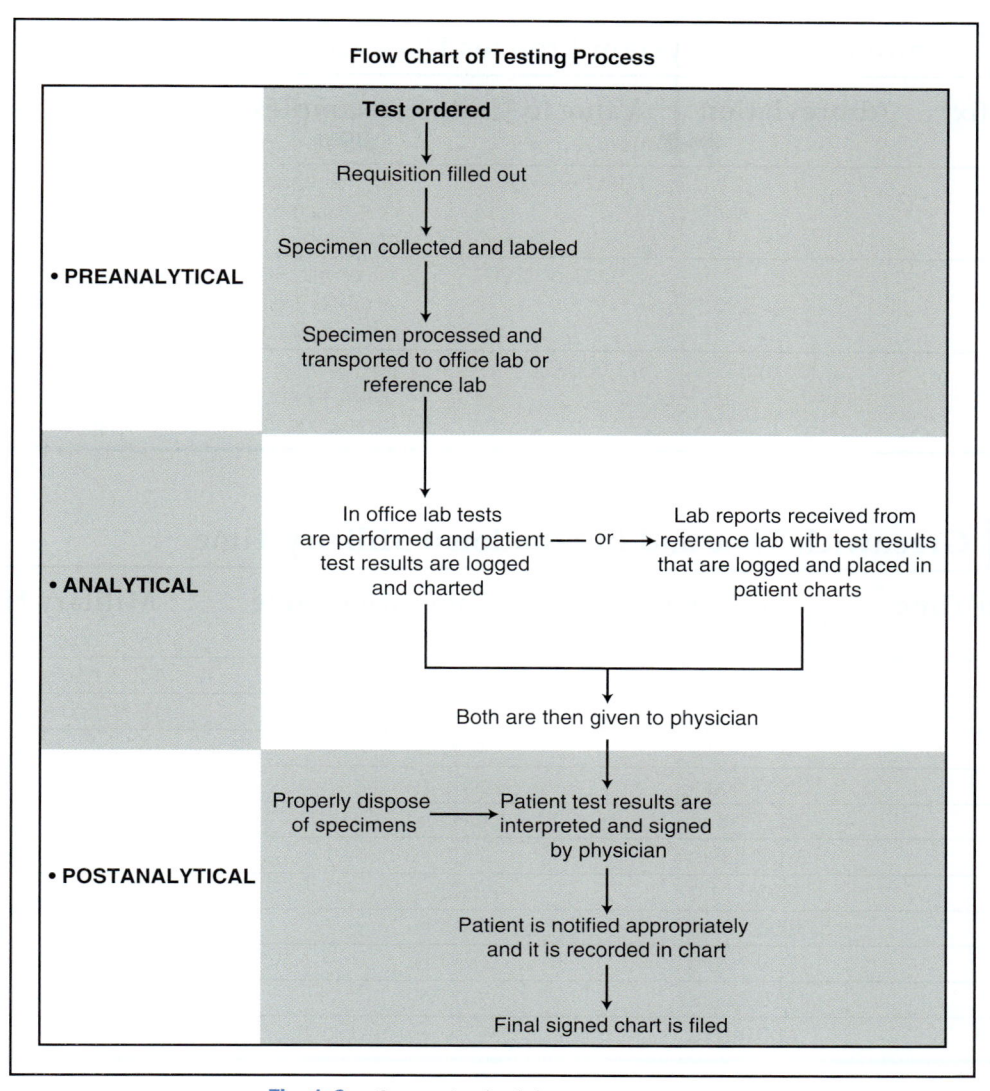

Flow Chart of Testing Process

- **PREANALYTICAL**
  - Test ordered
  - Requisition filled out
  - Specimen collected and labeled
  - Specimen processed and transported to office lab or reference lab

- **ANALYTICAL**
  - In office lab tests are performed and patient test results are logged and charted — or → Lab reports received from reference lab with test results that are logged and placed in patient charts
  - Both are then given to physician

- **POSTANALYTICAL**
  - Properly dispose of specimens → Patient test results are interpreted and signed by physician
  - Patient is notified appropriately and it is recorded in chart
  - Final signed chart is filed

Fig. 1-9. Stages in the laboratory process.

TABLE 1-2 Metric Units of Measurement

Measurement	Metric Unit	Abbreviation	Relative Comparison to American Units
Weight	Gram	G, g, or gm	1 g is approximately the weight of a raisin and is used in place of 1 oz. 1 kg (the weight of 1000 g) is used in place of 1 lb.
Volume	Liter	L or l	1 L is a little more than a quart (used in place of the liquid measurements cup, quart, and gallon). 1 mL (1/1000 of a liter) is used in place of a liquid ounce or teaspoon.
Length	Meter	M or m	A meter is a little longer than a yard. Centimeters (1/100 of a meter) are used in place of inches. Kilometers (1000 meters) are used in place of miles.
Temperature	Centigrade (Celsius)	°C	0° C = freezing; 100° C = boiling (Fahrenheit: 32° F = freezing; 212° F = boiling) 4°-8° C = refrigerator temperature storage 15°-30° C = room temperature storage 37° C = body temperature

TABLE 1-3 Common Metric System Prefixes Used in Laboratory Reports

Metric Prefix	Abbreviation	Value to Unit	Examples in Laboratory Reports
Deci-	d	1/10 or 0.1	dL or dl = deciliter (one tenth of a liter)
Centi-	c	1/100 or 0.01	cm = centimeter, cc = cubic centimeter (which is the same volume as a milliliter, one-thousandth of a liter)
Milli-	m	1/1000 or 0.001	ml or mL = milliliter (one thousandth of a liter, which is the same as a cubic centimeter); mg = milligram (one thousandth of a gram)
Micro-	μ (or mc)	1/1,000,000	μg (or mcg) = microgram (one millionth of a gram) (NOTE: When handwriting, use "mc" for micro, not the Greek letter μ.)

TABLE 1-4 Greenwich Time and International Military Time

Greenwich Time	Military Hours	Greenwich Time	Military Hours
1:00 AM	0100 hours	1:00 PM	1300 hours
2:00 AM	0200 hours	2:00 PM	1400 hours
3:00 AM	0300 hours	3:00 PM	1500 hours
4:00 AM	0400 hours	4:00 PM	1600 hours
5:00 AM	0500 hours	5:00 PM	1700 hours
6:00 AM	0600 hours	6:00 PM	1800 hours
7:00 AM	0700 hours	7:00 PM	1900 hours
8:00 AM	0800 hours	8:00 PM	2000 hours
9:00 AM	0900 hours	9:00 PM	2100 hours
10:00 AM	1000 hours	10:00 PM	2200 hours
11:00 AM	1100 hours	11:00 PM	2300 hours
12:00 PM (noon)	1200 hours	12:00 AM (midnight)	2400 or 0000 hours

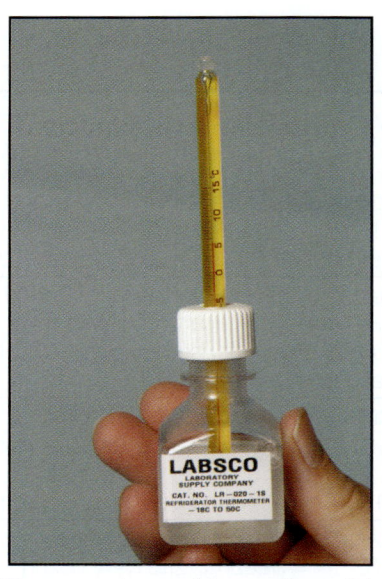

Fig. 1-10. Thermometer used to monitor refrigerator temperature. The reading of 6° C, an acceptable refrigerator temperature, would be logged.

Safety Training in the Laboratory

Potential hazards are present in the medical laboratory setting. Various government agencies have evaluated the most common laboratory dangers and created regulations and guidelines to help protect and prevent harm to laboratory employees. These agencies continually monitor potential hazards and periodically update their regulations. Checking their websites and staying current with the latest changes and required dates of implementation are wise practices.

The hazards found in medical laboratories are divided into the following categories:
- **Biohazards**—dangers related to exposure to infectious or **bloodborne pathogens** (infectious microorganisms that are transmitted by the blood or bloody body fluid from an infected host into the blood of another)
- **Chemical hazards**—dangers related to exposure to toxic, unstable, explosive, or flammable materials

Safety Training in the Laboratory

- **Physical hazards**—dangers related to electricity, fire, weather emergencies, bomb threats, and accidental injuries

The basic means by which diseases are spread must be understood before beginning laboratory work. Laboratory personnel must also learn how to prevent the spread of disease to themselves and others according to the regulations of two federal agencies: the Centers for Disease Control and Prevention **(CDC)** and the Occupational Safety and Health Administration **(OSHA).**

Transmission and the Chain of Infection

For a disease to spread, the following conditions must exist (Fig. 1-11). A pathogen must be present in a **reservoir host** (an infected person who is carrying an infectious agent). The pathogen must then find a **portal of exit** (a means of leaving the infected host's body, e.g., through the mouth, broken skin, rectum, or body fluids). Next, each pathogen has a particular transportation mode or **transmission** (a means of transporting itself from the infected individual to another person, by direct or indirect contact, e.g., by air, food, hand to hand, insects, or body fluids). The pathogen must then find a **portal of entry** (a body opening or break in the skin) in another person. Once inside the new person, the pathogen will not cause disease unless the person is a **susceptible host** (an individual who is unable to protect himself against the infectious agent). A susceptible person who becomes infected becomes a reservoir host, and the cycle begins again.

Health care workers must understand the chain of infection and endeavor to break the chain whenever possible to stop the spread of disease. If a disease is spread within a health care facility, it is referred to as a **nosocomial infection** (also referred to as **HCAIs** [health care associated infections]).

CDC Standard Precautions for Infection Control

The CDC has issued a list of **Standard Precautions** for infection control within health care facilities (Fig. 1-12). The most important way to stop the transmission of infectious disease, and first on the list, is hand washing. Next on the list is wearing various barriers referred to as personal protective equipment **(PPE),** which is "specialized clothing or equipment worn by an employee for protection against infectious material." Examples of PPE are gloves, goggles,

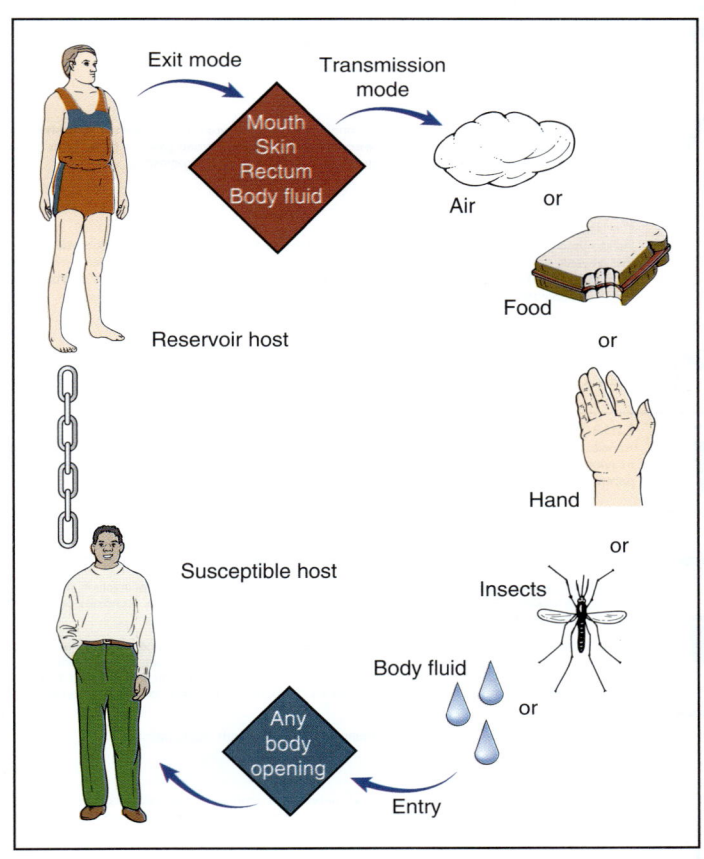

Fig. 1-11. Transmission and chain of infection. (From Stepp CA, Woods M: *Laboratory procedures for medical office personnel*, Philadelphia, 1998, Saunders.)

fluid-impermeable gowns, face shields, and masks. The remainder of the Standard Precautions list consists of equipment disinfection, environmental control, linen disposal, bloodborne pathogen guidelines, and patient placement (e.g., in isolation within a hospital setting). The serious occupational hazard of bloodborne pathogens has been further defined and regulated by OSHA and is discussed later in the chapter.

Hand Hygiene

The most common mode of transmission of pathogens is by the hands. The major cause of nosocomial infections (HCAIs) is the transmission of pathogens from health care workers' hands. These infections can also spread bacteria that may become resistant to antibiotics, which makes infections more difficult to bring under control.

Proper hand hygiene has proved to be the primary factor in infection control. Research has shown, however, that many health care workers do not practice routine hand washing. Their reasons have been as follows:

- Irritation and dryness caused by hand washing agents
- Inconvenient location of sinks
- Lack of soap and paper towels

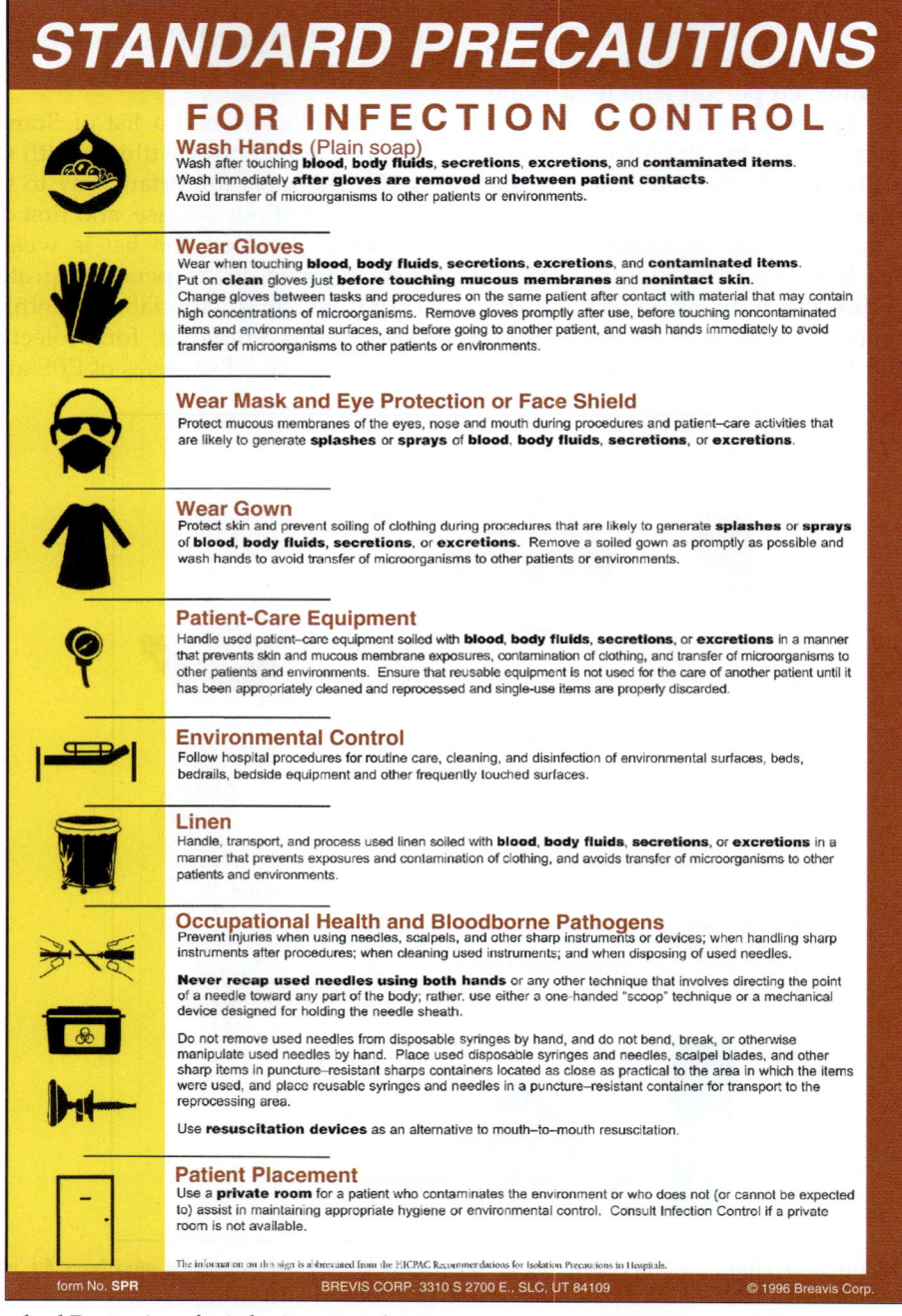

Fig. 1-12. CDC Standard Precautions for infection control. (From Zakus SM: *Clinical skills for medical assistants,* ed 4, St Louis, 2001, Mosby.)

Safety Training in the Laboratory

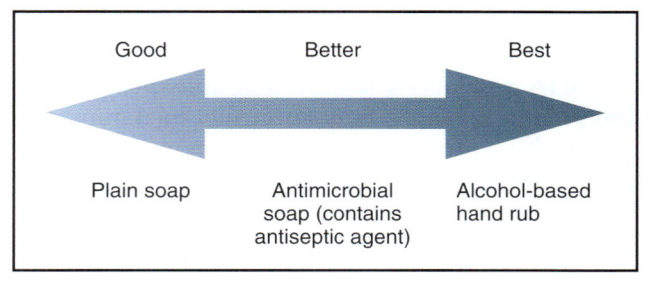

Fig. 1-13. Effectiveness of hand hygiene preparations in killing bacteria.

- Too busy/insufficient time
- Understaffing/overcrowding
- Priority of patient needs
- Misinformation about risk of acquiring infection from patients

In response, new guidelines developed by the CDC and infection-control organizations now recommend that health care workers use an alcohol-based hand rub (gel, rinse, or foam) to routinely clean their hands between patient contacts as long as their hands are not visibly soiled. Alcohol-based hand rubs require less time, are more effective than soap for routine hand washing, are more accessible than sinks, reduce bacterial counts on hands, and improve skin condition. The following three ways to clean the hands are now recommended (Fig. 1-13):

1. Washing with plain soap—good for removing microorganisms and dirt
2. Washing with antimicrobial detergent soap—better for removing and killing microorganisms
3. Using an alcohol-based hand rub—best for destroying transient microorganisms obtained from patients, specimens, and objects that are **contaminated,** that is, likely to have been in contact with materials or environmental surfaces where infectious organisms may reside

Laboratory employees' hands should be washed with *antimicrobial soap* (Fig. 1-14) at the beginning and end of work, before eating, after using the rest room, and whenever hands have visible dirt or are visibly contaminated with blood or body fluids. Effective washing with soap and water involves the following process:

1. Remove all hand jewelry.
2. Wet the hands with warm water (avoid hot water)
3. Apply 3 to 5 mL of liquid antiseptic soap to the hands. Use a towel on the pump dispenser to keep from contaminating the dispenser with soiled hands.
4. Rub the hands together for at least 15 seconds, covering all surfaces of the hands and fingers with soap.
5. Clean the fingernails with a brush if necessary.

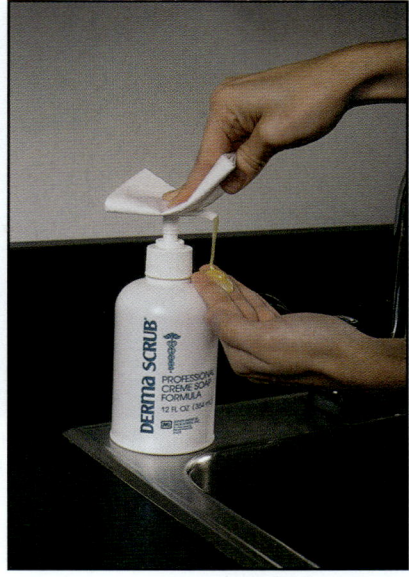

Fig. 1-14. Hand washing with antimicrobial soap. Note the use of a paper towel while pumping the dispenser. (From Bonewit-West K: *Clinical procedures for medical assistants,* ed 7, St Louis, 2008, Saunders.)

6. Rinse the hands with water and dry thoroughly.
7. Use a clean, dry paper towel to turn off the water faucet.
8. Apply appropriate hand lotion or cream provided by employer.

Healthy, intact skin acts as a barrier against **cross-contamination** (transmitting a pathogen from one individual to another) and harbors fewer pathogens. When the skin is damaged, **transient microorganisms** (organisms from contaminated objects or infectious patients that adhere to the skin and can be transmitted to others) are harder to remove.

An *alcohol-based hand rub* should be routinely used between patients and after having direct hand contact with patients, their wounds, broken skin, or body fluids (specimen containers) or after touching equipment used on the patient. Some patients may harbor "colonies" of infectious microorganisms on their skin with no sign of infection. Therefore the Standard Precautions pertaining to the use of gloves and proper hand hygiene apply to *all* patients. Use an alcohol-based hand rub routinely before putting on gloves and after removing gloves.

The following are tips on how to use an alcohol-based hand rub:

1. Apply 1.5 to 3 mL (or manufacturer's recommended amount) of an alcohol gel or foam to the palm of one hand, then rub the hands together (Fig. 1-15).
2. Cover all surfaces of the hands and fingers, including the areas around and under the fingernails.
3. Continue rubbing the hands together until the alcohol dries (15 to 25 seconds).

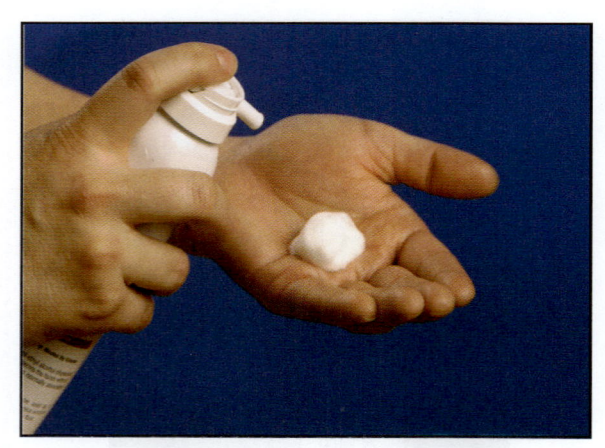

Fig. 1-15. Dispensing an alcohol-based foam hand rub. (From Bonewit-West K: *Clinical procedures for medical assistants,* ed 7, St Louis, 2008, Saunders.)

4. Make sure the hands are completely dry before putting on gloves.
5. Wash the hands with soap and water when a buildup of emollients can be felt on the hands.

Fingernail hygiene consists of maintaining natural nail tips at ¼ inch in length and using no polish. Artificial nails should not be worn by employees who have contact with any patients.

Personal Protective Equipment

Along with hand hygiene recommendations, the CDC also recommends when and how to use PPE. (OSHA also specifies and regulates the circumstances in which PPE must be used. These circumstances are discussed later in the chapter.)

OSHA Biohazard Training in Bloodborne Pathogens Standard

The federal Department of Labor has charged OSHA with finding ways of promoting worker safety and health in every workplace in the United States. On the basis of the history of hazards to health care workers, OSHA has developed a rigorous standard of policies and procedures called the **Bloodborne Pathogens Standard (BBPS)** to protect employees who work in occupations where they are at risk of exposure to blood or other potentially infectious materials **(OPIM). Occupational exposure** is defined as skin, eye, mucous membrane, or parenteral contact with blood or OPIM in the workplace. **Parenteral contact** means the blood entered the body through the skin or mucous membrane by means of a needle, bite, cut, or abrasion. Those who work in a medical laboratory or perform **venipuncture** (removal of blood from a vein) are at an increased risk for occupational exposure to bloodborne pathogens.

OSHA regulations require that an **exposure control plan** be provided by your facility to eliminate or minimize your occupational exposure to bloodborne pathogens. It is a key document developed to assist the employer in implementing and ensuring compliance with the Bloodborne Pathogens Standard, thereby protecting employees. It consists of the following elements:

- Determination of employee risk of exposure
- Implementation of methods of exposure control, including **Universal Precautions** (the assumption that the blood or body fluid containing blood from *any* patient or test kit could be infectious) when dealing with all patients, engineering and work practice controls to improve safety of employees, PPE for employees, and safe housekeeping practices
- Hepatitis B vaccination for employees at risk of bloodborne pathogen exposure
- Postexposure evaluation of patient and employee immediately after an exposure incident
- Evaluation of circumstances surrounding exposure incidents
- Communication of hazards by annual training of employees
- Documentation showing compliance to all the above

New employees of a laboratory receive initial training in the Bloodborne Pathogens Standard and subsequent annual training to learn of any changes in the standard. The following OSHA training session is divided into three sections:

1. Education on the causes, symptoms, and transmission of bloodborne pathogen diseases
2. Instruction on preventative measures to minimize exposure
3. Actions and procedures to follow when exposed to blood or OPIM

Diseases Caused by Bloodborne Pathogens

Three main bloodborne pathogens pose a threat to health care workers: HIV, hepatitis B, and hepatitis C. A fourth disease, hepatitis A, is not caused by a bloodborne virus but is similar to hepatitis B and C in that it is a viral infection of the liver.

The **human immunodeficiency virus (HIV)** is a retrovirus that attacks the immune system by destroying the white blood cells known as CD4+ T lymphocytes. An HIV infection has four stages:

1. An acute stage after exposure characterized by flu-like symptoms with swollen glands
2. An asymptomatic period in which no symptoms are readily apparent but the person is still infectious

3. Symptomatic stage with the appearance of **opportunistic infections** (infections that occur because of the body's inability to fight off pathogens normally found in the environment)
4. The AIDS (acquired immune deficiency syndrome) stage, when the immune system is so deficient that the following conditions start to appear: Kaposi's sarcoma, *Pneumocystis carinii* pneumonia, cytomegalovirus infection, herpes simplex 1 and 2, mycobacterial infection (e.g., tuberculosis), candidiasis (yeast infection), cryptosporidiosis, toxoplasmosis, and cryptococcosis. Currently no preventive vaccination for HIV or any cure for the infection exists. Treatment consists of reducing the growth rate of the virus and its effect on the body.

Hepatitis B virus (HBV) is the most prevalent bloodborne virus. It first infects the liver with acute flulike symptoms and possible jaundice. Most people recover and become immune to the virus, but approximately 2% enter the chronic stage and develop cirrhosis of the liver, cancer, or both. The good news is that a vaccine is available to produce immunity against the virus before an exposure incident. OSHA requires employers to provide the hepatitis B vaccine series free of charge to all health care employees who may be exposed to blood or OPIM. (Some health care employees who work only with medical records would not need the vaccination.)

Hepatitis C virus (HCV) is another bloodborne virus that attacks the liver. It is not as prevalent as HBV, but it is much more likely to reach the chronic stage. In fact, 75% to 85% of infected HCV individuals will reach the chronic phase with cirrhosis of the liver, cancer, and death. Because no vaccine for HCV exists, the health care worker cannot build up an immunity against the disease. Health care workers exposed to HCV are at risk.

Hepatitis A virus (HAV) is not a bloodborne virus, but it does attack the liver as HBV and HCV do. It is highly contagious and is transmitted by direct or indirect contact through the gastrointestinal tract. Patients with HAV are generally placed in isolation during their illness.

Table 1-5 summarizes the comparative information on the three bloodborne viruses and the infectious HAV virus, including the following facts:
- The average health care professional is more likely to contract HBV or HCV than HIV.
- Although all these diseases have initial flulike symptoms, HIV attacks the immune system, causing swollen glands, whereas HBV and HCV attack the liver, causing jaundice (a yellowing of the skin caused by excess bilirubin levels).
- HCV is becoming a threat because many individuals are chronic carriers and no vaccination is available.

Preventive Measures to Minimize Exposure

Practicing universal precautions is the most important way to prevent exposure incidents. The most common exposure to bloodborne pathogens in health care is from accidental puncture wounds with contaminated needles, glass, or other sharp items. All sharp items should be treated with respect.

The HBV vaccine should be made available to all health care employees who have the potential of being exposed to blood and OPIM. Employers must provide a three-vaccination series, and new employees should begin their series within the first 2 weeks of employment. Any employee who does not wish to be vaccinated must sign a Hepatitis B Vaccine Declination form. Health care students should also begin the series if they will be working with blood and blood products.

Engineering controls are efforts and research aimed at isolating and removing bloodborne pathogens from the workplace. Some examples of engineering controls involve the use of the following:
- Biohazard bags for blood-contaminated paper and plastic products and biohazard sharps disposal containers made of puncture-resistant material that will safely receive contaminated needles, syringes, and other sharp implements immediately after use
- Safer medical devices to cover contaminated needles immediately after use (Fig. 1-16), self-sheathing needles, and needleless systems when performing intravenous (IV) therapy
- Plastic supplies and equipment to replace breakable glass supplies when collecting and processing blood

The OSHA standard requires that everyone in the workplace explore new procedures and products regularly to provide greater safety to the health care worker while providing comfort and quality of care to the patient.

Work practice controls are policies that are recorded, monitored, and evaluated to protect employees from exposure to the pathogens in blood or body fluids. Various individuals (both administrators and front-line workers) are assigned the task of identifying, evaluating, and implementing changes in work behavior to reduce the risk of exposure. The implementation and commitment to adhere to work practice controls is required of each individual.

Examples of safe practices in the medical laboratory include the following:
- Do not eat, drink, smoke, or apply makeup or contact lenses in areas with a reasonable likelihood of exposure.
- Sanitize the hands before putting on and after removing gloves.

TABLE 1-5 Three Bloodborne Pathogens and Hepatitis A Virus

	Human Immunodeficiency Virus (HIV)	Hepatitis B Virus (HBV)	Hepatitis C Virus (HCV)	Hepatitis A Virus
Transmission	Contact with infected blood or blood products, semen, vaginal secretions; perinatal transmission. Must get into the bloodstream by direct entry into a vein, break in the skin, or mucous linings.	Found in body fluids, spread by blood transfusions, contaminated needles, and sexual contact. HBV is the most common bloodborne pathogen.	Intravenous drug use, body piercing, organ and blood transfusions, contaminated needles. Contaminated needles carry a tenfold greater chance of causing HCV than HIV.	Not bloodborne. Usually spread by contaminated food.
Symptoms	Flulike symptoms, fever, diarrhea, swollen glands, and fatigue. HIV infection leads to AIDS and an inability to fight off infections.	Flulike symptoms generally do not appear until 6 months after viral infection. They can include jaundice, fatigue, and abdominal and joint pain.	Milder than HBV; symptoms (if appearing) occur generally 1-2 months after exposure. They include jaundice, fatigue, dark urine, abdominal pain.	Jaundice, fatigue, abdominal pain, flulike symptoms.
Effects	Once infected, HIV is not curable. The majority of infected individuals do not develop AIDS until many years after infection.	Most people recover and become immune. Death can result in the 2% who become chronically infected.	85% of infected individuals acquire chronic form. Of those, cirrhosis of the liver develops in 1%-15%.	Infection results in immunity. Symptoms can last 6-9 months.
Prevention	No vaccination available.	HBV vaccination.	No vaccination available.	HAV vaccination, good hygiene
Treatment	Postexposure prophylaxis must start in 1-2 hours. Zidovudine reduces HIV infection, but it is never cured.	Postexposure treatment with immunoglobulins should begin as soon as possible—within 24 hours and no later than 7 days.	Treated with immunoglobulin, Heptazyme (inhibits viral synthesis), and alpha interferon.	Treatment consists of immunoglobulins and isolated bed rest to prevent spread.
Trends	Health care workers are more likely to contract HBV and HCV infections than HIV, although the incidence of HIV infection is rising.	10- to 49-year-olds most affected. Approximately 1.25 million are chronically infected.	2.7 million have the chronic form. This number is expected to triple in the next 10-15 years.	

- Bandage cuts and other lesions on the hands before gloving.
- Label all biohazard containers and appliances.
- Place all biohazard waste in appropriately labeled biohazard containers (e,g., sharps versus bag containers).
- If mucous membranes (eyes, mouth, nose) come in contact with blood, flush them with water as soon as possible.
- Do not store food or drink with biohazardous materials.
- Wear and use appropriate protective barriers and closed-toe shoes when working with blood or OPIM.
- Use mechanical means to pick up broken contaminated glass.
- Double-package specimens with a biohazard label when sending them to another laboratory.

In the medical laboratory gloves and fluid-impermeable gown barriers are routine requirements when dealing with blood or OPIM. Each procedure should be evaluated to determine if face shields or goggles are also necessary to protect the mucous membranes. This equipment should be used if the procedure is likely to generate splashes or sprays of blood, body fluids, secretions, or excretions.

Housekeeping guidelines in the laboratory consist of several measures:

- Disinfect counters at the beginning and end of each day with an OSHA-approved disinfectant such as freshly diluted 10% bleach solution. Fig. 1-17 shows a double-bottle system that dilutes the bleach with water on demand and a CaviWipe container with tissues to thoroughly disinfect contaminated surfaces. NOTE: Always wear protective gloves when working with either of these products.

Safety Training in the Laboratory

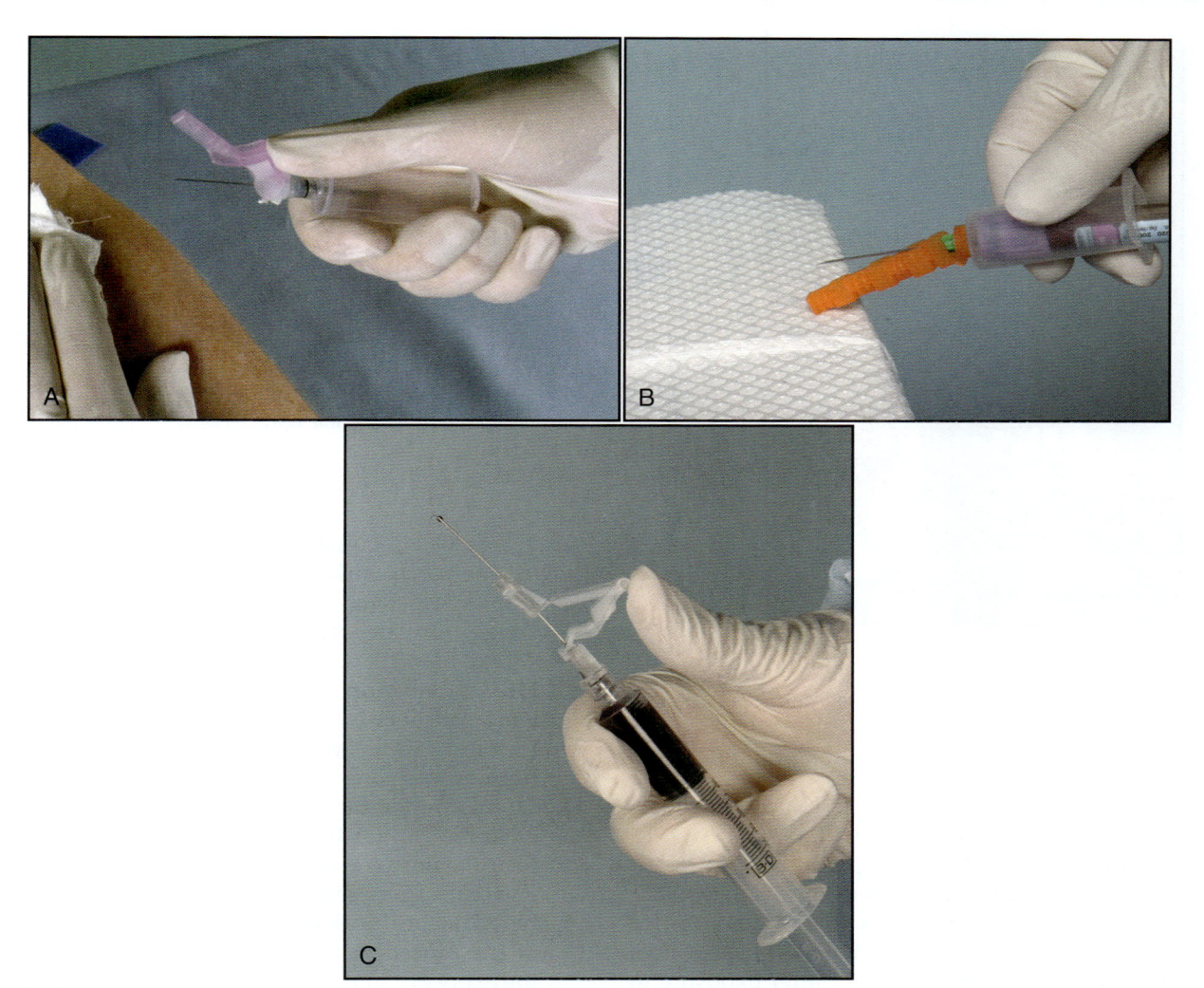

Fig. 1-16. Examples of needle safety devices being activated immediately after drawing blood. **A,** One-hand, thumb-activated device. **B,** One hand using surface to activate device. **C.** One-hand, thumb-activated spring device.

- When a waste receptacle contains biohazardous material, it must be red or contain the universal symbol for biohazard or both (Fig. 1-18). An understanding of the various waste receptacles and their functions is vital (Fig. 1-19).
  1. Regular wastebaskets should be used for paper wrappers, paper towels, and other materials that do not have blood or body fluids on them.
  2. Biohazard wastebaskets containing red plastic liners and bags with biohazard labels should be used for contaminated gloves, gowns, gauze, and soft plastic supplies.
  3. Biohazard sharps containers with biohazard labels should receive only sharp items such as needles and glass that could cut or break through a soft biohazard bag. They should be snapped closed when they are approximately three-fourths full.
  4. Biohazard-labeled bags and sharps containers are gathered into large cardboard boxes supplied by a regulated waste facility. The boxes are picked up and incinerated twice at a cost based on the total weight of the waste. Do not throw unnecessary items in biohazard receptacles.
- If a biohazard spill of blood or OPIM occurs, it should be cleaned up with a spill kit specifically designed to protect the person during the cleanup process (gloves and cleanup tools), the area should be decontaminated using the absorbent material and chemicals, and everything should be disposed of properly (biohazard-labeled bag or box).

Procedure After Exposure to Blood

If exposed to blood by a **percutaneous** (through the skin) injury or a splash on the mucous membranes of the eyes or mouth, the following postexposure steps must be taken immediately:
1. Flush with water, and wash the exposed area.
2. Report the incident immediately to your supervisor.
3. File an incident report that includes detailed information about how the exposure occurred. (See the

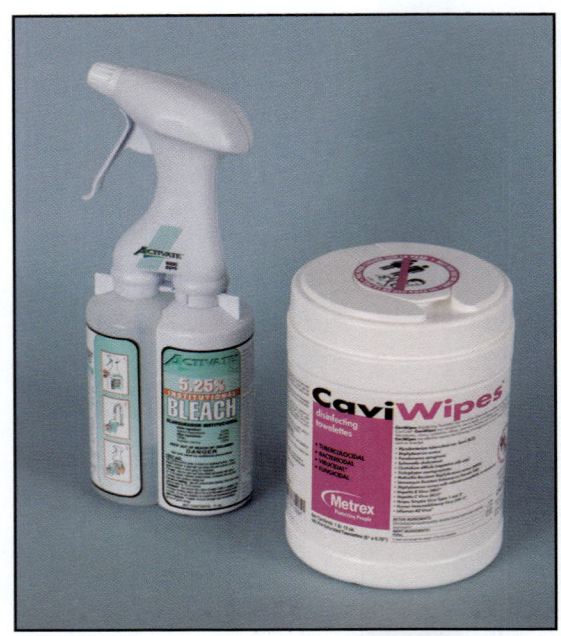

Fig. 1-17. A bleach/water dispenser automatically delivers a freshly diluted 10% bleach solution and CaviWipes for thorough disinfecting of contaminated surfaces. (Courtesy Zack Bent.)

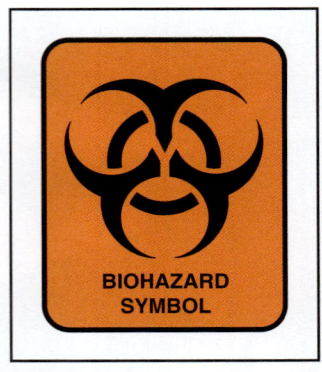

Fig. 1-18. Biohazard label. (From Stepp CA, Woods M: *Laboratory procedures for medical office personnel*, Philadelphia, 1998, Saunders.)

Sample Blood and Body Fluid Exposure Report form in the workbook appendix.)
4. Seek medical attention and permission to determine if the patient was infected with HIV, HBV, or HCV, then determine baseline blood defenses for each of the viral infections. If HIV is suspected, retest at 6, 12, 24, and 52 weeks after exposure to see if any change indicates infection.
5. Because a possibility always exists that the blood contained infectious viruses, a postexposure prophylaxis **(PEP)** (preventive treatment after being exposed to blood or OPIM) must begin as soon as possible. The PEP for each of the viral infections is based on the risk evaluation of a qualified health care professional and may consist of the following:
   - Hepatitis B: Passive HBV immune globulin and active HBV vaccine should be administered within 72 hours.
   - Hepatitis C: Immunoglobulin, Heptazyme, and alpha interferon should be administered as soon as possible.
   - HIV: Zidovudine, if administered within 1 to 2 hours, decreases the risk of percutaneous infection by 81%. Zidovudine and new antiretroviral drugs are also proven to reduce HIV infection, although they do not eliminate it.
6. Counseling and confidentiality are also available and required by OSHA.

Compliance with all the steps involved in OSHA's Bloodborne Pathogens Standard must be proven by each facility's documentation of its exposure control plan. The paperwork that must be presented during an OSHA inspection includes the following:
- Written job categories of employees at risk of exposure to blood
- HBV vaccination guidelines and records for each employee at risk
- Record of initial and annual Universal Standards training sessions for bloodborne pathogens and safety training for each employee
- Definition and listing of safe work practices
- Sharps injury log of all work-related needle sticks and cuts from sharp objects contaminated with blood, including date and time of exposure, details of the procedure being performed, the exposure, the exposure source, the exposed person, and postexposure follow-up
- A written plan to maintain the privacy of employees
- Documentation showing the evaluation of new technology by employees and their selection of safety devices based on effectiveness in decreasing injuries, acceptance by users, and ability to not adversely affect patient care

Chemical Hazard Training

Hazardous chemicals in the workplace are also regulated by OSHA in a federal document referred to as the **Hazard Communication Standard.** The document states that employees have the right to know about the dangers of all the hazardous chemicals to which they may be exposed under normal working conditions. As with the Bloodborne Pathogens Standard, the employer must develop a program that consists of taking an inventory of hazardous chemicals in the workplace, labeling the chemical hazards, collecting and maintaining a Material Safety Data Sheet **(MSDS)** for each hazardous chemical, properly storing and disposing of hazardous chemicals, and providing employees with

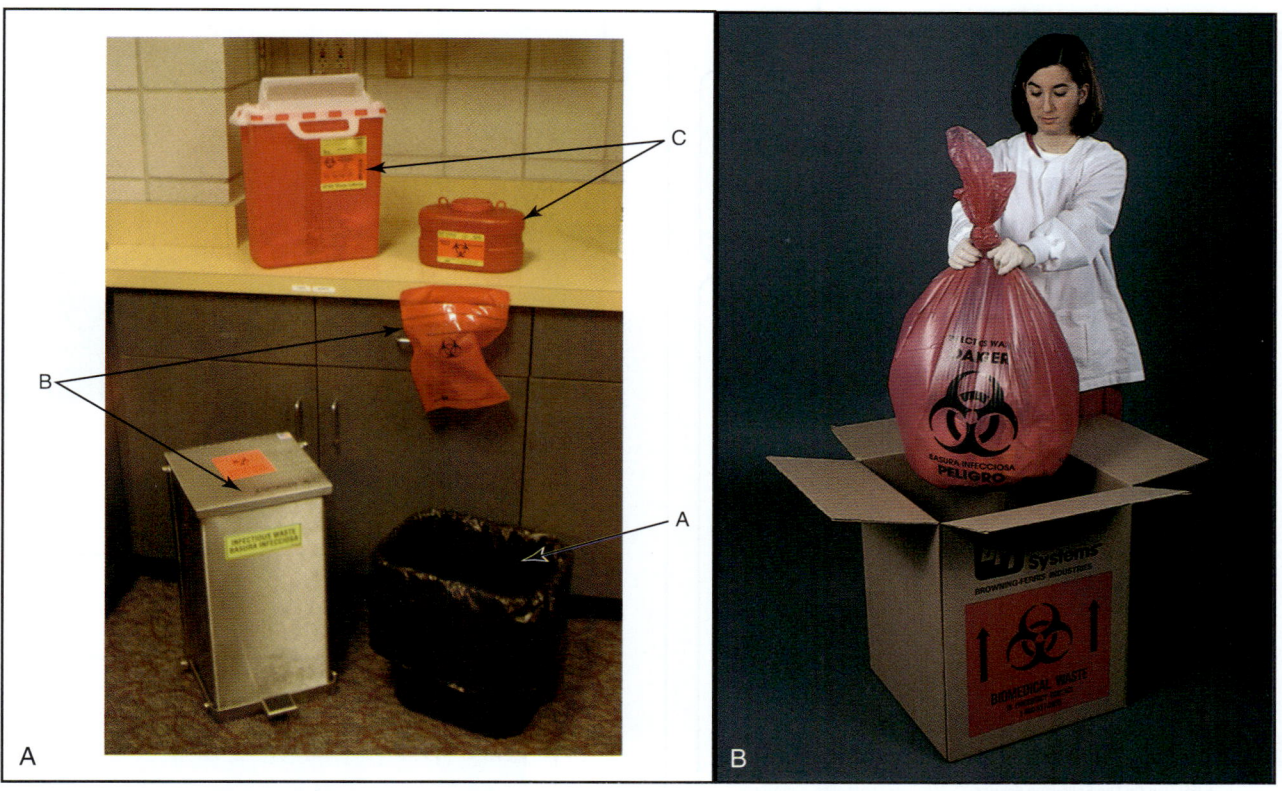

Fig. 1-19. **A,** Waste containers in the laboratory. *A,* Regular waste receptacle; *B,* nonsharps biohazard waste receptacles; and *C,* biohazard sharps containers. **B,** Biohazard waste is collected in boxes for managed-waste pickup. (*C,* from Bonewit-West K: *Clinical procedures for medical assistants,* ed 7, St Louis, 2008, Saunders.)

information and training. Examples of chemical hazards are dangerous acids, caustics, flammables, and inhalants.

In small medical laboratories, most of the chemicals used are fortunately in small, prepackaged quantities. The most common chemical hazard is the bleach used to disinfect counters. All labels on chemicals such as bleach should be read to understand their hazards. Fig. 1-20 shows a bleach label with the following eight container label requirements provided by the manufacturer:

1. Brand name of the chemical
2. Common or chemical name
3. Amount of the contents
4. Signal words such as *danger* (if flammable, corrosive, or highly reactive with other substances), *poison* (if toxic when ingested or inhaled), *warning,* or *caution* (if any other hazardous condition is present)
5. Instructions for the safe use of the chemical (storage, usage, and disposal)
6. Manufacturer information
7. Description of possible hazards such as physical hazards (will it explode, catch fire, react with other chemicals?), health hazards (will it irritate tissue or cause cancer?), toxicity (is it toxic if swallowed or inhaled?), and safety precautions (does it require protective clothing, gloves, or eye protection?)
8. First-aid instructions if necessary

Along with being properly labeled, each hazardous chemical must be listed on a chemical hazard inventory sheet and have its own MSDS. The sheets are compiled in an inventory notebook available to all employees (Fig. 1-21).

On the basis of the information in the MSDS or the manufacturer's label, chemical hazard labels must be placed on all containers holding hazardous chemicals. The National Paint and Coatings Association (NPCA) and the Hazardous Materials Information System **(HMIS)** are two of the most popular systems for labeling hazardous chemicals. The systems use standard labels to communicate hazards through the use of colors, numbers, letters, and symbols (Fig. 1-22).

The HMIS is a five-part rectangle that provides identification of the chemical using the information that appears on the MSDS in four categories:

- Blue: health hazards (e.g., if inhaled or ingested, skin irritants, carcinogens)
- Red: flammability (is it explosive, will it catch fire?)

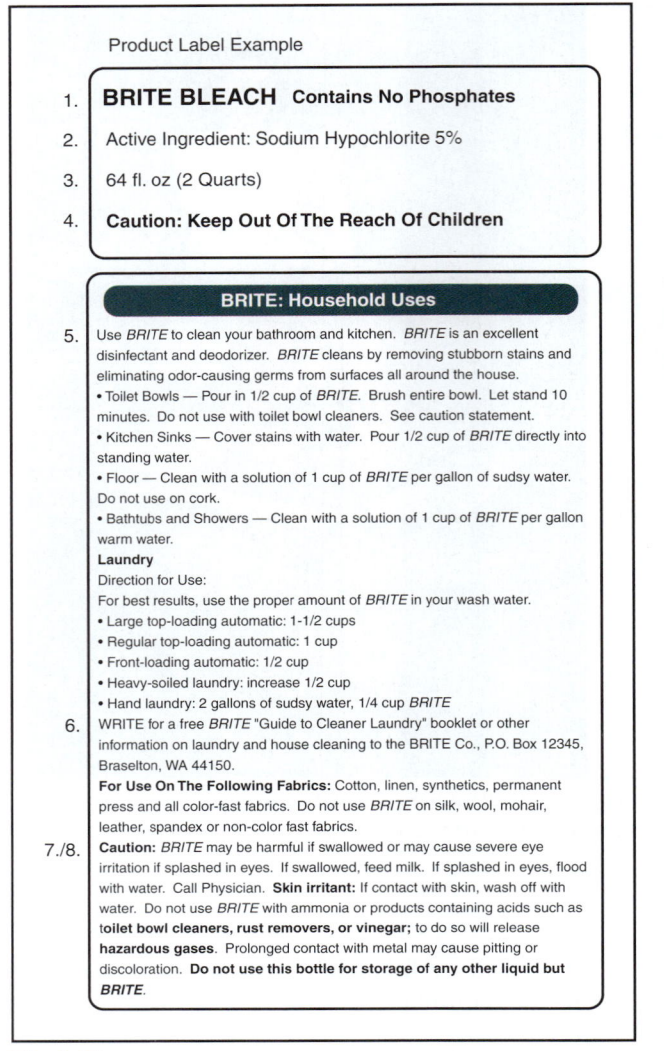

Fig. 1-20. Product label. Note the eight required elements for labeling a hazardous chemical.

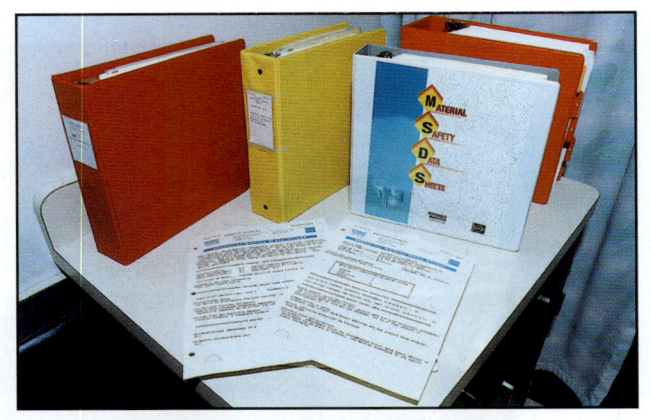

Fig. 1-21. Safety procedure manuals and MSDS manual. (From Stepp CA, Woods M: *Laboratory procedures for medical office personnel*, Philadelphia, 1998, Saunders.)

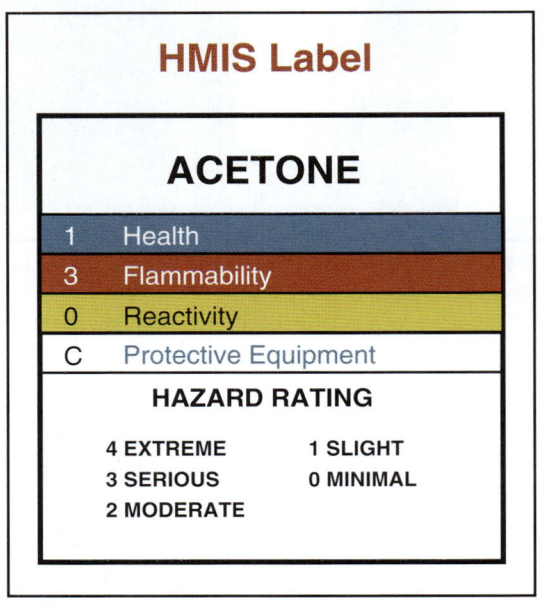

Fig. 1-22. HMIS system showing the labeling of acetone (used in staining procedures).

- Yellow: reactivity (is it stable, does it react with other chemicals?)
- White: the need for PPE (gloves, masks, gowns, etc.)

The numerical ratings range from 0 for no hazard to 4 for extreme hazard. An alphabetical designation is used to denote recommended PPE.

Another way to label hazardous chemicals is the National Fire Protective Association (**NFPA**) coding system (Fig. 1-23). The label uses the same four colors in a diamond pattern and a similar rating system of 0 to 4. Examples of typical NFPA-labeled solutions found in the laboratory are shown in Fig. 1-24.

Each facility must use a labeling system that everyone understands. Another way of identifying extremely hazardous chemicals is to use icons representing each chemical hazard: flammable, explosive, corrosive, poisonous, radioactive, compressed gas, and carcinogenic (Fig. 1-25).

Physical Hazard Training

The third area requiring safety awareness involves potential physical hazards. This area relies on common sense and physical hazard orientation in areas such as lifting, weather alerts, bomb threats, and electrical dangers.

- Make sure electrical instruments are grounded and the wires are intact when working with electrical instruments. Never operate electrical equipment with wet hands. Note the electrical hazard icons in Fig. 1-26.
- Run periodic drills for physical safety (fire drills, emergency weather protocol, terrorist attacks, etc.).
- Lift with the legs, not the back, and avoid twisting the back when carrying something heavy from one place to another.

Safety Training in the Laboratory

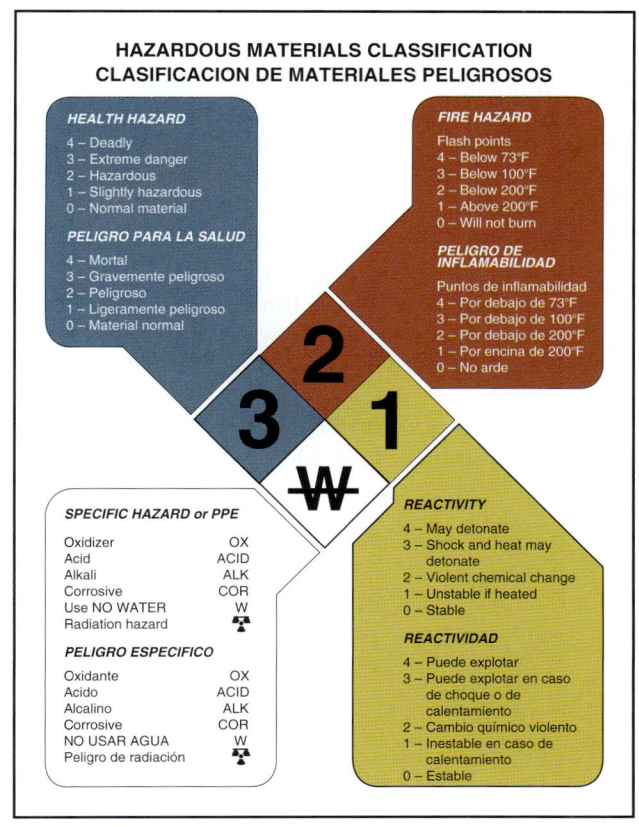

Fig. 1-23. NFPA coding system. (From Mahon CR, Manuselis G: *Textbook of diagnostic microbiology,* ed 3, St Louis, 2006, Saunders.)

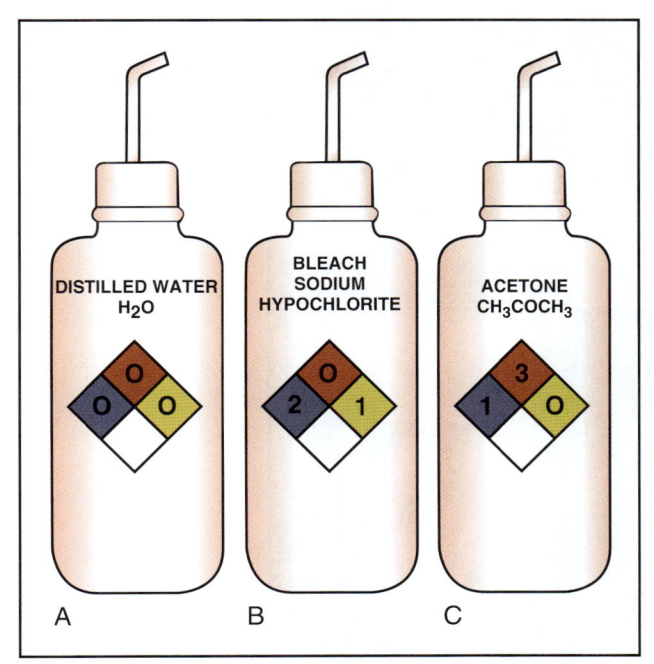

Fig. 1-24. Laboratory dispenser bottles with NFPA labels indicating acetone and bleach hazards. Compare the label for acetone with the HMIS label in Fig. 1-22, and compare the bleach (sodium hypochlorite) with the BRITE manufacturer label in Fig. 1-20.

- Keep hair shorter than shoulder length, or tie it back to avoid contamination or getting it tangled in moving instruments.
- Never push waste down into a wastebasket with the hands or reach into a biohazard disposal container.
- Learn **ergonomic practices** (proper movements and conditions that make you less prone to work-related injuries) such as proper positioning of seat and computer to prevent carpal tunnel syndrome, leg cramping, and undue stress on back and neck.

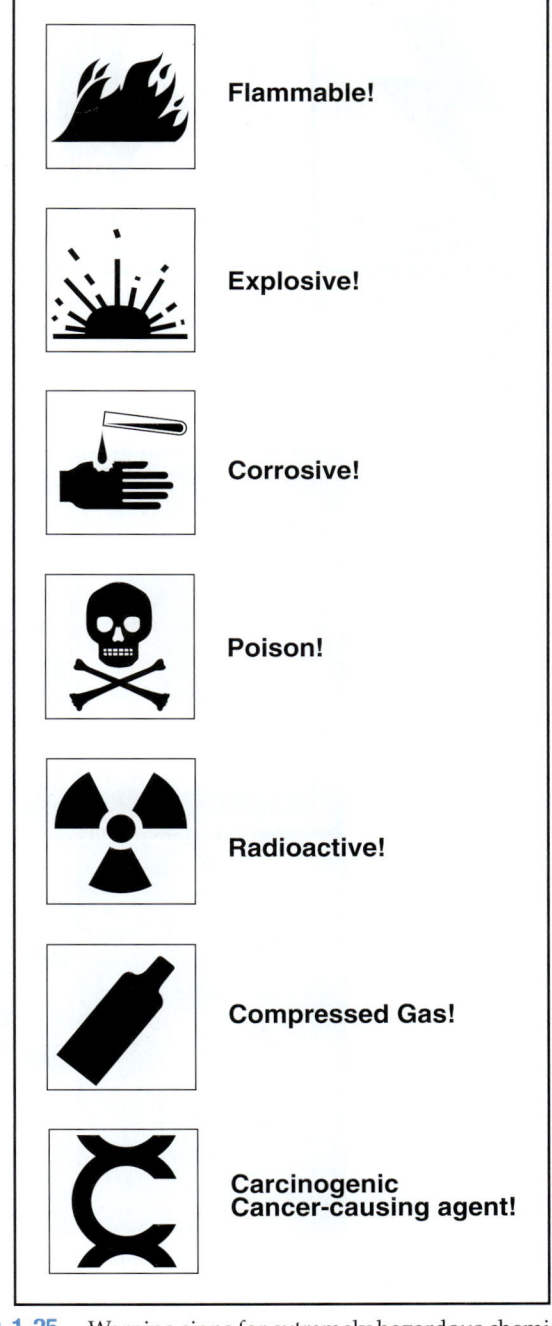

Fig. 1-25. Warning signs for extremely hazardous chemicals.

Laboratory Safety Evaluation

Laboratory safety training is completed by performing the following:
1. Complete the Chapter 1 review section in text and the workbook questions.
2. Complete the following on-line interactive exercises for Chapter 1:
    - Introductory terminology exercises
    - Exercise on ordering laboratory tests
    - Exercise on matching laboratory departments with their functions
    - On-line videos and training activities Units 1 through 5
3. Tour the laboratory using the Laboratory Safety Checklist at the end of Chapter 1 in the workbook. Be sure to locate and be familiar with how to use the biohazard spill kit (Fig. 1-27), the eye wash station (Fig. 1-28), and the chemical spill kit (Fig. 1-29).
4. Turn in the OSHA Blood Borne Pathogen Quiz at the end of Chapter 1 in the workbook and a mock exposure incident form in the appendix of the workbook.
5. Observe and perform Proper Use of Personal Protective Equipment found in Procedure 1-1.

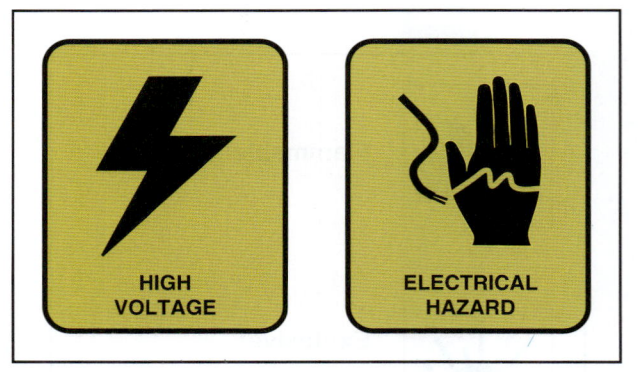

Fig. 1-26. Warning signs for electrical hazards. (From Stepp CA, Woods M: *Laboratory procedures for medical office personnel*, Philadelphia, 1998, Saunders.)

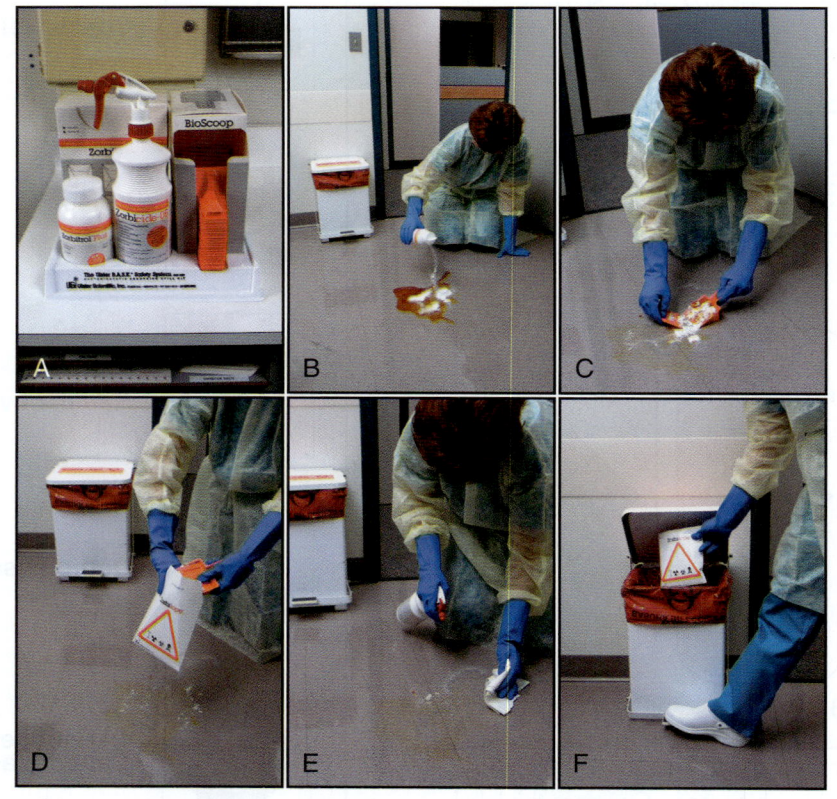

Fig. 1-27. Biohazard spill kit and cleaning procedure. (From Young AP, Kennedy DB: *Kinn's the medical assistant: an applied learning approach*, ed 10, St Louis, 2007, Saunders.)

Safety Training in the Laboratory

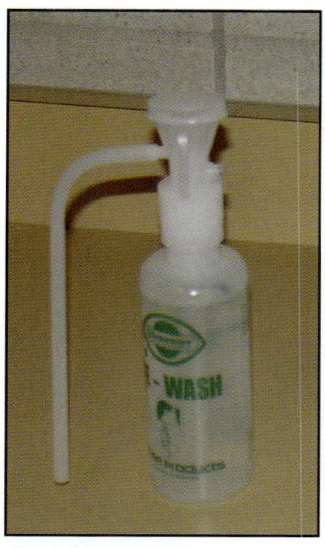

Fig. 1-28. Eye wash station.

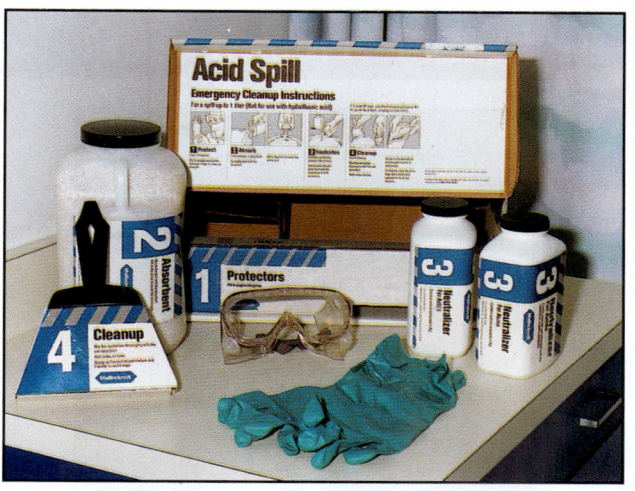

Fig. 1-29. Chemical spill kit. (From Stepp CA, Woods M: *Laboratory procedures for medical office personnel*, Philadelphia, 1998, Saunders.)

PROCEDURE 1-1 Proper Use of Personal Protective Equipment

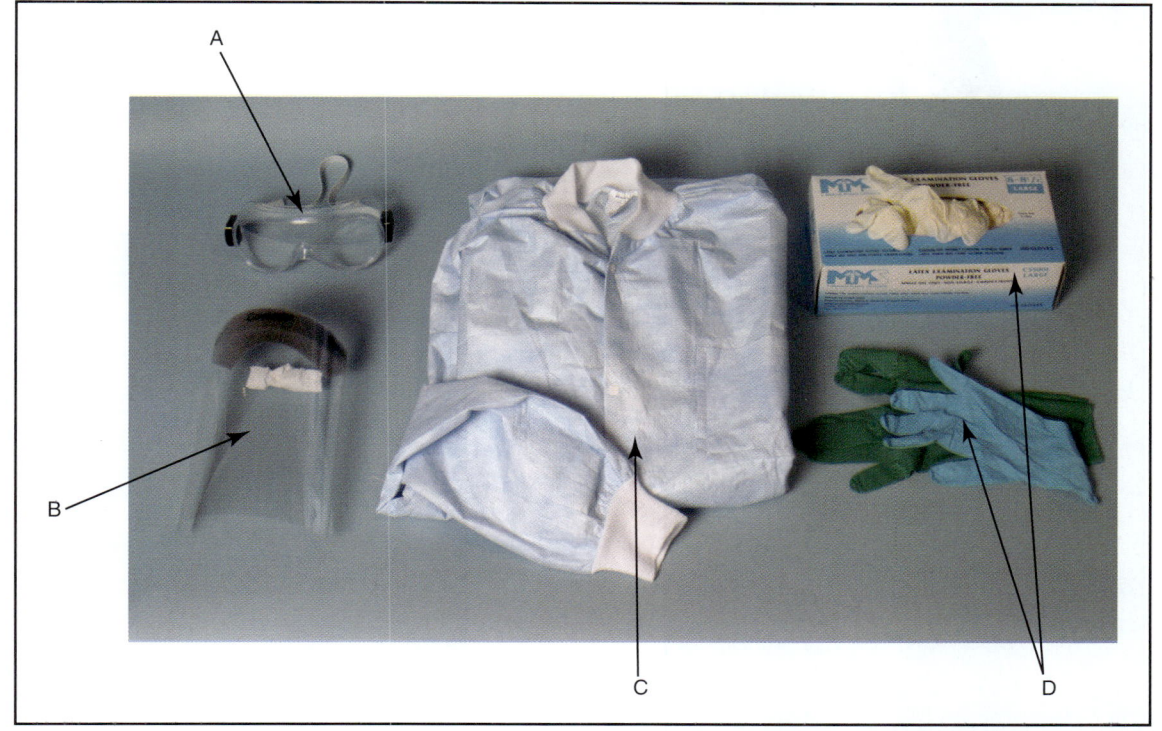

A. Examples of PPE. *a*, Goggles; *b*, face shield; *c*, fluid-impenetrable gown with elastic wrist bands; *d*, box of latex gloves and two pairs of colored nonlatex gloves.

(Continued)

28 CHAPTER 1 Introduction to the Laboratory and Safety Training

PROCEDURE 1-1 Proper Use of Personal Protective Equipment—cont'd

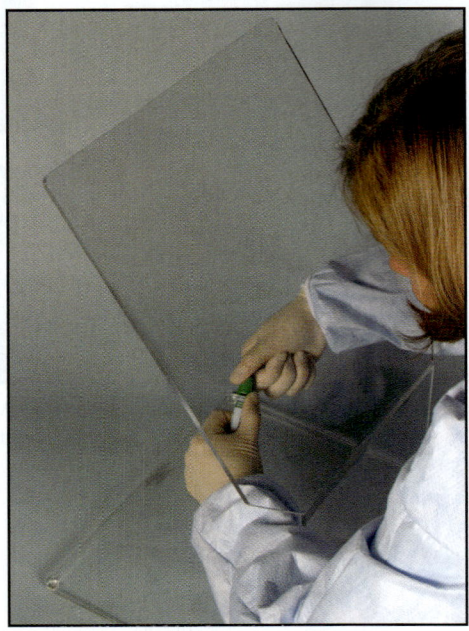

B. A Plexiglas shield provides splash protection in place of goggles and face mask when performing laboratory procedures.

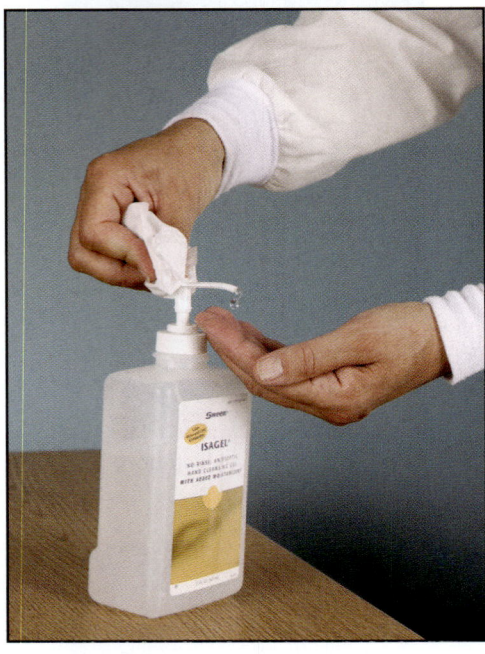

C. Sanitize hands before donning personal protective equipment.

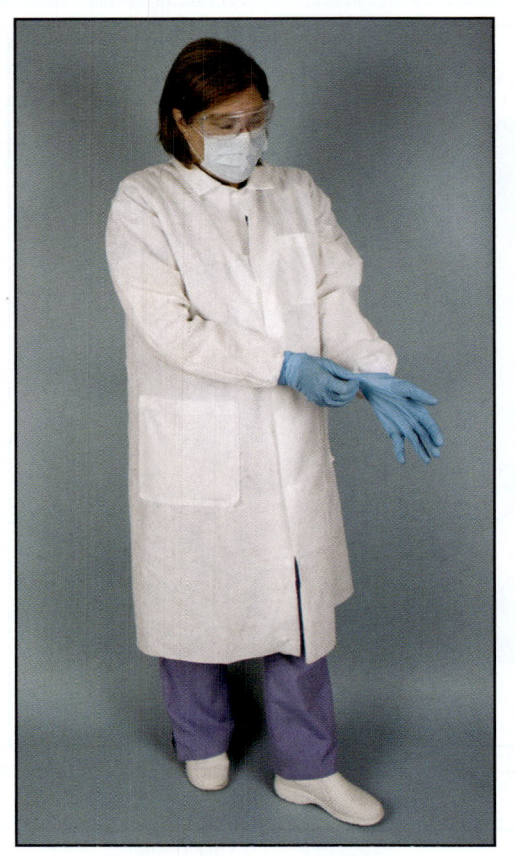

D. Order of donning PPE: (1) fluid impermeable coat, (2) face protection, (3) gloves.

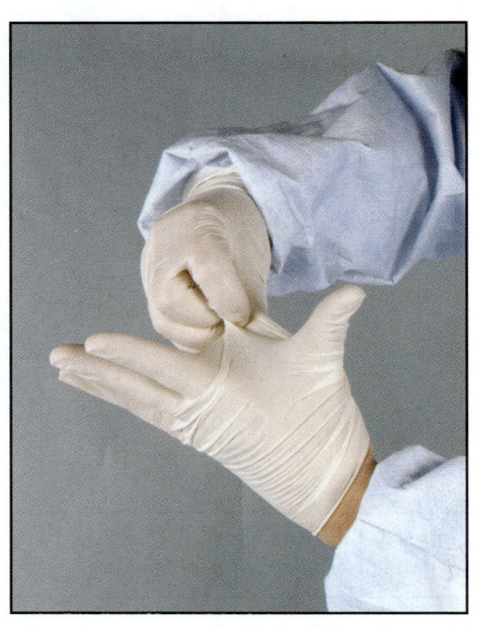

E. Removing gloves correctly. Pull off the glove with the nondominant hand.

Safety Training in the Laboratory

PROCEDURE 1-1 Proper Use of Personal Protective Equipment—cont'd

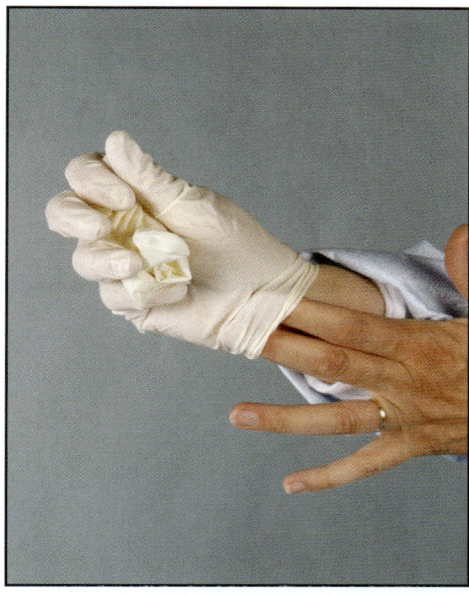

F. Hold the dirty glove in the dominant hand while slipping the nondominant fingers under the cuff.

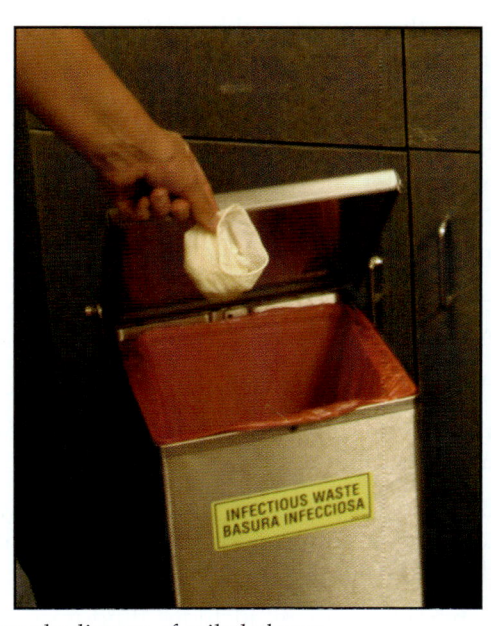

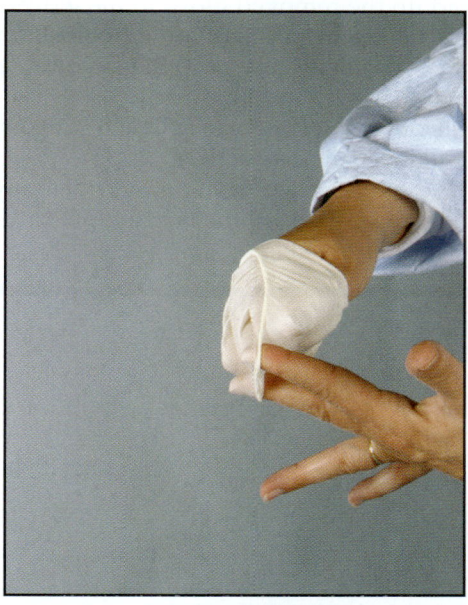

G. Flip the glove inside out while holding the other glove on the inside.

H. Properly dispose of soiled gloves.

PPE used in health care settings is displayed in Fig. A. In the laboratory nonpowdered gloves (d) and fluid-impenetrable gowns with cuffs at the wrists (c) are typically worn to protect the clothes and hands from direct contact with specimens. Latex gloves are not recommended because of potential allergic reactions. Vinyl, nitrile, and other nonlatex gloves are now available in a variety of sizes and colors. A Plexiglas shield can also be placed between you and your work area (Fig. B).

Procedure

1. Before **donning** (putting on) PPE, remember to perform either the hand wash or hand rub appropriately. (See Fig. C.)
2. If the procedure to be performed has the potential of splashing, eye goggles (a) or a face shield (b) or both will be required to protect the mucous membranes of the eyes, nose, and mouth.
3. Follow the proper sequence for donning PPE: (1) put on the gown, (2) put on any face protectors, and (3) don disposable nonsterile, nonpowdered, nonlatex, well-fitting gloves. Extend the gloves over the gown cuffs. (See Fig. D.)
4. Keep gloved hands away from the face.
5. Remove gloves if they become torn. (Perform hand hygiene before donning new gloves.)
6. Avoid touching other surfaces and items not involved in the testing process.
7. The outside of the front of the gown is considered contaminated. The clean areas of the gown and gloves are on the inside and the back of the gown.
8. The sequence for removing PPE is take off (1) gloves, (2) then face shield, (3) then gown.
9. The proper removal and disposal of gloves is as follows:
10. Remove one glove by grasping the outside with the other gloved hand and pulling it off. (See Fig. E.)

PROCEDURE 1-1 Proper Use of Personal Protective Equipment—cont'd

11. Wad up the removed glove in the gloved hand. Slip an ungloved finger under the cuff and fold it over until you can grasp the inside area of the second glove. (See Fig. F.)
12. Pull off the second glove inside out with the first glove still inside. (See Fig. G.)
13. If the gloves have visible blood or body fluid on them, dispose of them in a biohazard waste receptacle. (See Fig. H.)
14. Next, remove the gogles and then the gown.
15. Close the gown with the clean inside protected before hanging it up. The gown must not leave the lab area.
16. Perform hand hygiene (hand wash or hand rub) immediately after removing PPE.

*Figs. C and D courtesy Zack Bent.

Review Questions

1. The head of a hospital laboratory is usually a _____.

2. Phlebotomists perform _____.

3. Two nonhospital locations of medical laboratories are _____ and _____.

4. The educational degree of a pathologist is _____.

5. Five qualities important in a laboratory professional are
   _____
   _____
   _____
   _____
   _____

6. Match the prefix on the left with the definition on the right.
   _____ milli-   a. one hundredth
   _____ centi-   b. one millionth
   _____ deci-   c. one tenth
   _____ micro-   d. one thousandth

7. Write the symbol or abbreviation for the following units.
   milliliter _____
   deciliter _____
   centimeter _____
   micrometer _____
   cubic centimeter _____

8. The three major types of hazards are _____, _____, and _____.

9. An example of a physical hazard is _____.

10. An example of a chemical hazard is _____.

11. What is an appropriate surface disinfectant for use in the laboratory? _____

12. Bloodborne pathogen precautions apply only to patients who are known to have infectious disease. True _____ False _____

13. Laboratory apparel includes fluid-impermeable laboratory coats and closed-toe shoes. True _____ False _____

Review Question Answers

1. pathologist
2. venipuncture, blood draw
3. POLs (physician's office laboratories) and reference laboratories
4. doctor of medicine or osteopathy
5. honesty, communication skills, efficiency, organizational skills, good eyesight, and dexterity
6. d, a, c, b
7. mL, dL, cm, μm, cc
8. biohazards, chemical hazards, and physical hazards
9. fire, tornado, bomb, and electrical dangers
10. acids, caustics, flammables, inhalants
11. 10% solution of 1 part bleach and 9 parts water, or 70% alcohol
12. false
13. true

Websites

HHS information on disease control:
http://www.hhs.gov/diseases/index.html

OSHA's Bloodborne Pathogens Standard:
www.osha.gov/SLTC/bloodbornepathogens/index.html

OSHA-approved antiseptic hand cleansers for bloodborne pathogens:
www.osha.gov/pls/oshaweb/owadisp.show_document?p_table=INTERPRETATIONS&;p_id=24389&p_text_version=FALSE

The International Health Care Worker Safety Center at the University of Virginia Health System, dedicated to the prevention of occupational transmission of bloodborne pathogens:
www.healthsystem.virginia.edu/internet/epinet/

Example of Bleach MSDS sheet:
www.sciencelab.com/xMSDS-Sodium_Hypochlorite_5_-9925000

CHAPTER 2
Regulations, Microscope Setup, and Quality Assurance

Objectives
After completing this chapter you should be able to:

Laboratory Regulations
1. Explain the purpose of CLIA 1988 and its benefit to the patient.
2. Cite the three levels of complexity listed in CLIA 1988 and describe the process of obtaining certification to perform CLIA-waived laboratory tests and provider-performed microscopy.
3. Locate the latest CLIA-waived tests on the Internet.

Microscopic Procedure
1. Label the parts of a compound microscope and explain the functions of each.
2. Perform a microscopic exercise according to the stated task, conditions, and standards listed on the Learning Outcome Evaluation in the workbook, including focusing a slide under low, high dry, and oil immersion and cleaning and maintaining a microscope.

Quality Assurance, Quality Control, and Risk Management
1. Discuss the 10 areas of Good Laboratory Practices.
2. List and describe the three analytical phases of laboratory testing requiring quality assessment.
3. Explain the difference between quality assurance and quality control.
4. Define accuracy, precision, and reliability when observing the results of standard controls.
5. Identify trends, shifts, random error, out-of-control, and patient panic values.
6. Discuss current risk management and HIPAA issues as they apply to the physician's office laboratory.
7. Understand the uses and benefits of electronic medical records and bar coding as they relate to medical laboratories.

Key Terms

accuracy (correctness) when controls consistently fall within two standard deviations of the mean

bar code a pattern of narrow and wide bars and spaces that is encoded with its own particular meaning, just like words in a language are made up of letters and symbols

calibration the process of setting an instrument to accurately respond to the test reagents or devices

certificate of waiver (CoW) CLIA document that allows a facility to perform only waived tests

CLIA-waived tests tests that provide simple, unvarying results and require a minimum amount of judgment and interpretation

control sample a manufactured specimen that has a known value of the analyte being tested

external controls liquid positive and negative controls that are tested before the patient specimen to check the reliability of the instrument and the testing technique

internal control built-in positive control used in qualitative tests to prove the device or test kit is working

kit all components of a test packaged together

Levy–Jennings chart a graph used to plot and visualize the results of control samples over time

mean the average test result of a series of control tests

medical office risk management overseeing the physical and procedural risks that may bring about an injury or legal action against the practice

optics check confirming that the light source and light sensor in optical analyzers are working properly

precision (reproducibility) ability to produce the same test result each time a test is performed

proficiency testing proving laboratory competency by testing a sample specimen from an outside accreditation agency and obtaining the correct result

protected health information (PHI) any health information in any form (written, electronic, or oral) that contains patient-identifiable information (e.g., name, Social Security number, telephone number) that must be kept confidential

qualitative test test that simply looks for the presence or absence of a substance

quality assurance (QA) overall process to aid in improving the reliability, efficiency, and quality of laboratory testing in general

quality control (QC) process in which known samples (controls) are routinely tested to establish the reliability, accuracy, and precision of a specific test system

Key Terms—cont'd

quantitative test test that produces a numerical value indicating the amount of a substance present
reagent substance or ingredient used in a laboratory test to detect, measure, examine, or produce a reaction
reliability when both accuracy and precision are accomplished
semiquantitative test determines the approximate quantity of an analyte

standard deviation (SD) statistical term describing the amount of variation from the mean in a data set
work practice controls policies that are recorded, monitored, and evaluated with a view to protecting employees from exposure to the pathogens in blood or body fluids

Abbreviations

CLIA	Clinical Laboratory Improvement Amendments	PPM	provider-performed microscopy
CMS	Centers for Medicare and Medicaid Services	PPMP	Certificate provider-performed microscopic procedures certification
FDA	Food and Drug Administration		
HIPAA	Health Insurance Portability and Accountability Act		

This chapter presents additional government regulations, microscope setup, and quality assurance procedures as they apply to the medical laboratory.

CLIA: GOVERNMENT REGULATIONS

Whenever a specimen is removed from a human body and an analysis occurs that translates to a result, that activity is considered a medical laboratory test. As stated earlier, physicians use test results for the following reasons: (1) to *screen* and detect possible diseases, (2) to confirm a clinical *diagnosis* and make treatment decisions, and (3) to *monitor* the progress of diseases and treatments. If testing is not performed properly, the incorrect results can pose a threat to the patient's overall care and treatment. For example, if a clinical laboratory misreads or misreports a patient's blood sample as having a normal cholesterol level when in fact the patient's cholesterol is abnormally high, that patient may not receive the necessary treatment to prevent a heart attack.

To protect patients from inaccurate test results, Congress passed the Clinical Laboratory Improvement Amendments **(CLIA)** in 1988. CLIA 1988 required that all laboratories examining materials derived from the human body for diagnosis, prevention, or treatment purposes be certified by the Secretary of Health and Human Services **(HHS).** Centers for Medicare and Medicaid Services **(CMS)** administers the certification process by requiring all medical laboratories to register and pay a certification fee based on the level of complexity of the tests they perform.

CLIA Levels of Complexity and Their Certification Requirements

There are four complexity levels: high complexity, moderate complexity, provider-performed microscopy **(PPM**; a subset of moderate complexity), and waived testing. The Food and Drug Administration **(FDA)** is involved in determining the level of complexity for all commercial medical laboratory tests on the market.

CLIA Certificate of Waiver

The CLIA **Certificate of Waiver (CoW)** is used predominantly by physician's office laboratories (POLs), ambulatory settings, and institutions with point-of-care testing (POCT).

According to CLIA, CoW laboratories can perform only tests that are determined by the FDA to be so simple that there is little risk of error. The CLIA-waived tests with their appropriate procedure codes are listed in Table 2-1.

The number and types of tests waived under CLIA have increased from the eight originally approved tests in 1992 to more than 40. The number of waived laboratories has also grown exponentially, from 20% to more than 55% of the total laboratories enrolled in CLIA.

To become a CLIA-waived laboratory, the physician or facility simply needs to enroll in the CLIA-waived program through CMS, pay an applicable certification fee of $150 every 2 years, and follow the manufacturer's instructions for each FDA-approved waived test.

CLIA High and Moderately Complex Laboratories

Hospital and reference laboratories are staffed with highly educated laboratory professionals who have been trained to perform the complex tests in the various laboratory departments, such as hematology, chemistry, microbiology, and blood bank. To be registered and certified by CLIA, laboratory professionals must obtain a Certificate of Registration, then be surveyed to receive a Certificate of Compliance and then a Certificate of Accreditation. They must maintain their accreditation status by being surveyed periodically to

TABLE 2-1　Tests Granted Waived Status Under CLIA

CPT Codes	Test Name	Use
Original Eight Tests Approved in 1988		
Hematology		
83026	Hemoglobin by copper sulfate—nonautomated	Monitors hemoglobin level in blood
85013	Blood count; spun microhematocrit	Screen for anemia
85651	Erythrocyte sedimentation rate—nonautomated	Nonspecific screening test for inflammatory activity, increased for majority of infections and most cases of carcinoma and leukemia
Chemistry		
82962	Blood glucose by glucose monitoring devices cleared by the FDA for home use	Monitoring of blood glucose levels
Urine and Feces		
81002	Dipstick or tablet reagent urinalysis—nonautomated for bilirubin, glucose, hemoglobin, ketone, leukocytes, nitrite, pH, protein, specific gravity, and urobilinogen	Screening of urine to monitor or diagnose various diseases and conditions such as diabetes, the state of the kidney or urinary tract, and urinary tract infections
81025	Urine pregnancy tests by visual color comparison	Diagnosis of pregnancy
84830	Ovulation tests by visual color comparison for human luteinizing hormone	Detection of ovulation (optimal for conception)
82270 GO 107 (Contact Medicare carrier for claims instructions.)	Fecal occult blood	Detection of blood in feces from whatever cause, benign or malignant (colorectal cancer screening)
Examples of More Recently Approved Waived Tests		
Hematology		
85014QW	STAT-CRIT/hematocrit	Screen for anemia
85018QW	HemoCue Hemoglobin system GDS Diagnostics HemoSite Meter	Measures hemoglobin level in whole blood
Blood Chemistry		
82365QW (Contact Medicare for claims instructions.)	Cholestech LDX	Measures total cholesterol, high-density lipoprotein cholesterol, triglycerides, and glucose levels in blood
82947QW	HemoCue B—glucose photometer	Measures glucose levels in whole blood
83036QW	Bayer DCA 2000—glycosylated hemoglobin (Hgb A1c)	Measures percent concentration of hemoglobin A1c in blood, which is used in monitoring the long-term care of people with diabetes
80053QW	Blood Chemistry Analyzer	Measures alanine amino transferase (ALT), aspartate amino transferase (AST), albumin, total bilirubin, total calcium, carbon dioxide, chloride, creatinine, glucose, alkaline phosphatase, potassium, total protein, sodium, and urea nitrogen in whole blood
Drug Screening		
80101QW	Multiple Drug Cup Test	Screening test to detect the presence of amphetamines, barbiturates, benzodiazepines, tetrahydrocannabinol (THC), cocaine metabolites, methadone, methamphetamines, opiates, oxycodone, and phencyclidine (PCP) in urine

TABLE 2-1   Tests Granted Waived Status Under CLIA—cont'd

CPT Codes	Test Name	Use
Immunology/Serology		
86308QW	Rapid whole blood mononucleosis tests	Qualitative screening test for the presence of heterophile antibodies to aid in the diagnosis of infectious mononucleosis
86318QW	Rapid whole blood test for *Helicobacter pylori* antibodies for determining the possible cause of peptic ulcers	Immunoassay for rapid, qualitative detection of immunoglobulin G antibodies specific to *H. pylori*
86618QW	Rapid whole blood test for *Borrelia burgdorferi* (causative agent of Lyme disease)	Qualitative detection of immunoglobulin G and M antibodies to *B. burgdorferi*
86701QW	OraSure OraQuick Rapid HIV-1 antibody test with whole blood	Qualitative immunoassay to detect antibodies to HIV-1 in fingerstick and venipuncture whole blood specimens
Microbiology		
87804QW	Quick influenza A and B test	Qualitative detection of influenza type A and B antigens in nasal wash and nasopharyngeal swab specimens
87889QW	Quick *Streptococcus* A test	Rapidly detects *Streptococcus* A antigen from throat swabs as an aid in the diagnosis of strep throat, tonsillitis, and scarlet fever
Urinalysis		
81003QW	Bayer Clinitek 50 Urine Chemistry Analyzer—qualitative dipstick for glucose, bilirubin, ketone, specific gravity, blood, pH, protein, urobilinogen, nitrite, leukocytes (automated)	Screening of urine to monitor or diagnose various diseases and conditions such as diabetes, the state of the kidney or urinary tract, and urinary tract infections
82044QW	Bayer Clinitek 50 Urine Chemistry Analyzer—microalbumin, creatinine	Semiquantitative measurement of microalbumin and creatinine in urine for the detection of patients at risk for developing kidney damage

validate that they are performing only tests within their level of complexity and that their personnel are qualified and sufficiently trained in the test procedures.

All testing procedures are continuously monitored by the following systems:

1. **Quality assurance (QA)**—the overall process to aid in improving the reliability, efficiency, and quality of all laboratory tests in general. QA has three major phases: preanalytical, analytical, and postanalytical. Each of these steps must be evaluated regarding the effectiveness of the laboratory's policies and procedures in producing and documenting the test results, the identification of any problems, and the correction of the problems. The policies must ensure the accurate and prompt performance and reporting of tests.
2. **Quality control (QC)**—a part of QA that takes place during the analytical phase. It uses samples with known values that are tested along with the patient samples to establish the reliability, accuracy, and precision of a specific test system.
3. **Proficiency testing program**—biannual confirmation of laboratory competency by testing specimens from an outside accreditation agency and obtaining the correct results.

Further details in high and moderate complexity testing may be found at the government websites for HHS, CMS, CDC, and FDA. The purpose of this text, however, is to explore the lesser-regulated CLIA certificates most commonly used in physicians' offices, ambulatory care, and point-of-care settings, specifically the CLIA-waived tests and the PPM tests.

CLIA: Provider-Performed Microscopy Procedures Certificate

The PPM Procedures **(PPMP)** Certificate allows qualified health care providers to do waived testing and basic microscopic examinations during the patient's visit. The microscopic tests are performed on specimens that are not easily transportable. To receive PPMP

TABLE 2-2 CLIA Approved Provider-Performed Microscopy Tests

Code	Description
Q0111	Wet mounts, including preparations of vaginal, cervical, or skin specimens
Q0112	All potassium hydroxide preparations
Q0113	Pinworm examinations
Q0114	Fern test
Q0115	Postcoital direct, qualitative examinations of vaginal or cervical mucus
81015	Urinalysis, microscopic only
81000	Urinalysis, by dipstick or tablet reagent for bilirubin, glucose, hemoglobin, ketones, leukocytes, nitrite, pH, protein, specific gravity, urobilinogen, and any number of these constituents; nonautomated, with microscopy
81001	Urinalysis, by dipstick or tablet reagent for bilirubin, glucose, hemoglobin, ketones, leukocytes, nitrite, pH, protein, specific gravity, urobilinogen, and any number of these constituents; automated, with microscopy (Note: This may be used only when the laboratory is using an automated dipstick urinalysis instrument approved as waived.)
81020	Urinalysis; two- or three-glass test
89055	Fecal leukocyte examination
G0027	Semen analysis; presence and motility of sperm, excluding Huhner test
89190	Nasal smears for eosinophils

certification, the physician or medical facility must enroll in the CMS program for PPMP certification, pay applicable certificate fees of $200 every 2 years, and maintain certain quality assurance (QA) and administrative requirements such as the following:

- Proficiency testing by an outside agency to evaluate microscopic accuracy twice a year
- Documentation of microscope/centrifuge maintenance
- Confirmation that competent personnel are interpreting the microscopic findings

Some of the microscopic tests that require proper preparation before being interpreted are presented in this text. The preparations for these microscopic tests include the following:

- Urine sediment preparation as part of a complete urinalysis
- Direct wet mount preparations for the identification of bacteria, fungi, parasites, and abnormal human cellular elements
- Potassium hydroxide preparations for identifying fungi
- Cellulose tape preparations for identifying pinworms

The actual reading and reporting of the microscopic findings must be done by the physician or a laboratory professional who is trained and certified to interpret the particular test. Table 2-2 lists the approved PPM tests and their numerical Current Procedural Terminology (CPT) codes.

MICROSCOPE PROCEDURE

If the physician chooses to perform basic microscopic examinations of specimens, his or her employees will need to learn how to set up a microscope slide for observation and how to focus and maintain the microscope for optimal performance. The procedure for using a clinical microscope is described in the following section. (A microscope procedure skill checklist can also be found in the workbook at the end of Chapter 2.)

Preparation: Identifying the Parts and Functions of a Microscope

The microscope can be divided into the following three basic functional areas:

1. *The foundational structures*—consisting of the base, arm, and stage
2. *The illuminating structures*—consisting of the light source and condenser
3. *The magnifying structures*—consisting of the objectives lenses, the ocular lenses, and the focus adjustment knobs. As you look at the picture of the microscope in Fig. 2-1, note the name of each lettered structure in the text as it is described in the three subsequent categories.

Foundational Structures and Their Functions

First, always carry the microscope with two hands—one under the *(a) base*, and the other holding the *(b) arm*. The slide with the specimen is placed on the *(c) stage* and clipped into place with the *(d) mechanical holder*, which can then precisely move the slide back and forth and side to side when the operator turns the *(e) mechanical controls* located under the stage.

Microscope Procedure

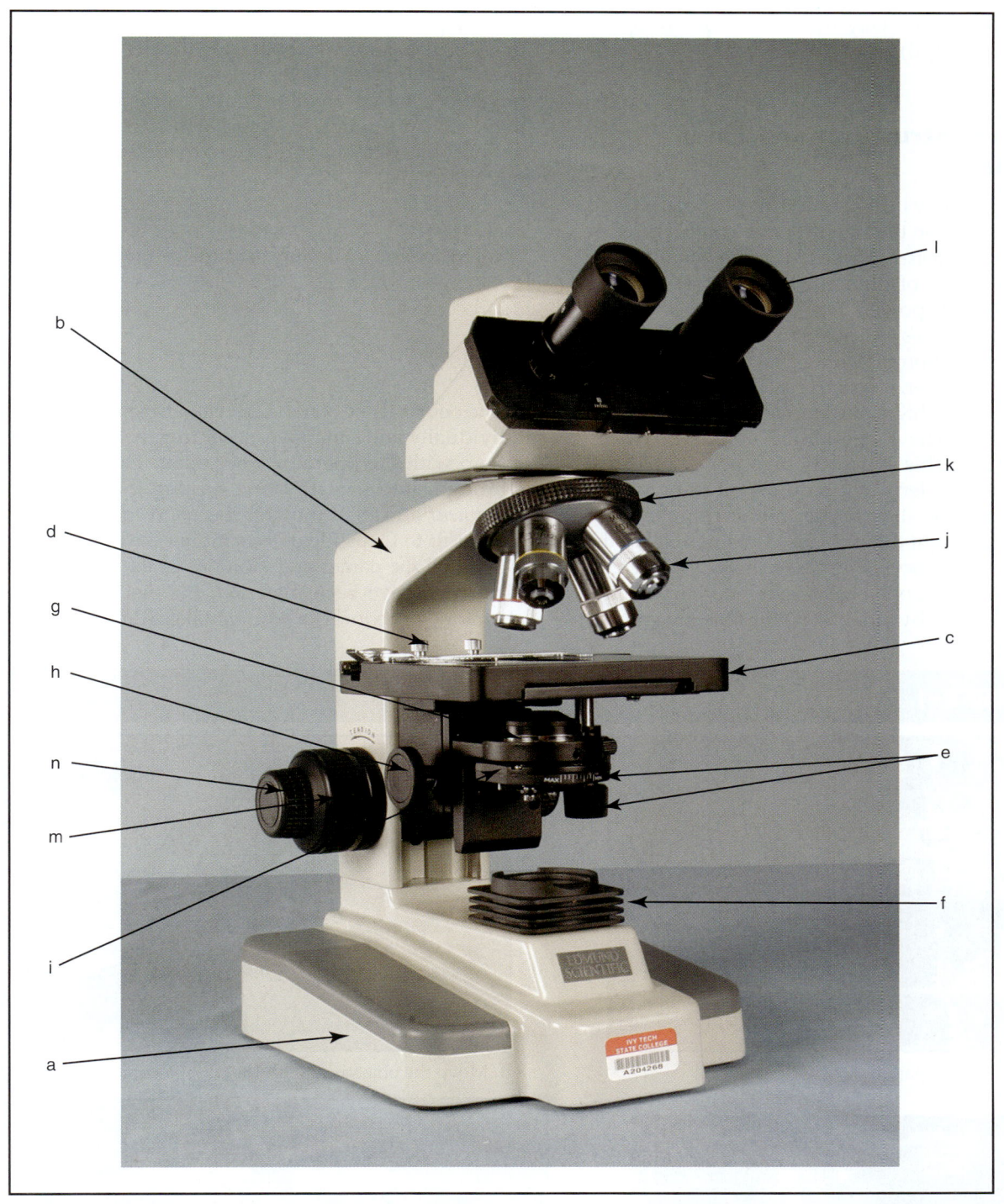

Fig. 2-1. Microscope. *a,* Base; *b,* arm; *c,* stage; *d,* slide holder; *e,* mechanical slide controls; *f,* light source; *g,* condenser; *h,* condenser adjustment; *i,* diaphragm lever; *j,* low power objective; *k,* nosepiece; *l,* ocular lens; *m,* coarse focus adjustment; *n,* fine focus adjustment.

Illuminating Structures and Their Functions

The slide is illuminated by the *(f) light source* in the base of the microscope. The light flows up into the *(g) condenser,* where it becomes highly concentrated. The condenser can be raised to a position just under the slide by using the *(h) condenser adjustment* when viewing densely stained specimens. The condenser can be lowered for more transparent wet mount specimens (slides that contain cells in water but no stain). The condenser also contains the *(i) iris diaphragm lever,* which opens up the iris for dense slides and closes down the light for more transparent slides (similar to the way the iris of the eye opens and closes the pupil).

Magnifying Structures and Their Functions

After the light flows up through the condenser and through the slide on the stage, it enters one of three or four *(j) objectives lenses*. These lenses are usually color coded, with tubes of different lengths marked with the magnification power. The shortest tubes are the low power objectives and are usually marked with 4× or 10× magnification, meaning they make the image 4 and 10 times larger, respectively. The middle-length tube contains the high power objective and usually magnifies 43×. The longest tube objective usually magnifies 100×. This extremely high power objective contains the only lens that requires oil to be placed between it and the slide to prevent air from bending (refracting) the light out of focus. Thus it is called the *oil immersion objective*. The *(k) revolving nosepiece* is used to move from one objective to another. (Do not turn the objectives by pushing on the objective tubes.)

After passing through the objectives, the lighted image strikes a mirror that sends the image through the *(l) ocular lenses* (eyepieces), where the operator can see the result. The ocular lenses enlarge the image an additional 10 times, which is multiplied by the objective magnification to determine total magnification.

Objective magnification	Ocular × magnification	=	Total magnification
Low power 10×	× 10×	=	100×
High power 43×	× 10×	=	430×
Oil immersion 100×	× 10×	=	1000×

The ocular lenses can be adjusted to focus each eye individually and can move closer together or apart to line up with the operator's eye span. The specimen is brought into focus by first turning the *(m) coarse adjustment* and then moving the hand to the *(n) fine adjustment* to focus the objects more clearly.

After all the names and locations of the parts of the microscope have been mastered, the first microscope laboratory procedure can be undertaken (Procedure 2-1).

PROCEDURE 2-1 Using a Microscope

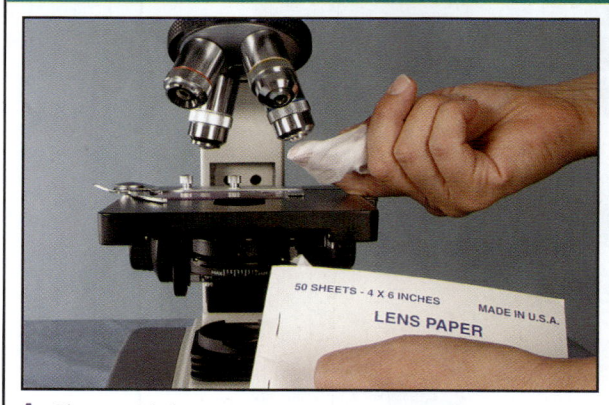

A. Clean with lens paper.

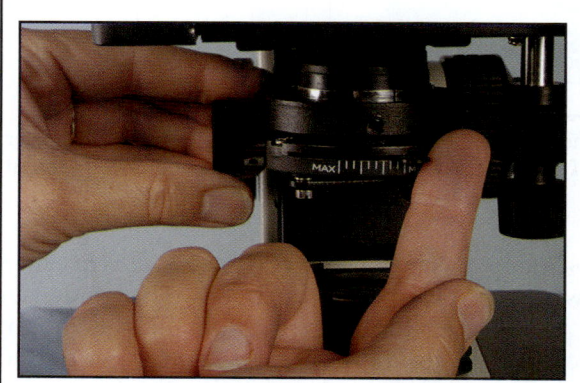

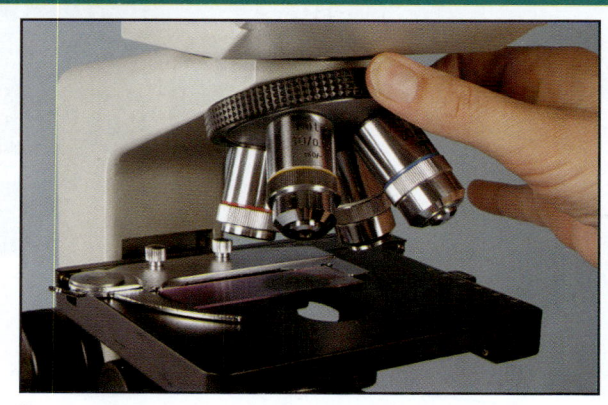

B. Move the objectives with the nosepiece.

C. The condenser height control is on the left, diaphragm control on the right.

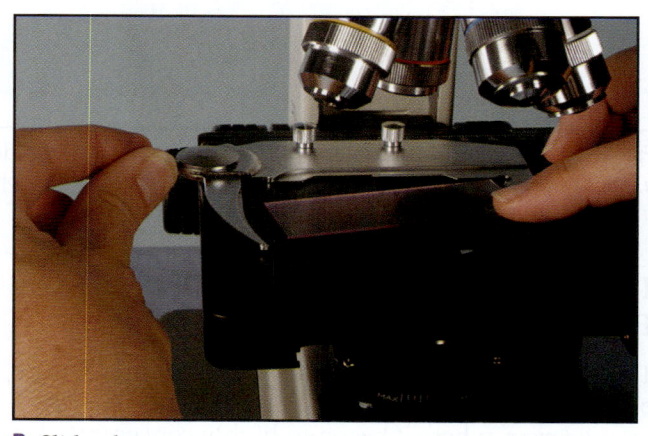

D. Slide placement on stage into the mechanical holder.

Microscope Procedure

PROCEDURE 2-1   Using a Microscope—cont'd

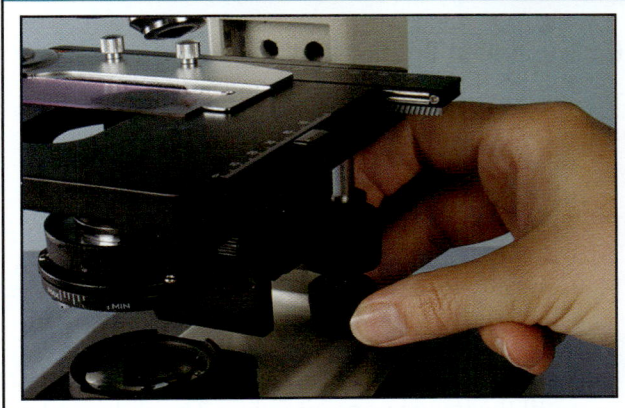

E. The mechanical stage control moves the slide up and down and back and forth.

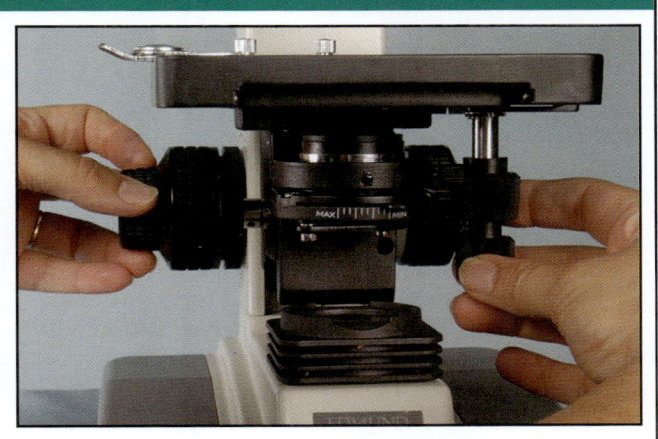

F. Fine focus while moving the slide slightly.

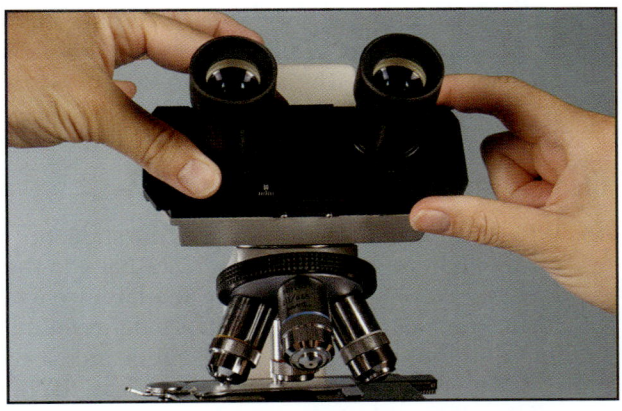

G. Adjust the oculars to your eyes' width and vision.

Equipment and Supplies

Microscope; lens paper; a stained slide; immersion oil; soft, lint-free tissue

Set Up the Microscope and Slide (see Fig. 2-1)

1. Always carry the microscope with one hand under the base (a) and the other grasping the arm (b) of the scope.
2. Clean the ocular (l) and objective (j) lenses with lens paper (clean the oil immersion lens last). Note that in Fig. A the soft part of the finger is used to clean the lens. Use a different part of the lens paper for each lens, and always clean the oil immersion lens last to keep from spreading the oil to the other lenses.
3. Turn the nosepiece (k) until the low power is directly above the stage (Fig. B). Do not push the objective tubes.
4. Turn the coarse adjustment (m) until the stage (c) and the low power objective (j) are farthest apart.

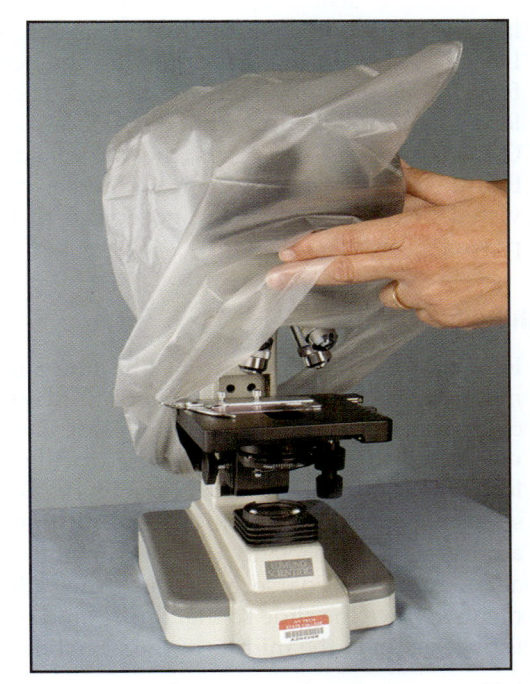

H. After cleaning, always store the microscope with its protective cover.

5. Turn on the light source (f), and turn the condenser adjustment (h) until the condenser (g) is all the way up for viewing stained slides. With the other hand, open the iris with the diaphragm lever all the way (i) to adjust for the maximum amount of light (Fig. C).
6. Place the slide in the slide holder (d) (Fig. D), and use the mechanical controls (e) to move the stained portion of the slide directly above the light source (Fig. E).
7. Adjust the ocular lens (l) to line up with your eyes.

(Continued)

PROCEDURE 2-1 Using a Microscope—cont'd

Low Power Focus

8. Always start with the low power objective in place, and initially focus using the coarse adjustment. While looking through the oculars, turn the coarse adjustment *(m)* until color starts to appear, then turn slowly to bring the image into coarse focus. (Fig. F). Tip: Moving the mechanical slide knob slightly back and forth with your right hand while finding the focus position with your left hand helps pick up movement.
9. Next, move the focusing hand to the fine focus adjustment *(n)* and turn it one way and then the other until the image becomes clear. Both eyes should see a clear image. If not, adjust the oculars by turning their individual focus controls. In Fig. G the left hand is adjusting the ocular focus while the right hand is pulling the ocular lenses apart to line up with the operator's eyes.
10. Once the image is in focus, move the slide so that the object of interest is in the center of the visual field. Then turn the nosepiece to high power.

High Power Focus

11. Refocus the image by turning the fine adjustment one way and then the other until you see color and then the clear image. (NOTE: Do not use the coarse adjustment because it will make too drastic a change and possibly break the slide. If you are unable to focus with the fine adjustment, go back to low power and start again with the coarse and fine focus adjustments.) Move the slide so that the desired object is once again in the middle of the visual field.

Oil Immersion Preparation and Focus

12. You are now ready to use the oil immersion lens for maximum magnification. Turn the nosepiece halfway between high power and the oil immersion objective.
13. Place a drop of oil directly on the slide where the condenser light is shining through the slide.
14. Carefully turn the nosepiece until the oil immersion lens dips into the oil and snaps into place.
15. Now, while looking into the oculars, move the small fine focus adjustment back and forth until the image pops into view. The slide can be moved and refocused by using the mechanical stage controls with one hand, while the other hand is turning the fine focus to continuously make adjustments while moving to different areas of the slide. The instructor or supervisor will verify the successful focused result.

Cleanup and Microscope Maintenance

16. When you are finished observing the slide, turn off the light and turn the nosepiece back to the low power objective. By using the large coarse focus knob, maximize the distance between the lens and the stage. Remove the slide, and clean the stage with soft, lint-free tissue. Clean the oil off the slide with tissue or xylene.
17. With a new piece of lens paper, clean off the ocular lenses, then the objective lenses. Always clean the oil immersion lens last.
18. Cover the microscope with a dust-proof cover (Fig. H), and store it in a clean, protected area.

PROCEDURE 2-1 Using a Microscope—cont'd

Keys to Proper Condenser and Objective Lens Settings Based on Three Common Slides

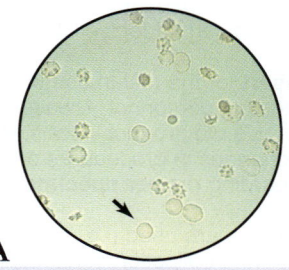

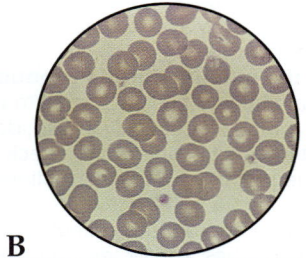

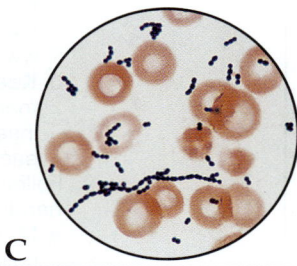

	A Liquid Urine	B Stained Blood Slide	C Stained Microbiology
Condenser Setting	Down with diaphragm almost closed	All the way up against the bottom of the slide with the diaphragm open	All the way up against the bottom of the slide with the diaphragm open
Objective Lens Setting	Low then high "dry" lenses only—no oil immersion (10×s and 43×s)	Start on low, then high, then oil immersion for identification	Start on low, then high, then oil immersion for identification

A from Stepp CA, Woods M: *Laboratory procedures for medical office personnel,* Philadelphia, 1998, Saunders; Zakus SM: *Mosby's clinical skills for medical assistants,* St Louis, 1998, Mosby.
B from Rodak BF: *Hematology: clinical principles and applications,* ed 2, St Louis, 2003, Elsevier.
C from Young AP, Kennedy DB: *Kinn's the medical assistant: an applied learning approach,* ed 10, St Louis, 2007, Saunders.

GOOD LABORATORY PRACTICES

The CLIA CoW is the least regulated category of laboratory testing. Waived tests can be performed by individuals with little or no previous experience in laboratory testing, and they do not require the rigorous QC, QA documentation, periodic surveys, and proficiency testing of the other CLIA categories. These facts, along with the ever-increasing number of approved waived tests, have raised the question: Are the waived test results accurate and reliable? The HHS, CMS, FDA, laboratory professionals, and test manufacturers are all looking for ways to better educate the personnel performing waived tests. Anyone performing a test on a specimen must know how to achieve accurate and reliable results to ultimately improve the quality of health care. This text is designed to follow the document by CMS entitled Good Laboratory Practices (Fig. 2-2).

Quality Assurance

As shown in Good Laboratory Practices, many factors contribute to the overall testing of specimens. How can the patient be assured that the results were obtained in a reliable, efficient, and well-monitored way? This is where QA comes in. Remember, QA is an overall process to aid in improving the reliability, efficiency, and quality of the laboratory as a whole. Also remember that QA has three major phases: preanalytical, analytical, and postanalytical.

Table 2-3 describes the QA that must be assessed and documented during the three phases of laboratory testing. Table 2-4 lists possible problems or variables that can occur within each phase. These tables are a good review of the concepts presented in this chapter. Everyone involved in the laboratory process must take personal responsibility for his or her part in providing safe, high-quality patient care.

Eight QA questions should always be asked:
1. Are the patients and specimens properly identified?

GOOD LABORATORY PRACTICES
QUALITY ASSURANCE RECOMMENDATIONS FOR
CERTIFICATE OF WAIVER (CoW) LABORATORIES

1. Upon receiving a **new test kit** (which contains all the components of a test that are packaged together):
    a. **Make sure it is CLIA-waived test** (this information may be printed on the box, printed in the package insert, in a letter to the manufacturer from HHS, or found on the web at www.accessdata.fda.gov/scripts/cdrh/cfdocs/cfCLIA/seardh.cfm or www.cms.gov/clia.)
    b. **Keep the manufacturer's product insert** for the test in use in a procedure manual that is readily available to the testing personnel. Always use the product insert for the kit currently in use; do not use old product inserts. Read the product insert each time a kit is opened to check for changes in procedures or quality control.
2. Follow the manufacturer's instructions regarding **proper specimen collection** and handling:
    a. Make sure appropriate collection containers are used (i.e., proper blood collecting tubes and/or test kit devices, urine collection containers, microbiology swabs, etc.)
    b. Make sure specimens are stored at the proper temperature and time interval (i.e., room temperature and/or refrigerated).
3. Be sure to **properly identify the patient.**
    a. Does the name on the **test requisition** (or prescription) match the patient's name?
    b. Does the name on the **patient's chart** match the name on the patient's identification?
    c. If more than one patient is present with the same first and last name, how do you determine which one is the **test patient**? (Look for possible gender differences, social security number, patient identification number, birth dates, different middle name, and relevance of the test to the patient's history.)
4. **Inform the patient** of any **test preparation** such as fasting, clean-catch urine, special diet, etc.
5. Be sure to **label the patient's specimen** for testing with an identifier unique to each patient.
6. Read the product insert completely prior to performing a test.
    a. Become **familiar with the test procedure.**
    b. **Study** each step and perform them in the proper order.
    c. Know the **time required** for performing the test and achieving the optimal result.
    d. Be sure to have all of the required **reagents and equipment ready** before actually performing the test.
    e. **Perform quality control testing** whenever a new test kit is opened to be sure that the kit works prior to testing the patient samples. For automated waived testing, quality control procedures must be consistent with manufacturer's recommendations, and are performed on each instrument used at least once on each day of patient testing. Control testing results must be recorded on a quality control log.
    f. Be able to **recognize when the test is finished** (e.g., will there be a blue plus or minus sign against a white background?)
7. Follow the **storage requirement for the test kit** (e.g., stored away from direct light, temperature requirements, open container expiration dates.) Also, if the kit can be stored at room temperature but this changes the expiration date, write the expiration date on the kit.
8. **Do not mix components of different kits!**
9. **Record the patient's test results** in the proper place, such as the patient's chart and the laboratory test log, but not on unidentified Post-it notes or pieces of scrap paper that can be misplaced.
    a. Record the results according to the instructions in the manufacturer's product insert.
    b. If it's a qualitative test, spell out **positive/negative** or **pos/neg** because the symbolic representations can be altered (the − can be altered to a +).
    c. Include the name of the test, the date the test was performed, and the initials of the testing personnel in the test record. Include the calendar year in the date.
    d. If the same test is performed on a patient multiple times in one day, include the time of each test.
10. Perform any **instrument maintenance** as directed by the manufacturer.

Fig. 2-2. Good Laboratory Practices. (From Centers for Medicare and Medicaid Services, http://www.cms.hhs.gov/CLIA/downloads/wgoodlab.pdf.)

Quality Assurance

TABLE 2-3 — Quality Assurance and the Three Stages of Laboratory Testing

Preanalytical Phase	Analytical Phase	Postanalytical Phase
1. Physician examines patient and **orders the tests** that need to be performed to (a) screen for possible disorders (b) confirm tentative diagnosis (c) monitor existing disorder 2. A **requisition** is filled out, and patient is instructed in any preparatory procedure, such as fasting (no eating) before some blood tests or first morning urine specimen (for some urine tests). 3. Appropriate **specimen is collected** in proper container: (a) urine (b) blood in proper tubes (c) specimen from infected site (d) fecal specimen 4. The **specimen is processed:** (a) labeled (b) stored at proper temperature (c) preservatives or additives added if needed 5. The specimen is transported to: (a) laboratory area in office (b) reference laboratory (c) hospital laboratory	6. If tested in the physician's office laboratory, **quality control** is run and logged before patient testing. (a) Instrument is calibrated daily and results are logged. (b) Controls provided by manufacturer are run and results are logged. (c) Proficiency test is run on sample from outside source twice annually and results are logged. 7. If all the preceding check out, the **patient specimen is tested.** 8. A **laboratory report** is produced showing the results of the tests. (a) In-office results are recorded directly on the patient's chart with reference ranges and on a patient log. (b) Reference laboratory reports are sent to the office by mail, phone, or fax or electronically. They are logged when received.	9. Specimen is properly **disposed of** in biohazard container and sent to a managed waste company. 10. **Quality control results are analyzed** to determine if test method is "in control" based on precision, accuracy, reliability, shifts, trends, and random errors. 11. **Patient reports are interpreted and signed** by (a) the ordering physician (b) laboratory pathologists (c) additional consulting physicians 12. **Patient is notified** in the proper confidential manner. Communication is documented in the patient record. 13. The **final signed report is filed** in the patient record.

TABLE 2-4 — Variables That Can Negatively Affect the Quality of Laboratory Results

Preanalytical Phase	Analytical Phase	Postanalytical Phase
• Improper patient identification • Improper patient instruction or compliance (e.g., did not fast, did not collect first morning urine specimen) • Improper collection of specimen (e.g., wrong time, wrong container, wrong volume, wrong site) • Improper labeling of specimen • Improper processing of specimen (e.g., spun versus unspun blood) • Improper storage of specimen (e.g., refrigerator or room temperature) • Improper transportation of specimen (e.g., timing, temperature, light) • Contamination	• Instrument not functioning correctly • Instrument not calibrated • Not running and observing controls before patient test • Reagents or test kit expired • Reagents or test kit not stored at the proper temperature • Reagents from one kit used with another kit • Poor testing technique of operator • Not following manufacturer's instructions regarding (1) amount of specimen (2) amount of reagents (3) steps involving time (4) proper temperature for testing (e.g., refrigerated test kit must first come to room temperature before testing)	• Incorrectly recording in-office results on patient log or patient record • Not identifying when controls are out of their range and problem-solve why • Not providing physician with reference range along with patient's results to aid in interpretation • Not notifying physician when results have arrived from outside reference laboratory • Not notifying patient in proper confidential manner regarding results of test • Results lost in mail or fax machine • Report filed in wrong patient chart

2. Are the patients' charts up to date, with the proper patient test information?
3. Is the QC performed and documented?
4. Did the laboratory get the right answers for the QC?
5. Do the waived test results correlate with the patient's history or symptoms?
6. Are there any complaints about the laboratory testing?
7. Are the testing personnel trained before performing laboratory testing?
8. Are there periodic discussions about laboratory concerns?

Quality Control

A major concern facing all medical laboratories is how to ensure that the test kit or test instrument is producing the correct results consistently. As mentioned earlier, if the patient's test result is *not* right, it can have a harmful effect on the patient's future course of diagnosis and treatment. The answer to the problem during the analytical phase is to implement QC for each test. This is done by testing a **control sample** (a manufactured specimen that already has a known value) before testing the patient specimen. If the control sample's test result is within the acceptable range of its known value, then the values from patients' specimens are surmised to also be reliable. When all the QC sample results are recorded on a dated log sheet, the overall performance of the test system can also be monitored over time.

In CLIA-waived laboratories, two different types of tests require QC: qualitative and quantitative.

Quality Control Monitoring of Qualitative Waived Tests

The method of simply testing for the presence or absence of an analyte is considered a **qualitative test**. Most qualitative test kits are designed to show two possible test results expressed as positive (the analyte is present) or negative (the analyte is not present). Fig. 2-3 shows three qualitative pregnancy test kits. These individual testing devices usually have a built-in positive control ("C") that produces a colored band to prove the device is working. If this built-in **internal control** does not show a positive result, the test would need to be repeated. If the repeated test also fails, the test system would be considered invalid and corrective action must be taken.

Check for these possible causes of an invalid test result:
1. Were the directions followed?
2. Were the **reagents** (substances used in a test to detect, measure, examine, or produce a reaction) added in the correct order and at the correct time?

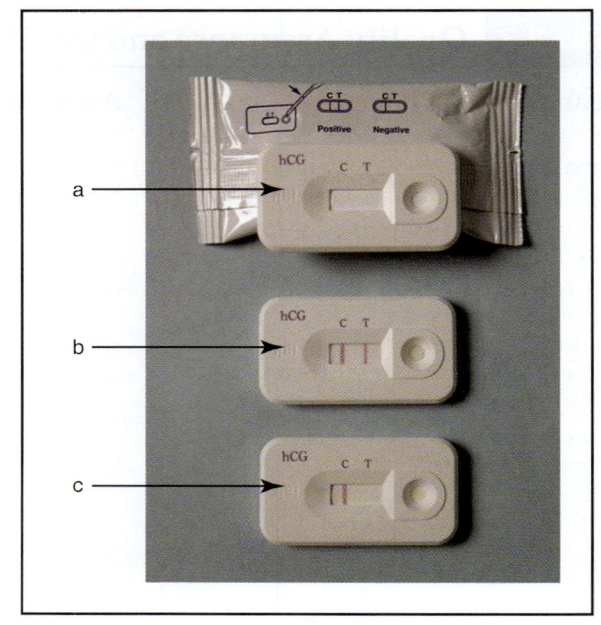

Fig. 2-3. Qualitative pregnancy tests. *a*, Test kit before adding urine specimen; *b*, a positive reaction in the test area *(T)* indicates that the pregnancy hormone, human chorionic gonadotropin (HCG), is present; *c*, a negative reaction in the test area indicates that no pregnancy HCG is present.

3. Were the reagents outdated or stored at the wrong temperature (e.g. room temperature, in the refrigerator)?
4. If everything seems accurate and problems still exist, contact the manufacturer and use a new kit.

Many manufacturers also supply and recommend **external controls** (liquid positive and negative controls that are tested the same way as the patient specimen to check the reliability of the instrument and the testing). These external controls must be run daily, weekly, or monthly as recommended by the manufacturer to further check the reliability of the test system. The dated results of these external controls must also be logged and evaluated. You will be using the qualitative log sheets in your workbook when doing immunology and microbiology tests.

Quality Control Monitoring of Semiquantitative Waived Tests

It is also possible to semiquantify the amount of an analyte by its color reaction with a particular reagent as seen when testing urine specimens (see Chapter 3). A urine test strip contains reagent pads that react specifically with each analyte, causing a variety of color changes. The more a particular analyte is present in urine, the darker the color will be on the reagent pad. This is referred to as *semiquantitative testing*. A *qualitative* test indicates if a particular analyte is present, whereas *semiquantitative* testing determines the approximate

Quality Control

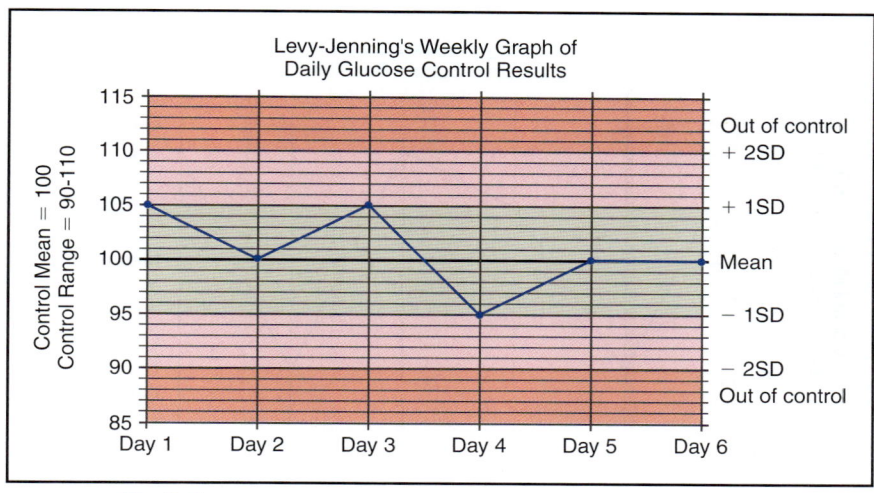

Fig. 2-4. Weekly glucose control results that are **in control**.

quantity of an analyte. Urine reagent strips provide both qualitative and semiquantitative measurements, with results recorded as negative and positive, or in ranges such as trace, 1+, 2+, and 3+; small, moderate, and large.

QC monitoring consists of running two manufactured liquid controls, one with normal results and a second with abnormal results. The manufacturer will provide the semiquantitative results of its control to be compared with the results obtained when running the test. If the results do not match, the same four questions listed in the preceding section should be addressed and the necessary corrections made.

Quality Control Monitoring of Quantitative Waived Tests

Quantitative test results have a numerical value indicating the amount of a substance present (for example, the glucose monitor in Chapter 1, Fig. 1-5, showed a numerical readout of 71). The quantitative result is compared with a population's reference range. A typical reference range for fasting glucose in the general population might be 70 to 110. If the patient's results are drastically below or above the reference range, it may be clinically significant. For example, if the glucose level in a diabetic patient is drastically low, the patient could go into insulin shock. If the glucose level is drastically high, the patient could go into a diabetic coma.

Optics

Monitors that measure the quantity of a substance often send a light through the specimen or reflect off the specimen to determine how much of the analyte is present. With this method of testing, an **optics check** (process of confirming that the light source and light sensor in optical analyzers are working properly) must be performed daily with the results logged. The manufacturer may refer to this process as *calibrating the instrument*. **Calibration** is the process of setting the instrument's optics to the test reagents or test devices that will be used. **Coding** the instrument may also be necessary after receiving a new set of testing supplies in order to reset the instrument's optics. Be sure to read the manufacturer's directions to determine if and when optic checks are necessary.

External Controls

Because quantitative test results indicate whether the analyte value is high or low, running two or three levels of control samples on the instrument may be necessary to ensure that all levels are being accurately detected (i.e., high, low, and normal controls). These QC samples are generally liquid and are tested in the same way as the patient's specimen. They, too, must be logged at specific intervals (daily, weekly, or monthly), dated, and evaluated over time.

External controls can be further evaluated by statistical means. For example, if a control specimen was tested 10 times, the results could be added together, then divided by 10 to arrive at a **mean** (average test result). Each result could then be compared with the mean, and a mathematic calculation could be made to determine how much each individual test varied from the mean. Another mathematical calculation could then be made to determine the **standard deviation (SD;** a statistical term describing the amount of variation from the mean in a data set). Once these figures are determined, a graph can be created showing the value of the mean and the value of one and two SDs above and below the mean (abbreviated as +1 SD, +2 SD, −1 SD, and −2 SD). When controls are being run, the goal is to make sure the results fall within ±2 SDs of the mean. In Fig. 2-4 the mean for a glucose

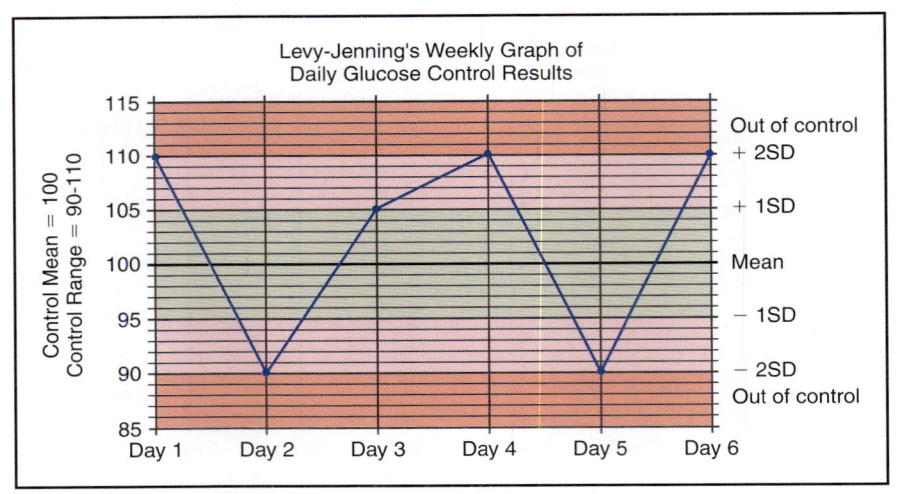

Fig. 2-5. Weekly glucose control results showing **excessive scatter.**

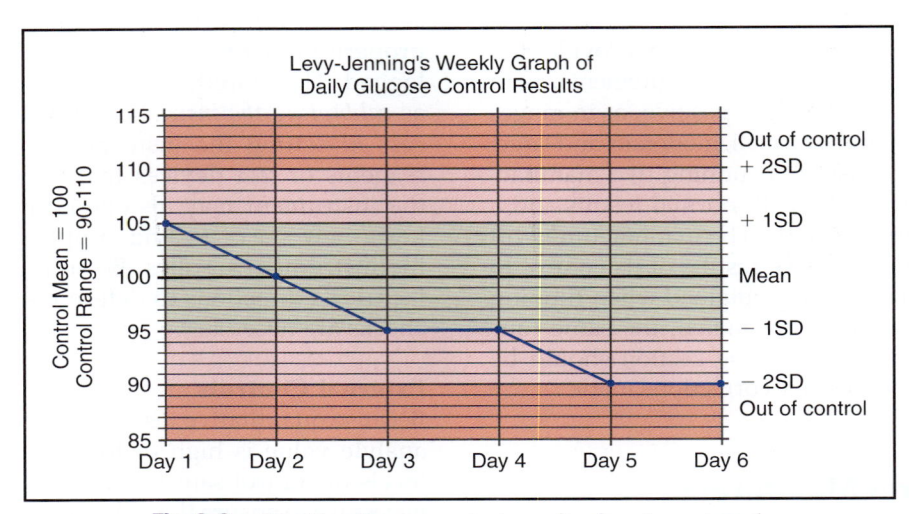

Fig. 2-6. Weekly glucose control results showing a **trend.**

normal standard is 100. If one SD is calculated to be 5, then ±1 SD would be 105 and 95. Two SDs would be equal to 10, and their values above and below the mean would be 110 and 90. In this example, six control results have been plotted and all the results fall within ±2 SDs. This indicates the test method is "in control." NOTE: CLIA-waived test controls have been statistically measured by the manufacturers and will be packaged with the control "range" already determined.

The graph in Fig. 2-4 is called a **Levy–Jennings chart,** which is used to plot the ongoing results of test control samples. If a control test result falls higher or lower than 2 SDs or outside the manufacturer's given range, it is considered "out of control" and corrective action must be taken before running and reporting patient samples.

By plotting quantitative results on a Levy–Jennings chart over time, the laboratory professional can identify possible problems and correct them before running patient samples. Examine each of the graphs in Figs. 2-5 to 2-7, and note the possible causes for each of the patterns. In all these cases, the control may be within 2 SDs, but reason for concern still exists. Here are some patterns seen in weekly control graphs and how they can be corrected:

Excessive scatter (Fig. 2-5): Values scatter widely above and below the mean. Possible cause: operator variability (e.g., days 2 and 4 were logged by technician A, and days 1, 3, 4, and 6 by technician B). Correction: Observe each technician's technique to see how he or she is performing the test and reading the results.

Trends (Fig. 2-6): Values move up or down incrementally in the same direction on each subsequent day. Possible cause: Reagents are outdated or instrument is losing its calibration. Correction: Use a new set of reagents, and run a calibration check.

Shift (Fig. 2-7): Values shift from a consistent set of results to another set of results. Possible cause:

Quality Control

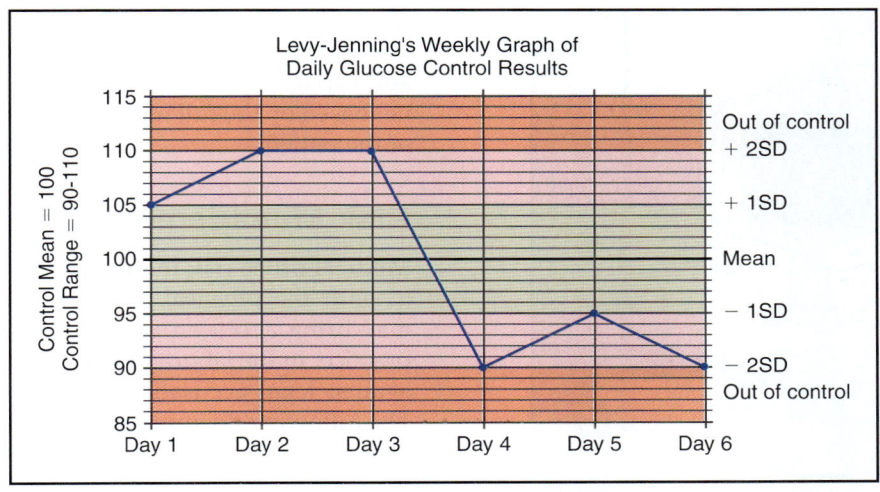

Fig. 2-7. Weekly glucose control results showing a **shift.**

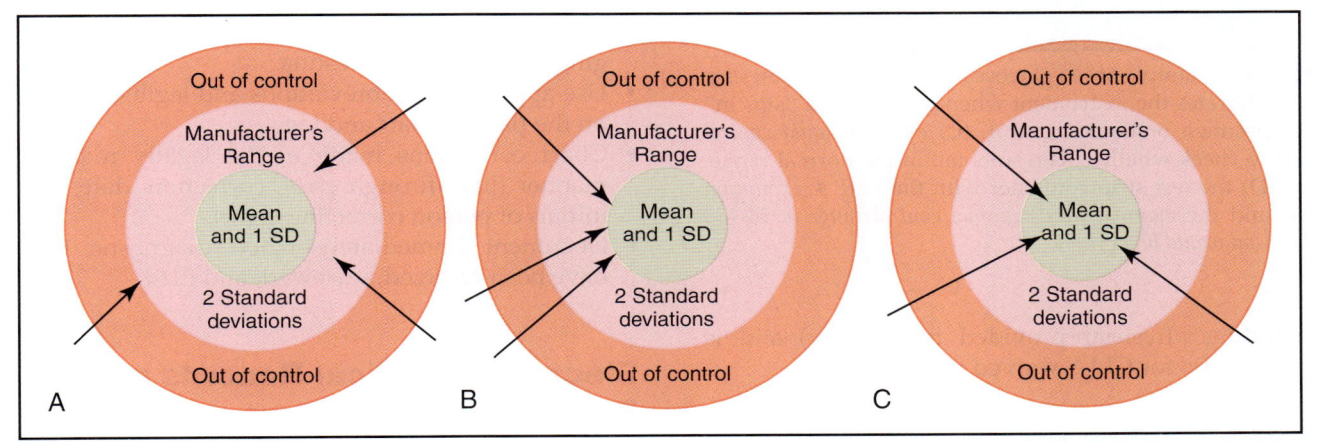

Fig. 2-8. Visual examples of quality control test results using a target to facilitate understanding of terms. **A,** Results are not *accurate* (not within required standard deviations, or the bull's-eye) and are not *precise* (not consistently reproducible, or hitting the same area). **B,** Results are precise but not accurate. **C,** Results are both precise and accurate and are therefore *reliable*.

new reagents, new person testing, or sudden deterioration of reagents. Check lot numbers and expiration dates on reagents, and observe new technician's performance.

Additional statistical terms must be understood when analyzing control results. **Accuracy (correctness)** occurs when control results consistently fall within 1 SD of the mean. **Precision (reproducibility)** is the ability to produce the same test result each time a test is performed. **Reliability** is the result when both accuracy and precision are accomplished. Reliability is the goal that must be achieved before testing patient specimens.

A way to visualize these three terms is to take the mean of a control and place it in the middle, or bull's-eye, of a target (Fig. 2-8). The two circles around the mean represent 1 SD and 2 SD. Any value beyond the 2 SD goal would be considered "out of control" and would miss the target. The goal for a *reliable* test system would be to have all the control values *accurate* (within the 1 SD circle) and *precise* (all showing a similar value). NOTE: These same terms apply when observing CLIA-waived control results. The controls should fall close to the manufacturer's stated mean (the bull's-eye), and they should also be within the manufacturer's stated range (the circle around the bull's-eye). See Fig. 2-9 for an example of the liquid control ranges for a glucose meter.

A **proficiency testing program** requires a lab to enroll in an accreditation organization that sends the lab unknown samples to test twice a year. The received samples must be run in exactly the same manner as patient specimens. The results are then sent back to the accreditation agency so it can confirm that the results agree with their known values. This method of QC is *required* for CLIA complex tests

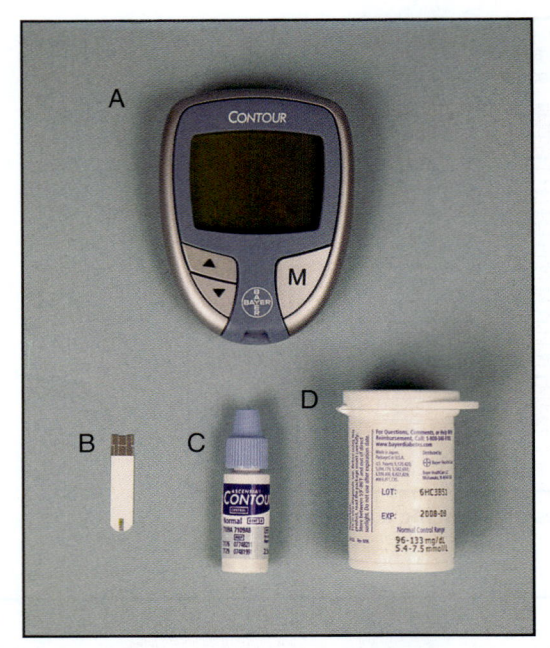

Fig. 2-9. Example of **(A)** glucose *meter* with its **(B)** *test strip* that calibrates the instrument when inserted and "sips in" the specimen or liquid control, **(C)** *external liquid control* used to check whether its results fall in the normal range, and **(D)** the test strip container with the *LOT #, expiration date*, and the *manufacturer's normal control range of 96-133 (the mean would be 114).*

(including physician-provided microscopy) and is *recommended* for CLIA-waived testing.

HIPAA Privacy Rule

Another area of concern that has generated governmental intervention in the medical community is that of patient confidentiality. On April 14, 2003, the Health Insurance Portability and Accountability Act **(HIPAA)** Privacy Rule went into effect. HIPAA is a federal law consisting of several components, one of which contains provisions to protect a patient's privacy. The privacy rule provides patients with more control over the use and disclosure of their health information. During the three phases of laboratory testing, many individuals handle what is referred to as **protected health information (PHI)**, which is any health information in any form (written, electronic, or oral) that contains patient-identifiable information, such as name, Social Security number, and telephone number. This information must be kept confidential. Because of this new approach to medical records and medical information, employees are trained regarding how their specific office uses, stores, maintains, and transmits laboratory testing information. No test result should be given to a patient or family member without the physician's permission. If a patient asks for his or her results or those of another person, you should explain that you are not authorized to disclose that information and that the physician will interpret and explain the results to the patient or family member based on the full medical findings and knowledge of the patient.

Risk Management

Medical office risk management is a term that refers to both the physical and the procedural risks that may bring about an injury or legal action against a practice. In the laboratory and office, the best defense against legal accusations is proper documentation. The following documentation recommendations contribute to sound risk management practices in the laboratory:

- Use written office procedures to inform patients of test preparation and results as well as to document this communication.
- Be accurate and consistent when charting and logging test and control results.
- Use appropriate abbreviations and legible writing on the patient chart and logs.
- Chart corrections made in the legally required manner (line through error, correction, date, and initials of person correcting error).
- Document immediately when diagnostic tests have been received, reviewed, and filed.

Electronic Medical Records and Bar Coding

As the demand for more laboratory and safety documentation increases, technological advancements in the area of electronic communications to ease this burden are increasing as well. These advancements will also make the process of test documentation more accurate. For example, electronic medical records are replacing patients' physical charts. These records will be accessible at each phase of the testing process by laptop computers or desktop computers located in the reception area, examination rooms, laboratory area, and reference laboratories. In most of the large reference laboratories and hospitals, the various departments are directly linked to a central computerized health information system. This system takes the test results directly from the laboratory's instruments to the patient's electronic medical record, then immediately alerts the physician about the results.

Another electronic aid to the laboratory is the use of bar code labels on all requisitions and specimens. Bar coding was introduced to the health care industry in the mid-1970s, when blood banks and blood collection centers began using the technology for error-free tracking, tracing, and positive patient identification

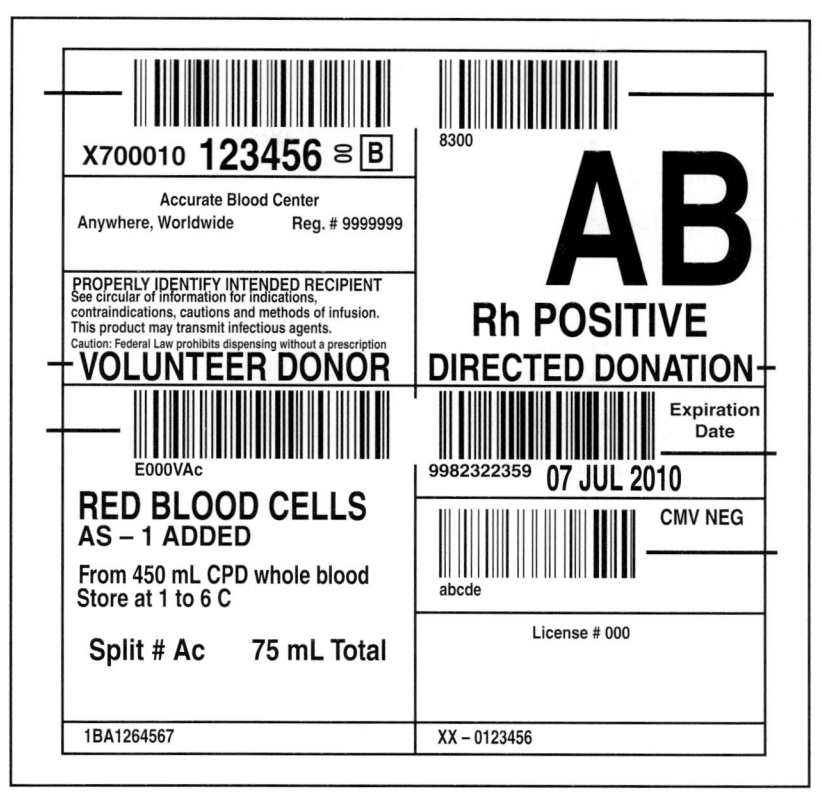

Fig. 2-10. Blood bank bar code label.

(Fig. 2-10). Today bar coding is used in virtually every hospital department to help improve accuracy and timely information management. Statistics show that the error rate for manual data entry is 1 in 300 characters compared with 1 in 3 million characters for bar code scanning.

So what exactly is a bar code? Without getting too technical, **bar codes** are a pattern of narrow and wide bars and spaces. Each pattern is encoded with its own particular meaning, just like words in a language are made up of letters and symbols. When a beam of light scans the bar code, the light reflects differences between the dark bar areas and the space areas. These differences are transformed into electrical impulses that are measured, decoded, and entered into a computer.

The single most important use of bar codes in the medical laboratory is for positive patient and specimen identification throughout the entire testing process. An understanding of an office's or reference laboratory's labeling system is important. A typical system consists of a specific bar code printer that prints out the bar code labels on the basis of typed input from a computer. As the operator types in the patient's name and the test ordered, a series of bar code labels are generated and then attached to the laboratory requisition and the collected patient specimens. Before the labels can be applied to the specimens, patients must be identified by at least two of the following patient identifiers, depending on specific office protocol:

1. Always ask the patient to give his or her name. Do *not* say, "Are you Mrs. Smith?"
2. Have the patient state his or her Social Security number, *or*
3. Ask the patient's birth date, *or*
4. Ask the patient's telephone number.

Once positive identification is made that agrees with the requisition and the bar code labels, have the patient print his or her name on the label that will be affixed to the requisition. The smaller bar code labels are then affixed to the tubes of blood after they have been filled.

Review Questions

1. What is the purpose of CLIA 1988?
2. What is the purpose of proficiency testing?
3. A slide is initially brought into focus by using the _____ power objective.
4. Ocular lenses have a magnification of _____.
5. The _____ directs and concentrates light through the slide and into the objective lens.
6. The revolving _____ contains the objectives.
7. The _____ objective usually has a magnification of 100×.
8. The total magnification is calculated by multiplying the 10× ocular lens by the magnification of the _____ lens.
9. Match each term on the left with its definition on the right.

    _____ standard deviation   a. uninterrupted rise or decline from the mean
    _____ trend   b. average value of a set of control tests
    _____ mean   c. variability from the mean in a dataset

Review Question Answers

1. All laboratories performing tests on specimens must register with CMS for permission to perform CoW, moderately complex, or highly complex tests based on the qualifications of the laboratory personnel and the difficulty of the tests performed to improve the accuracy and reliability of patient testing.
2. Laboratories performing moderately complex and complex tests must prove their proficiency by running specimens from an outside accreditation agency twice a year and obtaining the correct results.
3. low
4. 10×
5. condenser
6. nosepiece
7. oil immersion
8. objective
9. c, a, b

Websites

FDA listing of CLIA-waived tests since 2000:
www.accessdata.fda.gov/scripts/cdrh/cfdocs/cfClia/testswaived.cfm

FDA information on CLIA waivers:
www.fda.gov/cdrh/clia/cliawaived.html

HHS brochure on how to obtain a Certificate of Waiver:
www.cms.hhs.gov/CLIA/downloads/HowObtainCertificateofWaiver.pdf

American Academy of Family Physicians information on proficiency testing CLIA-waived tests:
www.aafp.org/pt.xml

FDA current list of CLIA-waived analytes with links to manufacturers:
www.accessdata.fda.gov/scripts/cdrh/cfdocs/cfClia/analyteswaived.cfm

CLIA-waived drug tests:
www.cliawaived.com/

CHAPTER 3

Urinalysis

Objectives
After completing this chapter you should be able to:

Fundamental Concepts
1. Demonstrate an understanding of the urinary system.
2. Describe urine formation, renal threshold, the flow of urine, and the composition of urine.
3. Discuss the importance of urinalysis.
4. Define medical terms related to the urinary system.
5. Explain the proper method of urine collection for voided urine, clean-catch midstream urine for bacterial studies, and timed urine specimens.
6. Properly handle and dispose of urine specimens according to the most current OSHA safety guidelines.
7. Educate the patient in the proper method of urine collection.

CLIA-Waived Tests
1. Describe the three parts of urinalysis: physical, chemical, and microscopic.
2. State the tests involved in physical urinalysis.
3. Recognize the diseases that cause abnormal results in a physical urinalysis.
4. Perform a physical assessment of an unknown urine sample according to the stated task, conditions, and standards listed in the Learning Outcome Evaluation in the student workbook.
5. List the 10 tests that can be performed with Multistix urine chemistry test strips.
6. Correlate various pathological conditions with abnormal results on chemistry strips.
7. Perform a chemistry Multistix test on an unknown sample according to the stated task, conditions, and standards listed in the Learning Outcome Evaluation in the workbook.
8. Describe the automated methods for performing chemical urinalysis, including microalbumin protein testing.
9. Apply the correct quality control for physical and chemical urinalysis testing.
10. Follow the most current OSHA safety guidelines when performing a physical and chemical urinalysis.

Advanced Concepts
1. Describe the standardized urine microscopic method (e.g., Kova).
2. Perform a microscopic urinalysis setup according to the conditions required.
3. Follow the most current OSHA safety guidelines when setting up a microscopic urinalysis.
4. Recognize the various elements in normal and abnormal urine microscopic sediment.
5. Correlate abnormal microscopic results with certain pathological conditions.
6. Correlate the results of the physical, chemical, and microscopic urinalysis.

Key Terms

anuria no flow of urine
Bence Jones protein protein found in the urine of patients with multiple myeloma
bilirubin waste product from the breakdown of hemoglobin
casts elements excreted in the urine in the shape of the renal tubules and ducts
diuresis increase in the volume of urine output
dysuria painful urination
electrolyte element or compound that forms positively or negatively charged ions when dissolved and can conduct electricity
glomerular (Bowman's) capsule cup-shaped structure surrounding the glomerulus that collects the glomerular filtrate
glomerulus structure in the renal corpuscle made up of tangled blood capillaries in which the hydrostatic pressure in the capillaries pushes substances through the capillary pores
glycosuria sugars (especially glucose) in the urine
hematuria intact red blood cells in the urine
hemolysis red cells breaking open and releasing hemoglobin
iatrogenic caused by treatment or diagnostic procedures
ketonuria ketones in the urine

Key Terms—cont'd

lipiduria lipids in the urine
lyse to break open
micturition expelling of urine, also referred to as *voiding* and *urination*
nephron functional unit of the kidney
nocturia excessive urination at night
oliguria decrease in the volume of urine output
pH scale that measures the level of acidity or alkalinity of a solution
polyuria passing abnormally large amounts of urine
porphyrin intermediate substance in the formation of heme (part of hemoglobin)
proteinuria proteins in the urine
pyuria white blood cells in the urine
reducing substance substance that easily loses electrons
renal corpuscle part of the nephron that contains the glomerulus and glomerular capsule
renal threshold level blood reabsorption limit of a substance and the point at which the substance is then excreted in the urine
renal tubules parts of the nephron composed of proximal convoluted tubules, the nephron loop (loop of Henle), and distal convoluted tubules
retroperitoneal located behind the peritoneal cavity
sediment the material at the bottom of the centrifuged tube of urine
specific gravity in urinalysis the weight of urine compared with the weight of an equal volume of water; measures the amount of dissolved substances in urine
supernatant the liquid portion of urine on top of the spun sediment
ureters slender, muscular tubes 10 to 12 inches long that carry the urine formed in the kidneys to the urinary bladder
urethra tube that carries urine to the outside of the body
urethral meatus urethral opening through which urine is expelled
urinary bladder hollow muscular organ that holds urine until it is expelled

FUNDAMENTAL CONCEPTS AND COLLECTION PROCEDURES

Anatomy of the Urinary System

Before the results of urine testing can be interpreted, the overall anatomy and function of the urinary system must be understood.

Function of the Urinary System

The urinary system has the following functions:
- It removes unwanted wastes.
- It stabilizes blood volume, acidity, and electrolytes.
- It regulates extracellular fluids of the body and the absorption of calcium ions by activating vitamin D.
- It secretes the hormone erythropoietin, which controls the rate of red blood cell (RBC) formation, and the hormone renin, which regulates blood pressure.

Structures of the Urinary System

The urinary system consists of the kidneys, ureters, urinary bladder, and urethra (Fig. 3-1).

Kidneys

Each person normally has two kidneys (Fig. 3-2), which are reddish-brown, bean-shaped organs. The kidneys are 4 to 5 inches long and are located in the **retroperitoneal** space (behind the peritoneal cavity) slightly above the waistline in the posterior wall of the abdominal cavity. The kidney is composed of three main sections: the cortex, which is the outer part; the medulla, which is the middle area; and the renal pelvis, which is the hollow inner area.

The functional unit of the kidney is the microscopic **nephron** (Fig. 3-3), located within the cortex and medulla of the kidney. Approximately 1

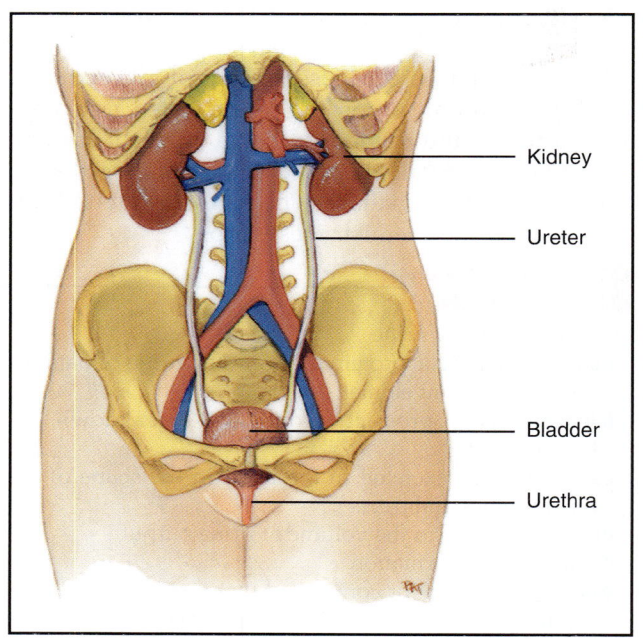

Fig. 3-1. The urinary system. (From Applegate EJ: *The anatomy and physiology learning system*, ed 3, St Louis, 2006, Saunders.)

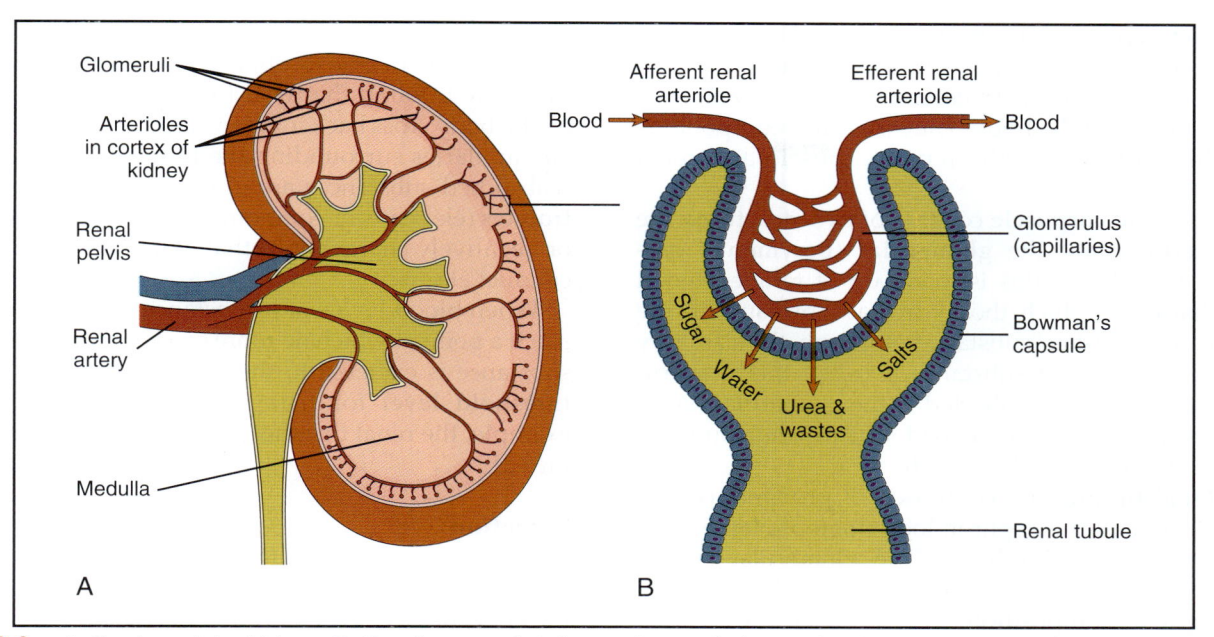

Fundamental Concepts and Collection Procedures

Fig. 3-2. **A,** Section of the kidney. **B,** Renal corpuscle, glomerulus, and glomerular (Bowman's) capsule. (From Chabner D: *The language of medicine,* ed 8, St Louis, 2007, Saunders.)

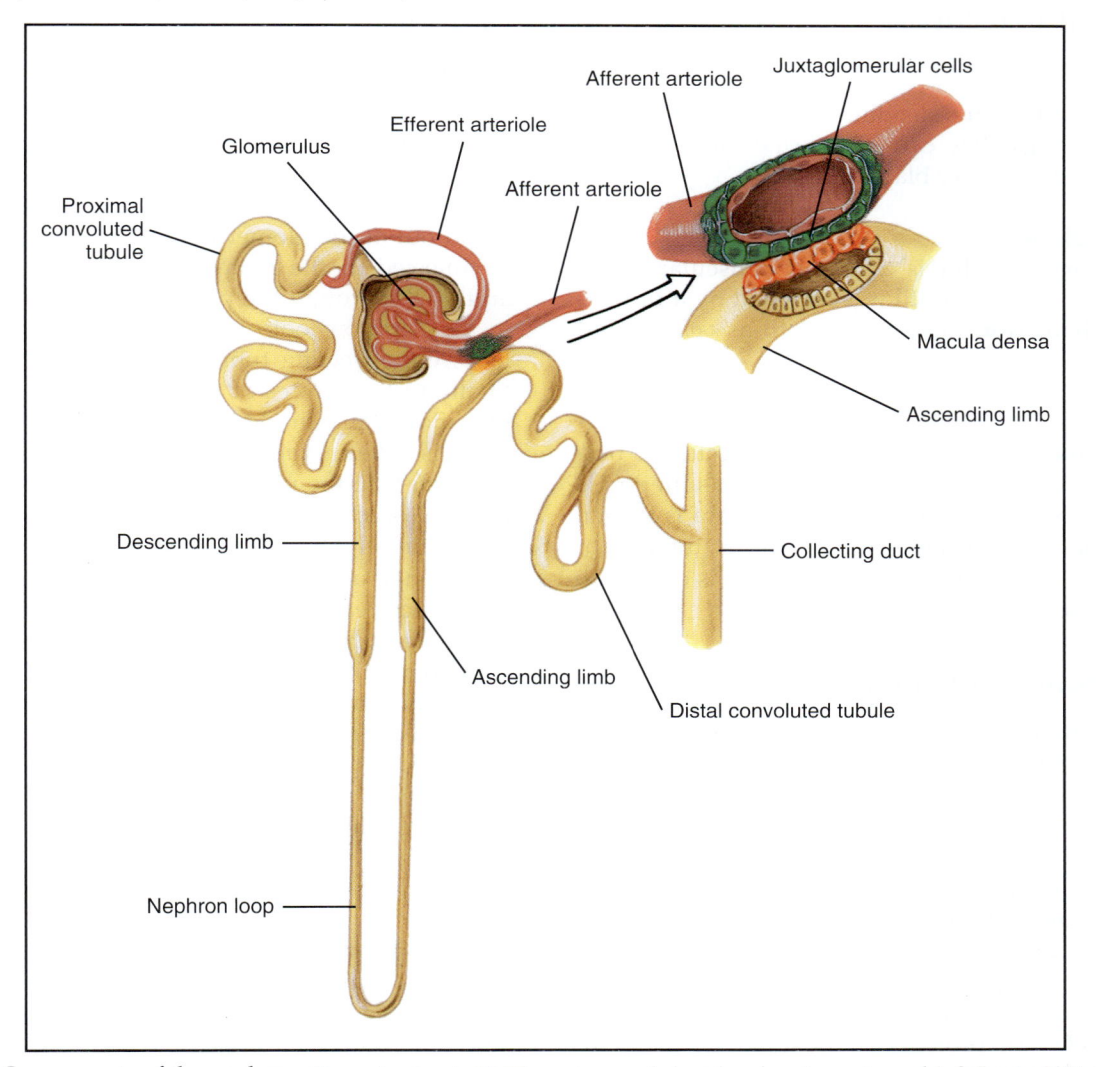

Fig. 3-3. Components of the nephron. (From Applegate EJ: *The anatomy and physiology learning system,* ed 3, St Louis, 2006, Saunders.)

million nephrons are in each kidney. The nephrons filter waste substances from the blood and simultaneously maintain the essential water and electrolyte balance of the body. The structural components of the nephron are the renal corpuscle and renal tubules.

The **renal corpuscle** consists of two structures: the **glomerulus** and the **glomerular (Bowman's) capsule.** The glomerulus is made up of tangled blood capillaries in which the hydrostatic pressure in the capillaries pushes substances through the capillary pores. The filtered substance is called the glomerular filtrate, and it is collected in the glomerular (Bowman's) capsule, a cup-shaped structure surrounding the glomerulus (see Fig. 3-2, *B*).

Renal tubules are composed of proximal convoluted tubules, the nephron loop (loop of Henle), and distal convoluted tubules. The glomerular filtrate fluid flows through these tubules and undergoes changes in composition. This process is discussed later in this chapter.

Also in the medulla of the kidney are collecting tubules and ducts that empty into the renal pelvis.

Ureters
The two **ureters** are slender, muscular tubes 10 to 12 inches long. They carry the urine formed in the kidneys to the urinary bladder.

Urinary Bladder
The **urinary bladder** is a hollow muscular organ that holds the urine until it is expelled by a process called **micturition** (also referred to as *voiding* and *urination*).

Urethra
The **urethra** is a tube that carries urine to the outside of the body. The length of a woman's urethra is approximately 1.5 inches. A man's urethra is longer, approximately 8 inches. The opening at the end of the urethra, where the urine is expelled, is called the **urethral meatus.**

Formation and Flow of Urine

In the nephron urine is formed by three mechanisms: filtration, reabsorption, and secretion.

Filtration
Filtration is the process by which fluids and dissolved substances in the blood are forced through the pores of the glomerulus into the glomerular capsule by hydrostatic pressure. Substances such as water, salts, sugar, and nitrogen waste products (urea, creatinine, and uric acid) can pass through the pores. Substances such as RBCs and proteins are too large and therefore remain in the blood.

Reabsorption
In the process of reabsorption, some of the substances that flow through the renal tubules that are needed by the body cross back into the blood by the peritubular capillaries surrounding the tubules. Examples of reabsorbed substances are glucose, water, and **electrolytes** (elements or compounds that form positively or negatively charged ions that, when dissolved, can conduct electricity).

When blood levels of a substance such as glucose reach a point at which no more can be reabsorbed, the substance is excreted in the urine. This is the **renal threshold level** for that particular substance. For example, the renal threshold for glucose is 160 to 180 mg/dL.

Secretion
The final process in the formation of urine is called *secretion,* in which substances are transported from the peritubular blood capillaries into the renal tubules. Metabolized drugs, potassium, and hydrogen ions are examples of substances that are secreted into the urine.

Flow of Blood and Urine Through the Kidney
Blood is carried into the kidney by the renal artery, which eventually branches into the afferent arterioles. The afferent arterioles carry blood into the capillaries of the glomerulus, and the efferent arterioles carry the blood out of the glomerulus. The glomerular filtrate is collected in the glomerular capsule (Bowman's) and flows through the proximal convoluted tubules to the nephron loop, then to the distal convoluted loop, the collecting tubule, the collection duct, and finally to the calyces of the renal pelvis. The filtrate then flows into the hollow renal pelvis and at this point is called *urine.* The urine then passes through the ureters to the urinary bladder, where it is stored until released by the process of urination or voiding. The main structures involved in the formation and excretion of urine, in sequence, are the following:
1. Bloodstream—renal afferent arterioles
2. Glomerulus
3. Glomerular (Bowman's) capsule
4. Renal tubules
5. Collecting ducts
6. Renal pelvis
7. Ureter
8. Urinary bladder
9. Urethra
10. Urinary meatus—urine is expelled

Composition of Urine
Water makes up 95% of urine. Urine also contains nitrogen waste products such as urea, uric acid, ammonia, and creatinine. Urea, uric acid, and ammonia are derived from the breakdown of protein, and

Fundamental Concepts and Collection Procedures

creatinine is a waste product of muscle metabolism. Other waste products found in urine include chloride, sodium, potassium, calcium, magnesium, phosphate, and sulfate.

Approximately 1200 mL of blood pass into the renal arteries per minute, with a daily output of 1200 to 1500 mL of urine per day. This amount varies depending on the amount of fluid intake and the amount of fluid lost from perspiration, feces, and water vapor from the lungs.

The following terms are related to urination:
1. **Oliguria**—decreased urine volume that can occur in the following situations:
   - Decreased fluid intake
   - Vomiting
   - Profuse sweating
   - Diarrhea
   - Kidney disease
2. **Diuresis**—increase in the volume of urine output, which can be caused by the following:
   - Intake of excessive amounts of fluids, especially those that contain caffeine
   - Some drugs, such as diuretics
   - Some types of diseases, such as diabetes mellitus, diabetes insipidus, and renal diseases that prevent the kidney from concentrating the urine
3. **Anuria**—no flow of urine
4. **Dysuria**—painful urination
5. **Nocturia**—excessive urination at night
6. **Polyuria**—frequently passing abnormally large amounts of urine

Urine Specimen Collection

The urine sample is usually easily obtained, but all types of urine collection methods have the following general requirements:
- The volume needed is usually between 25 and 50 mL.
- The outside of the filled container should be cleaned with a disinfectant.
- The specimen container must be correctly labeled with the patient's name, the collection date and time, and the type of specimen (e.g., random specimen, first morning specimen, clean-catch midstream, or catheterized). Do not label the lid because it can be separated from the specimen.
- Use the correct urine containers (Fig. 3-4). The physician's office should provide the patient with a urine container. Containers from the patient's home, such as glass jars, should not be used because their previous contents can affect the accuracy of

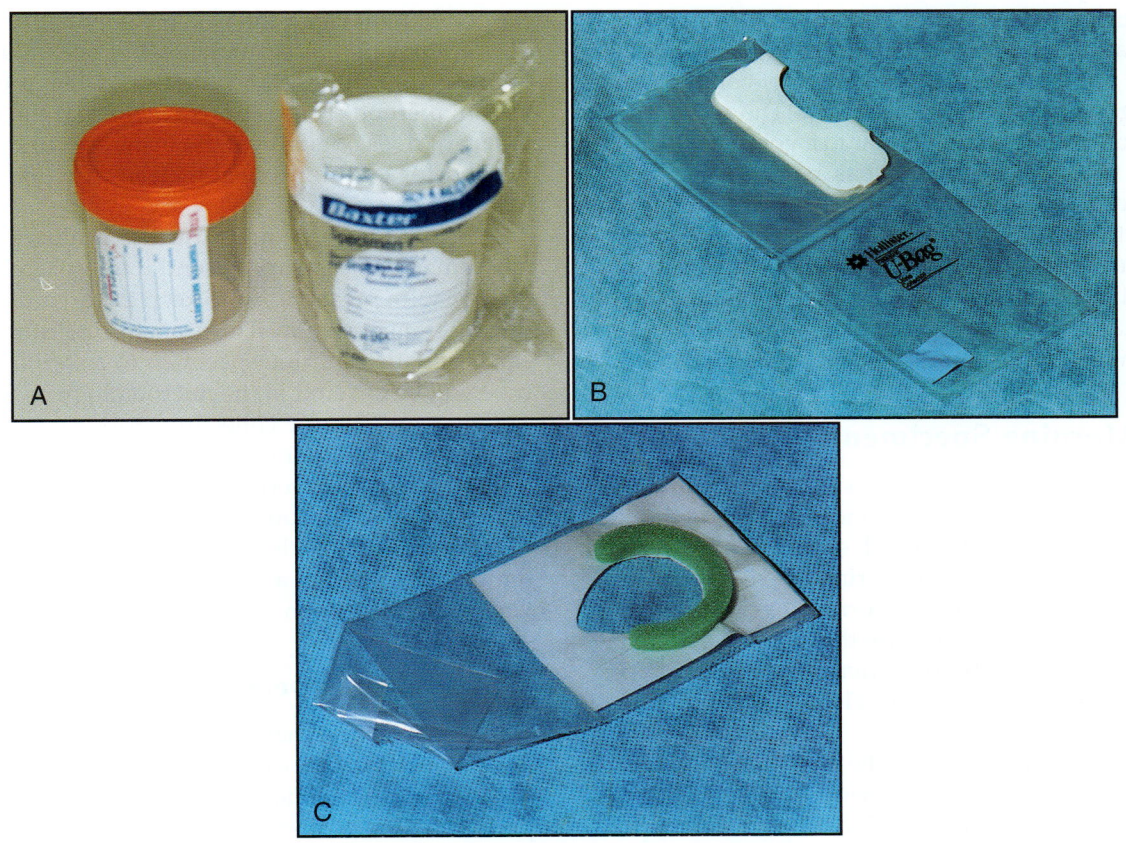

Fig. 3-4. **A,** Adult urine specimen container. **B** and **C,** Pediatric urine specimen containers. (From Stepp CA, Woods M: *Laboratory procedures for medical office personnel,* Philadelphia, 1998, Saunders.)

the tests. The most common types of containers are disposable, nonsterile plastic cups with lids. For infants and children who are not toilet trained, special pliable polyethylene bags are available that contain an adhesive section to stick to the skin. If urine is being collected for microbiological studies, a sterile urine container should be used.
- If a woman is having a menstrual period, collection of a urine sample should be postponed. If this is not possible and a urine specimen must be collected immediately, the requisition must note that the patient is menstruating.
- The urine should be tested as soon as possible after collection. If it is going to sit for more than 1 hour, it must be refrigerated or preservatives must be added.

The method of collection for urine specimens is dictated by the type of test being ordered. For example, special collection procedures are performed if the urine will be cultured for bacteria or if a 24-hour test is ordered. Documentation of the method used to collect the specimen should be noted on the specimen container, the requisition, and the patient's chart.

Random Specimen

A random specimen is usually collected in the medical office. The patient should collect the midstream portion of urine when voiding. The patient is instructed to void a small amount of urine into the toilet to flush the area around the urinary opening of contaminants and to get a steady midstream flow. The second portion is collected in the container to a volume of at least 25 mL. Once the specimen has been collected, the remaining urine in the bladder can be emptied into the toilet. A specimen collected this way is more representative of the contents of the bladder. The lid should be tightly placed on the container, and the outside of the container should be disinfected. The sample container (not the lid) should be appropriately labeled.

First Morning Specimen

The first morning specimen is usually the specimen of choice because it is the most concentrated and has the greatest amount of dissolved substances. Provided the patient has not voided during the night, the first morning urine specimen has formed over an approximately 8-hour period. Because this urine is more concentrated, the probability of detecting abnormalities increases and the microscopic elements remain intact for a longer period.

The patient must collect the first morning specimen soon after rising and preserve it by refrigeration until it is brought into the office. The collection procedure is the same as that described for the random specimen.

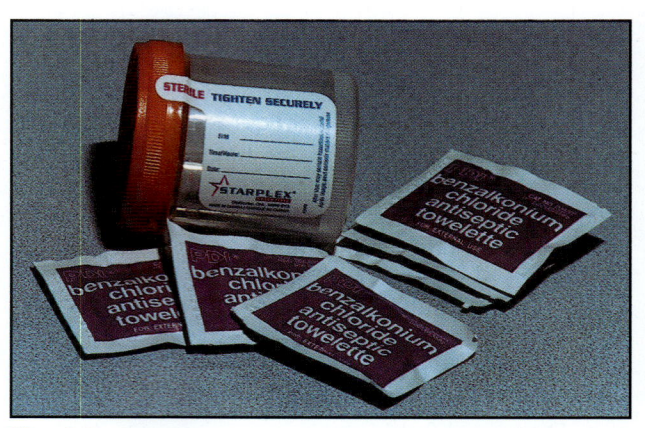

Fig. 3-5. Midstream clean-catch specimen equipment. (From Stepp CA, Woods M: *Laboratory procedures for medical office personnel*, Philadelphia, 1998, Saunders.)

Clean-Catch Midstream Urine Specimen

The urethra and urinary meatus harbor many microorganisms. Therefore, when a urine specimen is collected for culture to determine the source of a urinary tract infection (UTI), only the organisms causing the infection should be cultured. To avoid contamination, the midstream clean-catch method of collection is used. This method consists of having the patient clean the urinary opening first using antiseptic wipes, as seen in Fig. 3-5. The patient then urinates into the sterile container by using the midstream method (Procedure 3-1.) NOTE: If the medical assistant does not know if the urine specimen will be needed for culture, collect a clean-catch midstream just in case.

When the urine requires further evaluation in the lab, it may be necessary to send it to the lab in a sterile tube with preservative to keep the organisms alive during transportation. This transferring of the clean-catch midstream urine specimen to a sterile vacuum tube will be covered in the microbiology chapter.

Other options for collecting urine specimens for culturing are bladder catheterization and suprapubic aspiration. In catheterization a sterile tube called a *catheter* is passed through the urethra into the bladder to remove urine. With suprapubic aspiration urine is removed by passing a needle through the abdominal wall into the bladder.

Timed Urine Specimen

Some tests require that a urine specimen be collected at a certain time. One example is a 24-hour urine specimen. Collecting all the urine produced over a 24-hour period allows greater accuracy of measurement for urinary components. Substances produced in the urine are affected over time by body metabolism,

Fundamental Concepts and Collection Procedures

exercise, and hydration. Substances measured in a 24-hour specimen include calcium, creatinine, lead, potassium, protein, and urea nitrogen. In addition, this type of specimen is used in the diagnosis of the cause, control, and prevention of kidney stones.

24-Hour Collection Procedure

Urine containers for 24-hour collection (Fig. 3-6) are quite large, holding approximately 3000 mL.

The following guidelines should be given to the patient:
- The specimen should be kept refrigerated.
- Some containers may contain preservative. Patients should be instructed about the possible hazards associated with these preservatives.
- The patient should be provided with verbal and written directions.
- The patient should be instructed to moderately limit the intake of fluids during the collection process. Also, the patient should not consume alcohol 24 hours before and during the collection procedure.
- The physician should determine whether medication should be discontinued during the procedure because some medications, such as thiazides, phosphorus-binding antacids, allopurinol, and vitamin C, could alter the results (Procedure 3-2).

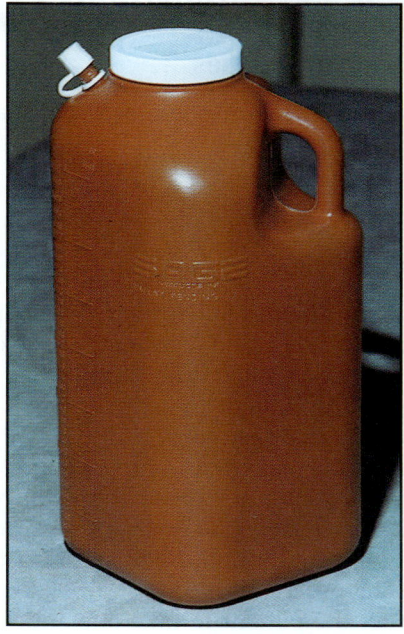

Fig. 3-6. A 24-hour urine container. (From Stepp CA, Woods M: *Laboratory procedures for medical office personnel*, Philadelphia, 1998, Saunders.)

PROCEDURE 3-1   Instructing Patients How to Collect a Clean-Catch Urine Specimen

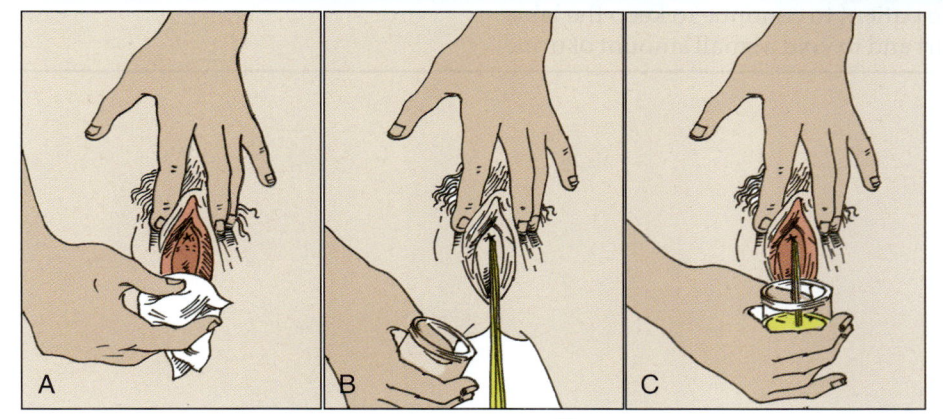

A to C. Procedure for female midstream clean-catch urine collection. **A.** Clean labia from front to back with antiseptic. **B.** Urinate in toilet first. **C.** Next, collect specimen in cup and then urinate in toilet.

(Continued)

PROCEDURE 3-1 Instructing Patients How to Collect a Clean-Catch Urine Specimen—cont'd

Equipment and Supplies

Sterile urine collection container, label, antiseptic towelettes

Procedure

For a Female Patient

1. Wash your hands, and gather the equipment.
2. Greet and identify the patient, and provide her with the clean-catch urine supplies.
3. Instruct the patient to sanitize her hands and remove her underwear.
4. Instruct the patient to spread apart her labia with one hand to expose the urinary meatus (Fig. A). Tell her to keep this area spread apart with her nondominant hand during the entire cleaning procedure.
5. Instruct the patient to take one antiseptic towelette and clean one side of the urinary meatus from front to back on one side. She should clean from front to back so that microorganisms in the anal region are not spread into the urinary meatus area.
6. Instruct the patient to repeat the same procedure with another antiseptic towelette, wiping from front to back on the other side of the urinary meatus.
7. Instruct the patient to use a third antiseptic towelette to wipe from front to back directly across the urinary meatus.
8. Instruct the patient to continue to keep the labia spread apart and to void a small amount of urine into the toilet to flush away microorganisms that may be around the urinary meatus (Fig. B). Tell her to be careful not to touch the inside of the sterile container at any time during the procedure.
9. Instruct the patient to collect the second part of the urine in the container (Fig. C). This is the midstream flow of urine.
10. Instruct the patient to urinate the last amount of urine into the toilet. This will ensure that the first and last sections of the urine flow are not in the container, only the midstream section.
11. Instruct the patient to dry the area with a tissue and wash her hands.
12. Instruct the patient to carefully cap the specimen container and put it in a specified place if collected in the office or refrigerate it if collected at home.
13. Gloves should be worn when receiving the specimen from the patient. The sample container (not the lid) should be labeled correctly, and a requisition should be completed if required.
14. The person receiving the sample should remove the gloves and sanitize his or her hands after the urine has been placed in the testing area.
15. The procedure should be charted correctly. The charting should document that midstream clean-catch urine collection instructions were given and that the specimen was received from the patient.

PROCEDURE 3-1 Instructing Patients How to Collect a Clean-Catch Urine Specimen—cont'd

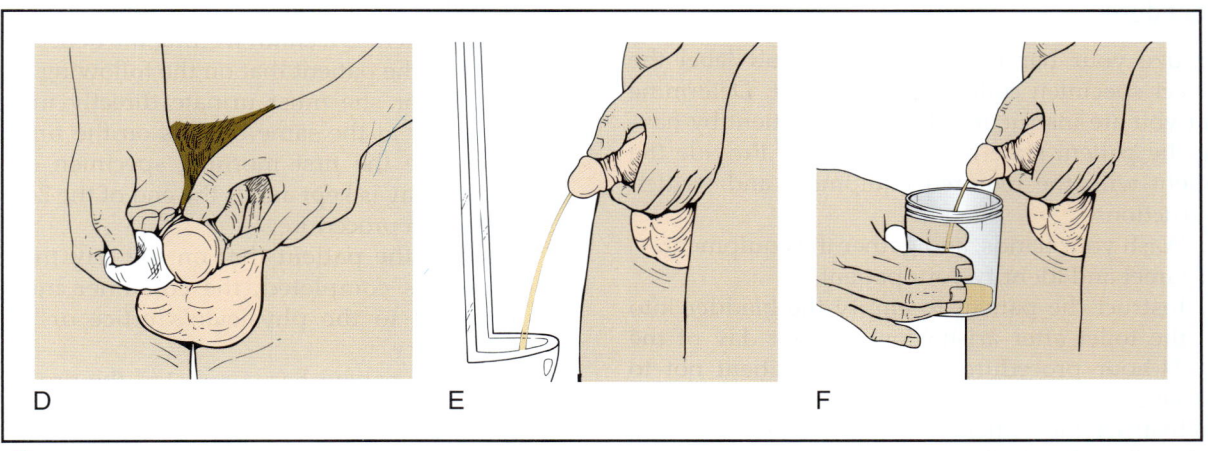

D to F. Procedure for male midstream clean-catch urine collection. (From Stepp CA, Woods M: *Laboratory procedures for medical office personnel*, Philadelphia, 1998, Saunders.)

For a Male Patient

1. Wash your hands, and gather the equipment.
2. Greet and identify your patient, and provide him with the clean-catch urine supplies.
3. Instruct the patient to sanitize his hands and remove his underwear.
4. If the patient is uncircumcised, instruct him to retract the foreskin, holding it back during the entire procedure.
5. Instruct the patient to clean the area around the penis opening (glans penis) by starting at the tip of the penis and cleaning downward (Fig. D), using a separate antiseptic towelette for each side.
6. Instruct the patient to use a third antiseptic towelette to clean directly across the meatus.
7. Instruct the patient to void a small amount (one third) of the urine into the toilet to flush away microorganisms that may be around the urinary meatus (Fig. E).
8. Instruct the patient to collect the second part of the urine in the container, being careful not to touch the inside of the container (Fig. F).
9. Instruct the patient to void the last amount of urine into the toilet so that only the midstream section is collected.
10. Instruct the patient to dry the area with a tissue if needed.
11. Instruct the patient to carefully cap the specimen container and place it in a specified place if collected in the office or refrigerate it if collected at home.
12. Gloves should be worn when receiving the specimen from the patient. The sample container (not the lid) should be labeled correctly, and a requisition should be completed if required.
13. The person receiving the sample should remove the gloves and sanitize his or her hands after the urine has been placed in the testing area.
14. The procedure should be charted correctly. The charting should document that midstream clean-catch urine collection instructions were given and that the specimen was received from the patient.

*Figs. A through C courtesy Gala Bent.

PROCEDURE 3-2: Instructing Patients How to Collect a 24-Hour Urine Specimen

Procedure

Sanitize your hands and assemble and label the correct specimen collection equipment. Determine that you are instructing the correct patient by having the patient state his or her name. Provide the patient with the required equipment and written instructions.

1. Wash your hands, and gather the equipment.
2. Greet and identify your patient.
3. Instruct the patient to empty the bladder into the toilet after arising on the first day of the 24-hour procedure. Inform the patient not to save this specimen but to record the time.
4. Instruct the patient that each time he or she urinates for the next 24 hours, the urine must be voided directly into the collection container. It might be necessary to give female patients a large sterile container that has a wide opening in which they can void; afterwards, they can pour the contents into the 24-hour jug.
5. Tell the patient to be sure to screw the lid on tightly each time and keep the container refrigerated. If at any time during the procedure some urine is not collected, the test must be started again. Examples include the patient forgetting to collect some urine; spilling some urine; and, if the patient is a child, wetting the bed.
6. Instruct the patient that on the following morning, he or she must urinate directly into the container at the same time as on the first day. Therefore the first morning specimen on the second day is kept and is the end of the 24-hour collection procedure.
7. Instruct the patient that on the day the procedure is completed, the container must be returned to the physician's office or to the laboratory.
8. After the patient has completed the procedure and returned the container, check the label for completeness and ask the patient whether any problems occurred during the collection procedure.
9. A requisition form must be completed and the 24-hour urine container transported to the laboratory that will perform the test.
10. Chart the instructions and equipment that were supplied to the patient. Also chart that the specimen was sent to the laboratory. Include the type of specimen that was sent, the date, the time, where it was sent, and the test that was ordered.

CLIA-WAIVED TESTS

Urinalysis

Urinalysis is the description and measurement of the substances found in urine. It is the most common test performed in the medical office. The specimen is easily obtained, and the testing is not difficult to perform. Urinalysis can be used for screening in a physical exam, to assist the physician in the diagnosis of pathological conditions, and to determine the effectiveness of a treatment. A routine urinalysis consists of three parts: physical analysis, chemical analysis, and microscopic analysis. Fig. 3-7 is an example of a urinalysis requisition/report form containing the test results for routine, microscopic, and quantitative analyses. NOTE: The quantitative tests in the right-hand column of the requisition are not CLIA waived and are generally performed on a 24-hour collected specimen in which the total volume of the urine has been measured and recorded.

Fresh or preserved urine can be used when performing a routine urinalysis. Preservatives are usually used for specimens being sent a long distance and requiring prolonged storage. Nonpreserved urine is preferred because some preservatives can interfere with the chemicals used in the testing. Urine should be tested within 1 hour of voiding, but if this is not possible, the urine should be refrigerated. Before the testing the urine must be brought to room temperature and mixed.

Urine that stands at room temperature for more than 1 hour may undergo the following changes:
- Bacteria will multiply, causing the urine to be cloudy. Some bacteria can break down urea to ammonia, which will change the **pH** (scale that measures acidity or alkalinity) of the urine to alkaline.
- Glucose that could be present in the urine decreases as it is metabolized by microorganisms.
- Cells in the urine will **lyse** (break open).
- **Casts** (elements excreted in the urine in the shape of the renal tubules and ducts) dissolve and disappear, and crystals may dissolve if the pH changes.
- **Bilirubin** (a waste product from the breakdown of hemoglobin that is metabolized by the liver), if present, will be oxidized with exposure to light.

CLIA-Waived Tests

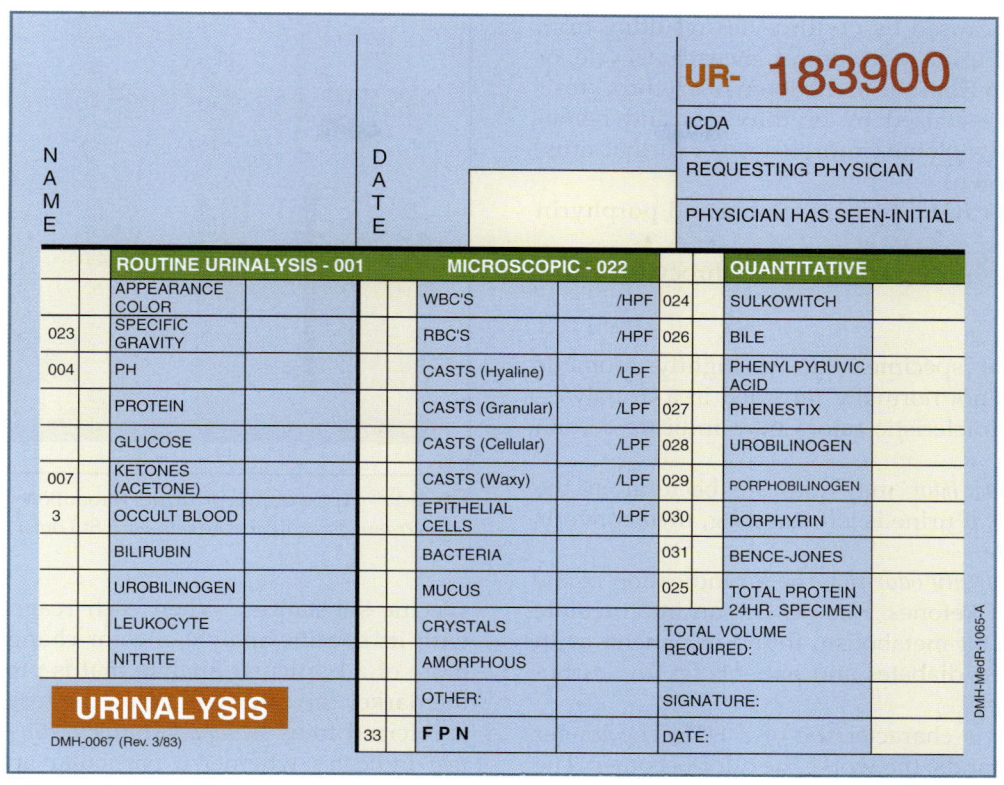

Fig. 3-7. Urinalysis laboratory form. (From Bonewit-West K: *Clinical procedures for medical assistants*, ed 7, St Louis, 2008, Saunders.)

Physical Routine Urinalysis

The physical part of a urinalysis consists of observing the color, odor, and appearance (transparency) of a urine specimen. To determine the color and appearance, the urine must be viewed through a clear container. NOTE: In the past, the urine would also be tested for pH and specific gravity during the physical analysis. These two tests are now included in the chemical analysis of urine because they are measured using the same test strips as the chemical analytes.

Color

The color of normal urine (Fig. 3-8) is typically described as *straw colored (light yellow)*, to *yellow*, to *amber (dark yellow)*. Varying amounts of a normal pigment called *urochrome* give the urine its characteristic shades of yellow. Concentrated urine with less water is dark yellow to amber, whereas a more diluted urine is a lighter yellow or straw color. The first morning specimen is most concentrated (dark yellow); the urine becomes more dilute (lighter in color) as the day progresses and more fluid is consumed.

Sometimes additional substances may cause a change in the color of urine, but this is not necessarily associated with disease. Such color changes may be caused by food dyes, some medications, and vitamins.

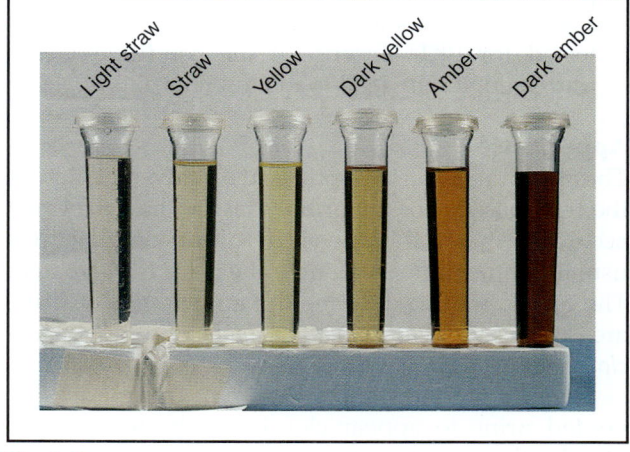

Fig. 3-8. Colors of urine. (From Bonewit-West K: *Clinical procedures for medical assistants*, ed 7, St Louis, 2008, Saunders.)

The colors in the following list, however, may be indications of a pathological condition. The following are abnormal urine colors and their possible causes:
- Yellow-brown—caused by bilirubin resulting from excessive RBC destruction or bile duct obstruction
- Orange-yellow—caused by bilirubin or urobilinogen resulting from a reduction in the functioning of liver cells or excessive RBC destruction
- Green—caused by biliverdin resulting from the oxidation of bilirubin

- Dark red—caused by erythrocytes resulting from bleeding of urinary structures, menstrual cycle, or hemoglobin from the breakdown of erythrocytes
- Red-brown—caused by erythrocytes and hemoglobin or myoglobin (from skeletal or cardiac muscle breakdown)
- Clear red—caused by hemoglobin and **porphyrin** products
- Cloudy red—caused by intact erythrocytes

Odor
A fresh urine specimen has a slightly aromatic odor. Odor is not normally recorded in a urinalysis, but some characteristic odors may indicate certain conditions.
- An *ammonia* odor may indicate bacteria in the urine. Also, if urine is left standing, urea converts to ammonia.
- A *sweet* or *fruity odor* may be an indication of the presence of ketones. Ketones are an intermediate product of fat metabolism found in patients with uncontrolled diabetes and patients on low-carbohydrate diets.
- A *foul odor* is characteristic of a UTI. The longer the urine stands, the worse the odor becomes. The decomposition of leukocytes causes the foul odor.
- A *musty odor* can be caused by certain foods, such as asparagus, or by an inherited metabolic condition, phenylketonuria (PKU), that occurs in newborns. The urine smells musty or mousy. Newborns are tested for PKU because if the condition is left untreated, it may lead to mental retardation.

Appearance
The appearance part of a physical urinalysis evaluates the transparency of the urine. This can be performed accurately only if the urine is in a clear container; it is usually done at the same time the color is evaluated. The terms used to describe the appearance of urine are *clear, hazy (slightly cloudy), cloudy,* and *turbid (very cloudy)* (Fig. 3-9).

Some of the substances that may cause a freshly voided urine to appear cloudy are bacteria, yeast, blood cells, casts, mucous threads, and sperm. These substances could be clinically important and are evaluated further in the chemical and microscopic parts of the urinalysis. Urine that is clear when voided may become cloudy as it is allowed to stand. Dissolved substances crystallize as urine cools, causing the cloudy appearance.

Chemical Urinalysis
The second part of a urinalysis is the chemical testing, which helps diagnose pathological conditions. A reagent strip is a thin plastic strip containing pads impregnated with chemical reagents that test for specific substances. When each reagent pad reacts with its specific analyte, a color change occurs. The more of a particular analyte that is present in urine, the darker the color will be on the reagent pad. This is referred to as *semiquantitative testing*. A *qualitative* test indicates whether a particular analyte is present, whereas *semiquantitative* testing determines the approximate quantity of an analyte. *Quantitative* testing measures the exact amount of a substance and usually requires more complex equipment and procedures that are not usually available in a physician's office. Reagent strips provide both qualitative and semiquantitative measurements, with results recorded in ranges such as trace, 1+, 2+, and 3+; small, moderate, and large; and negative and positive.

Reagent strips are also time dependent, which means that each test on a strip must be read at a particular time. The tests on the strips are referred to as *screening tests*. If a result is abnormal, then additional testing may be performed to confirm the presence of the abnormal analyte. Some of these confirmatory tests will be reviewed when individual analytes are discussed.

Urinalysis chemistry strips (Fig. 3-10, *A* and *B*) have multiple reagent pads on each strip. The most commonly used testing strip consists of reagent pads for specific gravity, pH, glucose, ketones, bilirubin, urobilinogen, blood, protein, nitrite, and leukocytes.

Chemical Urinalysis—Quality Assurance
The following guidelines help ensure high-quality results when performing urinalysis testing with a reagent strip:
- The reagent strip bottle must be kept tightly closed when not in use because moisture from air, light, and aerosols can affect the accuracy of the testing.
- The pads on the strip should not be touched or placed on any surface.

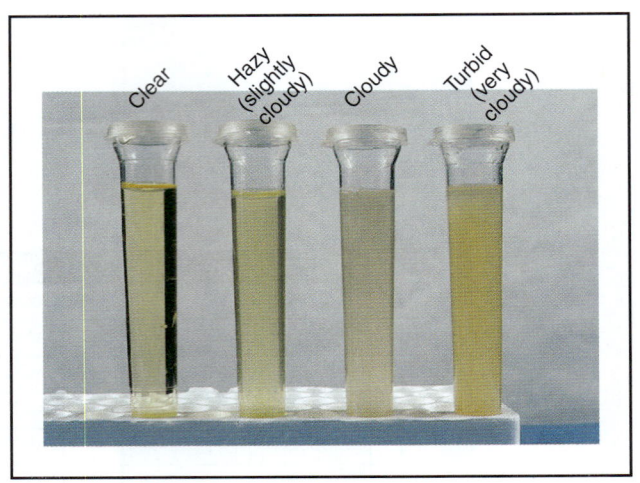

Fig. 3-9. Appearance of urine. (From Bonewit-West K: *Clinical procedures for medical assistants,* ed 7, St Louis, 2008, Saunders.)

CLIA-Waived Tests

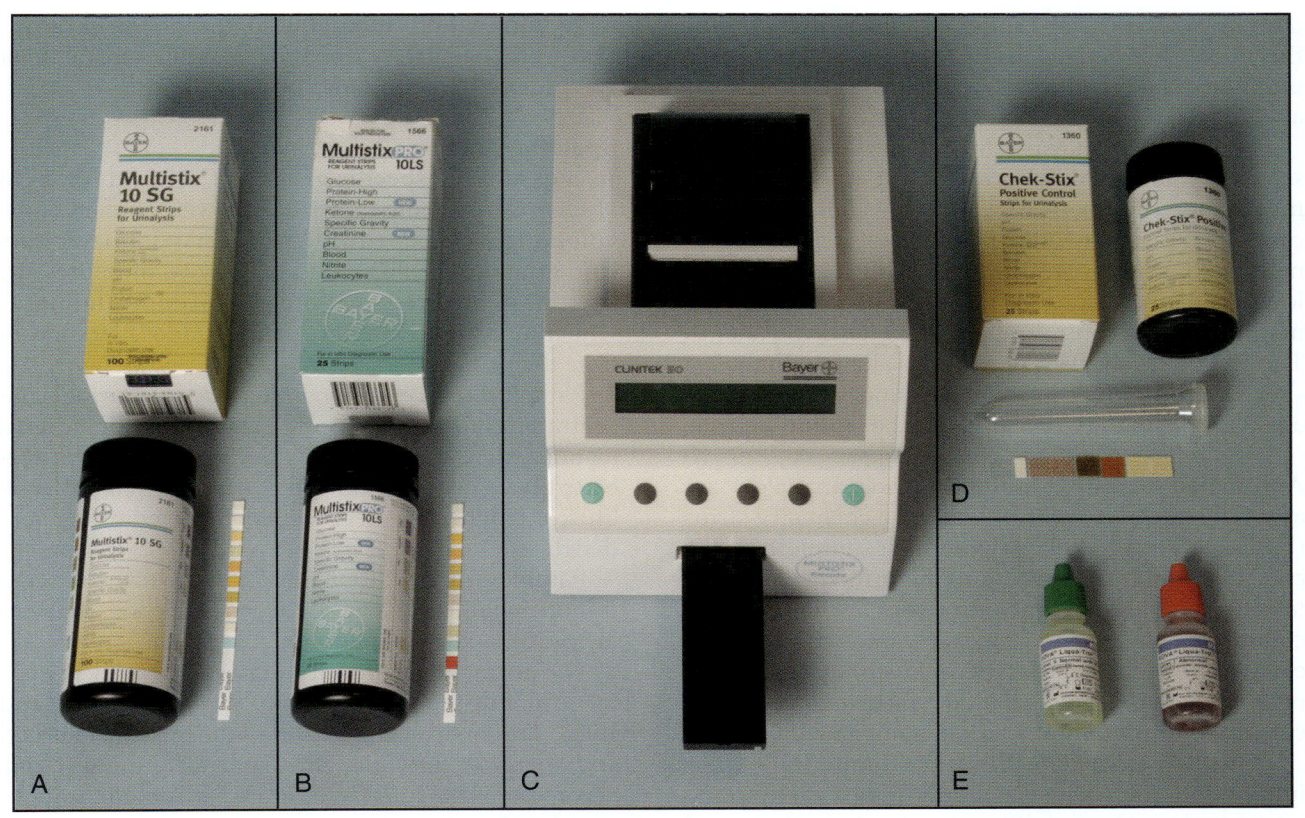

Fig. 3-10. Urinalysis chemistry supplies. **A,** Multistix 10 SG urinalysis chemistry reagent strips; **B,** Multistix Pro10LS urinalysis chemistry reagent strips; **C,** Clinitek instrument; **D,** Chex Stix positive control strips; **E,** Kova normal and abnormal controls.

- Keep the strips in a cool, dry place but do not refrigerate them.
- Do not use an expired bottle (the expiration date is displayed on the bottle).
- Any bottle that has been open longer than 2 months should not be used. Repeated exposure to air can change the accuracy of the strips. Be sure to note the date a bottle is opened.
- Do not combine strips from different bottles.
- Follow all directions from the manufacturer.
- Mix the urine specimen well, and bring it to room temperature before testing.
- Make sure that all pads are covered with the specimen.
- Do not leave the strip in the urine too long because this can cause the chemical in the pads to leach (wash out) into the urine.
- When taking the strip out of the urine, remove excess urine by pulling the back side of the strip against the container and then briefly blot the side of the strip against absorbent paper.
- Hold the strip horizontally to keep the colors on one pad from running into another while you are comparing the colors to the reference testing chart. Do not touch the bottle with the strip while comparing (see Procedure 3-4). NOTE: There are plastic charts available from the manufacturer that can be cleaned and disinfected should they become contaminated.
- Record observed results for each analyte on lab log and requisition/report.

Reagent Strip Quality Control. To ensure the accuracy of results, quality control procedures must be followed when performing chemical tests on urine. Quality control determines whether the reagent strips are working properly and whether the test is being correctly performed and accurately interpreted.

Several reagent control methods can be used (see Fig. 3-10, *D* and *E*). One method is to use a control strip containing synthetic ingredients (*D*). The strip is placed in water to dissolve the ingredients, and this solution is then tested as a urine specimen. Another method is to use a dehydrated urine control, which can be purchased from the manufacturer in normal and abnormal levels (*E*). The controls are rehydrated according to the manufacturer's directions, and then a chemical examination is performed in the same way a urine sample would be examined.

With any quality control method, the results obtained must be compared with the manufacturer's ranges that accompany the controls and the results must be logged in quality control record books. If the results do not fall within the quality control ranges, then appropriate steps must be taken to determine the cause. No patient testing should be performed until the quality control results fall within the acceptable ranges.

Proficiency checklists (also referred to as *procedure sheets*) for any new laboratory test must be documented for each person performing the test. In this case, each person would run the test using the urinalysis controls, write the results on the laboratory log, and then check to see if the results fall within the manufacturer's control range before testing patients. The procedure sheets for urinalysis along with the log sheets for both the control results and patient results are available in the workbook and the on-line website.

Automated Clinitek Method. Urine analyzers are available that automatically read the chemistry strips (Fig. 3-11). The Clinitek Analyzer, for example, runs the chemical analysis according to the principle of reflectance photometry. A microprocessor in the machine controls the movement of the strip into the reflectometer, where a light of specific wavelengths is beamed onto the strip. The light that is reflected is measured, converted into a digital reading, and printed.

In the automated method, the timing and color interpretation are consistent and do not vary among individual readers as the visual interpretation of color does. A disadvantage of this method is that if the urine contains a large amount of pigment, the machine cannot recognize this and will give false-positive results.

Urine Test Strips

The routine tests included in a chemical examination of urine are specific gravity, pH, glucose, ketones, bilirubin, urobilinogen, blood, protein, nitrite, and leukocytes. These tests can provide the physician with information about the status of the patient's acid–base balance, carbohydrate metabolism, liver and kidney functions, and possible UTIs.

Specific Gravity

To measure the **specific gravity** of urine, the weight of the urine is compared with the weight of an equal volume of water, which has a standardized specific gravity of 1.000. Specific gravity measures the amount of particles that are dissolved in the urine, which indicates the ability of the kidneys to concentrate the urine.

Pathological conditions that *increase* urine concentration and raise specific gravity include adrenal insufficiency; congestive heart failure; hepatic disease; **glycosuria** (sugars in the urine) of diabetes mellitus; and dehydration caused by fever, vomiting, and diarrhea.

Pathological conditions that *decrease* urine concentration include chronic renal insufficiency, diabetes insipidus, and malignant hypertension.

The normal range for urine specific gravity is 1.003 to 1.030, but the range is usually between 1.010 and 1.025. The first morning urine is more concentrated and therefore has a higher specific gravity. Urine becomes more dilute as fluids are consumed throughout the day, so subsequent urine samples have a lower specific gravity.

pH. The pH of a substance measures its level of acidity or alkalinity (Fig. 3-12). A pH of 7 is neutral, 0 to 6 is acid, and 8 to 14 is alkaline. The lungs and kidneys are responsible for maintaining the body's acid–alkaline balance in the blood. The blood pH must be in a range of 7.35 to 7.45. If the blood pH is below 7.35, acidosis occurs, and if the pH is above 7.45, alkalosis occurs.

Normal urine pH has a variable range of 5.0 to 8.0. The average is 6.0, slightly acidic. The pH of urine is determined by measuring the amount of hydrogen ions present. The pH should be measured by using a freshly voided specimen because urea is converted to ammonia by bacteria in urine that has been standing at room temperature. This conversion causes the urine to become alkaline. Freshly voided urine that is alkaline, however, may indicate a bacterial UTI.

Glucose. Glucose is not normally found in urine. In the glomerulus of the nephron, glucose is filtered into a glomerular filtrate, and in the renal tubules this substance is reabsorbed into the blood. However, if a large amount of glucose is present in the blood, glucose in the tubules cannot be reabsorbed because the renal threshold level has been reached. For glucose this is between 160 and 180 mg/dL.

When sugars are found in the urine (glycosuria), glucose is the most likely to be present (glucosuria). Other sugars that can be found are lactose, fructose,

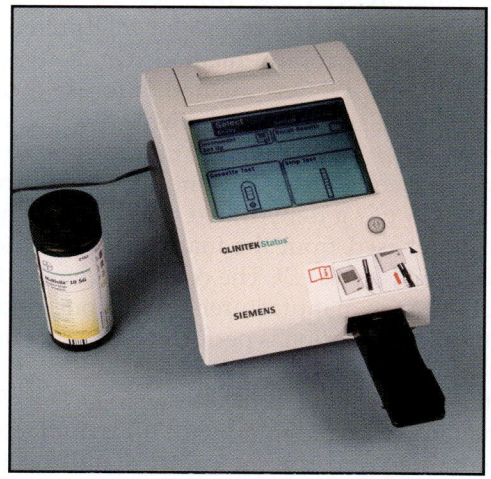

Fig. 3-11. Clinitek urine analyzer with tray for measuring reagent strips. (Courtesy Zack Bent.)

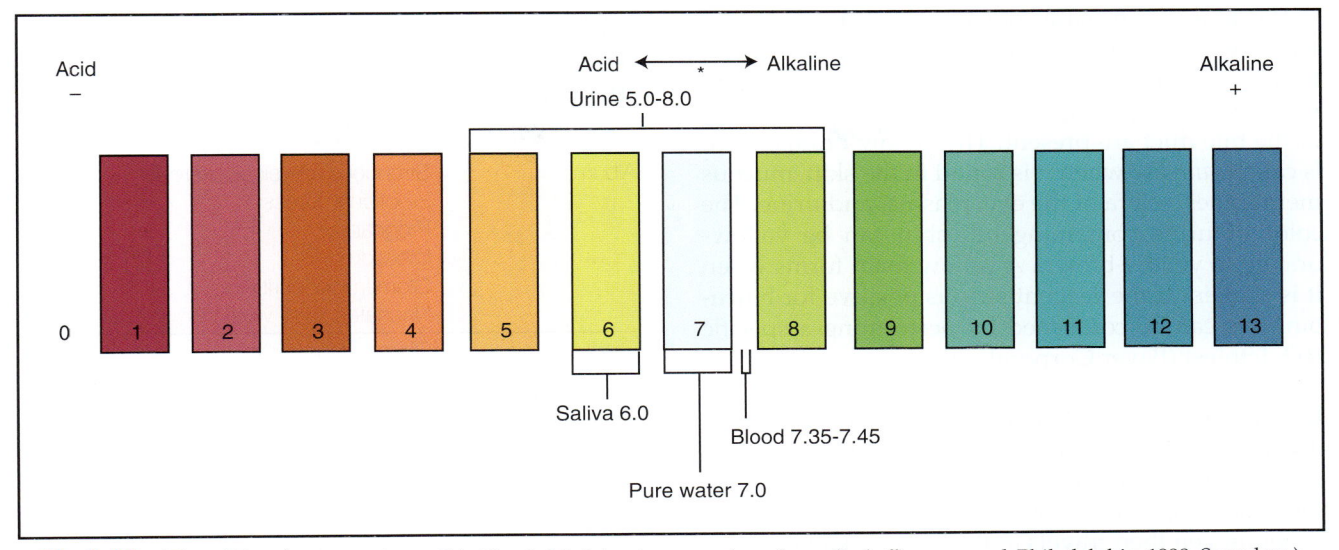

Fig. 3-12. The pH scale. (From Stepp CA, Woods M: *Laboratory procedures for medical office personnel*, Philadelphia, 1998, Saunders.)

galactose, and pentose. The reagent strip method of testing is an enzymatic reaction using the enzyme glucose oxidase that is specific for glucose. The presence of glucose in the urine may indicate diabetes mellitus, but it may also occur after vigorous exercise or in acute emotional stress. False-positive results can also be obtained in the presence of large quantities of aspirin, ascorbic acid (vitamin C), and any medication containing levodopa.

The Clinitest (Bayer Corporation) is a confirmatory test to determine if other sugars or **reducing substances** (substances that easily lose electrons) in addition to glucose are present in urine.

Galactosemia is a rare metabolic condition in which the body is not able to convert galactose to glucose, resulting in the excretion of galactose in the urine. In infants this condition results in the failure to thrive because of anorexia, vomiting, and diarrhea. In addition, enlargement of the liver and spleen; cirrhosis; cataracts; mental retardation; and, in extreme cases, permanent brain damage or even death can occur. A positive Clinitest and a negative glucose strip test in a pediatric urine analysis could indicate galactose in the urine.

Lactose may be found in the urine of pregnant women, and in rare instances fructose and pentose can be found in urine because of high consumption of honey or fruit (see Procedure 3-5).

Ketones. Ketones are products of fat metabolism that are then oxidized by the muscles. The body normally uses carbohydrates for energy, but if the body is low on these, it metabolizes fats. Excessive fat metabolism can lead to large amounts of ketones that the muscles cannot oxidize. The excess ketones accumulate in tissues and blood and subsequently in the urine, a condition called **ketonuria.**

Ketones and glucose in the urine may be associated with uncontrolled diabetes mellitus. The glucose levels in the blood and urine of a diabetic person are high because insulin is either absent or not working correctly and the glucose cannot be burned for energy. Fats are then metabolized for energy, and ketone blood levels increase, causing ketones to spill over into urine. In addition, ketones are acid compounds; therefore ketonuria is correlated with a low pH (acid) urine. If glucose, ketones, and acidity are all present in the urine, this may indicate a condition known as *ketoacidosis*, which may lead to diabetic coma.

Other conditions that may lead to ketonuria are fevers, starvation, anorexia, prolonged vomiting, and diets high in fat and low in carbohydrates. NOTE: These conditions generally do not have glucose present.

Ketones evaporate at room temperature; therefore the urine specimen must be tested immediately or capped tightly and refrigerated. If the reagent strip is positive for ketones, the confirmatory test Acetest (Bayer Corporation) can be performed to confirm the presence of ketones.

Bilirubin. The life span of a RBC is 120 days, after which the red cell lyses and releases hemoglobin. Heme, a product of hemoglobin decomposition, subsequently breaks down to form bilirubin. Bilirubin is an intensely yellow (yellow-orange) pigmented substance that is not soluble in water and must attach to a protein, usually albumin, to be transported through blood. Attached to protein, bilirubin does not pass through the glomerulus because of its large size. Instead, it enters the liver. In the liver it becomes water soluble, enters the gallbladder, and is excreted into the intestines, where it becomes a substance called *urobilinogen*. (See Fig. 5-8 for a graphic representation of this process.)

Bilirubin is normally not found in urine. Bilirubin levels are elevated if conditions such as hepatitis, excessive **hemolysis** (red cells breaking open and releasing hemoglobin), liver damage, and obstruction of the bile duct are present. The yellow-orange color is called *jaundice* when it is found in the skin, mucous membranes, sclera of the eye, plasma, and urine. The color of urine containing bilirubin can be yellow-orange to yellow-brown. A yellow foam forms when it is shaken. If the reagent strip is positive for bilirubin, this can be confirmed by performing a specific test, Ictotest (Bayer Corporation).

Urobilinogen. Urobilinogen results from the breakdown of bilirubin in the intestines by bacteria. The circulatory system reabsorbs approximately half of the urobilinogen that forms in the intestines, and the urobilinogen then travels to the liver, where it is sent to the intestines and excreted in the feces. It either remains as is or is further oxidized to urobilin by intestinal flora. Feces derive their color from urobilin, a pigmented substance. Small amounts of urobilinogen may be present in the urine (approximately 1%), but most is excreted in the feces.

Urine urobilinogen levels may be increased in conditions such as excessive hemolysis of RBCs, cirrhosis, infectious mononucleosis, and congestive heart failure.

Blood. Three types of blood components give a positive reagent strip reaction for blood: intact RBCs (nonhemolyzed), hemoglobin, and myoglobin. The presence of intact RBCs in urine is called **hematuria** and usually occurs in UTIs associated with bleeding, such as cystitis and urethritis. Kidney stones, tumors, and lesions may also cause bleeding.

If a female patient is having a menstrual period, a clean-catch, midstream urine is recommended and her menstrual status should be noted on the requisition. In general, if a small amount of blood and protein are detected on the urine dipstick, it may be necessary to repeat the urinalysis in a week or so to rule out possible infection.

Hemoglobin in the urine, hemoglobinuria, is caused by transfusion reactions, malaria, drug reactions, snakebites, and severe burns. Because it is the result of hemolyzed RBCs that are no longer visible, it is referred to as "occult blood." Myoglobin, an oxygen-storing pigment of muscle tissue, can be found in urine after massive muscle injury, physical trauma, or electrical injury.

Protein. Protein molecules are normally too large to pass though the glomerulus. One of the first signs of renal disease is **proteinuria,** the presence of large amounts of protein in the urine. Sometimes protein is temporarily found in the urine and may not be pathogenic—for example, during fever, exposure to heat or cold, excessive exercise, and emotional stress. However, large amounts of protein repeatedly excreted in the urine over a period of time indicate renal disease. In pathological conditions, albumin is the protein found in urine. The types of protein that can be found in urine are listed in Table 3-1. Proteinuria may occur because of damage to the glomerulus or an imperfection in the reabsorption ability of the renal tubules.

In addition, pregnant women are routinely checked for protein in the urine because it may be a sign of preeclampsia. Correlating protein with specific gravity is important because urine with a low specific gravity (very dilute) showing a trace or small amount of protein may be significant.

A microalbumin test determines if small amounts of albumin are excreted, 30 to 300 mg a day, and is performed if the routine strip is negative for protein or shows trace amounts. Annual screening for microalbuminuria helps identify patients with nephropathy at an early stage. Because urine concentration is so variable, it is recommended that the urine be standardized by performing a ratio of microalbumin to the creatinine concentration, which is excreted at a constant rate. Less than 3.4 mg/mmol (millimole) is considered negative, and levels between 3.4 and 33.9 mg/mmol indicate microalbuminuria. Bayer Corporation has developed microalbumin/creatinine ratio test strips that can be visually read or measured on the Clinitek instrument. The Multistix Pro10LS is a urinalysis strip that measures a protein/creatinine ratio.

TABLE 3-1　Proteins Found in Urine

Protein	Associated Causes/Conditions
Albumin	Strenuous physical exercise Emotional stress Pregnancy Infection Glomerulonephritis Neonates (first week)
Globulins	Glomerulonephritis Renal tubular dysfunction
Hemoglobin	Hematuria Hemoglobinuria
Fibrinogen	Severe renal disease
Nucleoprotein	White blood cells in urine Epithelial cells in urine
Bence Jones	Multiple myeloma Leukemia

From Stepp CA, Woods M: *Laboratory procedures for medical office personnel,* Philadelphia, 1998, Saunders.

Patient:						Date/Time Spec. Collected:					
Doctor:			DOB:			Date/Time Spec. Completed:					

	TEST	REFERENCE	RESULT	TEST	REFERENCE	RESULT		TEST	REFERENCE	RESULT	TEST	REFERENCE	RESULT
☐ VOID	Color	Yellow		Blood	Neg			WBC	0-5 HPF		Bact.	0-5	
☐ CC	Char.	Clear		pH	5.0-8.0			RBC	0-3 HPF		Mucus	0	
☐ CATH	Glucose	Neg		Protein	Neg		MICRO	Epith.	D		Casts	0	
☐ TURBID	Bilirubin	Neg		Urobili	0.2-1.0 EU			Cryst.	0-3 HPF				
☐ HAZY	Ketone	Neg		Nitrite	Neg			OTHER:					
☐ CLEAR	Sp. Gr	1,000-1,030		Leuk	Neg								

Fig. 3-13. Example of a urinalysis form to be completed and inserted into the patient record. NOTE: The physician or laboratory technician will fill out the microscopic results on the right side of the report form.

Microalbumin screening is critical for the following conditions: diabetes mellitus, hypertension, heart attack, stroke, and pregnancy.

Bence Jones Protein. Bence Jones protein is another protein found in the urine of patients with multiple myeloma, a malignant cancer of the bone marrow. Bence Jones protein coagulates at temperatures between 45° and 55° C and then redissolves when boiled.

Nitrites. Some urinary tract bacteria can convert nitrate, which is found normally in the urine, to nitrite. The first morning specimen is recommended for this test because the urine must stay in the bladder for at least 4 to 6 hours to allow any bacteria that may be present sufficient time to convert nitrates to nitrites. Urine should not be left standing because bacterial contamination may convert nitrate to nitrite and give a false-positive reaction. A negative nitrite test does not necessarily mean that no bacterial infection is present. Some bacteria cannot convert nitrates to nitrites, or possibly the urine did not stay in the bladder for 4 to 6 hours. A positive nitrite test is correlated with a positive leukocyte test and then confirmed with a bacterial culture to determine the quantity and identification of the organisms. The most common organism that causes UTI, *Escherichia coli*, does convert nitrates to nitrites.

Leukocytes. Another test on the reagent strip determines the presence of leukocytes, or white blood cells (WBCs). The strip tests for esterase, which is produced by lysed granulocytic WBCs (cells broken open). The presence of WBCs usually indicates a UTI and should be correlated with a nitrite test.

Becoming Proficient at Urinalysis Physical and Chemical Testing

Now that you have learned how to describe the physical characteristics of urine and how to measure the specific gravity, pH, and various urine analytes, you are ready to perform a urinalysis and record your results on a form such as that in Fig. 3-13. NOTE: The doctor or laboratory technician will fill out the microscopic results on the right side of the report form. The proficiency check-off sheets, report forms, and logs are located in your workbook.

The following are additional ways to increase your knowledge:
1. Answer the questions at the end of this chapter and in the workbook (Chapter 3).
2. View the videos on-line to see demonstrations of the skills.
3. Perform the on-line exercises designed to reinforce your terminology and reagent strip performance.
4. Study the *Procedure Sheet 3-3 Manual Chemical Reagent Strip Procedure* before your laboratory class.
5. Also study *Procedure Sheet 3-4 Clinitek Analyzer Method for Chemical Reagent Strip* and *Procedure Sheet 3-5 Clinitest Procedure for Reducing Substances Such as Sugars in the Urine* before class.

PROCEDURE 3-3 Manual Chemical Reagent Strip Procedure

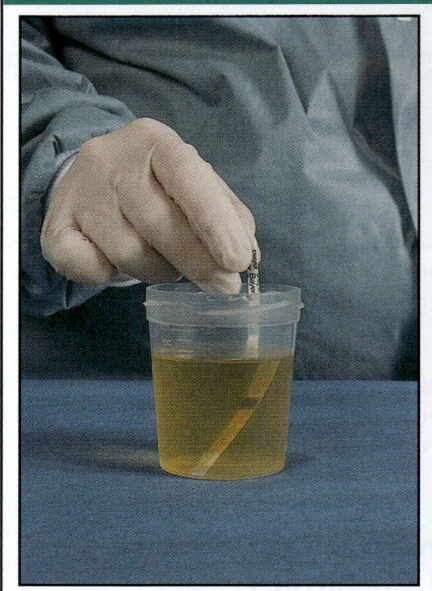

A. Urinalysis chemistry procedure. Dip the reagent strip in the urine. (From Bonewit-West K: *Clinical procedures for medical assistants,* ed 7, St Louis, 2008, Saunders.)

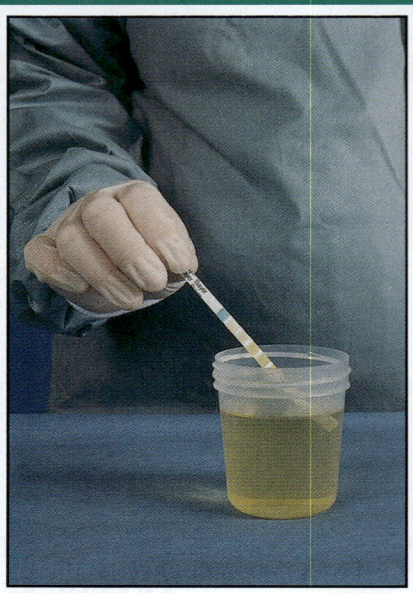

B. Slide the back of the reagent strip on the urine cup as it is removed to remove excess fluid. (From Bonewit-West K: *Clinical procedures for medical assistants,* ed 7, St Louis, 2008, Saunders.)

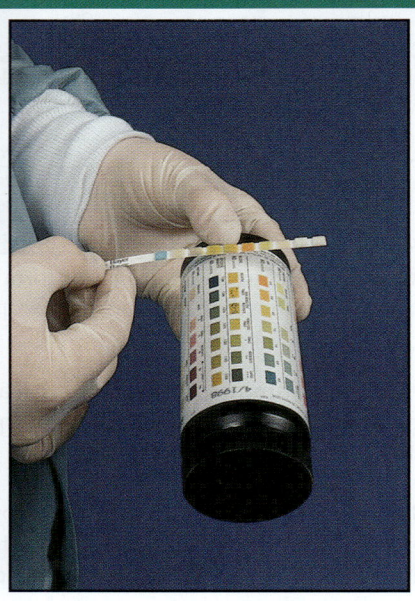

C. Compare each color pad on the strip to the reference chart starting with the first pad (glucose) and its corresponding row. (From Bonewit-West K: *Clinical procedures for medical assistants,* ed 7, St Louis, 2008, Saunders.)

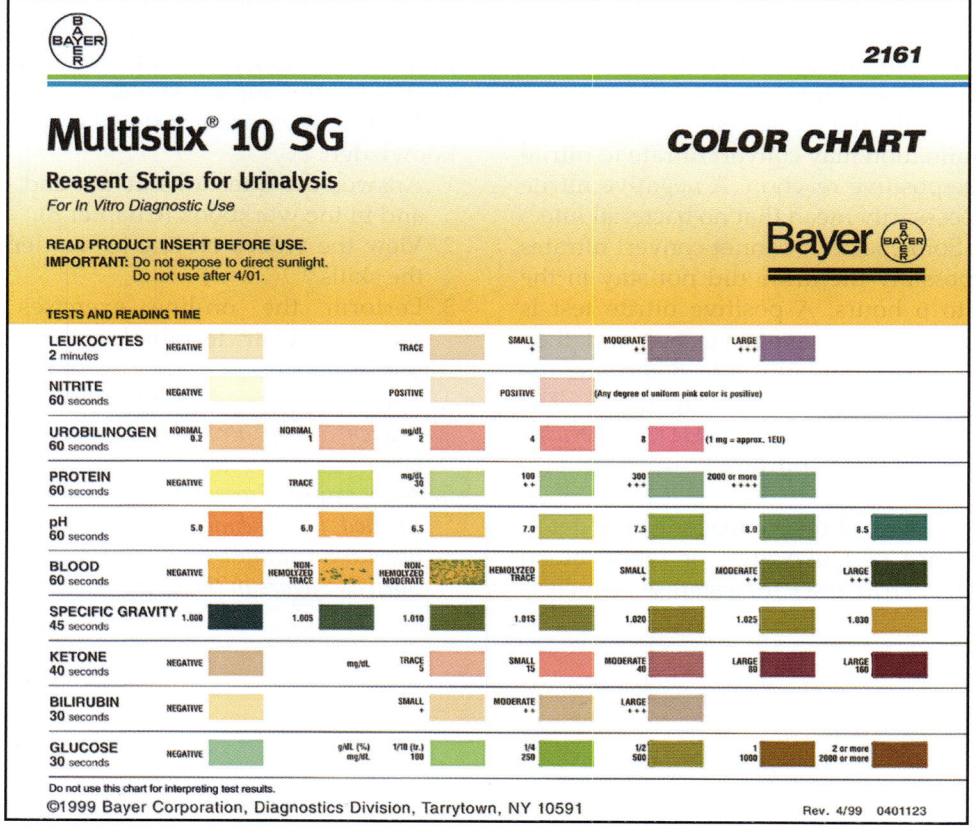

D. Multistix 10 SG chart showing each analyte with its reading time and possible reactions, beginning on the left with "normal" results and moving to the right as the analyte increases. (Courtesy Bayer Corporation.)

PROCEDURE 3-3 Manual Chemical Reagent Strip Procedure—cont'd

Purpose

Testing for chemical substances in a urine specimen.

Equipment and Supplies

Gloves, reagent strips, timing device, reference chart, requisition

Procedure

1. Sanitize and glove your hands, and assemble the equipment. Check the expiration date on the reagent strip bottle.
2. Have the patient produce freshly voided urine in the appropriate container. The sample must come to room temperature, if necessary. Be sure to mix the urine sample before testing. (NOTE: Urine is usually poured into a conical tube to make it easier to determine the color and appearance. This type of tube is used for centrifugation in the microscopic part of the urinalysis and also keeps the original container sterile if a urine culture is necessary.)
3. Perform quality control measures, and record the results to ensure accuracy.
4. After you remove the strip from the bottle, close it immediately. Do not touch the pad.
5. Make sure the pad is completely covered with urine, but do not immerse it too long (Fig. A)
6. Pull the nonpad side of the strip along the container (Fig. B), and then briefly blot the side of the strip against absorbent paper.
7. Hold the strip parallel to the color chart (horizontal position) so that the reagents in the pads do not run together (Fig. C). To keep from contaminating the chart, do not place the strip on it.
8. The reagents in the pads are time dependent, so read each test on the strip at its particular time and compare it to the reference chart (Fig. D). Start with the pad that corresponds with the bottom row of the color chart. The 10 tests on Multistix 10 SG reagent strips and their reading times are as follows:
   - Glucose: 30 seconds
   - Bilirubin: 30 seconds
   - Ketones: 40 seconds
   - Specific gravity: 45 seconds
   - Blood: 60 seconds
   - pH: 60 seconds
   - Protein: 60 seconds
   - Urobilinogen: 60 seconds
   - Nitrite: 60 seconds
   - Leukocytes: 2 minutes
9. After you have read all the pads, discard the strip in a biohazard bag.
10. Remove the gloves, and sanitize your hands.
11. Chart the procedure, indicating the results, the brand name of the test used, the date, the time, and the name of the person testing and charting (or record results on the preprinted requisition/report).
12. If no further testing is needed, discard the strips and supplies in the appropriate biohazard waste containers. Pour the remaining urine down the sink, and place the container in the biohazard waste container. Be sure to have a stream of water started before pouring the urine down the sink to keep from splattering the sample.

PROCEDURE 3-4 Clinitek Analyzer Method for Chemical Reagent Strip

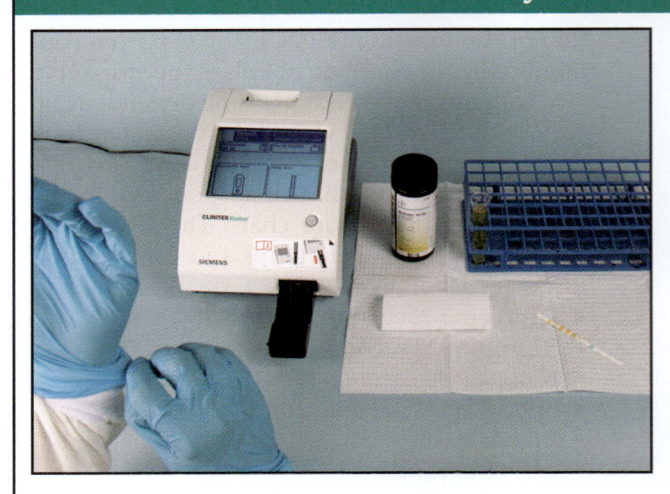

A. Prepare the following: gloves, Clinitek analyzer, absorbent paper, Multistix 10 SG reagent strips or MultistixPro10SL strips, urine and/or control specimen.

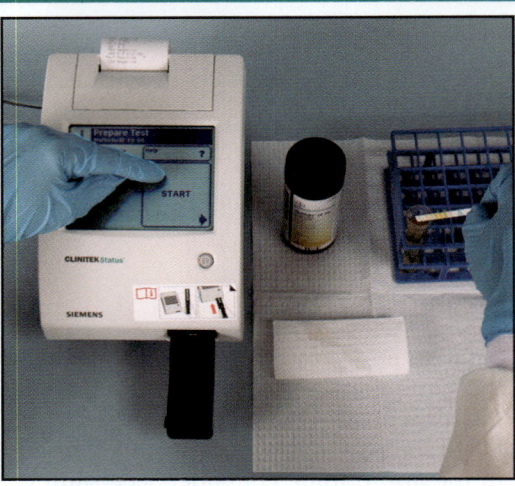

B. Follow the prompts on the instrument monitor and/or the manufacturer's flow sheet. IMPORTANT NOTE: Before pressing the "start" command, have your test strip ready to dip into the urine.

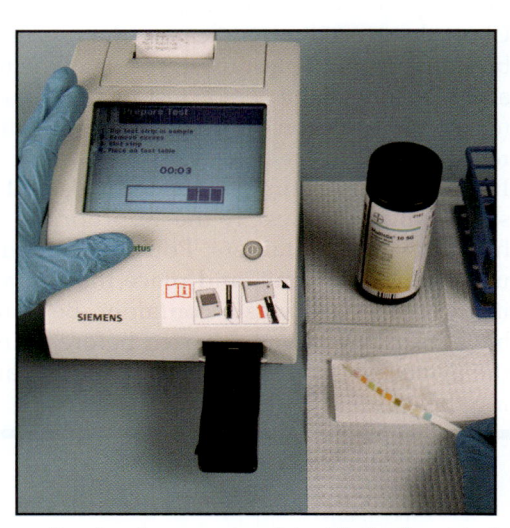

C. Immediately after pressing "start," dip the strip in the urine, remove excess urine from the back of the strip, turn the strip sideways, and blot on the paper.

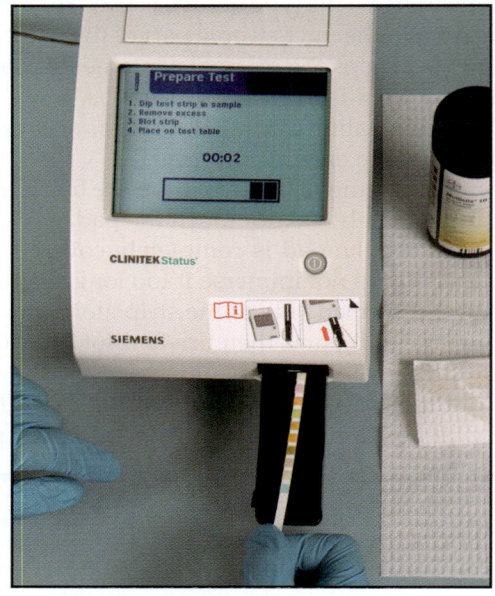

D. Place the strip in the proper position on the tray within 8 seconds.

PROCEDURE 3-4 Clinitek Analyzer Method for Chemical Reagent Strip —cont'd

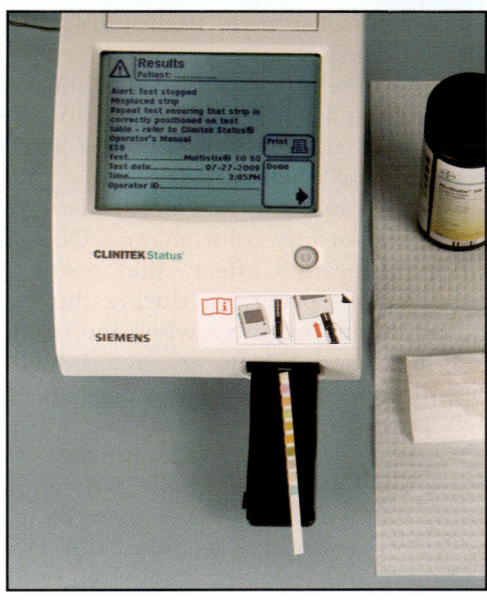

E. If the reagent strip was placed incorrectly, an error message will appear and the tray will push the sample out.

Equipment and Supplies

Gloves, Multistix 10SG reagent strips or Multistix-Pro10SL strips, absorbent paper, Clinitek analyzer, (Fig. A)

Procedure

1. Assemble the equipment. Sanitize and glove your hands. Check the expiration date on the reagent strip bottle.
2. Be sure to mix the room-temperature urine sample, and pour it into a conical tube before testing.
3. Perform quality control measures using a manufacturer's liquid control, and record the results to ensure accuracy.
4. After you remove the strip from the bottle, close it immediately. Do not touch the reagent pads.
5. Follow the instructions on the instrument monitor or the manufacturer's flow sheet.
   - Enter technician identification.
   - Enter patient information.
   - Before pressing the "start" command, have your test strip ready to dip into the urine (Fig. B)
6. After pressing start, you will have 8 seconds to do the following:
   - Dip the strip into the urine, making sure all the pads are completely covered with urine, but do not immerse it too long.
   - Remove excess urine from the strip by pulling the nonpad side of the strip along the edge of the container.
   - Blot the side of the strip against absorbent paper briefly (Fig. C).
   - Place the strip in the Clinitek tray, making sure it is placed correctly (Fig. D).
7. When the instrument completes its 8-second countdown, it will pull the specimen into the analyzer. NOTE: If the reagent strip was placed incorrectly, an error message will appear and the tray will push the sample out (Fig. E). The reagent strip must be discarded, the instrument will need to be reset, and a new reagent strip will be necessary to run the test again.
8. While the instrument is measuring each of the timed reagent pads, you will be prompted to record the color and transparency of the urine specimen.
9. When the test is complete, the analyzer will push out the sample tray and print out the date, the time, the patient's name, the name of the person testing, the results of the 10 tests, the color, and transparency.
10. Discard the strip in the appropriate biohazard waste containers. Gently wipe off the tray with gauze or paper towel. Pour the remaining urine down the sink, and place the container in the biohazard waste container. Be sure to have a stream of water started before pouring the urine down the sink to keep from splattering the sample.

*Figs. A through E courtesy Zack Bent.

PROCEDURE 3-5: Clinitest Procedure for Reducing Substances Such as Sugars in the Urine

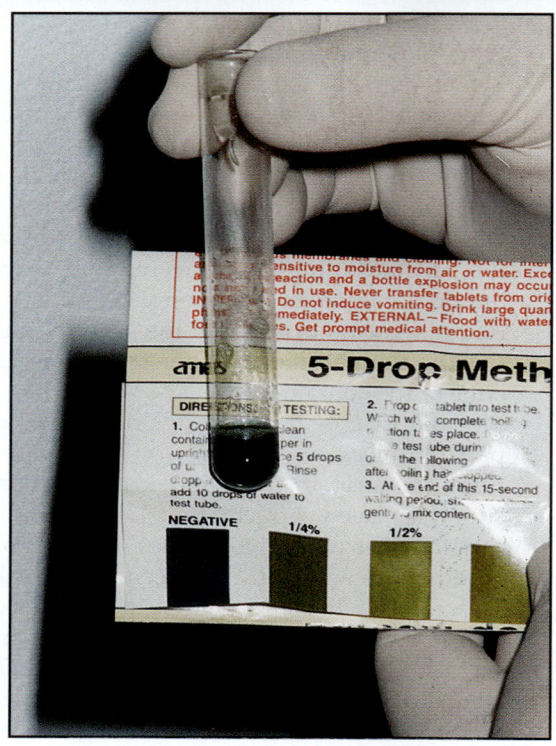

A. Comparison chart for measuring the color results of the Clinitest sugar test. The sample is blue, which would be negative for sugar. (From Young AP, Kennedy DB: *Kinn's the medical assistant: an applied learning approach,* ed 10, St Louis, 2007, Saunders.)

Equipment and Supplies

Bottle of Clinitest tablets, Clinitest glass tube, tube of water with pipette, urine sample with pipette, Clinitest reference chart

Procedure

1. Gather equipment, sanitize your hands, and put on gloves.
2. Add 5 drops of urine to 10 drops of water in a Clinitest tube.
3. Place the tube in a rack. Put a Clinitest tablet into the lid of the bottle so that you do not touch it; the tablet could become caustic if it becomes moist. Tap the tablet into the tube.
4. The boiling reaction that occurs is very hot. Observe it for any color change. Observe for the "pass-through effect" that results, with color changes occurring during the reaction and appearing negative when the reaction is completed and results are determined. The pass-through effect occurs as a result of very high concentrations of reducing substances in the urine. If this does occur, results should be recorded as greater than 2% if using the 5-drop method or as greater than 5% if using the 2-drop method. The final color of either method should not be compared with the color chart when the pass-through effect takes place.
5. Mix the tube 15 seconds after the boiling has stopped to blend the contents.
6. Compare the color of the reaction with the Clinitest chart (Fig. A) for the 5-drop method, and record the results. If the rapid pass-though effect has occurred and you briefly see an orange color, the test must be reported as positive.
7. Discard the equipment in the appropriate biohazard waste container. The remaining urine should be rinsed down the sink, and the container should be placed in biohazard waste container. Be sure to have a stream of water started before pouring the urine down the sink to keep from splattering the sample.
8. Disinfect the work area.
9. Remove gloves, and sanitize your hands.
10. Correctly chart the results.

ADVANCED CONCEPTS

Microscopic Urinalysis

A microscopic examination of urine consists of examining, counting, and categorizing the solid material seen under the scope. A standardized method called the *Kova System* is used to prepare the microscopic slide. It consists of centrifuging a standard amount of urine for a specific time with a specific centrifugal force. After centrifugation the urine separates into **sediment**, the material at the bottom of the centrifuged tube of urine, and **supernatant**, the liquid portion of urine on top of the spun sediment. The supernatant is poured off, and the sediment is stained and poured onto a slide or transferred into a Kova slide chamber. The slide is then placed under the microscope and focused in preparation for the analysis by the physician or trained professional (see Procedure 3-6).

Medical assistants prepare the urine microscopic slide, and either medical technologists or physicians interpret the results. The medical assistant should be familiar with the terminology of the microscopic findings and the basic shapes of the elements found in the urinary sediment in order to understand the complete urinalysis report. The sediment is examined under the microscope for the presence of cells, casts, and crystals. First, the presence of casts is viewed using the low power objective of the microscope; then all other substances are observed on high power.

Cells

The following cells may be found and reported during a microscopic examination.

Red Blood Cells

Hematuria is the abnormal presence of RBCs in the urine (Fig. 3-14). RBCs are round, biconcave, non-nucleated, colorless discs. They are highly refractile in unstained urine and can be difficult to differentiate from other structures, such as yeasts and oil droplets. Yeast usually shows budding, whereas RBCs do not. RBCs shrink in concentrated urine and are referred to as *crenated*. RBCs will swell and hemolyze in diluted urine. If the RBCs have been hemolyzed, they will not be seen on the microscopic examination, but the hemoglobin will be detected on the blood pad of the chemical strip test. A few RBCs, 1 to 2 per high power field (hpf), can be normal. Bleeding, damage to the glomerulus (e.g., inflammation of the glomerulus, or glomerulonephritis), and vascular injury are associated with the presence of RBCs in the urine.

White Blood Cells

The condition **pyuria,** or WBCs in the urine, usually indicates the presence of an infection in the genitourinary system (Fig. 3-15, *B*). WBCs are larger than RBCs, approximately 12 μm in diameter. The most common WBC found in the urine is the neutrophil, which possesses a multilobed nucleus and granules. A urine microscopic examination normally contains 0 to 5 WBCs/hpf. Pyuria can be temporary or caused by fevers or strenuous exercise, but the presence of WBCs can be a factor in pyelonephritis, cystitis, prostatitis, and urethritis.

Epithelial Cells

Another type of cell that can be found in the urine is the epithelial cell. Several types exist.

Squamous epithelial cells (see Fig. 3-15, *A*) are the most frequently seen and least significant of the epithelial cells found in urine. They are derived from the lining of the vagina and the lower portion of the male and female urethra. These cells are large and have abundant, irregular cytoplasm with a central nucleus the size of an RBC.

Transitional or *caudate epithelial cells* (Fig. 3-16) come from the lining of the renal pelvis, bladder, and upper urethra. They are spherical, polyhedral, or caudate (having a tail), with a central nucleus, and are smaller than squamous epithelial cells. They can be found in pairs and small clumps after catheterizations. The presence of large numbers of transitional epithelial cells may indicate a pathological condition.

Renal tubular epithelial cells (RTEs) (Fig. 3-17) are the most significant of the epithelial cells. The presence of increased amounts (more than 2/hpf) indicates tubular necrosis. The size and shape of these cells vary depending on their origin. These cells are round to oval, sometimes rectangular to columnar, slightly larger than WBCs, and can be distinguished from leukocytes by the presence of a single round, eccentric nucleus. Renal tubule cells are present in microscopic urine in conditions such as pyelonephritis, toxic reaction, viral infections, allograft rejection, and secondary effects of glomerulonephritis.

Casts

Casts are formed primarily within the lumen of the distal convoluted tubules and the collecting ducts. They provide a microscopic view of conditions within the nephron. Their shapes usually contain parallel sides and rounded ends. The main component of a cast is a gel-like protein. Four factors can lead to cast formation: decreased urine flow, increased acidity (low pH), increased concentration (high specific gravity), and increased plasma protein. When these factors are present, a cast is formed in the following manner:

1. Protein aggregates into individual protein fibrils that attach to renal tubule cells.
2. The protein fibrils interweave, forming a loose fibril network that becomes a solid structure.
3. Urinary components may attach to the solid structure.
4. The protein fibril structure detaches from the epithelial cells and is excreted as a cast.

Casts are observed and counted on low power, but they are identified on high power. They tend to migrate to the edges of the slide, so this area must be examined. Fresh urine should be examined because casts dissolve in alkaline urine that has been standing.

Hyaline Casts

The hyaline cast (Fig. 3-18) is the most frequently seen cast. It consists almost entirely of protein and appears colorless in unstained urine. Because the hyaline cast has a refractive index very similar to that of urine, it must be examined with the light subdued. This cast can normally be found in the urine (zero to two per low power field).

Conditions such as strenuous exercise, dehydration, heat exposure, and emotional stress can cause hyaline casts to be present in the urine. These casts can also be found in pathological conditions such as acute glomerulonephritis, pyelonephritis, chronic renal disease, and congestive heart failure.

Red Blood Cell Casts
An RBC cast (Fig. 3-19) contains RBCs, is refractile, and is yellow-orange to orange-red in color. RBC casts are primarily associated with glomerulonephritis. As they age, the RBCs lyse and the cast becomes a hemoglobin cast. A hemoglobin cast has the same color as an RBC cast but without visible intact cells.

White Blood Cell Casts
WBC casts (Fig. 3-20) most frequently contain neutrophils that are refractile because of the presence of granules and multilobed nuclei. They indicate infection or inflammation within the nephron, mostly seen in pyelonephritis.

Renal Epithelial Cell Casts
Renal epithelial cell casts (Fig. 3-21) contain renal tubule epithelial cells and can be very difficult to differentiate from WBC casts. They are found in conditions such as heavy metal and chemical- or drug-induced toxicity, viral infection, and allograft rejection.

Granular Casts
Granular casts (Fig. 3-22) contain granules throughout the matrix. They can appear as coarse or finely granular, but distinguishing between the two is not necessary. With urinary stasis present, a granular cast may form as a result of the disintegration of cellular casts and tubule cells or protein aggregates filtered by the glomerulus. Granular casts result from stress and strenuous exercise but can also be found in conditions such as nephrotic syndrome, orthostatic proteinuria, and congestive heart failure.

Waxy Casts
Waxy casts (Fig. 3-23) are very refractile and are homogenously smooth, with ends that are blunt and cracked. These casts appear dark pink, if stained, and represent extreme urine stasis, signifying chronic renal failure.

Crystals

Crystals are formed by the precipitation of urine salts when changes in pH, temperature (crystals form readily at low temperatures), or concentration occur. The most important aid in the identification of urine crystals is the urine pH. Although most crystals are normal, the few abnormal crystals that may represent disorders such as liver disease, inborn errors of metabolism, or renal damage caused by the crystallization of **iatrogenic** compounds (caused by treatment or diagnostic procedures) must be detected. Crystals are counted and identified under high power and reported as few, moderate, and many.

Acid Urine Crystals
The most common crystals seen in acid urine are uric acid crystals, amorphous urates, acid urates, sodium urate, and calcium oxalate.

Uric acid crystals (Fig. 3-24) are typically four-sided and flat yellow to reddish-brown. They can be seen in a variety of shapes, such as rhombic, wedge, and rosette. Although these crystals are usually normal, they can be seen in patients with leukemia who are receiving chemotherapy and sometimes in patients with gout.

Amorphous urates (Fig. 3-25) are yellow-brown granules often found in clumps that give the urine a macroscopic (i.e., sufficiently large to see with the eyes) pink "brick dust" color. Amorphous urates are found in urine at pH levels below 7 and are frequently seen in urine that has been refrigerated.

Calcium oxalates (Fig. 3-26) are frequently found in acid urine but can also be found in neutral and rarely in alkaline urine. They are commonly seen as colorless octahedron crystals that resemble envelopes (they have the appearance of an × on them). The presence of calcium oxalate crystals in fresh urine may indicate the formation of renal calculi. They are also associated with foods high in oxalic acid, such as tomatoes and asparagus, and ascorbic acid (oxalic acid is an end product of ascorbic acid).

Alkaline Urine Crystals
The majority of crystals seen in alkaline urine are phosphates and include triple phosphate, amorphous phosphate, and calcium phosphate.

Triple phosphate crystals (Fig. 3-27) resemble coffin lids and have no clinical significance. They are found in very alkaline urine that contains urea-splitting bacteria.

Amorphous phosphate crystals (Fig. 3-28) are found in urine with a pH greater than 7. They are yellow-brown granules with no distinctive shape. These crystals, which form when urine cools to room temperature, have a macroscopic appearance of white turbidity.

Abnormal Crystals
Most abnormal crystals are found in acid urine and only rarely in neutral urine.

Cystine crystals (acid pH) appear as colorless, refractile, hexagonal plates and can be confused with uric acid crystals. Differentiation can be made by the fact that uric acid crystals are very birefringent under a polarized microscope. However, only thick cystine crystals have polarizing abilities. Positive identification can be made with a cyanide–nitroprusside test.

Leucine crystals (acid or neutral pH) are oily-appearing spheres with radial and concentric striations. These crystals are often found with tyrosine crystals in patients who have severe liver disease.

Tyrosine crystals (acid or neutral pH) resemble fine needles in sheaves or rosettes and are found in conjunction with leucine. They may occur in patients with inherited disorders of amino-acid metabolism.

Bilirubin crystals are seen in hepatic disorders and appear as clumped needles or granules with the characteristic yellow color of bilirubin.

Cholesterol crystals (acid pH) are rarely seen because lipids do not usually crystallize, but they can be found in urine that has been refrigerated. They appear as rectangular plates with a notch in one or more corners (Fig. 3-29). Along with fatty casts and oval fat bodies (discussed later in this chapter), cholesterol crystals are characteristic of disorders such as nephrotic syndrome.

Sulfonamide (Fig. 3-30) and *ampicillin* crystals are formed after inadequate hydration in patients being treated with these antibiotics.

Other Substances

Bacteria

Because bacteria (Fig. 3-31) are normally not found in the urine, the presence of bacteria could indicate either contamination or a UTI. WBCs present with bacteria could signify a UTI. Because contaminant bacteria reproduce rapidly if the urine is kept at room temperature for a prolonged period, testing and microscopic examination should be done on fresh urine. Bacteria are very tiny and must be viewed on high power. They appear as either rod shaped (bacilli) or round (cocci) and are reported as few, moderate, or many or as 1+, 2+, 3+, or 4+.

Yeast

Yeasts (Fig. 3-32) are small, oval organisms that may bud. Differentiating them from RBCs is sometimes difficult, but the budding characteristic is helpful. *Candida albicans* is a yeast that may be found in the urine of women who have a vaginal infection (candidiasis), in patients with diabetes mellitus, and in immunocompromised patients. Yeasts are reported in the same way as bacteria.

Parasites

Trichomonas vaginalis (Fig. 3-33) is the most frequently seen parasite in urine specimens. It is a pear-shaped flagellate with an undulating membrane and a characteristic rapid darting movement that helps identify it in a wet preparation. *T. vaginalis* is a sexually transmitted parasite that causes vaginal inflammation in women and infection of the urethra and prostate in men. It is reported as rare, few, moderate, or many per high power field.

Sperm

Spermatozoa, or sperm, can be found in both male and female urine after sexual intercourse. They have oval, slightly tapered heads and long, flagella-like tails. Spermatazoa are reported as 1+, 2+, 3+, or 4+.

Mucus

Mucus (Fig. 3-34) is a protein whose major constituent is Tamm–Horsfall protein. It is produced by the glands and epithelial cells of the lower genitourinary tract and renal tubular epithelial cells. Microscopically, mucus appears as threadlike structures. To see mucus, the microscope light must be subdued. The presence of mucus in the urine has no clinical significance.

Artifacts

Artifacts that may be found in the urine may include fecal contamination (Fig. 3-35), starch granules from gloves, air bubbles, pollen grains, hair (Fig. 3-36), and clothing and diaper fibers (Fig. 3-37).

Calculating a Microscopic Urinalysis

Although medical assistants do not read microscopic urinalysis, they must understand how the calculation and interpretation of this test are performed. NOTE: There are excellent videos on-line that show moving examples of the cells, casts, and crystals seen under the microscope. Between 10 and 15 fields are examined under low power for casts. Casts are observed and counted under low power, but they must be identified under high power. Between 10 and 15 fields are then viewed under high power. Each substance that is seen in each of the high power fields is counted. When all the fields have been counted, the results for each substance are averaged and reported. Casts are reported as the average number seen per low power field (lpf), whereas cells are reported by using numerical ranges based on the average per high power field (hpf). Other substances are reported as rare, few, moderate, or many (or 1+, 2+, 3+, 4+) per hpf. Standard counting and reporting systems must be used by everyone in the same laboratory. Table 3-2 shows an example of how a microscopic urinalysis is calculated and reported.

Cells

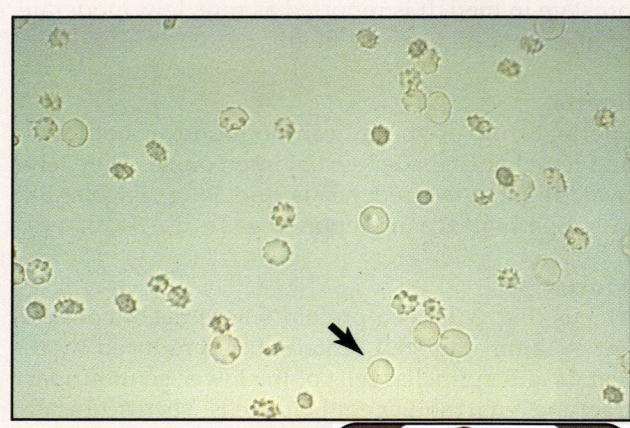

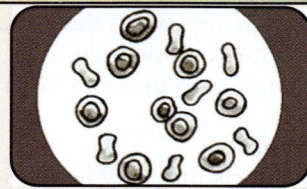

Fig. 3-14. Red blood cells in urine. (From Stepp CA, Woods M: *Laboratory procedures for medical office personnel*, Philadelphia, 1998, Saunders; and Zakus SM: *Mosby's clinical skills for medical assistants*, St Louis, 1998, Mosby.)

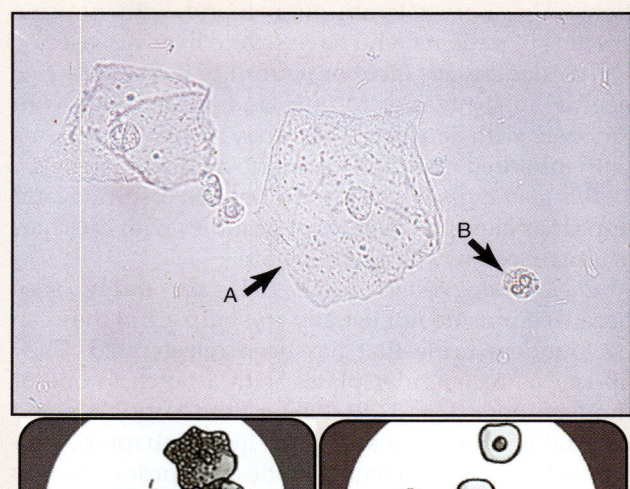

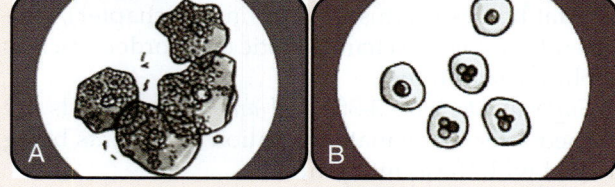

Fig. 3-15. Squamous epithelial cell **(A)** and white blood cell **(B).** (From Stepp CA, Woods M: *Laboratory procedures for medical office personnel*, Philadelphia, 1998, Saunders; and Zakus SM: *Mosby's clinical skills for medical assistants*, St Louis, 1998, Mosby.)

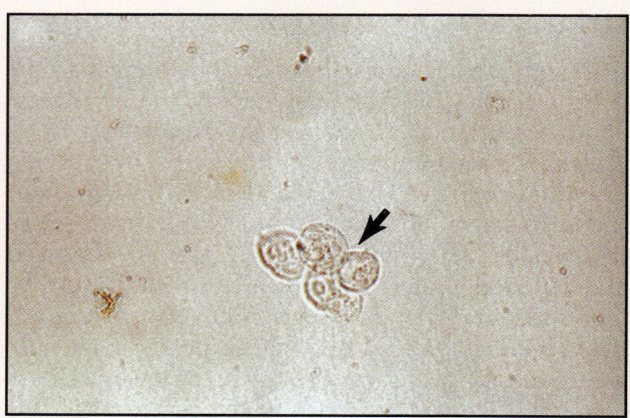

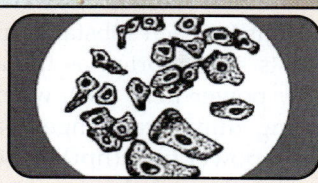

Fig. 3-16. Transitional epithelial cells. (From Ringsrud KM, Linne JJ: *Urinalysis and body fluids: a color text and atlas*, St Louis, 1995, Mosby; and Zakus SM: *Mosby's clinical skills for medical assistants*, St Louis, 1998, Mosby.)

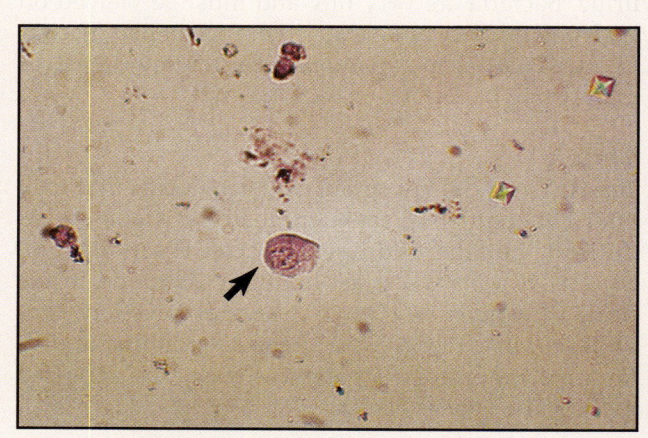

Fig. 3-17. Renal tubular epithelial cell. (From Ringsrud KM, Linne JJ: *Urinalysis and body fluids: a color text and atlas*, St Louis, 1995, Mosby; and Zakus SM: *Mosby's clinical skills for medical assistants*, St Louis, 1998, Mosby.)

Casts

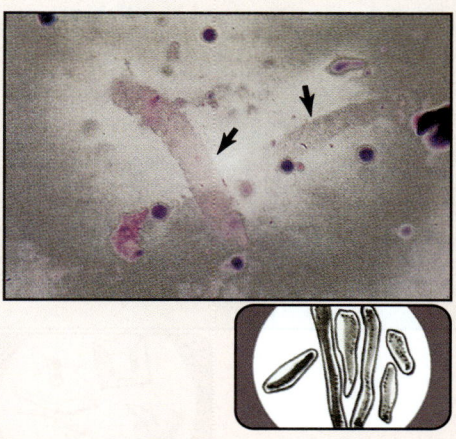

Fig. 3-18. Hyaline casts. (From Ringsrud KM, Linne JJ: *Urinalysis and body fluids: a color text and atlas*, St Louis, 1995, Mosby; and Zakus SM: *Mosby's clinical skills for medical assistants*, St Louis, 1998, Mosby.)

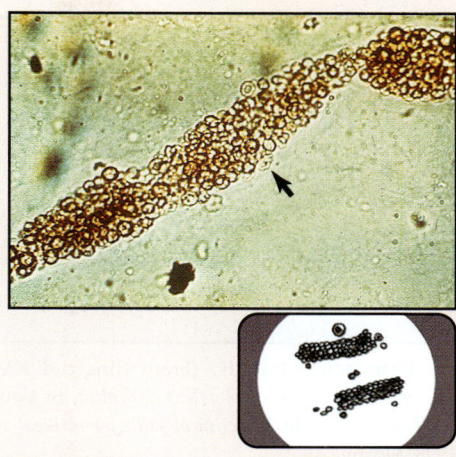

Fig. 3-19. Red blood cell casts. (From Stepp CA, Woods M: *Laboratory procedures for medical office personnel*, Philadelphia, 1998, Saunders; and Zakus SM: *Mosby's clinical skills for medical assistants*, St Louis, 1998, Mosby.)

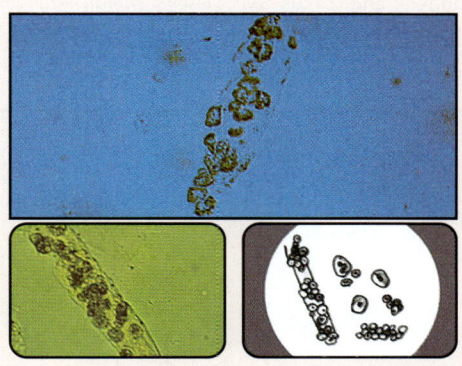

Fig. 3-20. White blood cell casts. (From Stepp CA, Woods M: *Laboratory procedures for medical office personnel*, Philadelphia, 1998, Saunders; and Zakus SM: *Mosby's clinical skills for medical assistants*, St Louis, 1998, Mosby.)

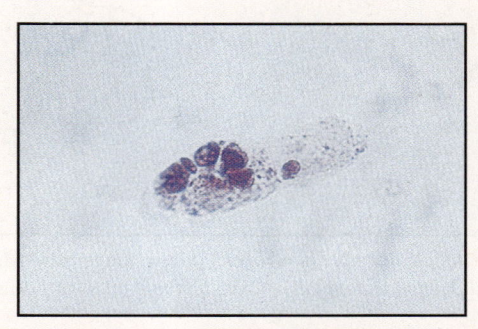

Fig. 3-21. Renal epithelial cast. (From Ringsrud KM, Linne JJ: *Urinalysis and body fluids: a color text and atlas*, St Louis, 1995, Mosby; and Zakus SM: *Mosby's clinical skills for medical assistants*, St Louis, 1998, Mosby.)

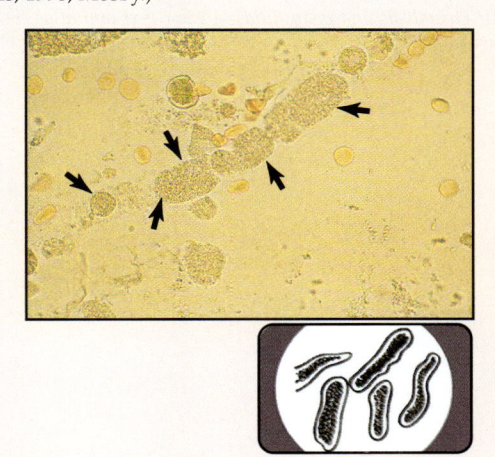

Fig. 3-22. Granular casts. (From Stepp CA, Woods M: *Laboratory procedures for medical office personnel*, Philadelphia, 1998, Saunders; and Zakus SM: *Mosby's clinical skills for medical assistants*, St Louis, 1998, Mosby.)

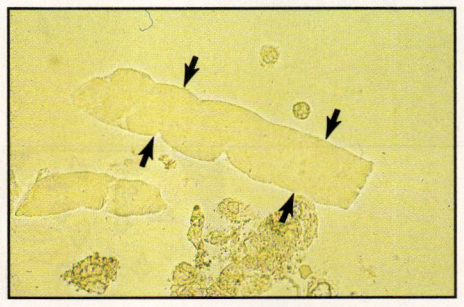

Fig. 3-23. Waxy casts. (From Stepp CA, Woods M: *Laboratory procedures for medical office personnel*, Philadelphia, 1998, Saunders.)

Crystals

Acid

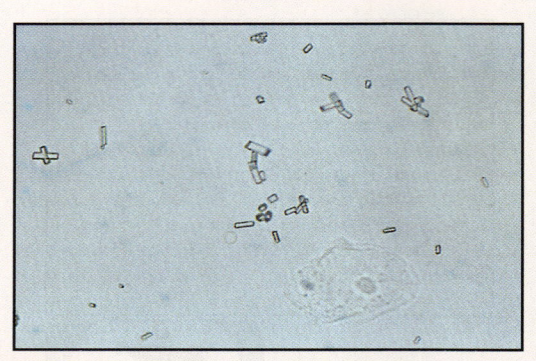

Fig. 3-24. Uric acid crystals. (From Ringsrud KM, Linne JJ: *Urinalysis and body fluids: a color text and atlas*, St Louis, 1995, Mosby; and Zakus SM: *Mosby's clinical skills for medical assistants*, St Louis, 1998, Mosby.)

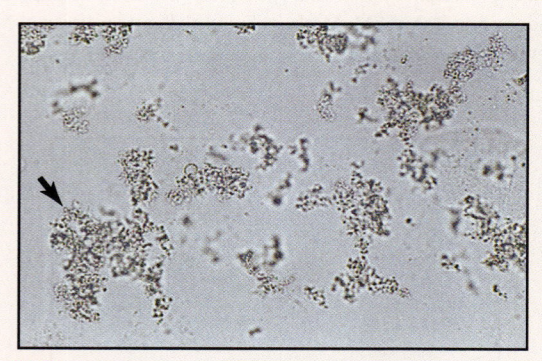

Fig. 3-25. Amorphous urates. (From Ringsrud KM, Linne JJ: *Urinalysis and body fluids: a color text and atlas*, St Louis, 1995, Mosby.)

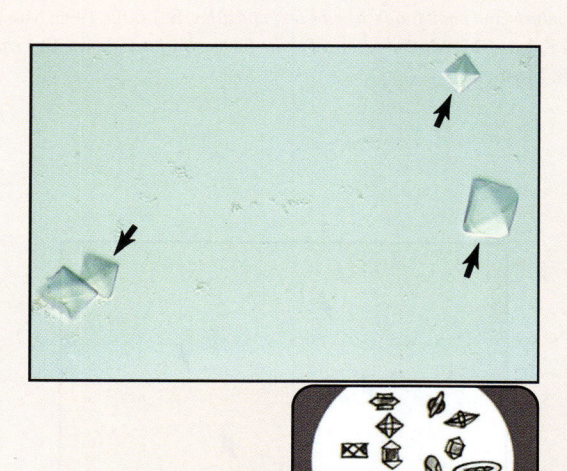

Fig. 3-26. Calcium oxalate crystals. (From Stepp CA, Woods M: *Laboratory procedures for medical office personnel*, Philadelphia, 1998, Saunders; and Zakus SM: *Mosby's clinical skills for medical assistants*, St Louis, 1998, Mosby.)

Alkaline

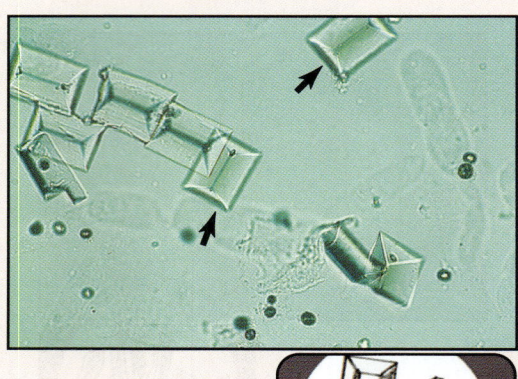

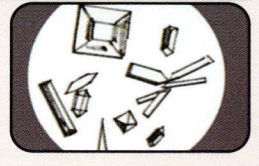

Fig. 3-27. Triple phosphate crystals. (From Stepp CA, Woods M: *Laboratory procedures for medical office personnel*, Philadelphia, 1998, Saunders; and Zakus SM: *Mosby's clinical skills for medical assistants*, St Louis, 1998, Mosby.)

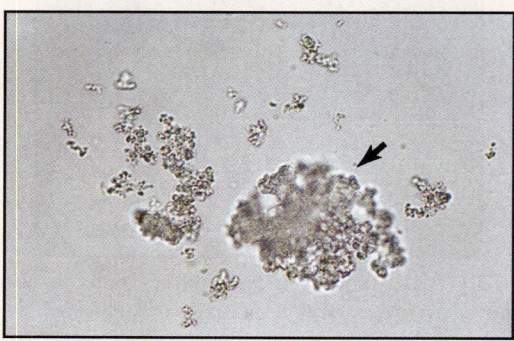

Fig. 3-28. Amorphous phosphates. (From Ringsrud KM, Linne JJ: *Urinalysis and body fluids: a color text and atlas*, St Louis, 1995, Mosby.)

Advanced Concepts

Abnormal Crystals

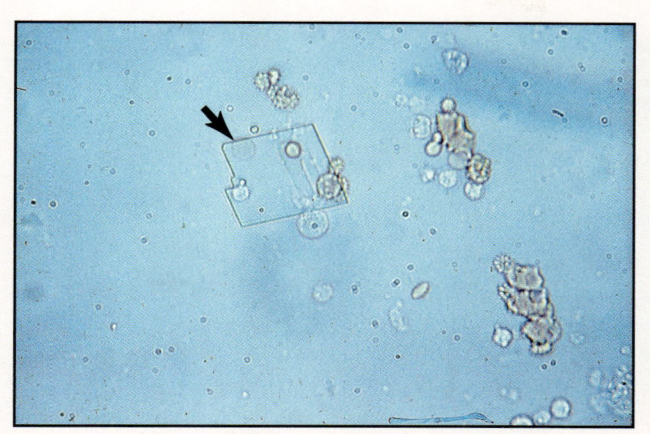

Fig. 3-29. Cholesterol crystals. (From Stepp CA, Woods M: *Laboratory procedures for medical office personnel*, Philadelphia, 1998, Saunders; and Zakus SM: *Mosby's clinical skills for medical assistants*, St Louis, 1998, Mosby.)

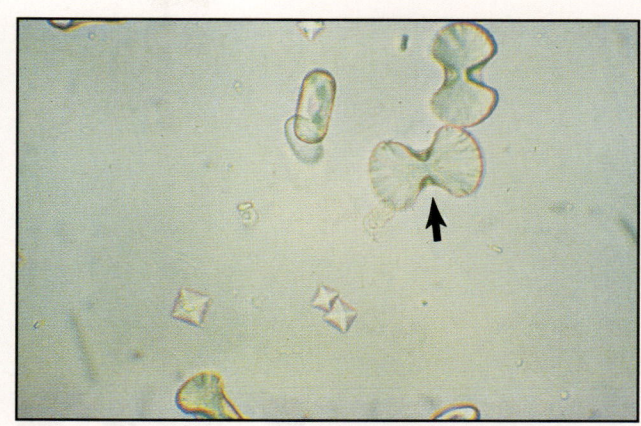

Fig. 3-30. Sulfonamide crystals. (From Stepp CA, Woods M: *Laboratory procedures for medical office personnel*, Philadelphia, 1998, Saunders; and Zakus SM: *Mosby's clinical skills for medical assistants*, St Louis, 1998, Mosby.)

Other Substances

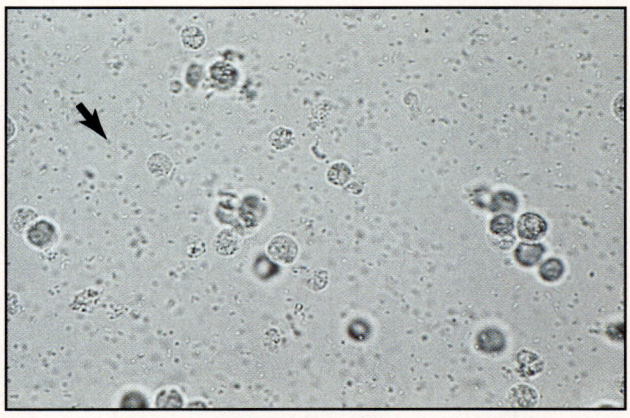

Fig. 3-31. Bacteria. (From Ringsrud KM, Linne JJ: *Urinalysis and body fluids: a color text and atlas*, St Louis, 1995, Mosby.)

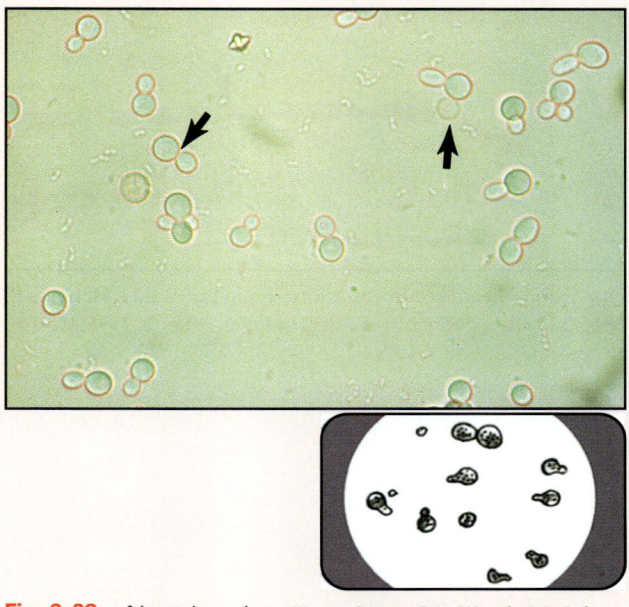

Fig. 3-32. Yeast in urine. (From Stepp CA, Woods M: *Laboratory procedures for medical office personnel*, Philadelphia, 1998, Saunders; and Zakus SM: *Mosby's clinical skills for medical assistants*, St Louis, 1998, Mosby.)

Other Substances cont'd

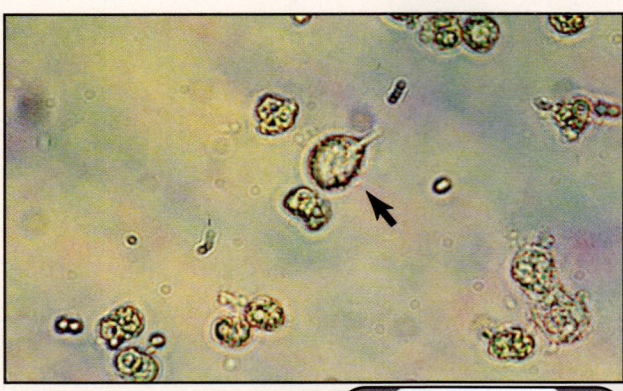

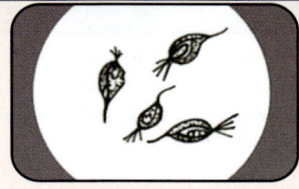

Fig. 3-33. Trichomonas vaginalis. (From Stepp CA, Woods M: *Laboratory procedures for medical office personnel*, Philadelphia, 1998, Saunders; and Zakus SM: *Mosby's clinical skills for medical assistants*, St Louis, 1998, Mosby.)

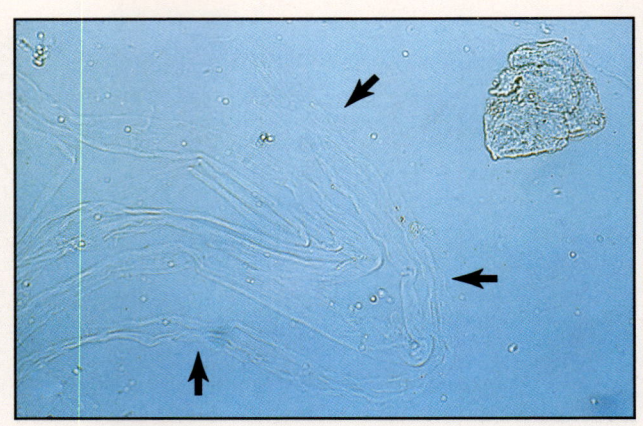

Fig. 3-34. Mucous threads in urine. (From Stepp CA, Woods M: *Laboratory procedures for medical office personnel*, Philadelphia, 1998, Saunders.)

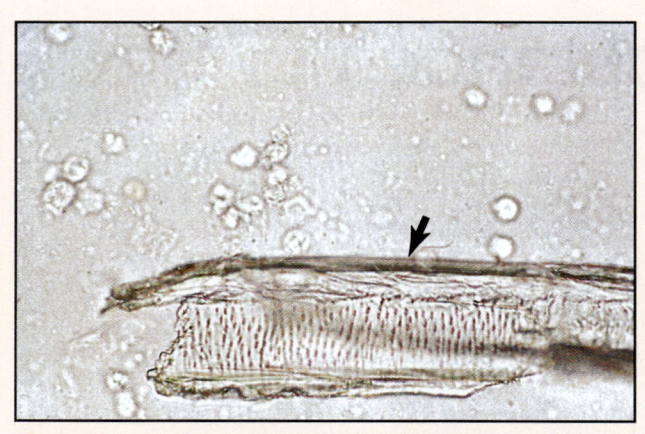

Fig. 3-35. Fecal contamination. (From Ringsrud KM, Linne JJ: *Urinalysis and body fluids: a color text and atlas*, St Louis, 1995, Mosby.)

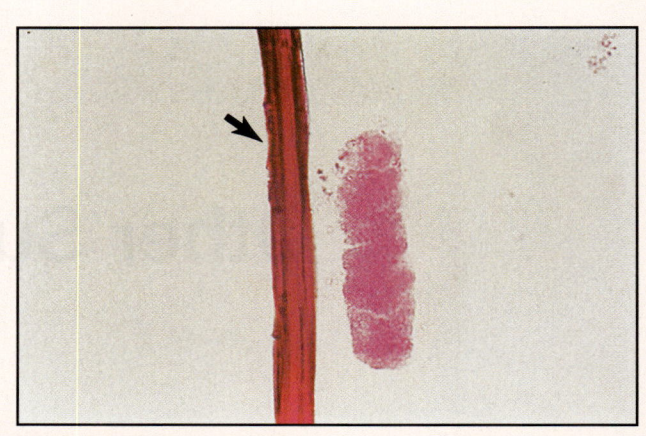

Fig. 3-36. Hair fiber. (From Ringsrud KM, Linne JJ: *Urinalysis and body fluids: a color text and atlas*, St Louis, 1995, Mosby.)

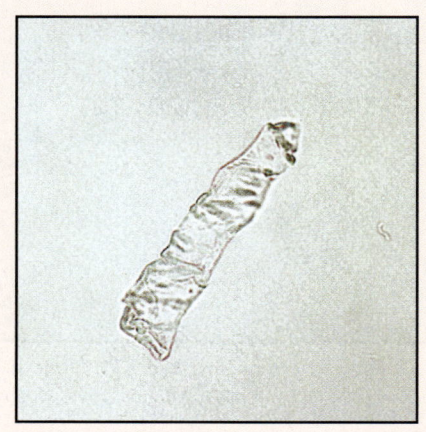

Fig. 3-37. Diaper fiber. (From Ringsrud KM, Linne JJ: *Urinalysis and body fluids: a color text and atlas*, St Louis, 1995, Mosby.)

TABLE 3-2 Calculating a Microscopic Urinalysis

	PER LOW POWER FIELD				PER HIGH POWER FIELD					
Field	Casts	Mucus	WBC	RBC	Squamous Epithelial	Transitional Epithelial	Round Epithelial	Bacteria	Crystals	Other
1	0	Few	16	1	1	0	0	Moderate (rods)	Calcium oxalate (few) Uric acid (few)	—
2	1 hyaline	Few	32	0	3	0	0	Many	Calcium oxalate (few)	Yeast
3	1 coarse granular	Moderate	21	2	3	0	0	Many	Calcium oxalate (few)	Yeast
4	1 coarse granular	Few	12	1	5	0	1	Moderate	Uric acid (few)	—
5	0	Few	25	0	4	0	0	Many	—	—
Total	1 hyaline 2 coarse granular	Few	106	4	16	0	1	Many	Calcium oxalate (few) Uric acid (few)	Yeast
Average	0.2 hyaline 0.4 coarse granular	Few	21.2	0.8	3.2	0	0.2	Many	Calcium oxalate (few) Uric acid (few)	Yeast
Report	hyaline 0-1 coarse granular	Few	20-30	0-1	Few	0	Occasionally	Many (rods)	Calcium oxalate (few) Uric acid (few)	Yeast

WBC, White blood cell; *RBC,* red blood cell.
From Young A, Kennedy D: *Kinn's the medical assistant: an applied learning approach,* ed 10, St Louis, 2007, Saunders.

PROCEDURE 3-6 Procedure for the Preparation and the Microscopic Examination of Urine

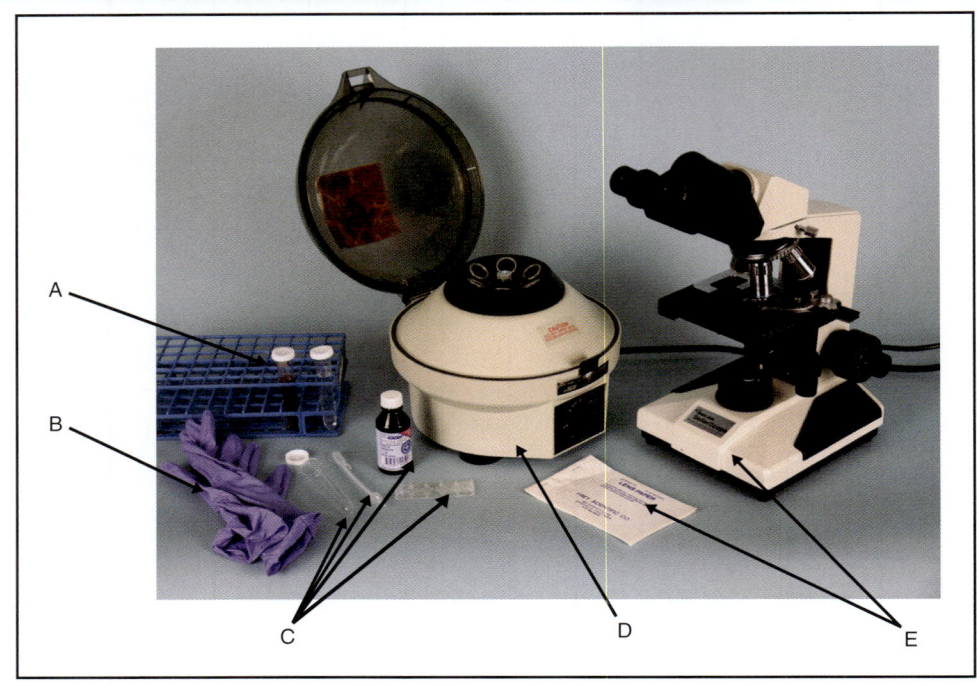

A. *a*, Specimen (freshly voided urine) in tube holder; *b*, gloves; *c*, Kova System (cap and tube, pipette, stain, slide); *d*, centrifuge; *e*, microscope and lens paper.

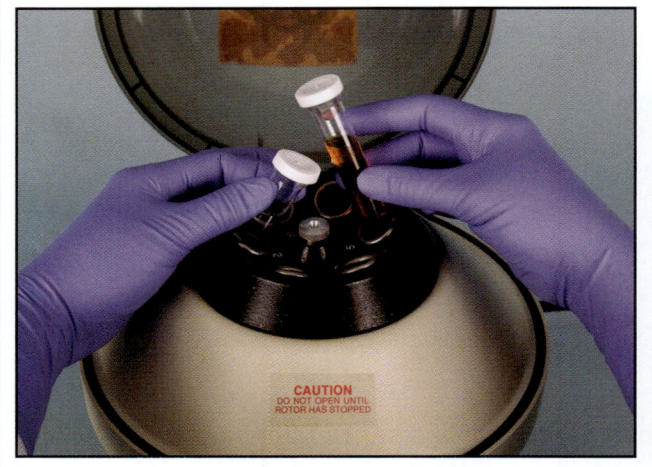

B. Place a centrifuge tube with urine and a centrifuge with water directly opposite each other to balance the centrifuge. Spin for 5 minutes at 1500 rpm.

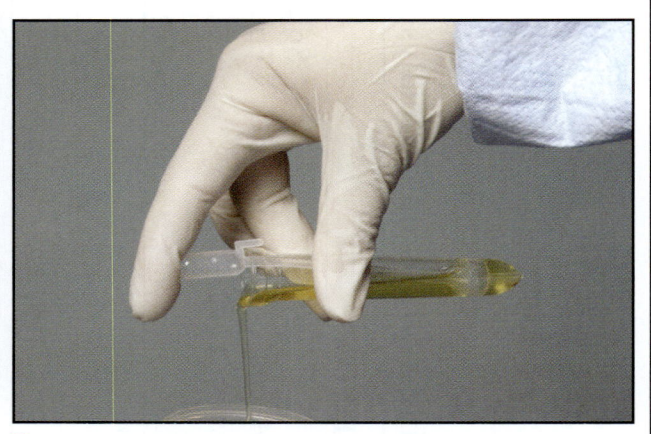

C. After centrifuging, place the pipette in the spun specimen and pour off the supernatant.

PROCEDURE 3-6 Procedure for the Preparation and the Microscopic Examination of Urine—cont'd

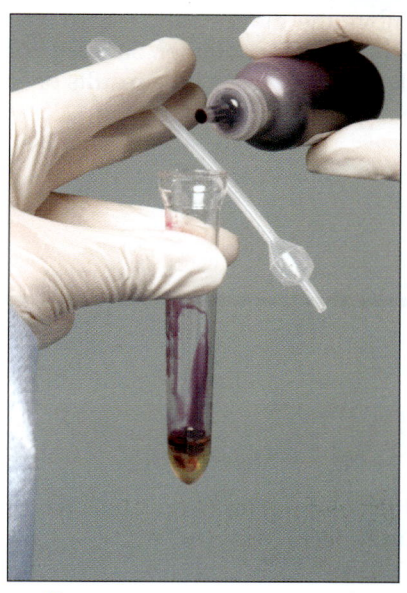

D. Add stain to the sediment.

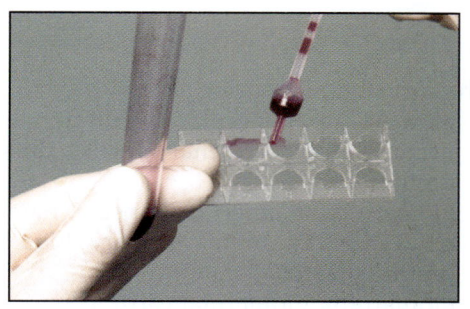

E. Fill the slide wells with the stained sediment.

Objective
To prepare a urine microscopic examination slide.

Equipment and Supplies
Specimen (freshly voided urine), Kova System (cap, pipette, slide, stain), test tube holder, centrifuge, microscope (Fig. A)

Preanalytical: Microscopic Setup

1. Sanitize your hands, and collect the equipment.
2. Put on gloves, and mix the urine. Allow it to come to room temperature if needed.
3. Pour the well-mixed urine specimen to the 12-mL mark in a urine centrifuge tube, and cap it.
4. Centrifuge the tube for 5 minutes at 1500 rpm, which will cause the solid particles in the urine, or sediment, to settle to the bottom of the tube (Fig. B).
5. After centrifugation is completed, carefully remove the spun tube centrifuge so that the sediment is not disturbed.
6. After removing the cap, place the Kova pipette into the bottom of the tube. Seat the tube firmly, hooking the clip on top of the pipette over the outside of the tube.
7. Pour off (decant) the supernatant by inverting the tube (Fig. C). With the Kova pipette method, approximately 1 mL of sediment will remain in the tube.
8. Remove the pipette from the tube, and add a drop of stain so that the structures are better viewed (Fig. D). Reinsert the pipette into the tube, and mix the urine sediment and stain by gently squeezing on the pipette bulb.
9. Transfer a drop of the stained sediment mixture to the Kova slide by placing the tip of the pipette onto the open area of one of the sections and squeezing the bulb until the well is filled (Fig. E). Do not overfill or underfill the well. Return the pipette to the urine tube after the well is filled. To allow the sediment to settle, let the filled well sit for 1 minute before performing the microscopic examination.
10. Place the filled well on the mechanical stage of the microscope and focus on low power with the coarse adjustment. With the fine adjustment knob, bring the specimen into sharp focus. Adjust the light source as needed for low power.

Analytical Interpretation of the Sediment on the Slide

11. The physician or laboratory technician scans the specimen under low power for casts, particularly at the edge of the slide.
12. Change the slide to high power by rotating to the high power objective and clicking it into place. Bring the specimen into sharp view by focusing with the fine adjustment. The coarse adjustment should not be used for focusing because the objective could strike the slide. The intensity of the light source will need to be adjusted for the high power objective.
13. Use high power to examine the specimen, viewing 10 to 15 fields. Casts are counted on low power but identified on high power. All other substances seen should be counted and identified on high power.
14. Record the results for each field.

(Continued)

PROCEDURE 3-6 Procedure for the Preparation and the Microscopic Examination of Urine—cont'd

Postanalytical: Cleanup and Recording of Results

15. The medical assistant may be asked to turn off the microscope and discard the plastic Kova slide, pipette, and capped centrifuge tube in the biohazard waste container. Rinse the remaining urine down the sink, and place the container in a biohazard waste container.

16. Remove the gloves and discard them in a biohazard waster container. Sanitize your hands.
17. Calculate and record the results of each field on the requisition and chart.

*Figs. A and B courtesy Zack Bent.

Review Questions

1. A patient's urine specimen is yellow-orange. Which of the following substances would be found in the urine?
   a. glucose
   b. ketones
   c. bilirubin
   d. nitrate

2. Which substance would be found in normal urine?
   a. hemoglobin
   b. urochrome
   c. porphyrin
   d. myoglobin

3. Which four conditions are conducive to cast formation?
   a. high pH, increased plasma proteins, decreased rate of urine flow, and low specific gravity
   b. low pH, increased plasma proteins, decreased rate of urine flow, and low specific gravity
   c. low pH, decreased plasma proteins, decreased rate of urine flow, and high specific gravity
   d. low pH, increased plasma proteins, decreased rate of urine flow, and high specific gravity

4. In a 24-hour urine specimen collection method, which of the following is correct?
   a. All the urine for a 24-hour period is collected, including the first morning sample of the first day.
   b. When the patient is collecting a urine sample, the first third should go into the toilet.
   c. The first specimen of a 24-hour urine is not collected.
   d. The last specimen of a 24-hour urine is not collected.

5. Which of the following values would represent a dilute specific gravity?
   a. 1.015
   b. 1.005
   c. 1.020
   d. 1.025

6. The correct flow of urine is
   a. glomerulus, glomerular capsule, renal tubules, urinary bladder, renal pelvis, ureter, and urethra meatus.
   b. glomerulus, glomerular capsule, renal pelvis, renal tubules, ureter, urinary bladder, and urethra meatus.
   c. glomerulus, glomerular capsule, renal tubules, renal pelvis, urinary bladder, ureter, and urethra meatus.
   d. glomerulus, glomerular capsule, renal tubules, renal pelvis, ureter, urinary bladder, and urethra meatus.

7. Which of the following substances is observed and counted on low power?
   a. crystals
   b. casts
   c. yeasts
   d. bacteria

8. Which casts are usually found in healthy people?
   a. renal epithelial casts
   b. white blood cell casts
   c. hyaline casts
   d. waxy casts

Advanced Concepts

9. Triple phosphate crystals resemble
   a. envelopes.
   b. dumbbells.
   c. rosettes.
   d. coffin lids.

10. Which is the most common parasite found in the urine?
    a. *Candida albicans*
    b. *Trichomonas vaginalis*
    c. *Enterobius vermicularis*
    d. *Escherichia coli*

Educating a female patient in the correct midstream clean-catch method of collection includes some of the steps below. Write "C" if the step is correct and "I" if the step is incorrect. If the step is incorrect, explain why.

11. The patient should wash her hands.

12. The patient should spread the labia and hold them apart during the procedure with her non-dominant hand.

13. The patient should clean one side with a towelette, wiping from back to front.

14. The patient should repeat step 3 on the other side with the same towelette.

15. The patient should urinate the first third of the urine into the toilet, catch the second third in the sterile cup, and urinate the last third in the toilet.

16. The medical assistant should disinfect the outside of the container.

Review Question Answers

1. c
2. b
3. d
4. c
5. b
6. d
7. b
8. c
9. d
10. b
11. C
12. C
13. I. This would contaminate the urethra opening with bacteria from the rectal area.
14. I. Besides contaminating the urethra opening with bacteria from the rectal area, this step would also contaminate the opening with organisms from the other side.
15. C
16. C

Websites

National Kidney Foundation:
www.kidney.org/

National Institute of Diabetes & Digestive & Kidney Diseases (NIDDK):
www.niddk.nih.gov/

National Kidney Disease Kidney Education Program (NIH):
www.nkdep.nih.gov/index.htm

"Bladder Diseases" from Medline Plus (NIH and the U.S. National Library of Medicine):
www.nlm.nih.gov/medlineplus/bladderdiseases.html

CHAPTER 4

Blood Collection

Objectives
After completing this chapter, you should be able to:

Fundamental Concepts
1. Identify the cardiovascular anatomical structures that relate to phlebotomy.
2. Explain the functions of the cardiovascular structures that relate to blood collection.
3. Correlate the positions of arteries and veins with the use of tourniquets.
4. Discuss the Needle Stick Safety and Prevention Act.
5. List the ways an employer complies with the Needle Stick Safety and Prevention Act.

Blood Collection Procedures
1. Describe the appropriate steps for patient preparation, emphasizing the importance of correctly identifying the patient.
2. Explain the proper procedure for capillary puncture, demonstrating an understanding of site selection, equipment, and complications of this procedure.
3. Perform a capillary puncture according to the stated task, conditions, and standards listed on the Learning Outcome Evaluation in the student workbook.
4. Describe or perform a simulated heel stick and neonatal blood screening collection on to a card.
5. Evaluate a patient's venipuncture site availability, and determine the correct venipuncture method to perform.
6. Describe the proper vacuum tube, syringe, and butterfly venipuncture methods.
7. Explain the order of draw for multiple-draw and syringe venipuncture.
8. Perform a Vacutainer venipuncture, syringe venipuncture, and butterfly venipuncture according to the stated task, conditions, and standards listed in the Learning Outcome Evaluation in the student workbook.
9. Explain the complications of venipuncture procedures and know what to do when they occur.
10. Relate the most current OSHA safety guidelines for capillary puncture and the various venipuncture methods.
11. Maintain a safe work environment by following the most current guidelines for disposing of used equipment and cleaning and disinfecting the working area.
12. Describe or perform the proper way to process a serum specimen and a plasma specimen in a plasma separator tube (PST).

Advanced Concepts
1. Discuss the importance of risk management as it pertains to blood collection procedures.
2. Identify complications that can occur with phlebotomy procedures, and discuss the appropriate steps to take when they occur.

Key Terms

antecubital space area in front of the elbow
arteries blood vessels that carry blood away from the heart
buffy coat narrow middle layer of white blood cells and platelets in a centrifuged whole blood specimen
capillaries microscopic blood vessels that contain a mixture of arterial and venous blood
capillary action process by which blood flows freely into a capillary tube in microcollection procedures
cyanotic a condition in which the skin and mucous membranes are blue; caused by an oxygen deficiency
edema abnormal collection of fluid in interstitial spaces

evacuate to remove air to produce a vacuum
hematoma tumor or swelling of blood in the tissues (resulting in bruising during blood collection procedures)
hemoconcentration condition in which blood concentration of large molecules such as proteins, cells, and coagulation factors increases
humors fluid or semifluid substances found in the body
interstitial fluid all the fluid except blood that is found in the space between tissues; also referred to as *tissue fluid*
lumen inner tubular space of a needle, vessel, or tube
microcollection collecting a small amount of blood

Key Terms—cont'd

osteomyelitis inflammation of the bone; caused by bacterial infection

palpating gently touching and pressing down on an area to feel texture, size, and consistency

petechiae tiny purple or red skin spots caused by small amounts of blood under the skin; found in those with coagulation problems; condition can lead to excessive bleeding during phlebotomy procedures

phlebotomy blood collection; derived from the Greek words *phlebo,* meaning vein, and *tomy,* meaning to cut

plasma liquid part of whole blood

serum liquid part obtained when blood is clotted; lacks the clotting factors

syncope fainting

veins blood vessels that carry blood toward the heart

FUNDAMENTAL CONCEPTS

One of the skills that medical assistants perform routinely is blood collection, or **phlebotomy.** The word *phlebotomy* means cutting into a vein, and *phlebotomist* is the term for the professional who performs phlebotomy. The history of blood collection dates to before the fifth century BC. At that time all medical treatment was based on four body **humors** (fluid or semifluid substances found in the body): blood, phlegm, yellow bile, and black bile. To reestablish health, techniques such as purging, starving, vomiting, and bloodletting were used. By the Middle Ages, barbers, along with surgeons, practiced the art of bloodletting. The red stripe on the barber's pole represented blood, the white stripe stood for the tourniquet, and the pole symbolized the stick squeezed by the patient to dilate the vein. Bloodletting flourished into the eighteenth and early nineteenth centuries. In 1799 George Washington died after 9 pints of blood were taken in a 24-hour period in an attempt to cure his throat infection.

Today phlebotomy is primarily performed by trained professionals. Before studying the procedures involved with blood collection, the function and structures of blood vessels must be understood.

Function and Structures of Blood Vessels

Blood vessels are part of the cardiovascular system. They make up a *closed circuit system* (Fig. 4-1) in which blood is carried from the heart to the blood vessels and back again. In general, all blood vessels except for capillaries have three layers (Fig. 4-2). These layers surround the area through which the blood flows and are called the *outer (tunica adventitia), middle (tunica media),* and *inner layers (tunica intima).*

Types of Blood Vessels

Blood vessels are classified as arteries, arterioles, capillaries, venules, and veins. **Arteries** have three layers, and their function is to carry blood away from the heart. Each artery has a thick middle muscle layer that allows the vessel to expand and contract as blood pressure rises and falls. Arteries have a pulse and are located deeper than veins. They branch into arterioles, which are smaller blood vessels. Arterioles also have three layers, but the layers are thinner than those in arteries. Arterioles then branch into capillaries. **Capillaries** are microscopic blood vessels composed of one layer of simple squamous epithelial cells. Substances are exchanged between blood and the surrounding tissue in the capillaries. Capillary blood is a mixture of arterial and venous blood. Capillaries join venules, which are composed of three thin layers, and the venules join together to form veins. **Veins** carry blood toward the heart and contain valves that prevent backflow of blood. Veins have three layers but thinner walls and less muscle than arteries.

A difference in the feel of veins and arteries can be detected when **palpating** (gently touching and pressing down on an area to feel texture, size, and consistency). Veins feel spongy, and arteries feel more elastic and have a pulse. Veins are the vessels most often used in blood collection because they are closer to the surface than arteries *and* are safer and easier to access.

Most blood tests are performed on venous or capillary blood. The differences in the blood composition of these vessels should be understood.

Comparison of Blood Substances

The composition of capillary blood is different from that of venous blood. Some of the differences are listed in Table 4-1. Capillary blood has higher amounts of hemoglobin and glucose than venous blood, whereas venous blood has higher amounts of potassium, calcium, and total protein.

Because capillary and venous blood specimens may yield different test results, performance of a capillary technique must always be reported. In addition, if an analyte from Table 4-1 needs to be retested, the same blood collection technique must be used (i.e., venipuncture versus capillary). This is especially significant when comparing glucose results during a glucose tolerance test that requires multiple glucose tests during a 2- to 3-hour time frame.

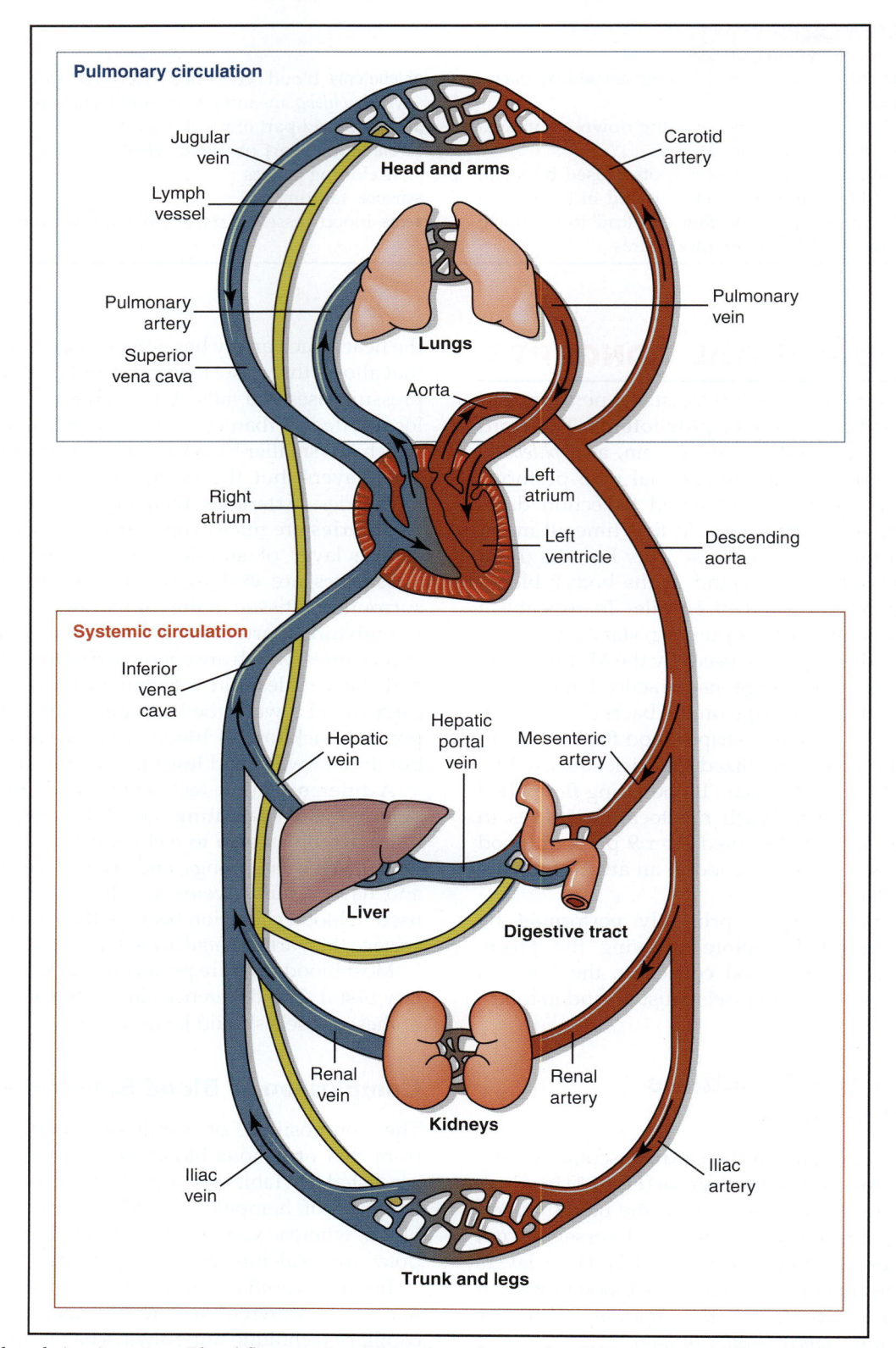

Fig. 4-1. Closed circuit system. Blood flows to the right atrium, then to the right ventricle, pulmonary artery, lungs, pulmonary veins, left atrium, left ventricle, aorta, arteries, arterioles, venules, veins, vena cava, and heart.
(From Warekois R, Robinson R: *Phlebotomy: worktext and procedures manual*, ed 2, St Louis, 2007, Saunders.)

Fundamental Concepts

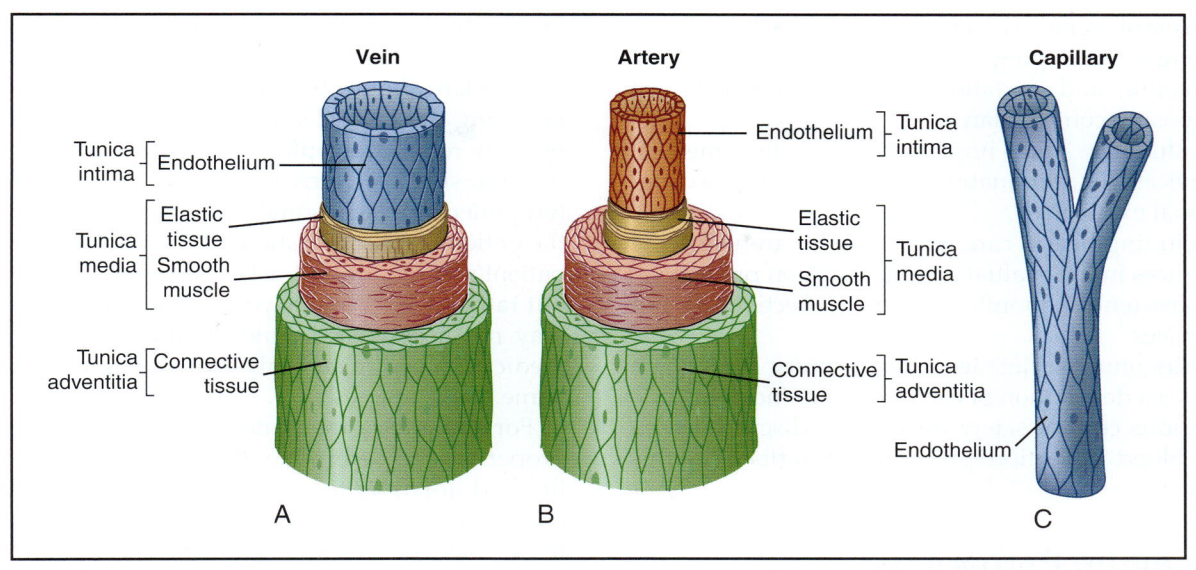

Fig. 4-2. Layers of the vein (**A**), artery (**B**), and capillary (**C**). (From Warekois R, Robinson R: *Phlebotomy: worktext and procedures manual*, ed 2, St Louis, 2007, Saunders.)

TABLE 4-1 Comparison of Capillary and Venous Blood Analyte Values

Capillary Blood	Venous Blood
Hemoglobin: higher	Potassium: higher
Glucose: higher	Total protein: higher
	Calcium: higher

Most Commonly Used Veins

The veins most commonly used when performing venipuncture are found in the **antecubital space** of the arm, the area in front of the elbow (Fig. 4-3). These veins are the median cubital vein, the cephalic vein, and the basilic vein. The median cubital is large and the most commonly used vein. It is located in the middle of the arm and is well anchored. The second choice is the cephalic vein, on the thumb side of the arm. This vein is not well anchored and may move, but in an obese person it may be the only vein that can be found. The basilic vein is the least well anchored and is the last choice of the three. It is located on the little-finger side near the brachial artery. Its position increases the risk of puncturing the artery if the needle is inserted too deeply.

Federal Law Concerning Safety Equipment

According to the Centers for Disease Control and Prevention, health care workers receive approximately 600,000 percutaneous injuries annually from contaminated sharps. Because of concern over this issue and the development of technologies for protection, the Needle Stick Safety and Prevention Act was passed by Congress, which directed the Occupational Safety and Health Administration (OSHA) to revise the Bloodborne Pathogens Standard to require employers to identify and use safer medical devices. Federal Bill HR 5178 was signed by President Bill Clinton on November 6, 2000, with an April 18, 2001, compliance date.

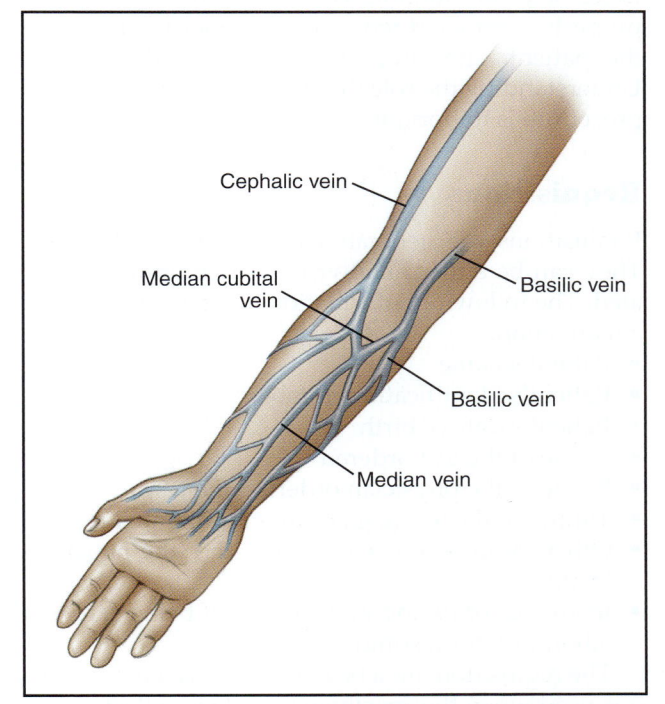

Fig. 4-3. The veins of the forearm. (From Hunt SA: *Saunders medical assisting*, St Louis, 2002, Saunders.)

An employer is in compliance with this law by performing the following actions:
- Creating and updating a bloodborne pathogen exposure control plan
- Evaluating and implementing safer medical devices for eliminating or minimizing occupational exposures
- Including health care workers who are using the devices in the evaluation and selection process
- Consistently monitoring the effectiveness of devices
- Maintaining a detailed sharps injury log, which gives a description of each exposure incident

Various current safety devices are discussed with each blood collection procedure described in this chapter.

Procedure Preparation

All blood-collecting procedures have the same preparation steps in common. These steps include having a properly completed requisition, properly identifying the patient, and properly positioning the patient. Understanding the role these steps play in the overall procedure is important.

Requisitions

Requisitions are generated by a physician's order. They can be either handwritten or computer generated. The following information must be included on a requisition:
- Patient's name
- Patient's identification number
- Patient's date of birth
- Name of the test ordered
- Name of the physician ordering the test
- Timing of the test (e.g., routine, stat, timed test)
- Other information, such as whether the patient is fasting
- Insurance or billing information (if being sent to a laboratory for testing)

The requisition must be filled out correctly because it is used when the specimen sample is collected and correctly identifies the patient.

Proper Identification of the Patient

The patient should always be greeted in a professional manner, and the medical assistant should introduce himself or herself to the patient. A brief explanation of the procedure being performed should be given. If the patient has any questions concerning the tests that have been ordered, the response should be that the patient will need to ask the physician.

One of the most important steps in any phlebotomy procedure is to identify the patient correctly. The most critical error is the misidentification of a patient. To protect against this error, a three-way identification system should be used. This system consists of matching the patient's name and date of birth with the test requisition, plus one more type of identification, such as a driver's license or chart number (outpatient) or a hospital identification number on the patient's wrist (inpatient). When determining the patient's name, do not ask, "Are you Mrs. Smith?" but rather ask, "What is your name?" Often patients may not hear what is said, or they may be taking medication and mistakenly answer yes to the wrong name.

For some tests the patient has to be fasting. The proper way to determine this is to ask if the patient has had anything to eat or drink for 12 to 14 hours before the phlebotomy procedure. Do not ask patients if they have fasted. Some patients do not understand this concept and may answer yes even if they have had coffee, chewed gum, or done other things that could affect the testing.

A patient has the right to refuse a blood collection procedure, in which case the physician should be notified.

Proper Patient Positioning

The patient must be properly positioned for a phlebotomy procedure. A reclining position is preferred. However, having the patient sit in a chair with an armrest (Fig. 4-4) is also appropriate. This position can help protect the patient from falling forward if he or she faints. Never have the patient sit on a stool or stand. In these positions the patient could be injured if fainting occurs.

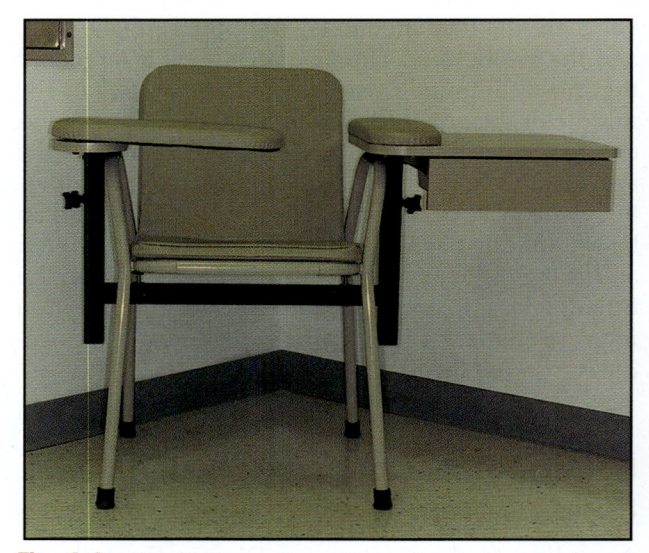

Fig. 4-4. Phlebotomy chair. (From Stepp CA, Woods MA: *Laboratory procedures for medical office personnel*, Philadelphia, 1998, Saunders.)

BLOOD COLLECTION PROCEDURES

Capillary Puncture

Although the venipuncture method is the most common blood collection method used, at times a capillary puncture is the procedure of choice. The phlebotomist typically determines if this method should be used.

Capillary puncture, also called *skin puncture* or "stick," is a method of collecting blood by puncturing the skin through the epidermis into the dermal layer. The composition of blood from a skin puncture is not the same as that of venous blood. Because capillaries are a bridge between arteries and veins, a skin puncture draws blood from arterioles, venules, and capillaries as well as **interstitial fluid** (all the fluid except blood found in the space between tissues, also called *tissue fluid*). Blood from skin punctures is more like arterial blood than venous blood because arterial pressure is greater in the capillaries than is venous pressure. Because of this difference in composition, the requisition must state that a capillary puncture procedure was performed.

The capillary puncture method is useful in the following situations:
- When only a small amount of blood is needed
- When the patient has burns, skin irritation, or small or fragile veins
- With cancer, geriatric, or obese patients, whose blood can be difficult to draw
- With children, because of the risks of venipuncture (e.g., anemia)
- When minimal blood volume reduction is desirable (a 10-mL sample of blood is 5% to 10% of the total blood volume in a neonate's body)

The capillary puncture procedure is being performed more often because of the increase in CLIA-waived testing in physicians' office laboratories, which do not require very much blood.

The capillary puncture method should *not* be used in the following circumstances:
- If the test requires a large amount of blood
- If the patient has poor peripheral circulation
- If interstitial fluid could dilute the test, causing inaccurate results

Coagulation studies (except CLIA-waived protime), blood cultures, and erythrocyte sedimentation rate testing cannot be analyzed by the capillary puncture procedure. Blood cultures and erythrocyte sedimentation rate require more blood than can be obtained by this technique. In the capillary puncture method, tissue fluid is released into the specimen. This fluid contains a clot-activating substance called *thromboplastin* that can interfere with coagulation tests. (The clotting process and coagulation studies are discussed more thoroughly in Chapter 5.)

Equipment Used in Capillary Puncture

Capillary Puncture Devices

Many types of capillary puncture devices are available. The safest and most current are *retractable nonreusable lancets* (Fig. 4-5) that are made with locks that prevent reuse. These retractable devices are colored coded by their manufacturers according to the depth of the puncture. Punctures performed on neonates and infants are performed with the lancet color coded for infants. The National Committee for Clinical Laboratory Standards (now CLSI) made a change in the standard that applies to the depth of a heel stick of an infant. The depth should not exceed 2 mm to prevent infection caused by puncturing a bone. For adults the average skin puncture depth should be 2 to 3 mm.

Automatic capillary puncture devices are used in home monitoring tests, but these usually do not result in a puncture sufficiently deep to collect the necessary amount of blood for point of care testing. Laser devices are also now available. They are used for glucose, hematocrit, and cholesterol screening. The laser concentrates on a small portion of the skin, makes a small hole 1 to 2 mm deep, and draws approximately 100 µL of blood. All capillary puncture devices must be discarded in a biohazard sharps container.

Point-of-Care Testing Collection Devices

Point-of-care testing (POCT) refers to testing that has expanded beyond the laboratory to include the hospital bedside, the home, the nursing home, and any other direct-contact patient setting. Examples of POCT capillary blood collection supplies in Fig. 4-6 consist of the following:
- Capillary tubes for four different test methods (see Fig. 4-6, *A*)
- Critoseal (Sherwood Medical) plastic sealant for capillary tubes (see Fig. 4-6, *B*)
- Microtainers with color-coded lids (see Fig. 4-6, *C*)

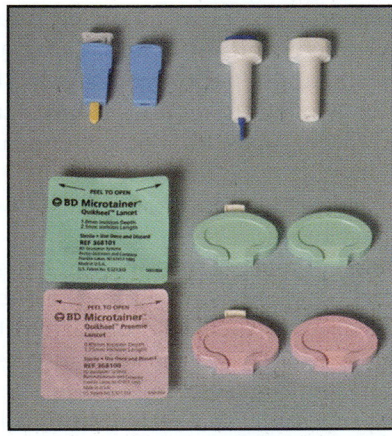

Fig. 4-5. Adult and pediatric safety lancets before and after use.

92 CHAPTER 4   Blood Collection

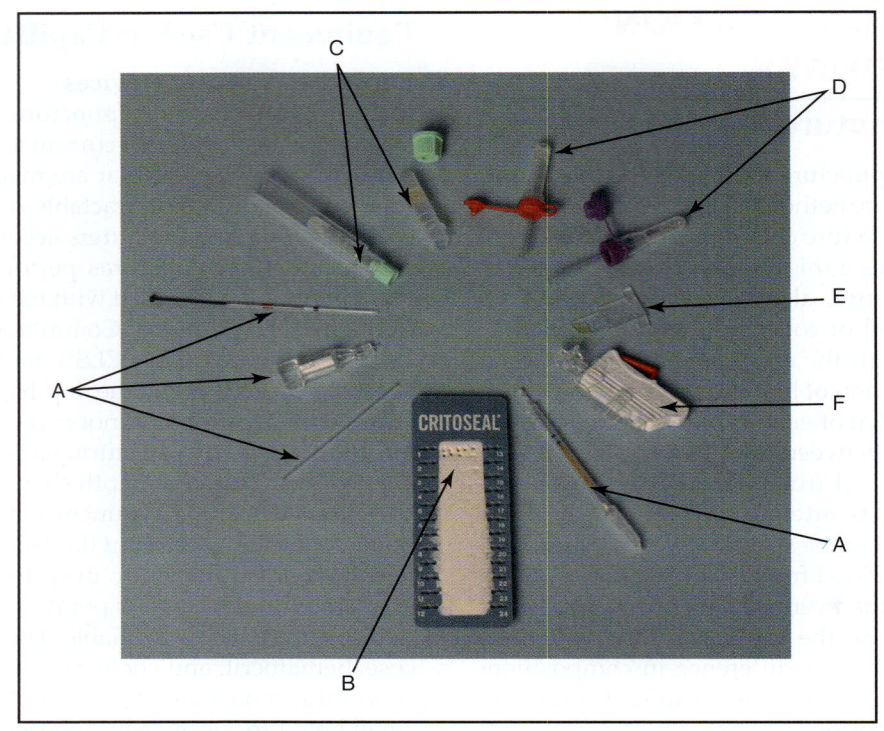

Fig. 4-6. Point-of-care testing equipment. **A,** Capillary collecting tubes; **B,** sealant for capillary tubes; **C,** Microtainers with color-coded lids; **D,** Microtainers with capillary tubes; **E,** cuvette; **f,** collection cup and lancet for protime testing.

- Microtainers with capillary tubes to aid in filling (see Fig. 4-6, *D*)
- Cuvette for collecting the blood specimen and placing it in the analyzer (see Fig. 4-6, *E*)
- Collection cup on the end of a lancet for protime testing (see Fig. 4-6, *F*)

Capillary Tubes

Capillary tubes are one type of device used to collect blood from a skin puncture site (see Fig. 4-6, *A*). These tubes can be glass or plastic, but the plastic tubes or plastic-covered glass tubes are recommended for safety reasons. Blood moves freely into the capillary tubes during **microcollection** (collecting a small amount of blood). The blood is pulled into the tube by a process called **capillary action.** Red-marked capillary tubes contain heparin, which keeps the blood from clotting. Mixing these tubes is important. Blue-marked capillary tubes do not contain anticoagulants, allowing the blood to clot naturally.

The following guidelines should be followed when using capillary tubes:
- Air bubbles in a capillary tube can cause erroneous results. The best way to prevent bubbles is to hold the capillary tube horizontally to the puncture site. Fig. 4-7 shows the tube incorrectly held downward, which results in bubbles.
- Capillary tubes may be sealed so that the specimen is less likely to be lost. Sealants may be clay, as seen in Fig. 4-6, *B,* and in the on-line video, or the

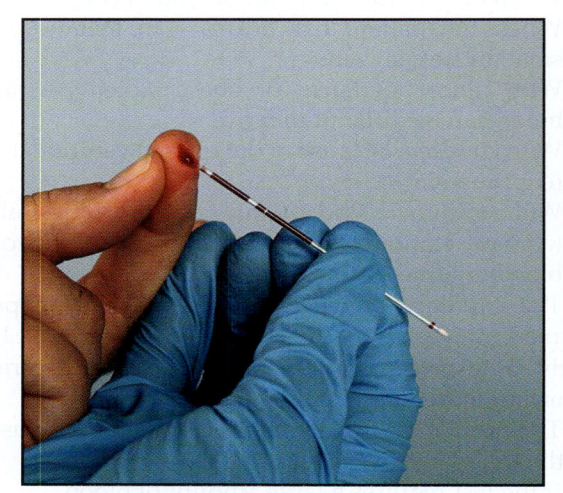

Fig. 4-7. The capillary tube is *improperly* held downward, resulting in air bubbles. (Courtesy Zack Bent.)

specimen may be contained in a self-sealing tube, as seen in Fig. 4-8.
- Capillary tubes are sometimes difficult to label. The recommended procedure is to place the sealed capillary tube into an unfilled vacuum tube and then label the vacuum tube. Tip: If the sealed capillary specimen is to be tested on-site, a sticky note with the patient's identification, technician's initials, and date may be used to hold the specimen against the sticky portion while transporting the specimen from the collection area to the testing

area. Another method is to thread the sealed capillary tube through two slits in a paper with the patient information written on it.

Microcollection Tubes

Microcollection tubes hold more blood than capillary tubes. Some tubes have a lip that allows the drop of blood to flow into the tube (see Fig. 4-6, *C*). The lids on these tubes are coded with various colors corresponding to the anticoagulant present (or absent) in the container. Collect the specimen into the Microtainer Tube by allowing the blood to run down the collection lip while holding at a 30- to 45-degree angle. Do not scrape the tube across the blood specimen. Another type of collection tube consists of a plastic capillary tube inserted into a microtube receptacle (see Fig. 4-6, *D*). Blood flows into the container because of the same capillary action that takes place within the capillary tube.

Order of Draw for Capillary Puncture

Because of the different types of anticoagulants in microcollection tubes, NCCLS (now CLSI) has recommended a specific order of draw for capillary punctures to prevent the transfer of substances from one tube to another and to allow for the clotting that takes place while collecting capillary specimens. According to NCCLS Standard H4-A3, "Procedures for the Collection of Diagnostic Blood Specimens by Skin Puncture," the order of draw for capillary skin puncture is as follows:

1. Lavender tubes containing ethylenediaminetetraacetic acid (EDTA), used for hematology tests, are filled first to keep any microclots from forming.
2. Other tubes with anticoagulation additives—green-topped tubes with the anticoagulant heparin—are next, followed by two blue (labeled 1 and 2) and then gray.
3. Nonadditive tubes (red-topped tubes that contain no anticoagulants, clot accelerators, or gels) are filled last because the capillary blood will clot in these tubes.

Blood normally clots in 2 to 6 minutes. Nonadditive tubes are filled last because clotting occurs in these tubes anyway (Table 4-2).

Appropriate Site Selection

The best site for capillary punctures is fleshy and vascular. A vascular site consists of a large capillary area without scars or calluses. Fleshiness helps protect against puncturing the bone. A bone puncture could lead to **osteomyelitis,** inflammation of the bone caused by bacterial infection. Sites that are swollen or callused should be avoided for skin puncture.

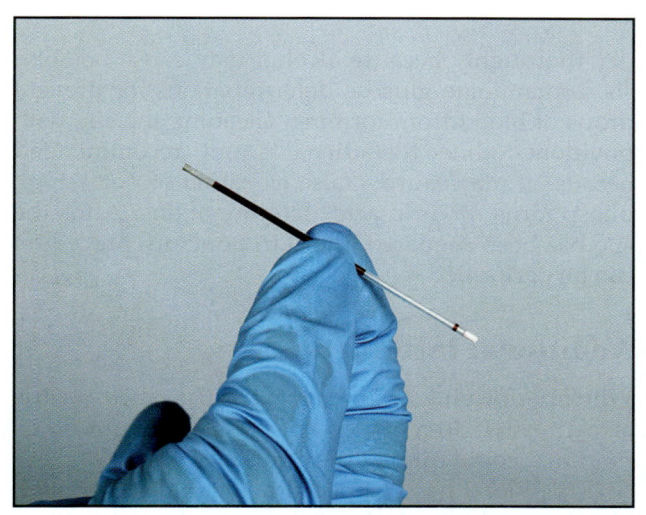

Fig. 4-8. Self-sealing capillary tube will seal itself when the specimen flows down the tube and connects with the clay at the end. NOTE: It then must be held vertical for 15 seconds so that sealing can take place. (Courtesy Zack Bent.)

TABLE 4-2 Order of Draw when Collecting More than One Microtainer by Capillary Puncture

Order	Microtainer Color	Rationale
First	Lavender	EDTA specimen is drawn first to ensure adequate volume and accurate hematology test results (e.g., CBC). Microclots will interfere with the blood cell counts and blood smears.
Second	Green, blue (two), gray	These "whole blood" tubes also contain anticoagulants that produce blood that is not clotted. The blue top needs two tubes to prevent any anticoagulant from the lavender or green tubes from entering the second blue tube, which will be used for coagulation studies.
Last	Gold (two), red	These tubes, which yield serum from a clotted specimen, are collected last. The two gold tubes that contain a gel are needed to ensure that sufficient blood is collected to run the blood chemistry tests.

EDTA, Ethylenediaminetetraacetic acid; *CBC,* complete blood count.

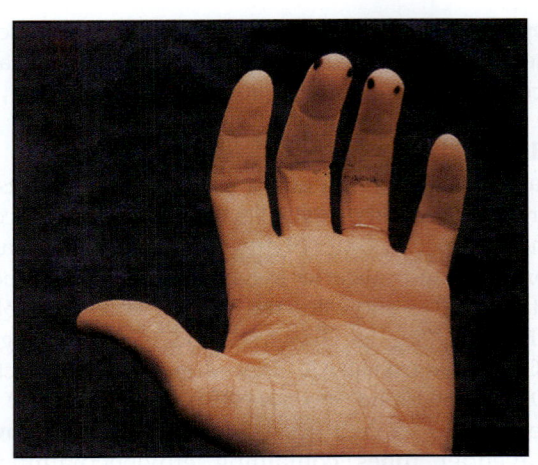

Fig. 4-9. Appropriate capillary puncture sites on the fingers. (From Young AP, Kennedy DB: *Kinn's the medical assistant: an applied learning approach,* ed 10, St Louis, 2007, Saunders.)

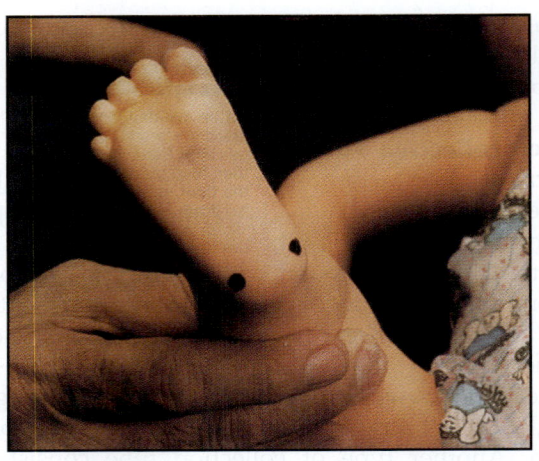

Fig. 4-10. Appropriate capillary puncture site for infant. (From Young AP, Kennedy DB: *Kinn's the medical assistant: an applied learning approach,* ed 10, St Louis, 2007, Saunders.)

Cyanotic sites, where the skin and mucous membrane are blue because of oxygen deficiency, should be warmed before use. A cyanotic site will not produce a good blood sample if it is not warmed up or massaged.

In adults and children, the appropriate skin puncture site is the middle or ring finger (Fig. 4-9). The pinkie finger should not be used because it is thinner and not very fleshy. The index finger and thumb are also not recommended. The index finger could be more sensitive or callused, making it difficult to obtain blood, and the thumb has a pulse. With the middle or ring finger, the puncture should be made on the lateral part of the fingertip (slightly to the side of the center) and perpendicular to the whorls of the fingerprint. A puncture performed parallel to the fingerprint whorls will cause the blood to travel down the troughs of the fingerprint, preventing the blood from forming a drop.

The appropriate skin puncture site for newborns and infants who are not yet walking is the medial or lateral plantar surface of the heel of the foot (Fig. 4-10). The puncture depth should not be more than 2 mm to prevent puncturing the child's bone or connective tissue.

Site Preparation

Blood flow can be increased seven times by warming the site. This can be accomplished by massaging the area five or six times or by applying a warmed towel, preemie diaper, or commercially available device to the site for 3 to 5 minutes. The temperature of the warmed device should not be higher than 42° C. Microwave heating is not advisable because heating may be uneven.

The site should be cleaned with 70% aqueous solution of isopropyl alcohol. Allow the cleaned site to dry thoroughly because alcohol may cause hemolysis, contaminate glucose determinations, or prevent drops of blood from forming. Cleaning the site with povidone-iodine (Betadine) is not recommended because it may cause a false elevation of potassium, phosphorus, or uric acid determinations. After the site has been prepared, the skin puncture procedure can be performed.

Additional Information

When performing a capillary puncture, always wipe away the first drop of blood because it contains tissue fluid that could dilute the sample.

If the blood has stopped flowing and not enough blood was obtained, the entire procedure should be repeated at a new site with a new sterile puncture device. Never stick the same puncture site more than once.

Bandages are not recommended for small children because they can irritate the skin and cause choking if swallowed. If an adhesive bandage must be used to control bleeding, inform the parent that it should be removed as soon as the bleeding has stopped. Adhesive strips should not be used on infants because their skin is very delicate and could macerate under this type of bandage or be damaged when it is removed. (See the video demonstration on-line and refer to Procedure 4-1 at the end of this section.)

Neonatal Screening

Neonatal screening for *phenylketonuria* (PKU) and *hypothyroidism* is mandated in the United States for all newborns. These are conditions in which the newborn lacks the enzymes needed for certain metabolic reactions. If these conditions are not discovered and treated early, abnormalities as severe as mental retardation could develop. Some states require screening for other conditions as well, such as galactosemia, sickle-cell anemia, cystic fibrosis, and human immunodeficiency virus (HIV). More about these requirements can be found at www.mchb.hrsa.gov, the website of the Maternal and Child Health Bureau of the Health Resources and Services Administration, and www.aap.org, the website of the American Academy of Pediatrics.

The PKU/newborn screening blood collection must be performed between 24 hours and 72 hours after birth. If screening is done before the child is 24 hours old, it must be repeated before the child is 14 days old, because many newborns have not yet had enough feedings to determine if a metabolic condition is present. The collection of blood for these tests is generally performed in the hospital, but sometimes the test samples are required in the outpatient setting. Be sure to read and follow the instructions for collecting these specimens properly and note the following guidelines.

- After warming the heel, a capillary puncture (no deeper than 2 mm) is done on the medial or lateral plantar surface of the heel of the foot.
- Wipe away the first drop of blood, then collect the blood in the appropriate microcontainer or on the screening card.
- Apply a drop of blood to each circle on the screening filter paper form, making sure to apply the blood to only one side of the paper (Figs. 4-11 and 4-12).
- All circles must be filled and completely saturated, but do not add a second drop to the same circle.
- Do not massage the foot of an infant with excessive force because this can cause bruising.
- Allow the screening forms to dry in a horizontal position for a minimum of 3 minutes.
- Do not stack wet forms.
- Mail the forms to the testing center (the state health department) in the provided envelopes within 24 hours of collection.

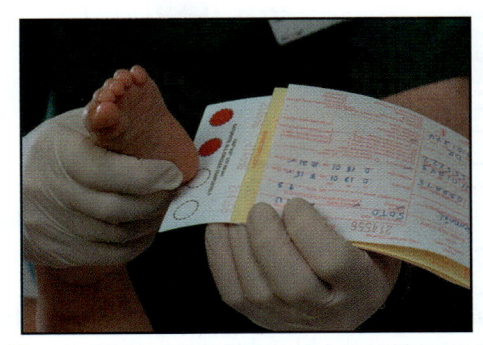

Fig. 4-11. Technique for placing a drop of blood from an infant's foot on the neonatal screening filter form. (From Sommer S, Warekois R: *Phlebotomy workbook and procedures manual*, Philadelphia, 2002, Saunders.)

Becoming Proficient at Capillary Puncture

Now that you have learned about the equipment, appropriate sites, site preparation, and the procedure for capillary punctures and neonatal screenings, you will want to reinforce your knowledge by doing the following:

1. Answer the capillary puncture questions in Chapter 4 of the workbook using your structured notes and text.
2. View the videos on-line to see demonstrations of the finger stick and the heel stick.
3. Perform the online Chapter 4 exercises designed to reinforce your knowledge of terminology and capillary puncture.
4. Study *Procedure 4-1: Capillary Puncture Procedure* at the end of this section.
5. Also study *Procedure 4-2: Neonatal Screening Procedure* before your lab.

Venipuncture

Another method of collecting blood samples is venipuncture, which involves extracting blood from a vein. Venipuncture can be accomplished in three ways: by the evacuated tube (or vacuum tube) method, the syringe method, and the butterfly method.

Equipment Used in Venipuncture

Vacuum Collection Tubes

The collection containers for venipuncture are called *vacuum tubes* (Fig. 4-13). These tubes are **evacuated** (the air has been removed to create a vacuum) so that a preset amount of blood will be collected. They are available in different sizes, ranging from 2 to 15 mL (5, 7, and 15 mL for adults and 2, 3, and 4 mL for children). The tubes are available in glass or plastic, but OSHA recommends that plastic tubes be used for safety reasons. The manufacturer's label on each tube indicates the type of anticoagulant or additive that is present, the expiration date of the tube, and the amount of blood it will hold. Hemoguard (Becton Dickinson, Franklin Lakes, NJ) plastic-covered tubes are designed with a special rubber stopper surrounded by a plastic closure that hangs over the outside of the tube and reduces the risk of blood splattering when the stopper is removed.

The expiration date should always be checked and the tubes examined for cracks and other damage before use. If air should get into the tube, the tube would be rendered useless because no blood would flow into it.

Each tube has a colored stopper and label that indicate whether anticoagulants or additives are present

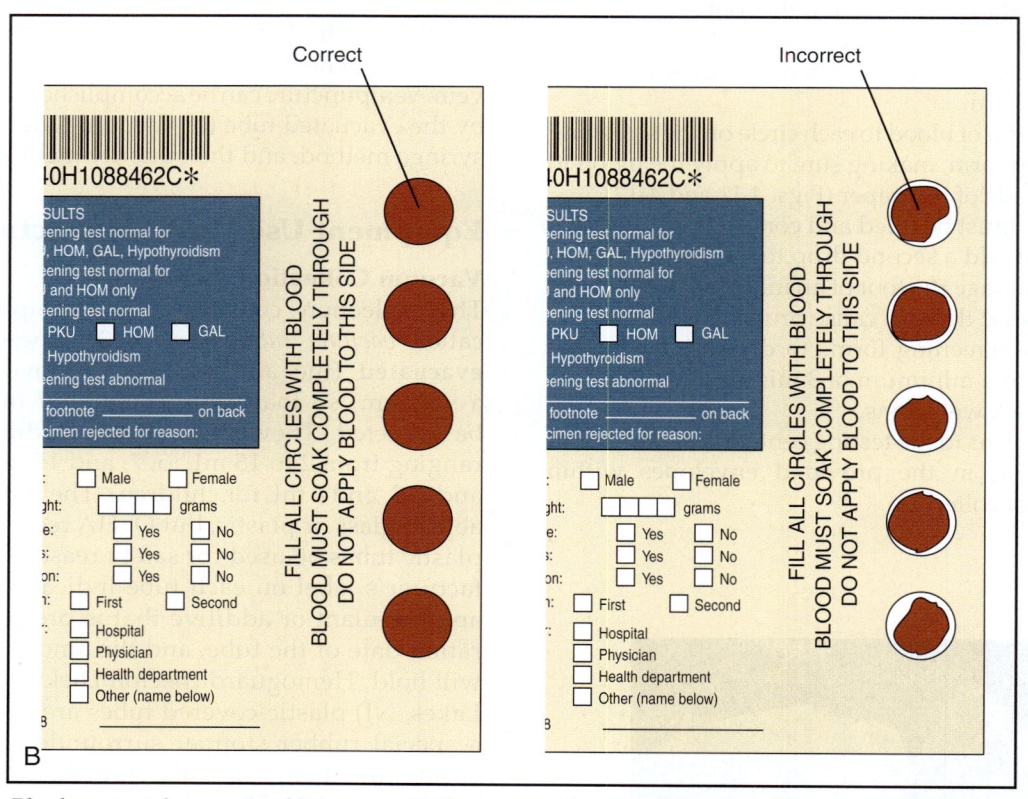

Fig. 4-12. **A,** Blank neonatal screening filter paper. **B,** Correct and incorrect completed screening forms. (Modified from Warekois R, Robinson R: *Phlebotomy: worktext and procedures manual,* ed 2, St Louis, 2007, Saunders; and Bonewit-West K: *Clinical procedures for medical assistants,* ed 7, St Louis, 2008, Saunders.)

and, if so, what type. When blood is extracted from the body and nothing is added to the specimen, the cells automatically clot, yielding a liquid called **serum** and clotted cells. When blood is prevented from clotting, the cells are suspended in liquid that is referred to as **plasma.** Anticoagulants are added to the collection tubes to prevent the blood from clotting.

Fig. 4-14, *A,* shows a blood specimen collected in the left gold-topped tube that allows the blood to clot. The recommended time to allow blood to clot is

Blood Collection Procedures

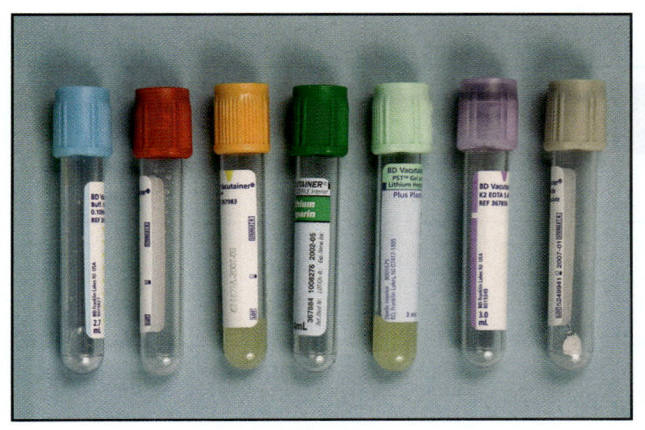

Fig. 4-13. Vacutainer Hemoguard tubes in the proper order of draw. (Courtesy Zack Bent.)

30 to 45 minutes, no longer than 1 hour, in an upright position at room temperature. NOTE: Tubes may also contain additives that accelerate clotting, such as silicone and glass beads. If the appropriate amount of time is not allowed for clotting, not enough liquid serum will be obtained. Also, fibrin clots could form in the serum if the clotting factors do not have time to settle into the clot. When the blood has clotted, the tube is spun in a centrifuge for 15 to 20 minutes. The clot becomes compressed on the bottom of the tube with the serum on top (see Fig. 4-14, *B*, left tube). The white gel in the tube acts as a barrier between the *serum* and the clot.

Blood collected in an anticoagulant tube, as seen in the right lavender tube in Fig. 4-14, *A*, will not clot and can be used for testing when *whole blood* is needed. When whole blood is centrifuged, the red cells pack into the bottom of the tube. The **buffy coat** is the narrow middle layer of white blood cells and platelets in the centrifuged whole blood specimen, and the liquid layer on top is referred to as *plasma* (see Fig. 4-14, *B*, right tube).

Anticoagulation occurs by using a variety of additives, such as oxalates, citrates, EDTA, and heparin. Oxalates, citrates, and EDTA bind with calcium, which is needed for clotting to occur. Heparin prevents clotting by inactivating thrombin and thromboplastin, the proteins needed in the blood-clotting mechanism.

Both serum and plasma are straw colored and contain essentially the same substances. The main difference between the two is that serum no longer has its clotting factors because they were used to form the clot.

Another common additive is the white gel that forms a barrier between the cells and the liquid (serum or plasma, depending on the tube) to stop further interaction between these layers. The gel has a lower density than the red blood cells or the clot and a higher density than the liquid part. After the

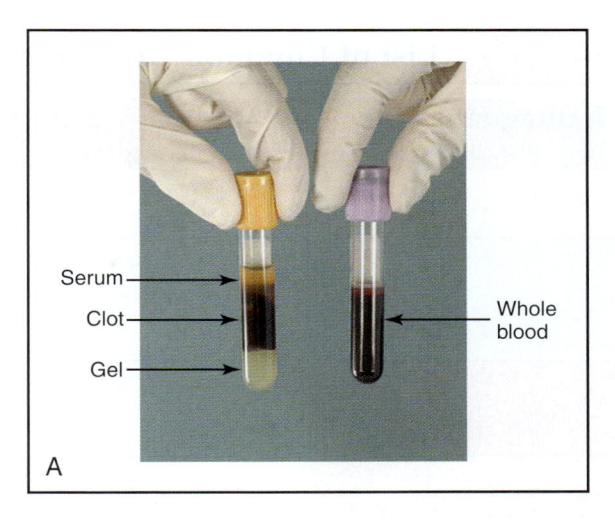

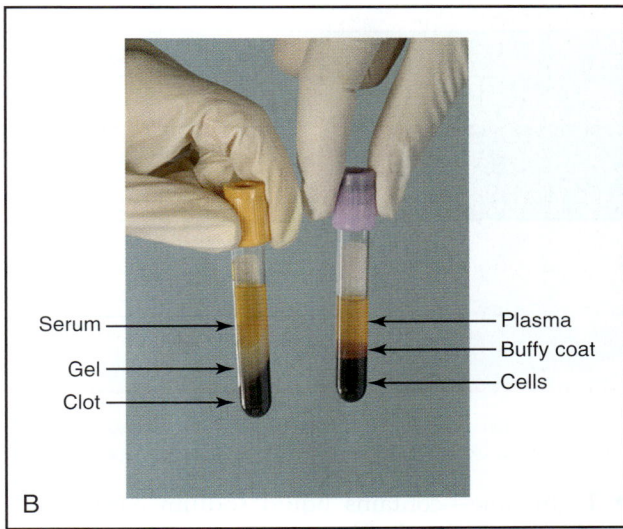

Fig. 4-14. **A,** Gold tube with clotted blood and lavender tube with whole blood before centrifuging. Note the composition of each. **B,** Clotted and whole blood after centrifuging. Note the layers in each tube.

blood is centrifuged, the clot or red blood cells will be on the bottom of the centrifuged tube, the gel in the middle, and the liquid portion on top. When this gel is in a "clot" tube, it is referred to as *SST*, which stands for "serum separator tube." When the gel is in a whole blood tube with anticoagulant it is referred to as *PST*, or plasma separator tube. In both cases the tubes must be centrifuged within 2 hours of the blood draw to prevent the living blood cells from metabolizing the chemicals in the serum or plasma.

Additives and Color-Coded Hemoguard Tubes

The different types of anticoagulants and additives within the vacuum tubes are differentiated by the following color-coded plastic stoppers (Table 4-3):

- Pale yellow—sterile tubes containing preservatives and/or nutrients, used for growing blood cultures

TABLE 4-3 List of Common Tube Stoppers

Hemoguard Color	Additive	Number of Inversions at Blood Collection	Laboratory Use
Yellow	Sodium polyanetholsulfonate (SPS)	8	Blood cultures
Light Blue	Sodium citrate	3-4	Coagulation studies PT APTT Factor assay
Red	None or clot activator	0	Serum chemistries Serology Blood bank
Gold	Thixotropic gel serum separator and clot activator	5	Most chemistry testing Not suitable for blood bank testing
Light Green	Thixotropic gel plasma separator and lithium Heparin	8	Potassium determinations
Green	Sodium heparin, or Lithium heparin, or Ammonium heparin	8 8 8	Plasma chemistries
Lavender	EDTA	8	Whole blood hematology cell count CBC
Gray	Sodium fluoride Potassium oxalate	8 8	Glucose testing (usually) Glucose tolerances

PT, Prothrombin time; *APTT*, activated partial thromboplastin time; *EDTA*, ethylenediaminetetraacetic acid; *CBC*, complete blood count. (Modified from Sommer S, Warekois R: *Phlebotomy workbook and procedures manual*, Philadelphia, 2002, Saunders.)

- Light blue—contains liquid sodium citrate anticoagulant, used for coagulation testing (e.g., prothrombin time)
- Red—contains no anticoagulants, which means the blood will automatically clot (NOTE: *Red plastic tubes contain a clot activator to accelerate the clotting process.*)
- Gold—contains a silicone coating to accelerate clotting and a gel barrier to separate the serum from the cells (SST tube). It contains no anticoagulant. The serum is typically used for blood chemistry tests.
- Green—contains a heparin anticoagulant: sodium heparin, lithium heparin, or ammonium heparin; used for chemistry specimens, especially when a test is stat, because waiting for the blood to clot is not necessary as it is with serum tubes. It is important to note the type of anticoagulant substance that is in a heparin tube (e.g., a sodium heparin tube would not be used if sodium testing and lithium heparin would not be used for a lithium test, because the sodium or lithium heparin would falsely raise the test results). Lithium heparin tubes are often used with the separating gel and are referred to as *PST*.
- Lavender—contains EDTA, which acts as a anticoagulant and preservative for blood cells; used for hematology studies and molecular diagnostic testing. EDTA prevents platelet aggregation and allows preparation of blood smears with minimal distortion of white blood cells
- Gray—contains potassium oxalate/sodium fluoride anticoagulant, which removes calcium to prevent clotting; used for glucose studies because the fluoride inhibits glycolysis (sugar breakdown)

Vacuum Tube Method Using the Vacutainer Collection System

The most commonly performed venipuncture method involves the use of vacuum tubes, which automatically fill with blood during the procedure. This method calls for Vacutainer tubes with Vacutainer holders and needles, as seen in Fig. 4-15.

Equipment Used in the Vacutainer Method

Vacutainer Needle. The *Vacutainer needle* is pointed at both ends (Fig. 4-16). The shorter end punctures the vacuum tube, and the longer end has a bevel that is inserted into the vein. For a smoother and less painful puncture, the bevel end should always be turned

Blood Collection Procedures

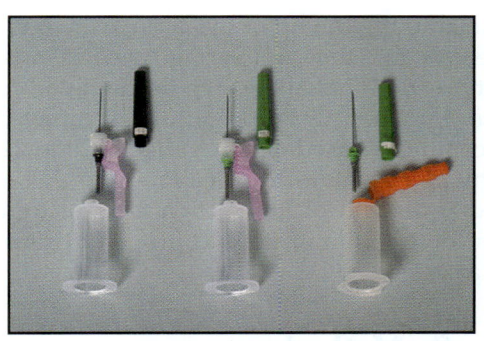

Fig. 4-15. Vacutainer safety needles with pink safety devices *(left, middle)*. Vacutainer holder with orange safety device *(right)*.

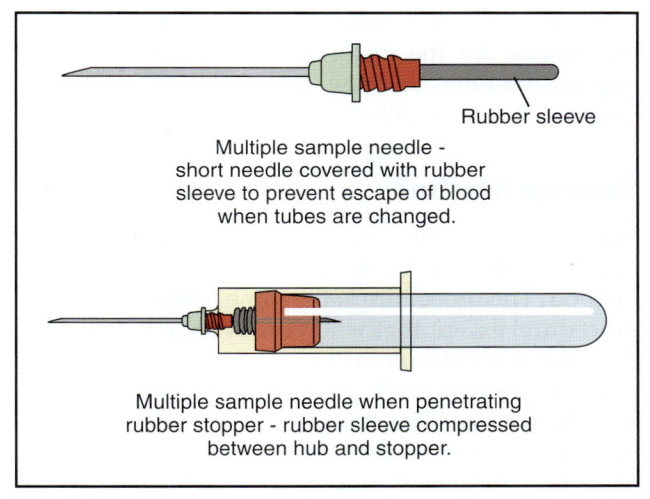

Fig. 4-16. Vacutainer multisample needles with rubber sleeves that allow blood to flow only when the sleeved needle is pushed into the vacuum tube. (From Hunt SA: *Saunders fundamentals of medical assisting*, Philadelphia, 2002, Saunders.)

upward. Safety needles are now required by law. Some types of safety needles are activated by a one-hand thumb mechanism (Fig. 4-17, *A* and *B*); another type is activated by pressing against a hard surface (Fig. 4-17, *C*).

The Vacutainer needle ranges in length from 1 to 1.5 inches. The space inside the needle is referred to as the **lumen** or *bore*. The diameter of the needle is called the *gauge*. The higher the gauge number, the smaller the diameter. The most frequently used gauges are 20 to 22. A high-gauge needle (e.g., 25) could cause hemolysis of the cells because the lumen is too small.

Vacutainer Holder. The *Vacutainer holder* is a plastic sleeve that allows the tube to connect to the needle (Fig. 4-18). The Vacutainer double needle screws into one end of the holder. After the needle has been inserted into a patient's vein, the tube is pushed all the way into the holder. The needle must be in the vein before pushing the vacuum tube all the way into the holder. An indentation is present approximately ½ inch down from where the needle attaches to the holder. Pushing the vacuum tube within this ½-inch space *before* the needle is in the vein will result in the tube being filled with air.

Two types of Vacutainer holders are available: one for adults and one for children. A plastic extension, or flange, is located at the large-opening end of the Vacutainer. The design of the flange prevents the holder from rolling and provides a lip on which to position the fingers as the tube is inserted and removed.

OSHA recommends that Vacutainer needles not be removed from the holder after use but instead be disposed of with the holder attached because the rubber-stoppered needle can expose health care workers to needle sticks.

Tourniquet. A *tourniquet* is used to make the vein more prominent and easier to puncture. The average tourniquet is approximately 1 inch wide and 15 to 18 inches long and should be placed 3 to 4 inches above the venipuncture site. A tourniquet that is too tight is uncomfortable for the patient and can give inaccurate results. It should be tight enough to restrict venous flow but not so tight that it stops arterial flow. It should be looped so that it can be easily released with one hand. Do not place a tourniquet over sores or burned areas on the skin.

The recommended time to leave a tourniquet on is 1 minute. If it is left on too long, results may be inaccurate because of **hemoconcentration,** a condition in which blood concentration of large molecules such as proteins, cells, and coagulation factors increases. The recommended tourniquet procedure is to take the tourniquet off after a vein has been chosen, clean the site, prepare the equipment, and then put the tourniquet back on before making the incision. Tourniquets should be cleaned after use or discarded if they are disposable. See Procedure 4-3 for the proper application of the tourniquet.

Site Preparation

Have the patient place his or her arm in a downward position to prevent reflux (backward flow of blood). For patients who do not want to feel the needle stick (e.g., children), a eutectic mixture of local anesthetics (EMLA) can be used to anesthetize the puncture area. EMLA is a topical cream that is a mixture of lidocaine and prilocaine. It is applied as a cream or patch and requires approximately 60 minutes for optimal anesthesia to occur. It may last as long as 2 or 3 hours. Some of the limitations to its use are cost, the need to wait 60 minutes, and the need to repeat the anesthetizing procedure if the venipuncture is not successful. Another topical anesthesia, IOMED "Numby Stuff" (IOMED, Inc., Salt Lake City, Utah), contains lidocaine HCl 2% with epinephrine. It penetrates to a depth of 10 mm and takes 10 minutes to take effect.

See *Procedure 4-3: Vacutainer Method* at the end of this section for the pictorial sequence and step-by-step instructions on how to perform a successful venipuncture using the Vacutainer method.

Syringe Method

The syringe method is used on fragile veins that might collapse under the pressure of the Vacutainer method. The procedure is the same as the Vacutainer procedure, except that when the syringe needle is in the arm, the phlebotomist pulls *back* on the syringe plunger, creating back pressure and drawing blood into the syringe. The syringe method allows control over the pressure exerted on the vein. This control helps keep the vein from collapsing, which makes the syringe method particularly useful for small, fragile veins.

Equipment Used in the Syringe Method

Syringe. The *syringe* consists of a barrel and a plunger (Fig. 4-19). The barrel is graduated into milliliters in sizes ranging from 2 to 20 mL and larger. The plunger should always be loosened by moving it back and forth several times before use (Fig. 4-20, *A* and *B*). When the plunger is pulled back when the attached needle is in the vein, a back pressure is produced and blood fills the syringe.

Syringe Needle. The *syringe needle* is also called a *hypodermic needle*. Like the Vacutainer needle, it has a shaft and a hub, but the hub attaches directly to the syringe with no opposing sheathed needle. Blood can be seen entering the tip of the syringe as soon as the needle goes into the vein. Syringe needles must have a safety section that allows the needle to be covered or blunted when the procedure is completed. The most commonly used needle gauge is 20 to 22, with a length of 1 to 1.5 inches. See *Procedure 4-4: Syringe Method* at the end of this section for a pictorial and written description of how to properly draw blood using a syringe.

Butterfly Method

The *butterfly method* is used on very small veins, such as those in the hand, and for pediatric draws. Hand veins collapse and bruise more easily because they have thin walls. More nerves are also present in this area, which makes a hand puncture more uncomfortable for the patient. The equipment for this method consists of a uniquely designed needle with a safety sheath and plastic wings (used to grip the needle as it is inserted into the vein), tubing, and devices to attach to either a syringe or a Vacutainer collection system. Fig. 4-21 shows the push-button butterfly needle, tubing, and connecting devices.

In the butterfly method, a crucial safety issue arises when the needle is pulled out of the vein. Two recommended safety methods are described in Procedure 4-5. Laboratory professionals should stay informed of the most current safety devices and how they are activated. It is also wise to practice on a training model before using a new safety device on a patient. (The student workbook contains a form to evaluate various safety devices.)

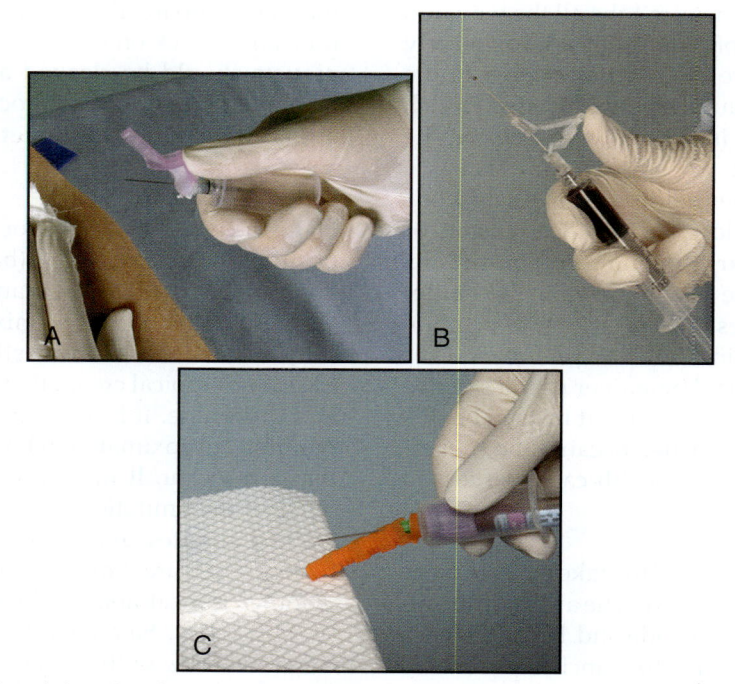

Fig. 4-17. *A*, One-hand thumb safety activation. *B*, One-hand spring device. *C*, One-hand surface activation.

Blood Collection Procedures

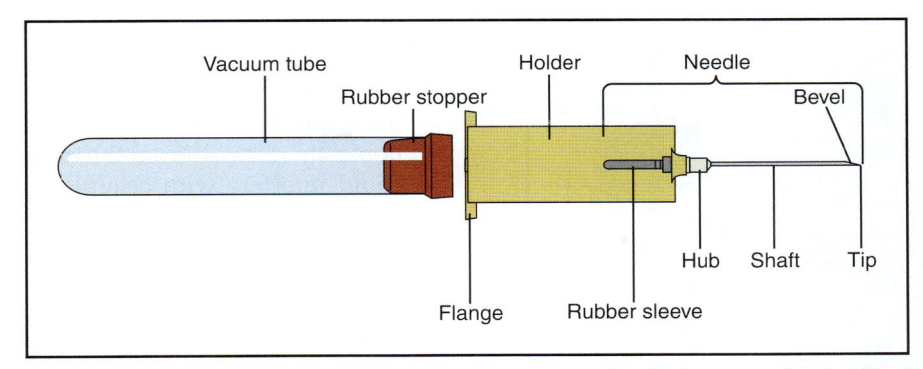

Fig. 4-18. Vacuum tube system. (From Hunt SA: *Saunders fundamentals of medical assisting,* Philadelphia, 2002, Saunders.)

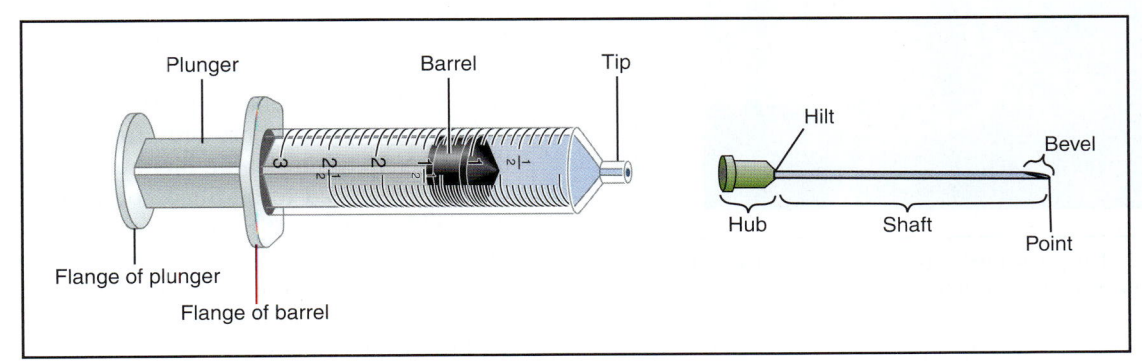

Fig. 4-19. Parts of a syringe and a hypodermic needle. (From Hunt SA: *Saunders fundamentals of medical assisting,* Philadelphia, 2002, Saunders.)

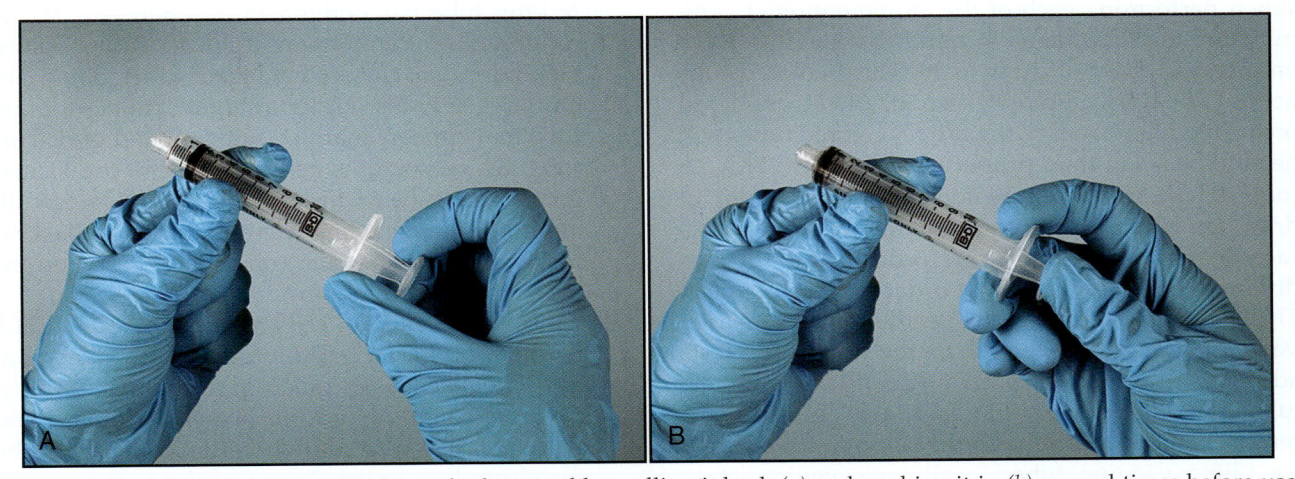

Fig. 4-20. **A,** The plunger should always be loosened by pulling it back *(a)* and pushing it in *(b)* several times before use. **B,** Make sure it is pushed in before connecting the needle. (Courtesy Zack Bent.)

If the Vacutainer method is used, a small adapter device (Luer adapter) is attached to the end of the butterfly tubing that will allow the tubing to attach to a Vacutainer holder. If the syringe method is used, the Luer adapter is removed and the end of the butterfly tubing fits directly onto the tip of the syringe. The syringe method allows more control of the pressure, which is necessary when working with fragile veins.

See *Procedure 4-5: Butterfly Method* to learn the steps for performing the butterfly method using both a Vacutainer method and syringe method. Also, both butterfly safety devices will be presented: the safety lock and the push button.

Fig. 4-22 displays all the supplies used in the three venipuncture procedures: Vacutainer, syringe, and butterfly methods. The vacuum tubes have also been placed in their correct order of draw from left to right.

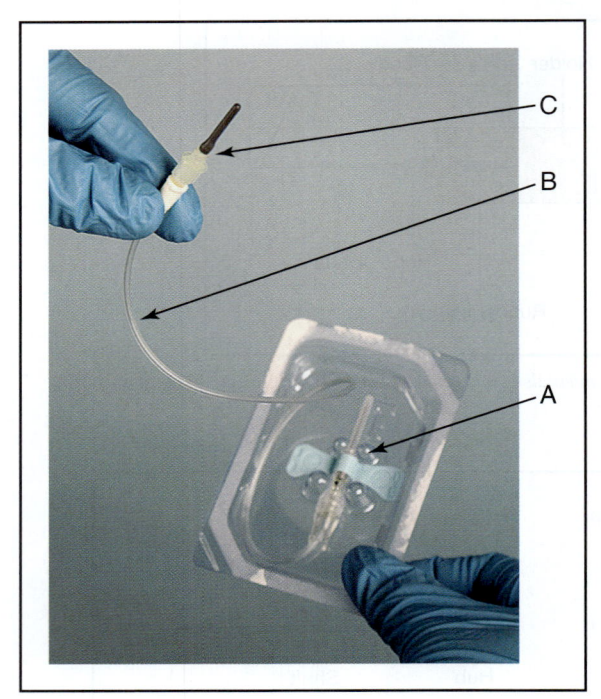

Fig. 4-21. The push-button butterfly needle **(A)**, tubing **(B)**, and connecting devices **(C)**. (Courtesy Zack Bent.)

Order of Draw for Vacutainer, Syringe, and Butterfly Methods

When performing each of the aforementioned venipuncture methods, keep in mind that there is a recommended order of draw as to which colored tube needs to be drawn up first, second, and so on. Based on the requisition order, the proper colored tubes will need to be set in their proper order of draw. NCCLS (now CLSI) has recommended a specific order of draw for venipuncture as it has for capillary puncture. NOTE: The venipuncture order of the tubes is different from the capillary order of microtainers. This is because the sheathed needle that enters each Vacutainer tube is exposed to the additives. Tests adversely affected by *additive contamination* from one tube to another are listed in Table 4-4. The most current guidelines recommend the same order of draw for filling vacuum tubes in all three venipuncture methods. The following reflects the recommendations by NCCLS ("Order of Draw," NCCLS H3-A5, Vol. 23, No. 32, 8.10.2):

- **Yellow** is drawn first. This is for blood cultures, which are always drawn first to maintain sterility. NOTE: When drawing up anaerobic and aerobic tube culture, always draw the aerobic tube first when using the butterfly method because the air from the butterfly tubing will enter the bottle.
- **Light blue** is next because anticoagulants and additives from the other tubes can interfere with coagulation testing. This tube must be completely filled to achieve accurate clotting results. In the past, when a coagulation study (light blue tube) was ordered, a plain red glass tube with no additives was drawn first to take up the tissue thromboplastin released from the traumatized tissue that could interfere with coagulation testing. The red tube was referred to as the "waste tube" because its only purpose was to collect the tissue thromboplastin caused by the venipuncture. However, the new recommendations no longer require this. The new standard does, however, recommend that a plain red waste tube be drawn before a light blue tube if the butterfly method is being used. The tubing in the butterfly system has dead space in the line that could reduce the volume of blood drawn, thereby resulting in an underfilled tube. An alternative, if a plain red tube is not available, would be to use two blue tubes, with the first tube considered a waste tube whose only function is to clear the butterfly tubing of air. Neither the red or blue waste tubes need to be filled completely because they will not be sent to the laboratory. Their only purpose is to pull the blood through the tubing before connecting the blue tube that will then be filled accurately (with no air from the tubing) and sent to the laboratory.
- **Red** "clot tube," with or without clot activators, and **Gold** SST with gel and clot activators are next. These tubes yield a serum/clot specimen. A glass red-top tube has nothing in it, whereas a plastic red-top tube often contains a clot activator because blood does not clot well in plastic tubes. Some laboratories may also order a **"tiger"** rubber-topped tube that appears marbled with red and gray. This tube, which contains gel, is similar to the Hemaguard gold tube and is also considered an SST. In all three cases, it is important to follow the laboratory's designated serum tube choice based on the tests they will be running.
- **Green** (plain and gel PST) are drawn *before* EDTA because the EDTA could interfere with some heparin chemistry tests, such as electrolyte testing. EDTA is usually bound to potassium or sodium. If an EDTA tube is drawn before a heparin tube for electrolyte testing, some of the EDTA anticoagulant could be mixed in with the green tube and cause inaccurate electrolyte results (see Table 4-4).
- **Lavender** (EDTA) is drawn next and is most commonly used for hematology testing.
- **Gray** is drawn last, after the EDTA tube, because the anticoagulant potassium oxalate can affect potassium results and red blood cell morphology. It is commonly used for glucose testing.

Table 4-5 details the correct order of drawing using the most common plastic Vacutainer (Becton Dickinson) tubes, their additives, and uses. A helpful way to remember the proper order is to visualize the

Blood Collection Procedures 103

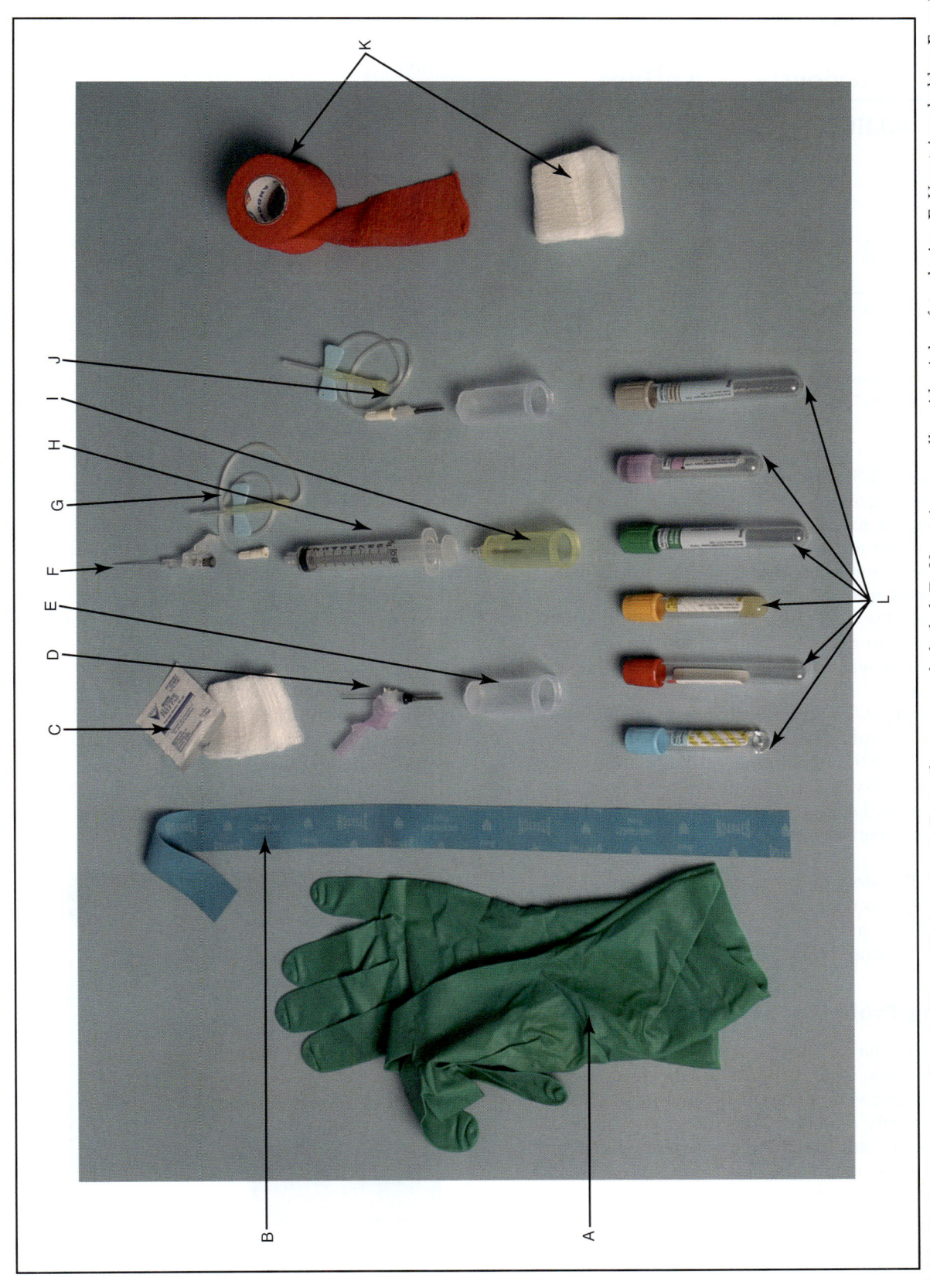

Fig. 4-22. Venipuncture supplies. **A,** Gloves; **B,** tourniquet; **C,** sterile gauze and alcohol; **D,** Vacutainer needle with pink safety device; **E,** Vacutainer holder; **F,** syringe needle with spring safety device; **G,** butterfly needle assembled to connect directly to tip of syringe; **H,** syringe; **I,** safety transfer device for transferring blood from syringe to vacuum tube; **J,** butterfly needle assembled to connect directly to Vacutainer holder; **K,** nonlatex pressure bandage and gauze to control bleeding; **L,** the six most commonly used Hemoguard Vacutainer tubes in the recommended order of draw.

TABLE 4-4 Tests Adversely Affected by Anticoagulant Additive Contamination from a Previously Drawn Tube

	Additive	Tests Adversely Affected
Lavender stopper	EDTA	Calcium, APTT, PT, sodium, potassium, serum iron
Green stopper	Heparin	PT, APTT, ACT
Gray stopper	Potassium oxalate	Potassium, APTT, ACT

EDTA, Ethylenediaminetetraacetic acid; *APTT*, activated partial thromboplastin time; *PT*, prothrombin time; *ACT*, activated clotting time.

picture in Table 4-5. Start at the top of the picture, and work your way down:

- Clouds at the top of the picture are for blood culture tests that must be the drawn first in order to maintain their sterility. (See Chapter 8 for the variety of blood culture tubes available.)
- Blue sky is the next layer. Blue is usually the first plastic tube to draw for coagulation studies. (Do not forget the waste tube if using a butterfly needle and tubing.)
- The *red* and *gold* rays of the sun are on the horizon. These "clot" tubes both must be drawn *after* the blue but *before* the remaining anticoagulant tubes.
- The *green* grassy hill is below the red and gold rays of the sunset. *Light green* is the PST heparin tube, and dark green is typically the lithium heparin tube.
- *Lavender* flowers are at the base of the hill below the green grass near the bottom of the picture.
- *Gray* rocks are at the bottom of the picture because the gray "glucose" tube is the last tube to draw.

Becoming Proficient at Venipuncture

Now that you have learned about the equipment, appropriate sites, site preparation, the four methods of obtaining venous blood (Vacutainer, syringe, and two butterfly methods), and the proper order of draw, you will want to reinforce your knowledge by doing the following:

1. Answer the venipuncture questions at the end of this chapter and in Chapter 4 of the workbook using your structured notes and text.
2. View the videos on-line to see Venipuncture with a Vacuum Tube and Venipuncture with Winged Infusion Set and Syringe.
3. Perform the Chapter 4 exercises on-line to reinforce your terminology and venipuncture skills.
4. Study *Procedure 4-3: Vacutainer Method* before your lab.
5. Study *Procedure 4-4: Syringe Method* before your lab.
6. Study *Procedure 4-5: Butterfly Methods* before your lab.

Preparing Blood Specimens for Laboratory Pickup

The last step in blood collection is the processing of the blood before the laboratory picks up the specimen for testing. Each laboratory has a specific protocol regarding the following:

- Log each collection on the laboratory log sheet, indicating date, time, patient identification, tubes drawn, tests ordered, and the phlebotomist's initials.
- Allow 30 minutes for gold, red, and tiger rubber-topped tubes to clot in a upright position in a test tube rack. They should be centrifuged within 2 hours of collection to separate the liquid from the clotted cells.
- Place the closed tubes in the centrifuge, creating a balanced load. Opposing centrifuge holders must be equally weighted with loaded samples that are the same size and equal in fill (Fig. 4-23).
- Fill a tube with water to match the weight of any unpaired sample, and place it across from the sample.
- The tubes should remain closed with their tops on at all times during the centrifugation process.
- Centrifuge the clotted specimens for 15 to 20 minutes depending on centrifuge speed and laboratory recommendations.
- PSTs should also be centrifuged for 15 to 20 minutes within 2 hours of collection, according to laboratory protocol.

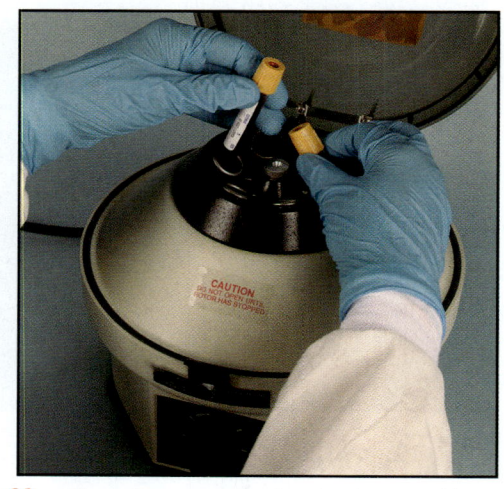

Fig 4-23. Place the capped tubes in the centrifuge, creating a balanced load. Opposing centrifuge holders must be equally weighted with loaded samples that are the same size and equal in fill. (Courtesy Zack Bent.)

Blood Collection Procedures

TABLE 4-5 Vacuum Tube Table

		Additive or Brief Descriptors	Laboratory Uses
Blue sky	(blue)	"Citrate tube"	Coagulation studies such as prothrombin time
Red and gold rays of sun coming from above the grassy hill	(red)	"Clot tube" Clot activator in plastic tubes (NOTE: Red glass tubes do not have clot activator.)	Both yield serum commonly used for testing blood chemistry analytes
	(gold)	"SST tube" Clot activator and gel to separate the serum from the clot	
Green grass of the hill	(light green)	"PST tube" contains heparin plus gel to separate the plasma from the cells	Special tests such as electrolytes and tests that need to be run immediately
	(dark green)	"Heparin tubes" (with lithium, ammonium, or sodium)	
Lavender flowers at the bottom of the hill	(lavender)	"EDTA tube"	Hematology tests such as CBC
Gray rocks under the flowers	(gray)	"Oxalate tube"	Glucose testing

SST, Serum separator tube; *PST*, plasma separator tube; *EDTA*, ethylenediaminetetraacetic acid; *CBC*, complete blood count.

- Store specimens at room temperature or refrigerate, according to laboratory guidelines.
- Place specimens in a biohazard specimen bag with their corresponding requisition placed in the front pocket of the bag.

Centrifuge Safety

- Do not spin uncovered specimen tubes, and always have the centrifuge lid cover closed when the centrifuge is running to prevent the vaporization of hazardous droplets.
- If an abnormal noise, vibration, or sound is noted while the centrifuge is in operation, immediately stop the unit by turning off the switch, and check for a possible load imbalance.
- Centrifuges must never be slowed down or stopped by grasping any part of the device with your hand or applying another object against the rotating equipment.
- Broken tubes or liquid spills must be cleaned according to OSHA standards. Clean the centrifuge daily with a disinfectant and paper towel.

Watch the online video: Preparing a Serum Specimen Using a Serum Separator Tube.

PROCEDURE 4-1 Capillary Puncture Procedure

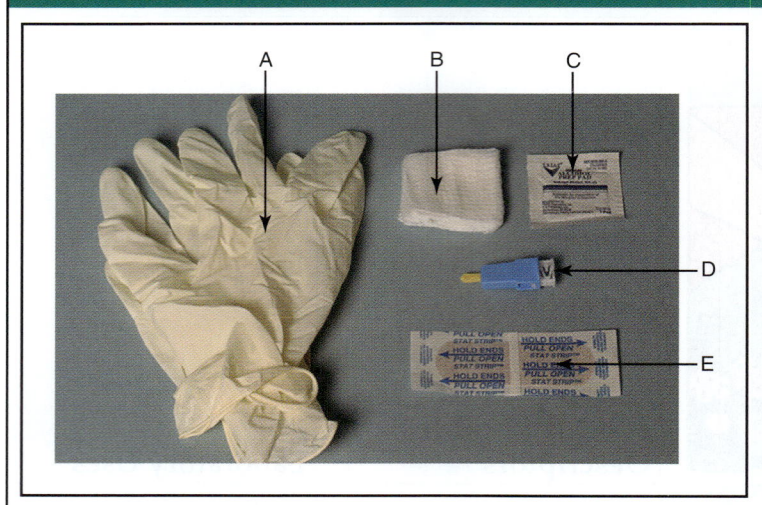

A. Capillary puncture setup. *a*, Sterile gloves; *b*, sterile gauze; *c*, 70% isopropyl alcohol pads in sterile packages; *d*, sterile, disposable, retractable, nonreusable lancet; *e*, latex-free bandage.

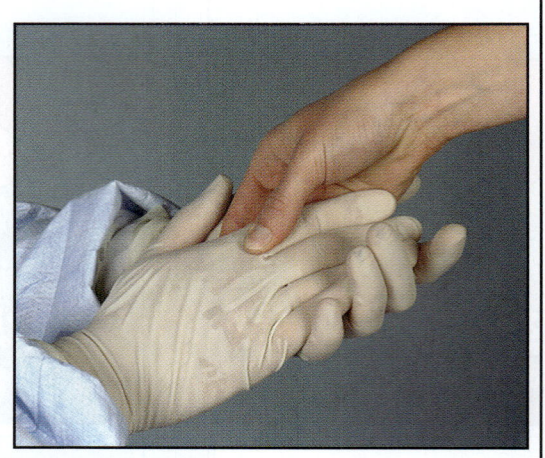

B. Warm the puncture site.

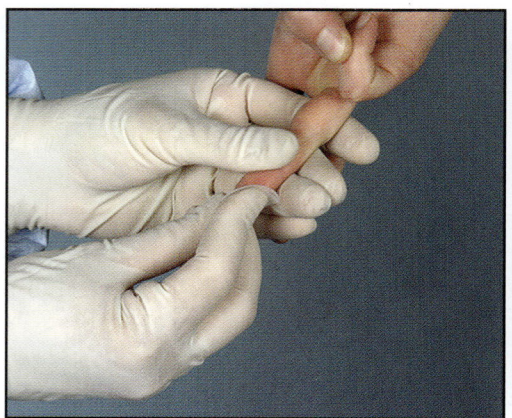

C. Disinfect with alcohol.

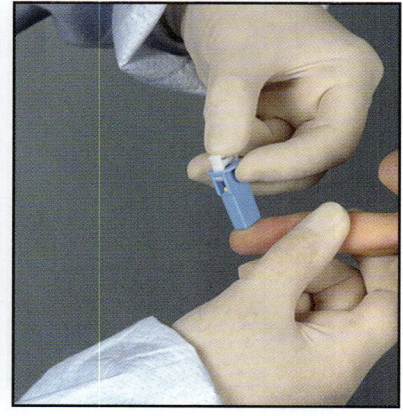

D. Perform the puncture with an incision-type safety lancet.

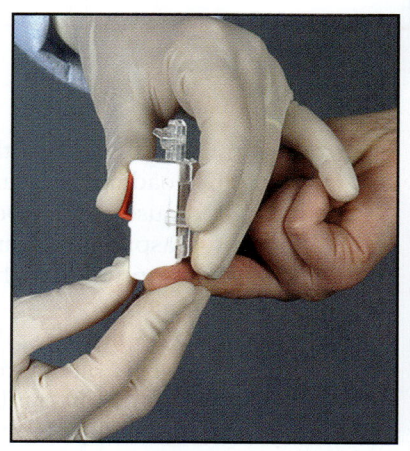

E. Alternatively, perform the puncture with a Tenderlett (ITC, Edison, NJ) safety lancet.

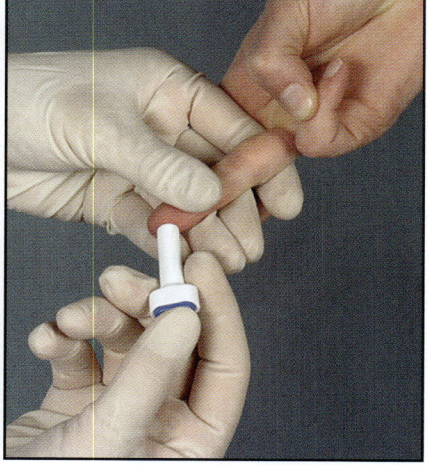

F. A puncture-type Safe-T-Pro Lancet (Roche Diagnostics, Indianapolis, Ind) can also be used.

Blood Collection Procedures

PROCEDURE 4-1 Capillary Puncture Procedure—cont'd

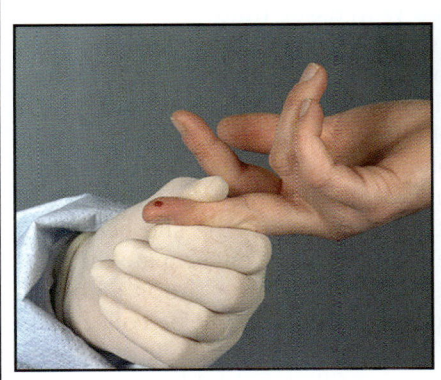

G. Wipe away the first drop of blood, then gently massage the finger to produce a large drop of blood.

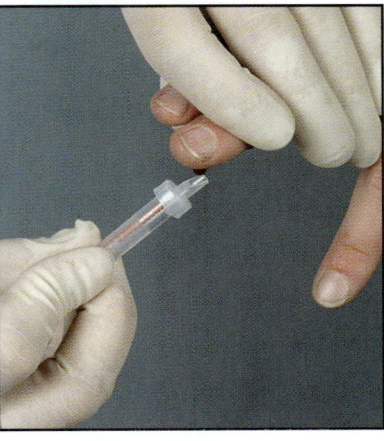

H. Collect the specimen in a microtainer.

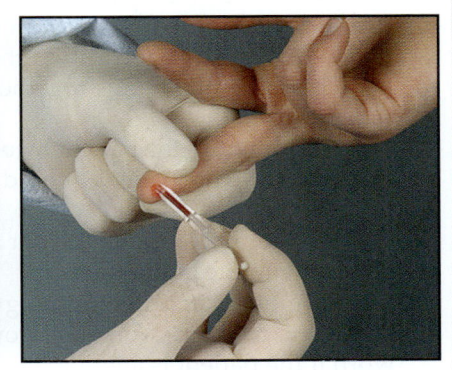

I. Alternatively, collect the specimen in a plastic pipette from a CLIA-waived test kit.

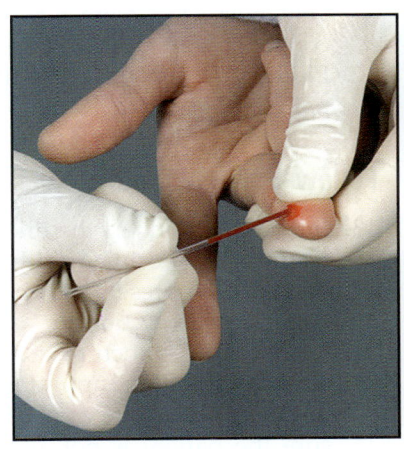

J. Alternatively, use a capillary tube for a hematocrit test.

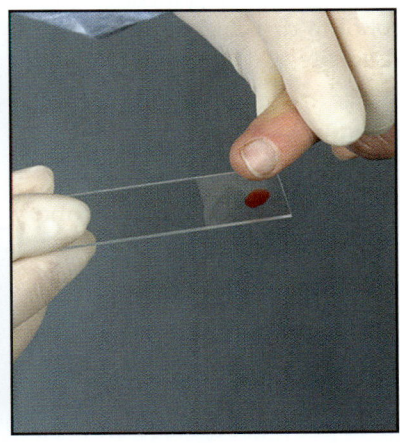

K. Alternatively, place the blood on a slide for a blood smear.

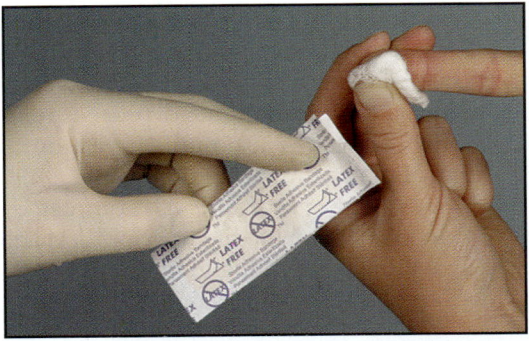

L. After 3 to 5 minutes of applying pressure to the puncture site, check for bleeding and apply a latex-free bandage.

Equipment and Supplies (Fig. A)

- Gloves (preferably nonlatex for latex-sensitive patients)
- Sterile gauze
- 70% Isopropyl alcohol pads in sterile packages
- Sterile, disposable, retractable, nonreusable lancets (varying lengths for the appropriate depth)
- Latex-free bandage

Additional supplies for collecting and processing the specimen (not pictured) are appropriate microcollection containers based on tests ordered, plastic capillary tubes (with and without anticoagulants) and sealers, glass slides to make hematology slides, biohazard puncture-resistant sharps container, warming devices (optional), and a marking pen.

(Continued)

PROCEDURE 4-1   Capillary Puncture Procedure—cont'd

Preparation—Preanalytical

1. Wash the hands if they are visibly soiled. If not, use an alcohol-based rub for routine decontamination. Apply the hand rub to the palm of one hand, and rub the hands together, covering all surfaces until dry.
2. Correctly identify the patient by using the three-way match. The patient should be sitting or lying down.
3. Choose the appropriate site for a finger stick according to the guidelines.
4. Put on gloves, first determining if the patient is allergic to latex. Nonlatex gloves should be worn if the patient is allergic.
5. Warm the site, if needed, by massaging the area or applying a warming device to the site for 3 to 5 minutes (Fig. B).
6. Clean the site with 70% isopropyl alcohol (Fig. C). Allow the alcohol to dry, and do not fan or blow on the cleansed site.

Blood Collection Procedure—Analytical

7. Determine the appropriate lancet device (Figs. D, E, F) according to the age of the patient and the amount of blood needed.
8. Open the lancet package, and keep the lancet sterile until used. Tell the patient, "You will feel a stick." Firmly hold the finger below the cleansed site, and puncture the site in the appropriate place. When making the puncture, be sure to press hard to get a good blood flow so that the patient does not have to be stuck again. Observe the hand positioning with each of the lancet devices in Figs. D, E, and F. Immediately after the puncture, discard the lancet into a biohazard sharps container placed nearby.
9. Wipe away the first drop of blood, which contains tissue fluid that could dilute the sample.
10. Gently massage the finger from the base of the finger to just below the puncture site to get a uniform drop of blood. Apply intermittent pressure below the site. You should be able to get an adequate drop to fill at least a capillary tube (Fig. G). NOTE: Do not squeeze excessively at the tip of the finger. Squeezing with too much force near the site could cause the blood sample to be contaminated with tissue fluid.
11. Collect the sample in the appropriate container for the test ordered: a microtainer (Fig. H), a plastic pipette from a CLIA-waived test kit (Fig. I), a capillary tube for a hematocrit test (Fig. J), or a slide for a blood smear (Fig. K). When collecting blood in a microcollection tube, do not scrape or scoop the container against the site because it could cause tissue fluid to contaminate the sample. Collect only free-flowing drops of blood. The microcollection tube should be collected in the order of draw for capillary puncture. If a capillary tube is being filled, hold it horizontally to prevent air bubbles from getting into the tube. Tubes with additives should be gently tapped or mixed during the collection procedure to prevent microclots from forming. Cap or seal the container when full.
12. Place gauze on the puncture site, and ask the patient to apply pressure to it.

Follow-Up—Postanalytical

13. Immediately invert the microtube 8 to 10 times to mix the specimen with any anticoagulants that may be present. Always follow the manufacturer's instructions.
14. Recheck the puncture site. If the patient has stopped bleeding, apply an adhesive bandage to the puncture site as necessary (Fig. L). Make sure the patient is not allergic to the bandage material. If bleeding does not subside after 5 minutes, contact the physician.
15. Label the tubes with the patient's name, identification number, the date and time the specimen was drawn, and your name (initials are sufficient in some facilities). When using capillary tubes, the recommended procedure is to place the filled tubes into unfilled vacuum tubes and label the vacuum tubes.
16. When the procedure is completed, discard blood-contaminated items in appropriate biohazard containers including gloves.
17. Remove gloves and sanitize hands.

Blood Collection Procedures

PROCEDURE 4-2 Heel Stick for Neonatal Screening Test Procedure

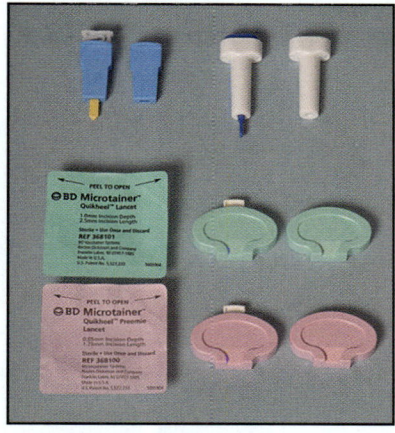

A. Neonatal safety lancets are the lower green and pink lancets designed to puncture the heel at a depth equal to or less than 2 mm.

B. Neonatal screening filter paper with five circles to saturate with the neonate's blood.

(Continued)

PROCEDURE 4-2 Heel Stick for Neonatal Screening Test Procedure—cont'd

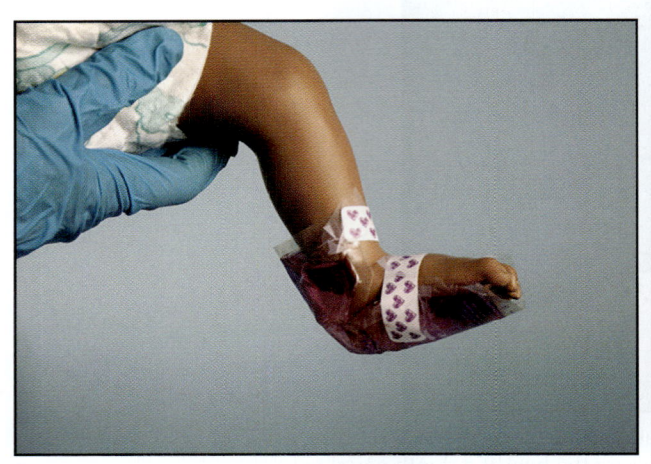

C. A commercial warming device designed for infant heels. After 3 to 5 minutes, the blood flow will increase 7 times.

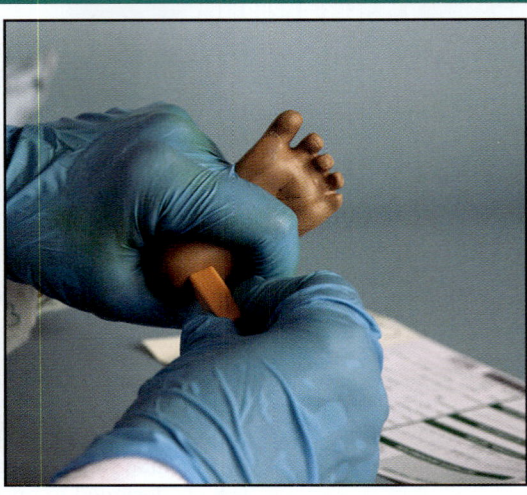

D. Note the hand position for holding the foot while the other hand performs the heel puncture on the lateral plantar portion of the heel.

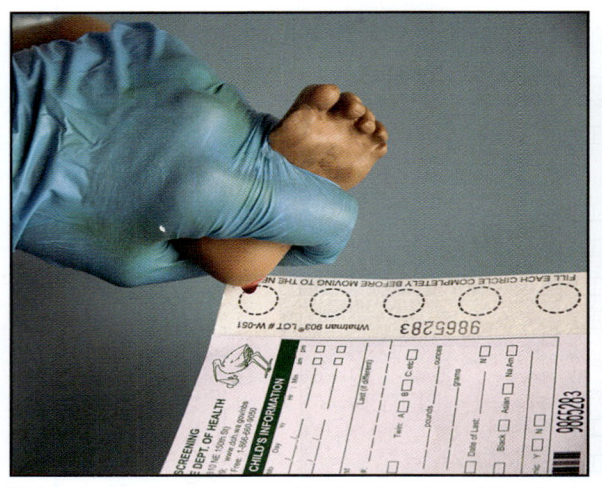

E. Apply gentle pressure with the thumb and forefinger and ease intermittently as drops of blood form.

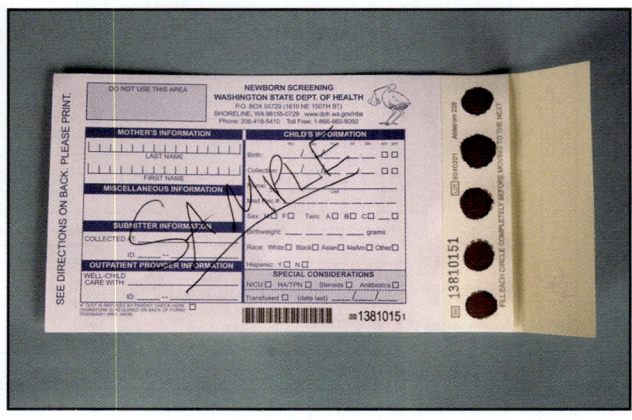

F. Example of a thoroughly dried card with all five circles saturated.

Equipment and Supplies (Fig. A)

- Gloves (preferably nonlatex for latex-sensitive patients)
- Sterile gauze
- Warming device
- 70% Isopropyl alcohol pads in sterile packages
- Sterile, disposable, retractable, nonreusable neonatal lancets with no more than 2 mm depth (Fig. A)
- Neonatal screening filter paper (Fig. B)

Preparation—Preanalytical

1. Wash the hands if they are visibly soiled. If not, use an alcohol-based rub for routine decontamination. Apply the hand rub to the palm of one hand, and rub the hands together, covering all surfaces until dry.
2. Correctly identify the newborn by using the three-way match, and fill out all the information required on the card.
3. Choose the appropriate site for the heel stick according to the guidelines.

PROCEDURE 4-2 Heel Stick for Neonatal Screening Test Procedure—cont'd

4. Put on gloves.
5. Warm the site by applying a warming device to the site for 3 to 5 minutes (Fig. C).

Blood Collection Procedure—Analytical

6. Clean the site with 70% isopropyl alcohol. Allow the alcohol to dry, and do not fan or blow on the cleansed site.
7. With a gloved hand, place the lancet against the medial or lateral plantar surface of the heel of the foot.
8. Place the blade slot area securely against the heel, and firmly and completely depress the lancet trigger (Fig. D).
9. After triggering the lancet, remove the lancet and discard it into a biohazard sharps container.
10. Gently wipe away the first drop of blood with sterile gauze or cotton ball.
11. Apply gentle pressure with the thumb and ease intermittently as drops of blood form. Be sure to apply pressure in such a way that the incision site remains open. Note the position of the hand in Fig. E.
12. The filter paper should be touched gently against the large blood drop, and in one step, a sufficient quantity of blood should soak through to completely fill a preprinted circle on the filter paper. Do not reapply additional drops in the same circle.
13. The paper should not be pressed or smeared against the puncture site of the heel.
14. Blood should be applied only to one side of the filter paper, but both sides of the filter paper should be examined to ensure that the blood uniformly saturated the paper.
15. After all five circles of blood have been collected from the heel of the newborn, the foot should be elevated above the body. NOTE: A minimum of three successful circles is needed by the laboratory to test for multiple metabolic disorders.
16. A sterile gauze pad or cotton swab should be pressed against the puncture site until the bleeding stops.
17. It is not advisable to apply adhesive bandages over skin puncture sites on newborns.

Follow-Up—Postanalytical

18. Wash the hands.
19. Log and chart the procedure.
20. Allow filter paper to dry thoroughly on a horizontal, level, nonabsorbent open surface for 3 hours at ambient temperature and away from direct sunlight.
21. Do not touch or smear blood on the filter paper, and do not contaminate the specimen card with cleaning chemicals or other substances.
22. Mail the thoroughly dried card (Fig. F) in the envelope provided by the health department.

*Figures C through F courtesy Zack Bent.

PROCEDURE 4-3 Vacutainer Method

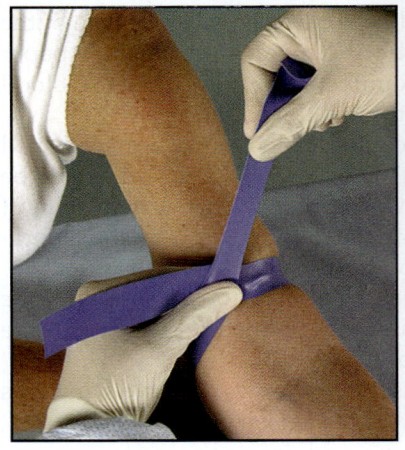

A. Apply the tourniquet. Pull the two ends of the tourniquet taut, then cross them in the front of the arm.

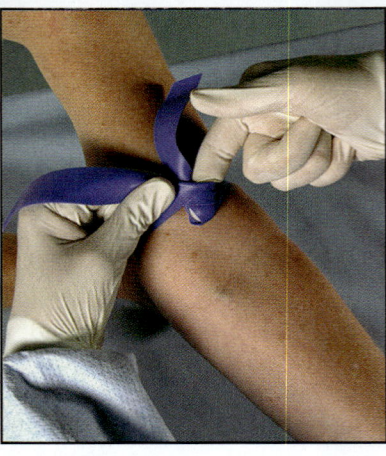

B. While holding the crossed area, tuck the top strap under the bottom strap so that the ends hang upward.

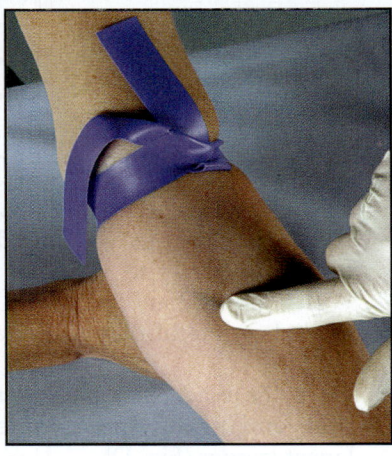

C. Palpate across the antecubital area, and visualize the size, depth, and direction of the vein.

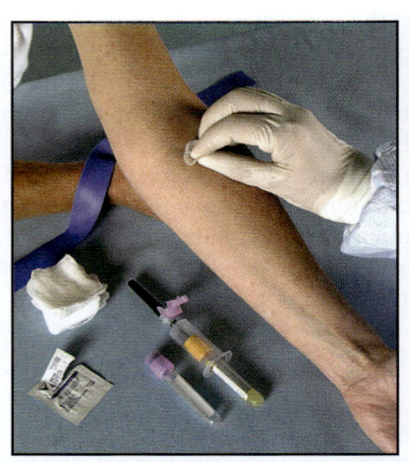

D. After taking off the tourniquet, disinfect the area and assemble equipment on the appropriate side of the arm.

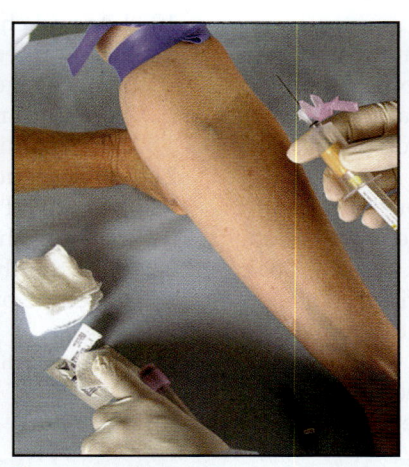

E. Reapply the tourniquet, apply alcohol to the finger if you need to recheck the position of the vein by palpation, and remove the needle cover.

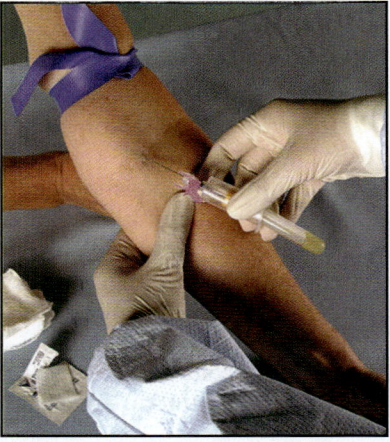

F. Anchor the vein with the nondominant hand, and insert the needle with the dominant hand.

Equipment and Supplies

- Disposable gloves
- Tourniquet
- 70% Isopropyl alcohol
- Vacutainer double-pointed needle
- Vacutainer holder
- Correct vacuum tubes for the requested tests
- Sterile gauze pads
- Adhesive bandages
- Test tube rack
- Biohazard sharps containers and bags

Preparation—Preanalytical

1. Wash the hands if they are visibly soiled. If not, use an alcohol-based hand rub. Apply the rub to the palm of one hand, and rub the hands together, covering all surfaces until dry.
2. Correctly identify the patient by using the three-way match.
3. Position the patient properly, such as in a reclining position or sitting in a chair with an arm support. Have the patient place his or her arm in a downward position to prevent reflux.
4. Determine if the patient is allergic to latex. Put on the appropriate type of gloves.

Blood Collection Procedures

PROCEDURE 4-3 Vacutainer Method—cont'd

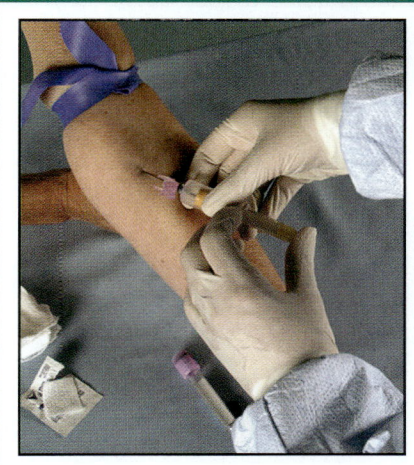

G. Push the Vacutainer tube into the needle holder with the thumb of the nondominant hand. Apply counterpressure on the flange of the Vacutainer holder with the fingers of the nondominant hand.

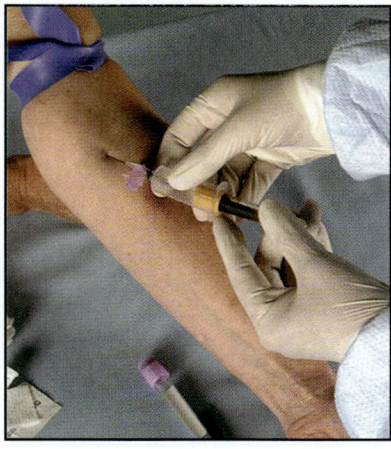

H. Pull out the tube with the fingers of the nondominant hand while applying counterpressure against the flange with the thumb.

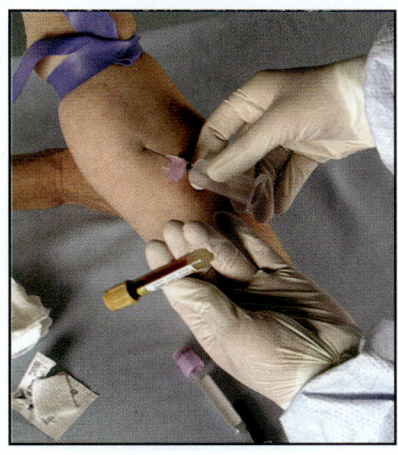

I. Mix the specimen by tilting the tube back and forth.

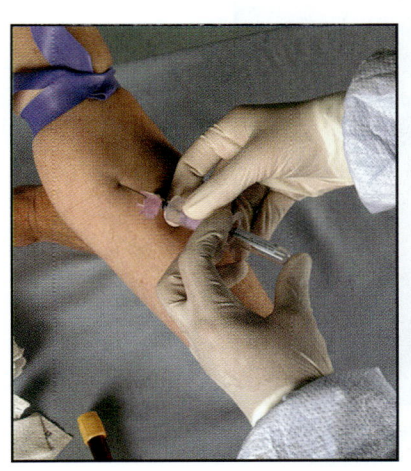

J. Insert the second tube with the nondominant hand.

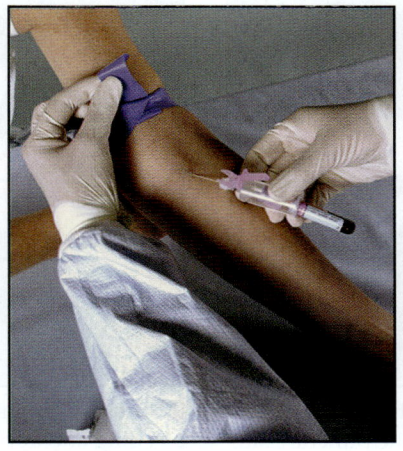

K. Remove the tourniquet as the last vacuum is filling.

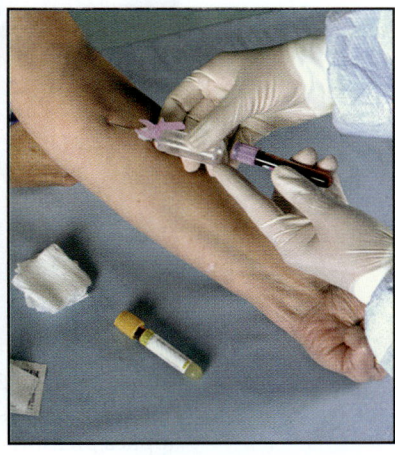

L. Remove the final tube from the holder.

5. Apply the tourniquet, and determine the appropriate site (Figs. A and B). Have the patient make a fist, and palpate the arm for a vein. Ask the patient to clench and unclench the fist a few times to push the blood from the lower arm to the veins, but the patient should avoid vigorous pumping, which could cause hemoconcentration.
6. Begin on one side of the antecubital space, and palpate across to the other side with the index finger (Fig. C). The vein will feel spongy. When the vein is found, determine its size and depth and follow it up and down to determine its direction.
7. Remove the tourniquet.
8. Clean the arm with 70% isopropyl alcohol (Fig. D). Rub the chosen site with the alcohol, working in concentric circles from the inside out, making sure not to backtrack. Allow the alcohol to dry without fanning or blowing on the cleansed site.
9. While the site is drying, assemble the equipment. Take the sheath off the holder end of the Vacutainer needle, and screw it into the holder. Determine which vacuum tubes are needed for the testing, and place them in a rack in the order of draw. Check the expiration date of the tubes and look for cracks. Be sure to tap the tubes that contain additives to release any additives that may be on the lids. Place the gauze, tubes, and

(Continued)

PROCEDURE 4-3 Vacutainer Method—cont'd

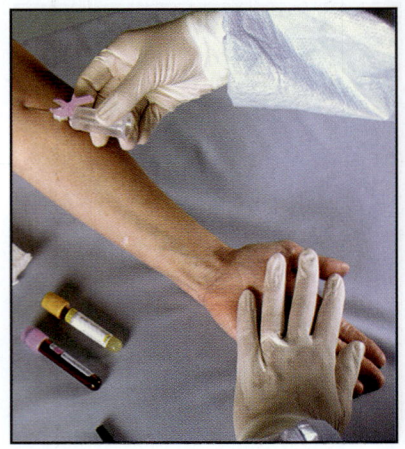

M. Have the patient relax his or her fist.

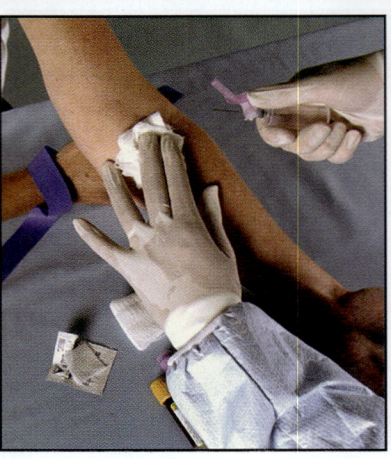

N. Place sterile gauze over the site. After the needle is removed, then apply pressure and activate the needle safety device.

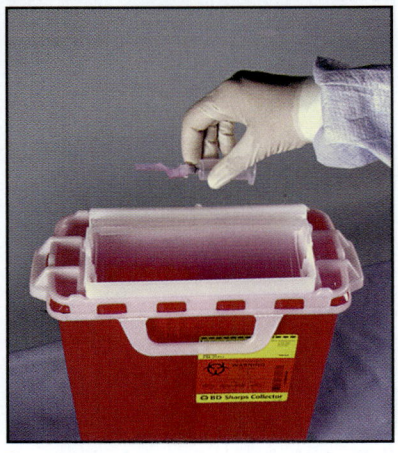

O. Immediately dispose of the needle/holder assembly in a biohazard sharps container.

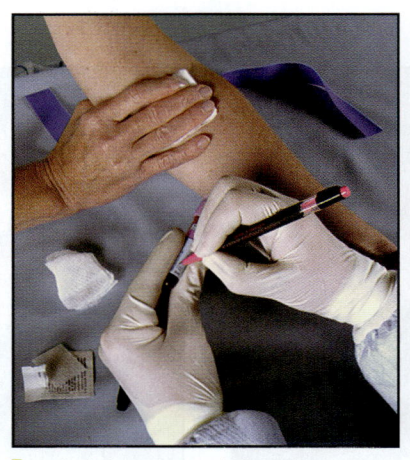

P. Label the tubes while the patient applies pressure to the puncture site.

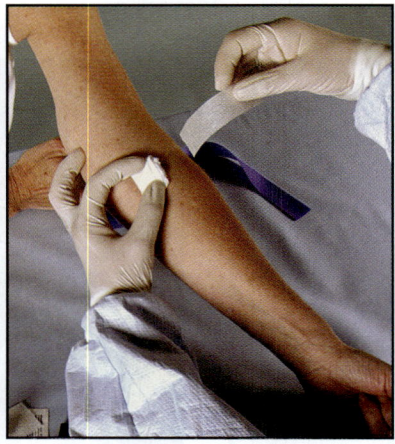

Q. After 3 to 5 minutes, check for bleeding and apply a pressure bandage.

all equipment close to the drawing station so they can be easily reached during the procedure.

Blood Collection Procedure—Analytical

10. The collection process begins after the alcohol has dried. Reapply the tourniquet, being careful not to contaminate the cleansed site. Have the patient make a fist. If you need to palpate the site again, clean your gloved finger(s) with 70% alcohol (Fig. E). Remove the needle sheath, exposing the needle.

11. Anchor the vein with the nondominant thumb, placing it approximately 1 to 2 inches below and to the side of the puncture site so that it is not in the way of the entry of the needle into the vein (Fig. F). Make the skin over the vein taut by pulling toward the patient's hand. This will help keep the vein from moving and allow the needle to enter more easily.

12. Approximately ¼ to ½ inch below the site and with the bevel up, insert the needle at a 15-degree angle with one swift, continuous motion to prevent tissue damage. Phlebotomist and needle should be positioned in the same direction as the vein. The correct angle will vary depending on the depth of the palpated vein. The common angle is 15 degrees. If the angle is less than 15 degrees, the needle may go above the vein; conversely, if the angle is greater than 15 degrees, the needle may go through the vein. Never stick unless a vein has been determined. The holder

Blood Collection Procedures

PROCEDURE 4-3 Vacutainer Method—cont'd

should be held steady with the dominant hand during the procedure so that the needle does not move through the vein or pull out.

13. Push the tube into the needle holder (Fig. G). Put the index and middle fingers of the nondominant hand on both sides of the flange of the holder, and push the tube into the Vacutainer needle with the thumb of the same hand.
14. Follow the order of draw for vacuum tubes when filling the tubes. To remove a tube from the holder, put the thumb of the nondominant hand against the flange of the holder and pull the tube out with the fingers of the nondominant hand (Fig. H). Gently invert the tube a few times to mix the blood with any additives (Fig. I).
15. Insert the next tube into the holder, and use the same method of pushing the tube into the holder with your thumb while applying counterpressure with the fingers of the same hand on the flange of the holder (Fig. J).
16. While the last tube is filling, remove the tourniquet (Fig. K). When the last tube is filled, remove it (Fig. L) and mix it by tilting. The last tube must be removed before removing the needle from the arm to prevent blood from dripping out of the needle.
17. Make sure the patient's hand is relaxed (Fig. M) and that the tourniquet is removed *before* you take the needle out of the arm. If this is not done, blood may leak into the tissues from the venous puncture site, causing a hematoma (literally, a tumor or swelling of blood in the tissues).
18. Place a sterile gauze or cotton ball over the needle as it is pulled out to prevent tissue damage. Do not press down on the gauze until the needle has been removed (Fig. N). Pressure on the needle is painful for the patient.
19. After exiting the vein, activate the needle safety device and discard the entire Vacutainer device (holder with attached needle) in a biohazard sharps container (Fig. O). Never recap a needle.

Follow-Up—Post Analytical

20. With the gauze over the site, ask the patient to apply pressure for 3 to 5 minutes with the arm straight or elevated above the heart. This pressure will help prevent a hematoma from forming. Bending the arm at the elbow can cause blood flow from the puncture site to increase.
21. While the patient is applying pressure, gently mix the tubes 8 to 10 times. Label them with the patient's name, identification number, the date and time that the specimen was drawn, and your name (or initials, if appropriate) (Fig. P). NOTE: Never prelabel tubes before the actual specimen is obtained—a prelabeled tube may end up with someone else's specimen!
22. During the entire process, assess the patient for signs of fainting. Check the site for bleeding. If bleeding has subsided, first determine if the patient is allergic to any type of bandage, then apply a pressure bandage if appropriate (Fig. Q). Tell the patient not to lift any heavy objects for approximately 1 hour. If the site is still bleeding, continue to apply pressure. If bleeding has not stopped after 5 minutes, contact the physician. During the entire process, make sure that the patient is feeling well.
23. Discard all materials in the appropriate containers.
24. Remove gloves in the appropriate manner discussed in Chapter 1, and discard in a biohazard bag.
25. Wash the hands.
26. Document the procedure in the patient's chart, making sure to include the following five items:
    When: date and time of collection
    Where: location on the body the blood was collected (e.g., right antecubital space, hand, finger) and where specimen is being sent (e.g. reference lab, hospital)
    What: types of tubes collected (e.g., gold and lavender)
    Why: what tests were ordered (e.g., blood chemistry profile, complete blood cell count)
    Who: person who collected the specimen (your name, credentials)

PROCEDURE 4-4 Syringe Method

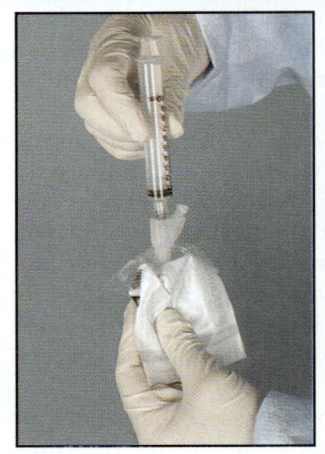

A. Assemble the sterile syringe and safety needle.

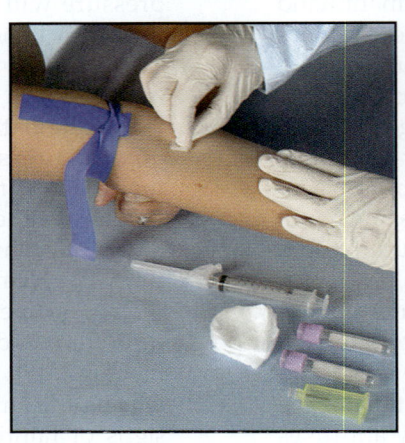

B. Apply the tourniquet as in the Vacutainer method, disinfect the site, and have supplies ready.

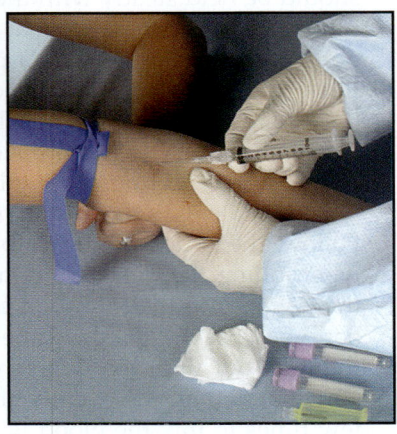

C. Anchor the vein with the non-dominant hand, and insert the needle.

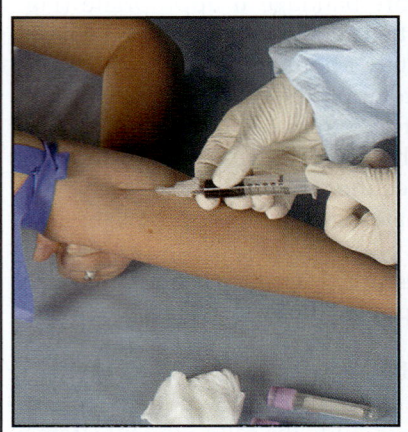

D. Withdraw blood by pulling back on the plunger.

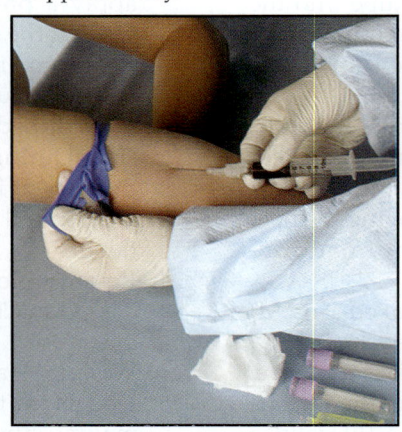

E. Instruct the patient to unclench the fist, and remove the tourniquet before collecting the last blood specimen.

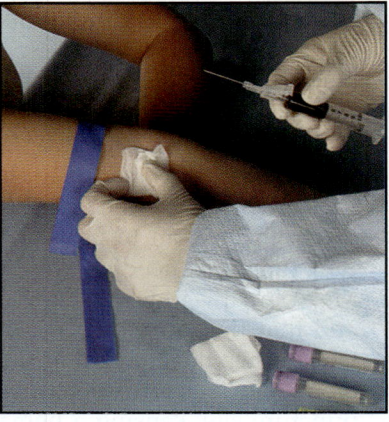

F. Place sterile gauze over the puncture site while removing the needle. After the needle is removed, apply pressure.

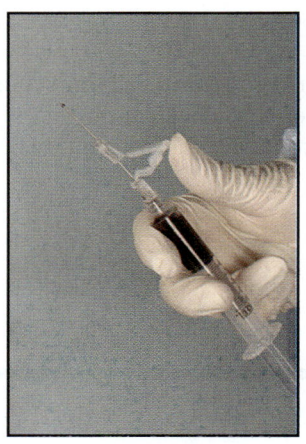

G. Immediately activate the needle safety device.

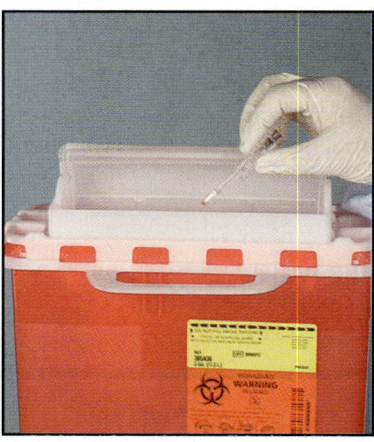

H. Remove the protected needle from the syringe, and discard the needle in a biohazard sharps container.

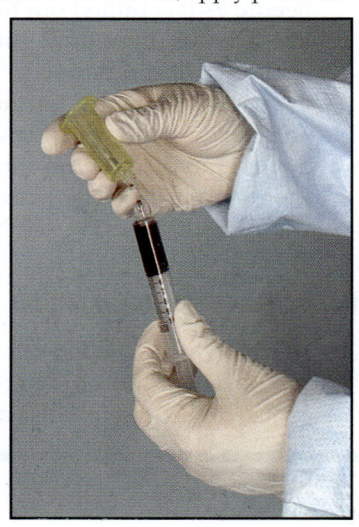

I. Attach the yellow safety transfer device to the tip of the syringe.

PROCEDURE 4-4 Syringe Method—cont'd

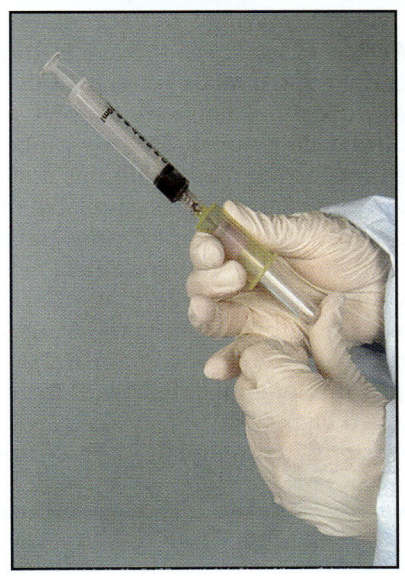

J. Invert the syringe above the device, and connect the proper vacuum tubes by pushing them into the transfer device from below. Mix each tube after it is filled.

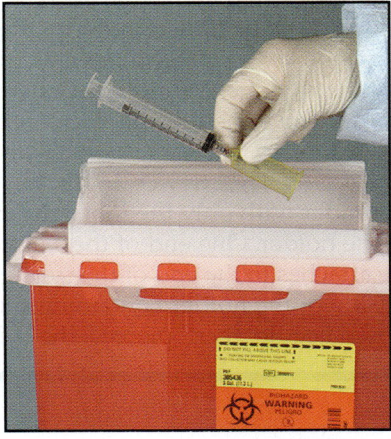

K. When the transfer is finished, discard the entire syringe/transfer device assembly in the biohazard sharps container.

Equipment and Supplies

- Disposable gloves
- Tourniquet
- 70% Isopropyl alcohol
- Syringe and needle in correct sizes
- Correct vacuum tubes for the requested tests
- Safety transfer device
- Sterile gauze pads
- Adhesive bandages
- Test tube rack
- Biohazard sharps containers and bags

Preparation—Preanalytical

1. Follow steps 1 through 8 of Procedure 4-3.
2. While the site is drying, assemble the equipment. Remove the sterile syringe and needle from their packages, keeping them sterile (Fig. A). Move the plunger back and forth several times to break the seal on the syringe. Screw the hub of the needle tightly onto the syringe. Determine which vacuum tubes are needed for the testing, and place them in a rack in the order of draw for vacuum tubes. Check the expiration date of the tubes, look for cracks, and tap the tubes that contain additives to release any additives that may be on the lids. Place all equipment close to the draw station so it is easily reached during the procedure.

Blood Collection Procedure—Analytical

3. Follow steps 10 through 12 of Procedure 4-3, including applying the tourniquet, disinfecting the site (Fig. B), and anchoring the vein while inserting the needle (Fig. C).
4. When the needle is in the vein, blood may be seen in the hub of the syringe. Gently pull back on the plunger to pull blood into the syringe (Fig. D). If the plunger is moved too fast, the blood may be hemolyzed or the vein may collapse. Be careful not to move the needle while it is in the vein, which could be painful for the patient. Also, do not withdraw the needle prematurely from the patient's arm while pulling back on the plunger.
5. When the syringe has filled with the required amount of blood, have the patient unclench his or her fist and release the tourniquet (Fig. E). Place sterile gauze over the puncture site as you remove the needle (Fig. F). Be careful to remove the needle in the same path it was inserted. Do not press down on the gauze until the needle has been removed; such pressure would be painful for the patient.
6. Activate the syringe needle safety device after the needle has been removed from the arm (Fig. G). Detach the needle from the syringe, and discard the protected needle in the sharps biohazard container (Fig. H).

(Continued)

PROCEDURE 4-4 Syringe Method—cont'd

Follow-Up—Postanalytical

7. With the gauze on the site, ask the patient to apply pressure for 3 to 5 minutes with the arm straight or elevated above the heart.
8. The blood must be transferred into the vacuum tubes as quickly as possible so that it does not clot in the syringe. While the patient applies pressure to the puncture site, transfer the blood from syringe to vacuum tubes with a *safety transfer device*. This device looks like a Vacutainer holder with only the inner sheathed needle in the holder. One end of the safety transfer device attaches to the end of the syringe (Fig. I). The inside of the holder containing the rubber-sheathed needle then pierces the Vacutainer tube when the syringe and holder are inverted (Fig. J). The blood in the syringe is drawn automatically into the tubes because of the vacuum in these tubes. To keep from hemolyzing the red blood cells, never push on the syringe plunger while transferring blood with this device.
9. Mix the tubes 8 to 10 times, and label them with the patient's name, identification number, the date and time that the specimen was drawn, and your name (or initials, if appropriate).
10. Discard the entire connected syringe/transfer device into the sharps container (Fig. K). Discard all other potential biohazard materials in a biohazard bag.
11. Follow steps 20 through 24 of Procedure 4-3.

PROCEDURE 4-5 Two Butterfly Methods from a Hand and Training Model

I. Butterfly Safety Lock Needle Using Vacutainer System

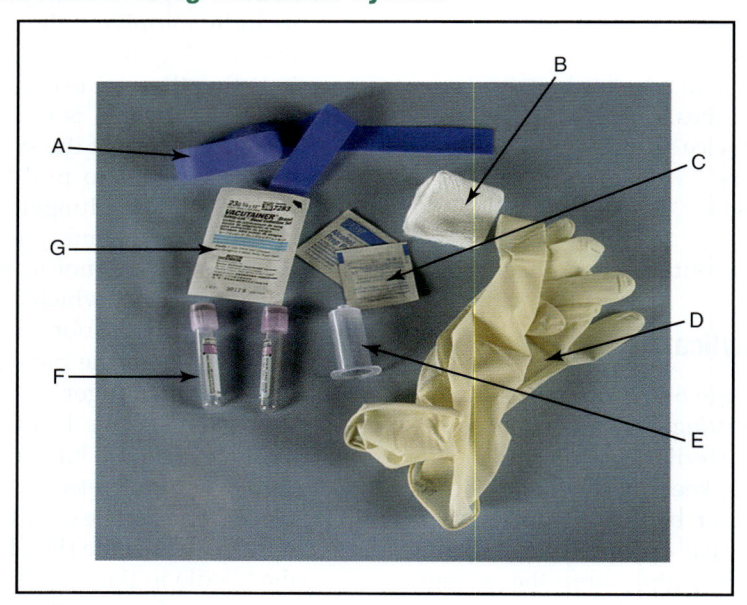

A. Butterfly setup. *a,* Tourniquet; *b,* sterile gauze pads; *c,* 70% isopropyl alcohol; *d,* disposable gloves; *e,* Vacutainer holder; *f,* Vacutainer tubes; *g,* winged infusion Safety Lock butterfly set with Vacutainer adapter to connect to Vacutainer holder.

Equipment and Supplies (Fig. A)

- Tourniquet
- Sterile gauze pads
- 70% Isopropyl alcohol
- Disposable gloves
- Vacutainer holder
- Vacutainer tubes
- Winged butterfly with Safety-Lock needle and Vacutainer adapter to connect to Vacutainer holder
- Biohazard sharps containers and bags

Blood Collection Procedures

PROCEDURE 4-5 Two Butterfly Methods from a Hand and Training Model—cont'd

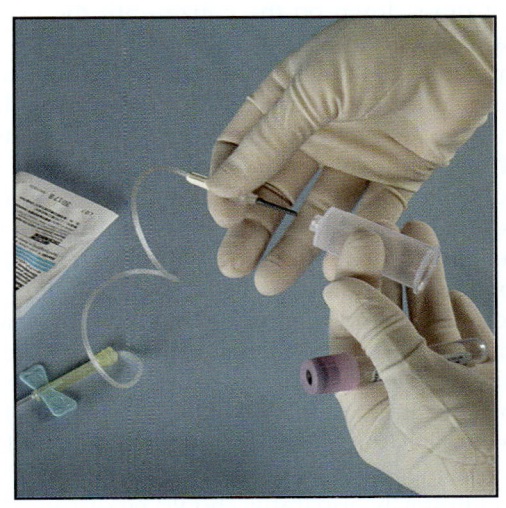

B. Attach the rubber-sheathed multineedle Vacutainer adapter to the butterfly tubing, then screw the needle into the Vacutainer holder.

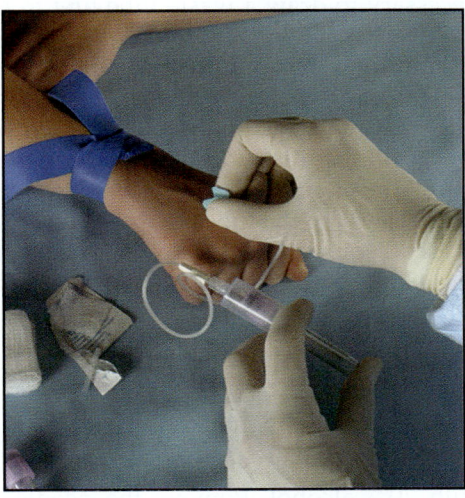

C. After disinfecting the hand, applying the tourniquet, and anchoring the vein, insert the butterfly needle into the vein. Push the vacuum tubes into the holder, which will draw the blood through the tubing into the tubes.

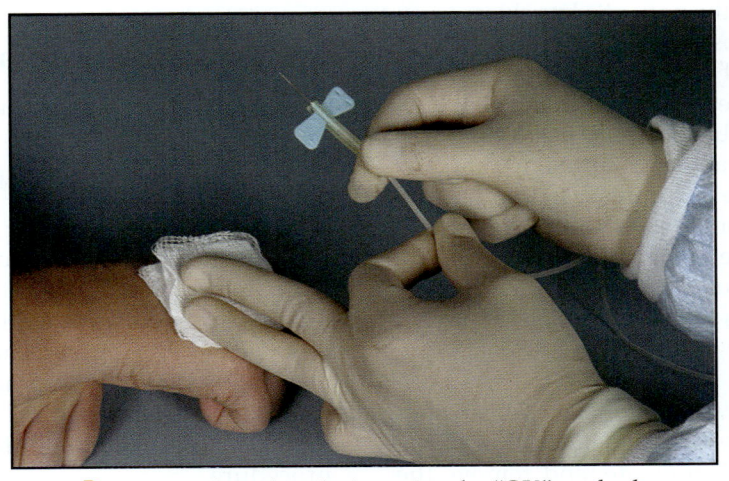

D. Activate the safety device using the "OK" method.

Preparation—Preanalytical

1. Follow steps 1 through 4 of Procedure 4-3. The procedure for entering a vein in the arm is the same as for the syringe and vacuum tube methods. If blood is being drawn from the hand, apply the tourniquet above the wrist and have the patient make a half fist.
2. Beginning on one side of the puncture area, palpate across to the other side with the index finger. The vein will feel spongy. When the vein is found, determine its size and depth and follow it up and down to determine its direction.
3. Remove the tourniquet.
4. Clean the hand with 70% isopropyl alcohol. Allow the alcohol to dry without fanning or blowing on the cleansed site.
5. While the site is drying, assemble the equipment. Remove the winged infusion set from the package, and stretch the tubing to straighten it. If you are using the Vacutainer method, attach a Luer adapter to the end of the tubing of the winged infusion, then screw the other end into a Vacutainer holder (Fig. B).
6. Determine which vacuum tubes are needed for the testing, and place them in a rack in the order of draw. NOTE: If a blue top is ordered, it is

(Continued)

PROCEDURE 4-5 Two Butterfly Methods from a Hand and Training Model—cont'd

necessary to draw a waste tube first to remove the dead space in the tubing. A red tube with no additives or an additional blue top may be used to clear the air in the tubing with blood. The waste tubes do not need to be filled because they will be discarded after the procedure. Check the expiration date of the tubes, look for cracks, and tap the tubes that contain additives. Place all equipment close to the draw station so it can be easily reached during the procedure.

Blood Collection Procedure—Analytical

7. When the alcohol has dried, reapply the tourniquet. If you need to determine the puncture site again, clean the gloved finger(s) you will use with 70% alcohol. Remove the needle sheath from the needle.
8. Anchor the vein by placing the nondominant thumb 1 to 2 inches below and to the side of the puncture site. Make the skin over the vein taut by pulling toward the patient's knuckles.
9. Grip the folded plastic wings to guide the needle into the vein (Fig. C). At approximately ¼ to ½ inch below the site and with the bevel up, quickly insert the bevel of the needle into the vein at a 5-degree angle. Continue to "thread" the needle with one continuous, swift motion to keep the needle from twisting out of the vein.
10. If you are using the Vacutainer holder/system, push the vacuum tubes into the holder (Fig. C). After each tube has filled with blood, remove it and gently mix it.
11. After the required amount of blood has been obtained, have the patient unclench his or her fist and release the tourniquet. Place a sterile gauze over the puncture site, and remove the needle by holding the "tail" of the butterfly. Do not press down on the gauze until the needle has been removed.
12. Immediately activate the safety device. One recommended safety procedure consists of pulling the needle out with the thumb and forefinger of the dominant hand, grasping the back of the butterfly device with the thumb up. The nondominant hand holds the gauze with three fingers and grabs the tubing with the thumb and forefinger forming the "OK" sign (Fig. D). The dominant hand then pulls the device forward, causing the sheath to cover the needle. (NOTE: Always keep both hands behind the needle tip to prevent an accidental stick.) After the safety device has been activated with the butterfly/Vacutainer method, the entire Vacutainer holder and butterfly apparatus should be discarded in a biohazard sharps container.
13. With the gauze on the site, ask the patient to apply pressure for 3 to 5 minutes with the arm straight or elevated above the heart.

Follow-Up—Postanalytical

14. Follow steps 20 through 26 of Procedure 4-3.

II. Butterfly Push-Button Needle Using a Syringe

This procedure is basically the same as the previously described Safety Lock butterfly procedure, with a few changes. The push-button butterfly needle is considered safer than the safety lock needle when used properly. The best way to learn any new safety device is to practice first on a training model. Figs. E through M* demonstrate the ways in which this method differs from the previous procedure.

Blood Collection Procedures

PROCEDURE 4-5 Two Butterfly Methods from a Hand and Training Model—cont'd

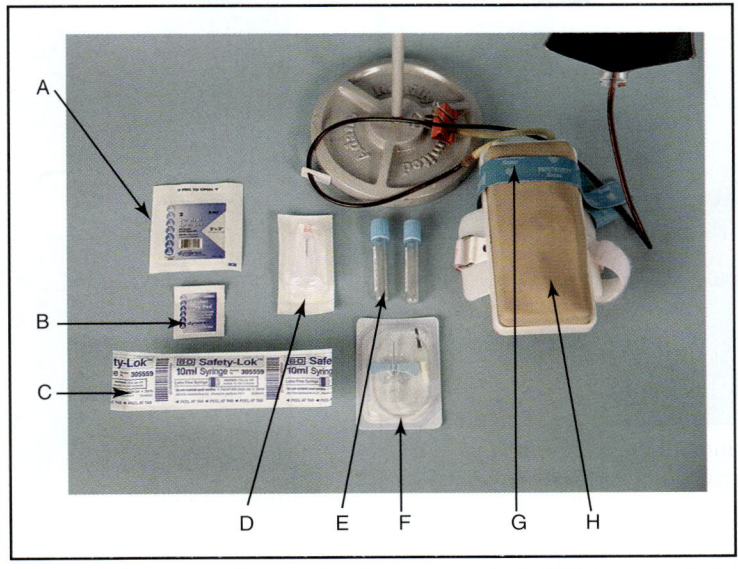

E. Equipment and supplies for push-button method: *a*, Sterile gauze pads; *b*, 70% isopropyl alcohol; *c*, sterile syringe; *d*, transfer device; *e*, Vacutainer tubes; *f*, butterfly with push-button safety needle; *g*, tourniquet; *h*, training model with artificial blood for practicing.

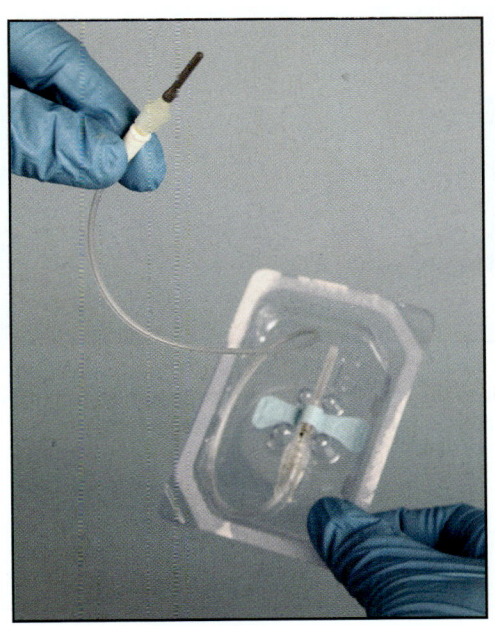

F. Proper removal of the butterfly from its container consists of pulling out the adapter end of the tubing to prevent accidental activation of the push button on the tail of the winged needle.

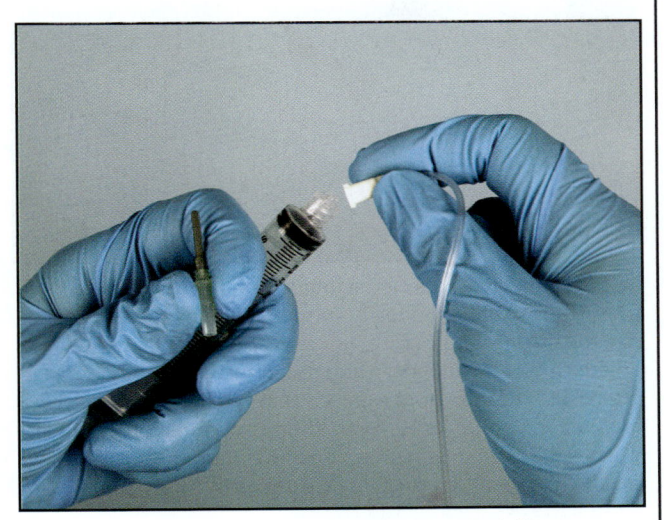

G. When using a syringe, remove the Luer-Lok Vacutainer holder adapter (on the left) and place the syringe adapter tightly on to the tip of the syringe. Also, remember to move the plunger back and forth several times to break the seal on the syringe.

(Continued)

PROCEDURE 4-5 Two Butterfly Methods from a Hand and Training Model—cont'd

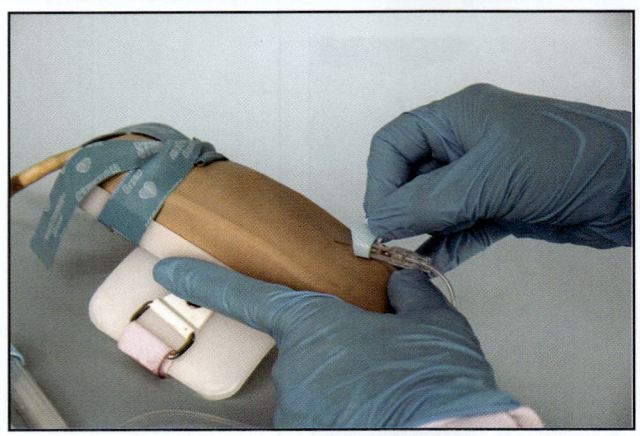

H. While anchoring the vein with the nondominant hand, quickly insert the bevel of the butterfly needle at a 5-degree angle and observe the flash of blood entering the tail of the butterfly. Continue to thread the needle along the lumen of the vein to anchor the needle.

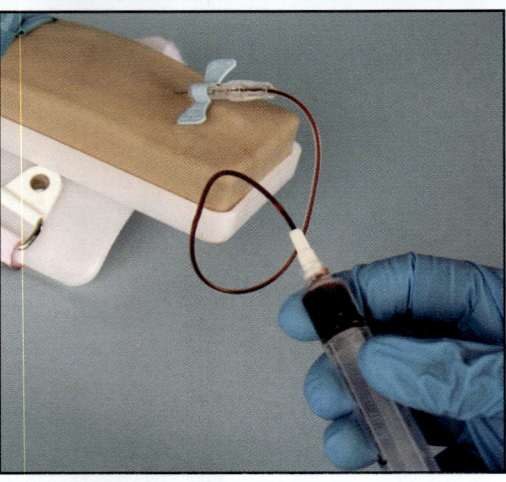

I. With the needle in place, both hands may be used to slowly pull up the blood into the syringe. It may be necessary to pull back the plunger a little at a time to keep the vein from collapsing.

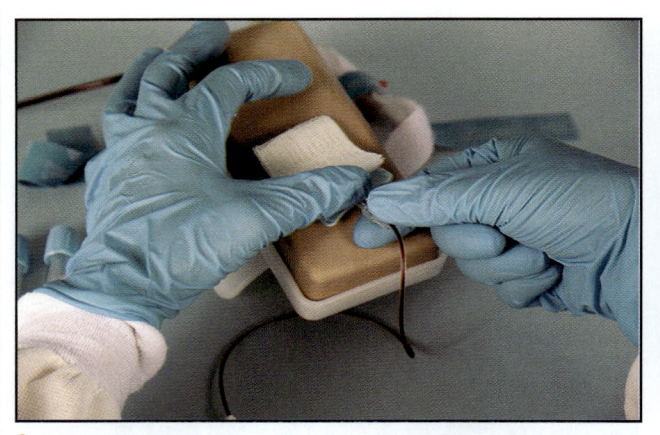

J. After you have collected enough blood in the syringe, grasp the tail of the butterfly, as seen in the picture, to stabilize the needle, and place a gauze over the needle to prevent splattering of the blood during the retraction of the needle NOTE: Tell the patient to expect a snapping sound that will indicate the procedure is over. The nondominant hand then pushes the button using the side of the thumb, causing the needle to instantly retract into the butterfly tail.

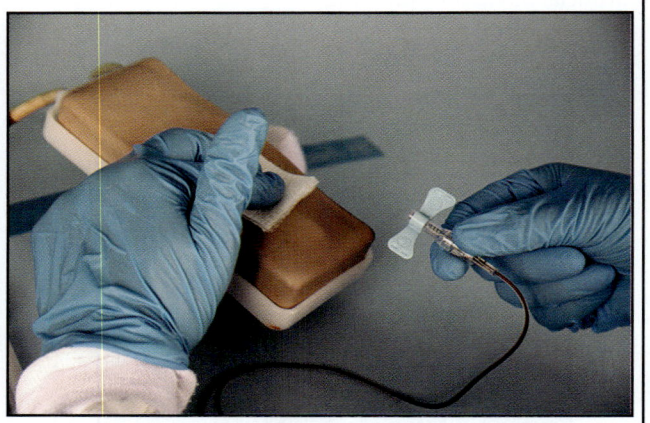

K. After the snap has been heard and the needle is safely tucked into the tail of the butterfly, the nondominant hand immediately applies pressure to the site.

Advanced Concepts

123

PROCEDURE 4-5 Two Butterfly Methods from a Hand and Training Model—cont'd

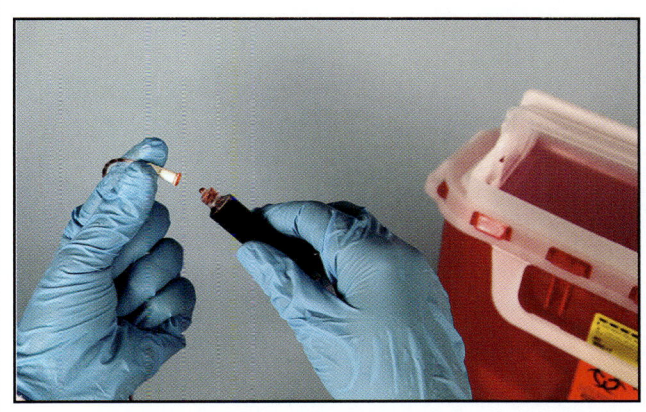

L. Remove the hub of the butterfly from the syringe, and throw the tubing into the sharps container.

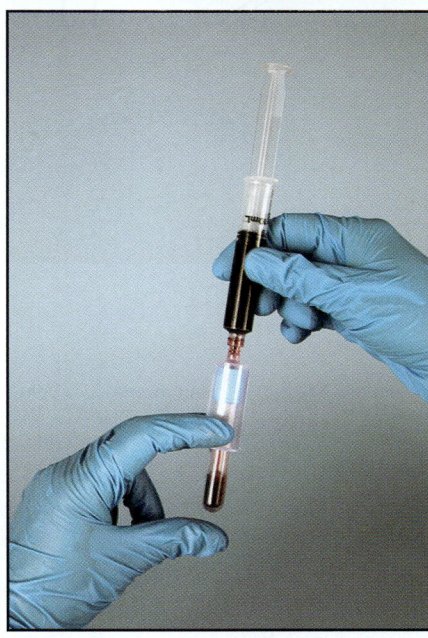

M. Using the transfer device, transfer the blood into the appropriate tubes in their correct order of draw. Hold the syringe above and the vacuum tubes below in an upright position. NOTE: It is still wise to draw a waste tube before filling the blue top tube because the syringe will contain the air that was first removed through the butterfly tubing. Also, keep pushing on the tubes as they are filling so they do not slip off the sheathed needle in the transfer device, causing an incomplete fill.

*Figs. E through M courtesy Zack Bent.

ADVANCED CONCEPTS

Complications

Complications may occur during a phlebotomy procedure. All complications and ways to prevent them, when possible, should be understood.

Hematomas

A **hematoma** is a bruising that results from a break in a blood vessel. It can occur around a puncture site when blood leaks from the vein into the surrounding tissue. A hematoma may result when any of the following occurs:
- The needle goes through the vein.
- The needle is only partially in the vein.
- Insufficient pressure is applied to the puncture site after the procedure is completed.

If a hematoma occurs, remove the tourniquet and needle immediately, in that order. Apply pressure for 3 to 5 minutes. If the bleeding continues, call for assistance.

Failure to Obtain Blood

If blood is not obtained, one of the following problems may have occurred:
- The bevel is against the wall of the vein (Fig. 4-24, *A*).
- The needle pierced all the way through the vein (Fig. 4-24, *B*). Insertion of the needle at an angle greater than 15 degrees is a likely cause.
- The needle is only partially inserted into the vein, possibly because the needle is inserted at less than a 15-degree angle (Fig. 4-24, *C*).

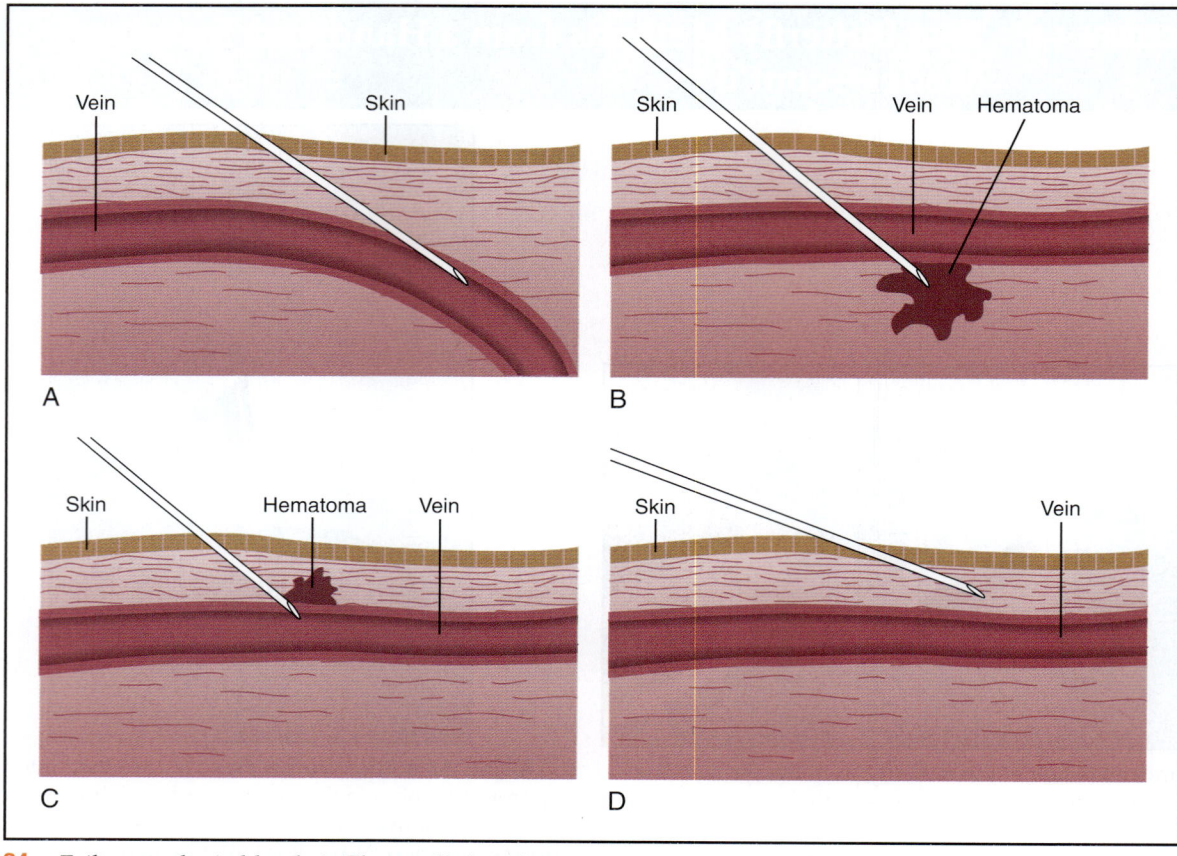

Fig. 4-24. Failure to obtain blood. **A,** The needle bevel is on the wall of the vein. **B,** The needle bevel has gone through the entire vein. **C,** The needle bevel is only partially inserted into the vein, which causes blood to leak into tissue. **D,** The needle bevel has completely missed the vein. (From Warekois R, Robinson R: *Phlebotomy: worktext and procedures manual*, ed 2, St Louis, 2007, Saunders.)

- The needle has missed the vein entirely (Fig. 4-24, *D*). Do not probe excessively if the vein is missed because this bruises the arm and could hemolyze the red blood cells.
- A defective tube has been used. Always inspect tubes before using them.
- A patient should never be stuck more than two times by the same phlebotomist.
- There is now an instrument that transilluminates the surface of the skin with infrared light to assist in locating difficult-to-find veins (Figs. 4-25 and 4-26).

Syncope

Some patients experience **syncope,** or fainting, during phlebotomy procedures. Signs of fainting include pallor, sweating, and hyperventilation. If a patient expresses concern about fainting, place him or her in a reclining position before starting the procedure.

If a patient feels faint, release the tourniquet and remove the needle. Be sure to activate the safety device. Have the patient lower his or her head and breathe deeply. Place a cold or wet towel on the forehead and back of the neck. Do not attempt to put anything in the patient's mouth. If possible, place the patient in a reclining position and stay with the patient for at least 15 minutes after the patient has recovered. Instruct the patient not to drive for at least 30 minutes. A glass of juice may be helpful. An incident report from your health care facility should be completed describing the fainting incident and any follow-up action taken.

Hemolysis

Hemolysis is the breaking open of red blood cells and the release of hemoglobin. Hemoglobin turns serum or plasma pink or red. Hemolysis can be caused by one of the following actions:
- Using a needle that is too small
- Collapsing the vein by putting too much pressure on it, either by using the Vacutainer method on a small vein or by pulling back the plunger too quickly with the syringe method

Advanced Concepts

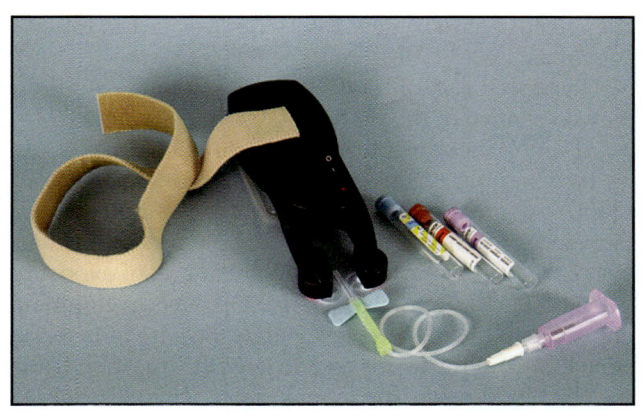

Fig. 4-25. The vein finder. Venoscope II Model VT 03 infrared light source displays vein. (Courtesy Zack Bent.)

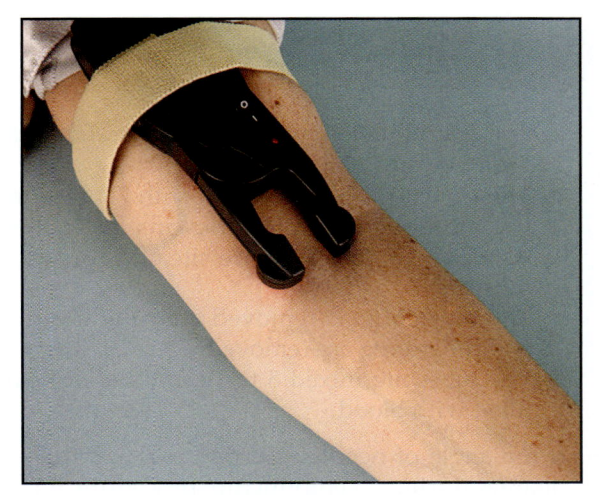

Fig. 4-26. Attaching venoscope to arm for assisting in blood draw. (Courtesy Zack Bent.)

- Vigorously shaking the filled tubes

Hemolyzed blood releases chemicals into the plasma and serum that adversely affect the test results for the following analytes:
- Potassium
- Magnesium
- Iron
- Lactate dehydrogenase
- Phosphorus
- Ammonia
- Total protein

Excessive Bleeding

A patient typically stops bleeding in 2 to 6 minutes. However, patients who take medications such as blood thinners and arthritis medications may bleed for a longer time. Even aspirin can act as a blood thinner. Patients may also have coagulation abnormalities such as platelet defects. In this case **petechiae** (small red or purple spots) may appear on the patient's skin. Petechiae are caused by small amounts of bleeding under the skin. Let the physician know if bleeding does not stop.

Neurological Problems

One neurological problem that could occur during a phlebotomy procedure is a seizure. If a patient has a seizure, remove the tourniquet and needle immediately and apply pressure to the puncture. Call for help, and do not attempt to put anything in the patient's mouth unless authorized to do so.

Another neurological problem may occur if the needle hits a nerve. The patient will probably experience a tingling sensation radiating down the affected nerve. Again, immediately remove the tourniquet and needle, and apply pressure to the site. Notify an authorized person, and file an incident report.

Obesity and Mastectomy

The veins on obese patients may be difficult to see and palpate, making them a challenge to find and penetrate. Caution must be taken not to probe the area excessively if a vein is missed.

Do not perform a venipuncture on the arm adjacent to a mastectomy (removal of the breast) site. A patient who has had a mastectomy may have no lymph flow to that arm because the axillary lymph nodes on the mastectomy side may have been removed. This condition carries a potential risk for infection, along with alterations in body fluids and blood analytes. In addition, the tourniquet may injure the patient's arm.

Intravenous Therapy and Edema

Drawing blood from a patient's arm in which there is an intravenous (IV) fluid running is not recommended because the fluid could dilute the results of the tests. A glucose drip could falsely increase glucose values. If an arm with an IV tube must be used, always draw on the arm *below* the IV insertion area.

Areas affected by **edema** (abnormal accumulation of fluid in interstitial spaces) should not be used for venipuncture because the fluid may contaminate and dilute the test results.

Other Areas to Avoid

Veins that are obstructed in some way—such as those that are sclerosed with plaque, scarred, or occluded—should not be used. Sites that are burned and susceptible to infection should also be avoided.

Risk Management

OSHA regulates the Bloodborne Pathogens Standard by requiring all health care facilities to have an exposure control plan in place to help reduce employee exposure. The most common exposure to bloodborne pathogens in health care results from accidental puncture wounds with contaminated needles, glass, or other sharp items. In an effort to reduce these percutaneous incidents in the workplace, the Bloodborne Pathogens Standard requires documentation of the selection and evaluation of any new safety technology used by employees. The goal is to determine the effectiveness of new safety devices in the following areas:

- Decreased risk of injuries
- Acceptance of the device by users
- Ability of the device to not affect patient care adversely

Two sample safety device evaluation forms from OSHA are included in the workbook: "Sample Device Preselection Worksheet" and "Sample Device Evaluation Form." All employees who are at risk of exposure must be alert and involved in finding ways to eliminate exposure to bloodborne pathogens. Be sure to take the time to fill out the forms and answer the questions during the blood-collecting laboratory practice sessions.

Review Questions

1. What is the *most critical* error a phlebotomist can make?
   a. not collecting enough blood
   b. not releasing the tourniquet before removing the needle
   c. misidentifying the patient
   d. collecting the blood in the wrong tube

2. A certified medical assistant is in the process of collecting a blood sample by the Vacutainer method. During the procedure a hematoma begins to form. Which of the following scenarios could explain why this occurred?
   a. The bevel is against the wall of the vein.
   b. The bevel is in the middle of the vein.
   c. The bevel was inserted above the vein.
   d. The bevel is only partially inserted in the vein.

3. Which of the following tubes is used for coagulation studies?
   a. lavender
   b. light blue
   c. green
   d. gray

4. A capillary puncture is performed on a newborn. All the following steps are correct *except*
   a. The puncture site is warmed before the puncture is made.
   b. The medial or lateral section of the plantar surface of the foot is the site of the puncture.
   c. A lancet no deeper than 3 mm is used for the puncture.
   d. The first drop of blood is wiped away.

5. A certified medical assistant is performing a Vacutainer blood collection. Which of the following techniques is incorrect?
   a. The tourniquet is placed 3 inches above the puncture site.
   b. The puncture site is cleaned with 70% isopropyl alcohol in a concentric circular motion, starting with the puncture site and spreading outward.
   c. The tourniquet is removed after the last tube and the needle are removed.
   d. The tubes are mixed 8 to 10 times after being filled with blood.

6. If the angle of needle insertion is lower than 15 degrees during a venipuncture procedure, which of the following may occur?
   a. The needle may enter above the vein.
   b. The needle may pierce completely through the vein.
   c. The vein may collapse.
   d. The needle bevel may stick to the bottom of the vein wall.

7. You are in the process of drawing blood when you notice that the patient is looking pale and sweating. Which of the following steps should you *not* do?
   a. Continue with the procedure until all the required blood is drawn.
   b. Call for help.
   c. Try to get the patient into a reclining position.
   d. Apply cold compresses to the patient's head and back of the neck.

8. What is the recommended maximum time to leave a tourniquet on?
   a. 4 minutes
   b. 3 minutes
   c. 2 minutes
   d. 1 minute

Advanced Concepts

9. Which of the following tests should *not* be done by the capillary puncture method?
    a. glucose
    b. complete blood count
    c. blood cultures
    d. cholesterol

10. The following tubes are being used in a Vacutainer venipuncture procedure: green, lavender, red (plastic), and light blue. Place them in the correct order of draw.

Review Question Answers

1. c
2. d
3. b
4. c
5. c
6. a
7. a
8. d
9. c
10. Light blue, red plastic (has clot activator—should not be drawn before the light blue), green, and lavender.

Websites

http://www.nlm.nih.gov/medlineplus/newbornscreening.html
http://kidshealth.org/parent/medical/genetic/newborn_screening_tests.html
http://www.marchofdimes.com/pnhec/298_834.asp
http://www.cincinnatichildrens.org/health/info/newborn/procedure/infant-screening.htm

American Academy of Pediatrics:
www.aap.org
Becton Dickinson site for safety needle and lancet supplies:
www.bd.com
Clinical and Laboratory Standards Institute (formerly NCCLS):
www.clsi.org/
Occupational Safety & Health Administration:
www.osha.gov
www.phlebotomypages.com/phlebotomist_skills.htm
www.marketlabinc.com/products/details/806
www.phlebotomy.com/index.html
www.cdc.gov/niosh/topics/bbp/safer/default.htm
www.bd.com/safety/products/b_collect/index.asp#b3

Maternal and Child Health Bureau of the Health Resources and Services Administration:
www.mchb.hrsa.gov
Website for vein finder: www.venoscope.com

CHAPTER 5

Hematology

Objectives
After completing this chapter you should be able to:

Fundamental Concepts
1. Define and match terms and abbreviations from the glossary.
2. Identify the proper specimen collection for hematology testing.
3. Identify the blood components found in bone marrow and peripheral blood, and describe their functions.
4. Describe and identify the basic formation of cells in the bone marrow.
5. Perform a blood smear and stain.
6. Identify typical blood cells from a stained blood smear.
7. Observe selected abnormal cells from visual aids.
8. Describe the basic principles of hemostasis (including the involvement of blood vessels, platelets, clotting factors, and anticoagulants).

CLIA-Waived Tests
1. Identify equipment and supplies used in waived hematology and coagulation tests.
2. Follow the most current OSHA safety guidelines when performing hematology and coagulation tests, and apply the correct quality control for the CLIA-waived hematology tests.
3. Perform the FDA-approved hemoglobin, hematocrit, erythrocyte sedimentation rate, and prothrombin time waived tests according to the stated task, conditions, and standards listed in the Learning Outcome Evaluations in the student workbook.
4. Describe the role of prothrombin in blood coagulation.
5. Explain the major use of the prothrombin time test.

Advanced Concepts
1. Describe the seven tests involved in the complete blood count.
2. Identify the red blood cell indices, and explain their significance in determining anemia.
3. Explain the significance of the white blood cell count and differential.
4. Discuss the moderately complex QBC method used in ambulatory settings. Compare the QBC method to the Coulter method of complete blood count testing.

Key Terms

anemia condition in which the red blood cell or hemoglobin level is below normal
anisocytosis abnormal variances in red blood cell size
band immature neutrophil whose nucleus has not segmented (also called *stab*)
baso- prefix meaning alkaline
basophil white blood cell with large granules that stain dark blue
cytoplasm fluid within cells between the nucleus and the outer cell membrane
differential count procedure for determining the distribution of the five types of leukocytes based on their staining characteristics, shapes, and sizes
embolus traveling clot
eosino- prefix meaning *acid*
eosinophil white blood cell with large granules that stain red
erythroblasts immature red blood cells (also called *rubriblasts*)
erythrocyte sedimentation rate (ESR) rate at which red blood cells settle out of an anticoagulated blood specimen after 60 minutes

fibrinogen (factor I) one of two plasma proteins involved in clotting
formed elements cells and cell fragments that can be viewed under the microscope
granulocytes white blood cells that contain granules in their cytoplasm: neutrophils, basophils, and eosinophils
hematocrit test that measures percentage of packed red blood cells compared with total blood volume
hematologist one who evaluates the cellular elements of blood microscopically and analytically by using a variety of test methods
hematology study of the visible cellular components in the bloodstream and bone marrow
hematopoiesis blood production
hemocytoblast stem cell that differentiates (changes) and becomes any of the seven visible blood elements found in circulating blood
hemoglobin oxygen-carrying reddish pigment in red blood cells
hemolysis (hemolyzing) destruction of the red blood cells

Key Terms—cont'd

hemostasis body's ability to initiate a clotting response to stop bleeding and at the same time prevent the blood from forming an unwanted stationary clot
hyperchromia increase in color (based on hemoglobin concentration)
hypochromic pertaining to less than normal color
hypoxemia lack of oxygen in the blood
immunoglobulins antibodies that destroy or render harmless foreign invaders containing antigens
leukemia various cancers of the white blood cells
leukocytosis abnormal increase in white blood cells
leukopenia abnormal decrease in white blood cells
lymphocyte small, nongranular white blood cell that develops from lymphoblasts in bone marrow
macrophages large, engulfing cells that come from monocytes when they enter the tissues
megakaryocyte large nuclear cell in the bone marrow that fragments its cytoplasm to become platelets
monocytes large, nongranular white blood cells that develop from monoblasts in bone marrow
myeloblasts stem cells that develop into the three kinds of granulocytes
neutro- prefix meaning *neither acid nor alkaline*
neutrophil white blood cells with fine granules that stain lavender/pink
nongranulocytes (agranulocytes) white blood cells that may have a few or no granules in their cytoplasm; lymphocytes and monocytes
normocytes young red blood cells that shed their nuclei before entering the bloodstream
nucleus central controlling structure in the cell
-phil suffix meaning *attraction*
poikilocytosis abnormal shapes in red blood cells
polychromia increase in color variation (based on hemoglobin concentration)
polycythemia abnormal condition of increased red blood cells
polymorphonuclear having a multishaped, segmented nucleus; sometimes abbreviated as *PMN* or *seg*
prothrombin (factor II) one of two plasma proteins involved in clotting
protime test test for monitoring coagulation times for patients taking anticoagulants
RBC indices mathematic ratios of the three red blood cell tests (hemoglobin, hematocrit, and red blood cell count)
reticulocytes newly released red blood cells in the blood that still contain some nuclear DNA
rouleaux formation arrangement of red blood cells resembling stacked chips
thrombocytes platelets; cellular fragments that gather at the site of a damaged blood vessel and release clotting chemicals to form a clot
thrombosis abnormal condition of clotting
thrombus unwanted stationary clot
vitamin K critical element in the production of prothrombin

Abbreviations

ALL	acute lymphocytic leukemia	**Hgb**	hemoglobin
AML	acute myelocytic leukemia	**INR**	international normalized ratio (for protime test results)
CBC	complete blood count		
CLL	chronic lymphocytic leukemia	**MCH**	mean cell hemoglobin
CML	chronic myelocytic leukemia	**MCHC**	mean (average) cell hemoglobin concentration
ESR	erythrocyte sedimentation rate	**MCV**	mean cell volume
g/dL	grams per deciliter (g/dL), which represents the weight of a substance (g) per volume (dL)	**PMN**	polymorphonuclear
		PT	prothrombin time (protime)
HCT	hematocrit		

FUNDAMENTAL CONCEPTS

Overview of Hematology and Blood

Hematology is the study of the visible cellular components in the bloodstream and bone marrow. The complete blood count **(CBC)** is one of the most commonly ordered "routine" tests for evaluating a person's internal health status. **Hematologists** work in the hematology departments of hospitals, reference labs, and private practices, where they evaluate the blood's cellular elements microscopically and analytically by using a variety of test methods. Hematologists may also evaluate **hemostasis,** the body's ability to initiate a clotting response to stop bleeding and at the same time prevent the blood from forming an unwanted stationary clot.

In the ambulatory setting, basic CLIA-waived hematology tests and coagulation (clotting) tests are performed on capillary blood. If a reference laboratory does the testing, the requisition and laboratory protocol must be checked to determine the proper tubes to draw and how they are to be processed. The blood for hematology tests is usually collected in lavender-topped vacuum tubes containing the anticoagulant ethylenediaminetetraacetic acid (EDTA), which also preserves cellular elements in their natural state.

The blood for coagulation studies is usually collected in blue-topped vacuum tubes that must be allowed to fill accurately because the blood and the liquid anticoagulant in the tube must be in the proper ratio. This is why a "waste" tube is needed when using the butterfly needle and tubing.

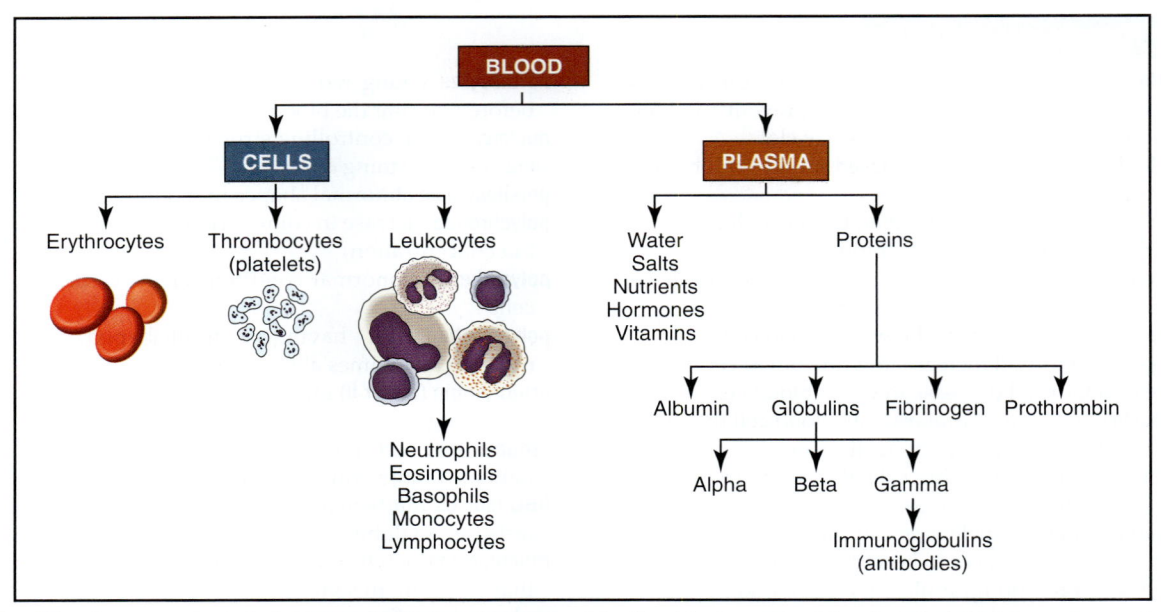

Fig. 5-1. Blood components. *Left*, Formed cellular elements; *right*, liquid plasma and its chemical divisions. (From Chabner D: *The language of medicine,* ed 8, St Louis, 2007, Saunders.)

Blood is a complex liquid connective tissue that is constantly circulating through the blood vessels. The **formed elements** within blood can be viewed under the microscope as cells and cell fragments (Fig. 5-1, *left*). These formed elements are suspended in the watery liquid called *plasma,* which contains hundreds of dissolved biochemical substances (see Fig. 5-1, *right*). (NOTE: Chapters 6 and 7 will focus on the biochemical substances located in the plasma.)

Blood cells are produced in the red bone marrow found in flat bones and at the ends of long bones (Fig. 5-2). All the cells originate from a stem cell, or **hemocytoblast,** that differentiates (changes) and becomes any of the following seven visible blood elements found in circulating blood (red blood cells, five types of white blood cells, and platelets):

- Red blood cells (RBCs, also called *erythrocytes*)
- White blood cells (WBCs, also called *leukocytes*):
  - Basophils
  - Neutrophils
  - Eosinophils
  - Monocytes
  - Lymphocytes
- Platelets (also called *thrombocytes*)

Fig. 5-3 is a simplified flow chart illustrating blood production, or **hematopoiesis.** Each of the seven formed elements is viewed and discussed as it is developed in the bone marrow and then released into the bloodstream or tissue, where it fulfills its function.

Red Blood Cells (Erythrocytes)

The bone marrow is constantly producing new RBCs. The beginning stages of RBC production in the bone marrow are shown in Fig. 5-4. **Erythroblasts**

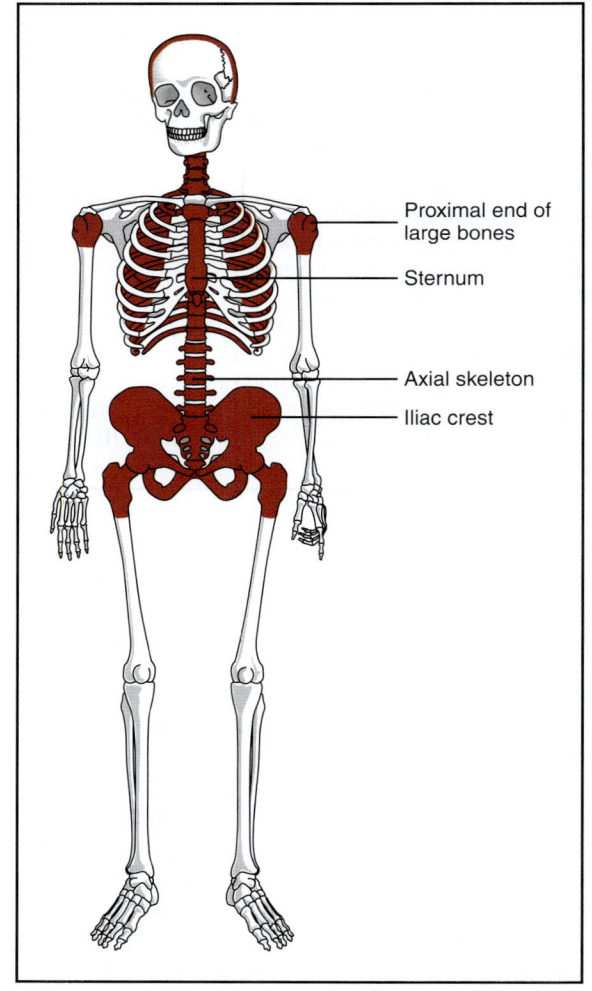

Fig. 5-2. Red bone marrow sites of hemopoiesis. (From Rodak BF: *Hematology: clinical principles and applications,* ed 3, St. Louis, 2007, Saunders.)

Fundamental Concepts

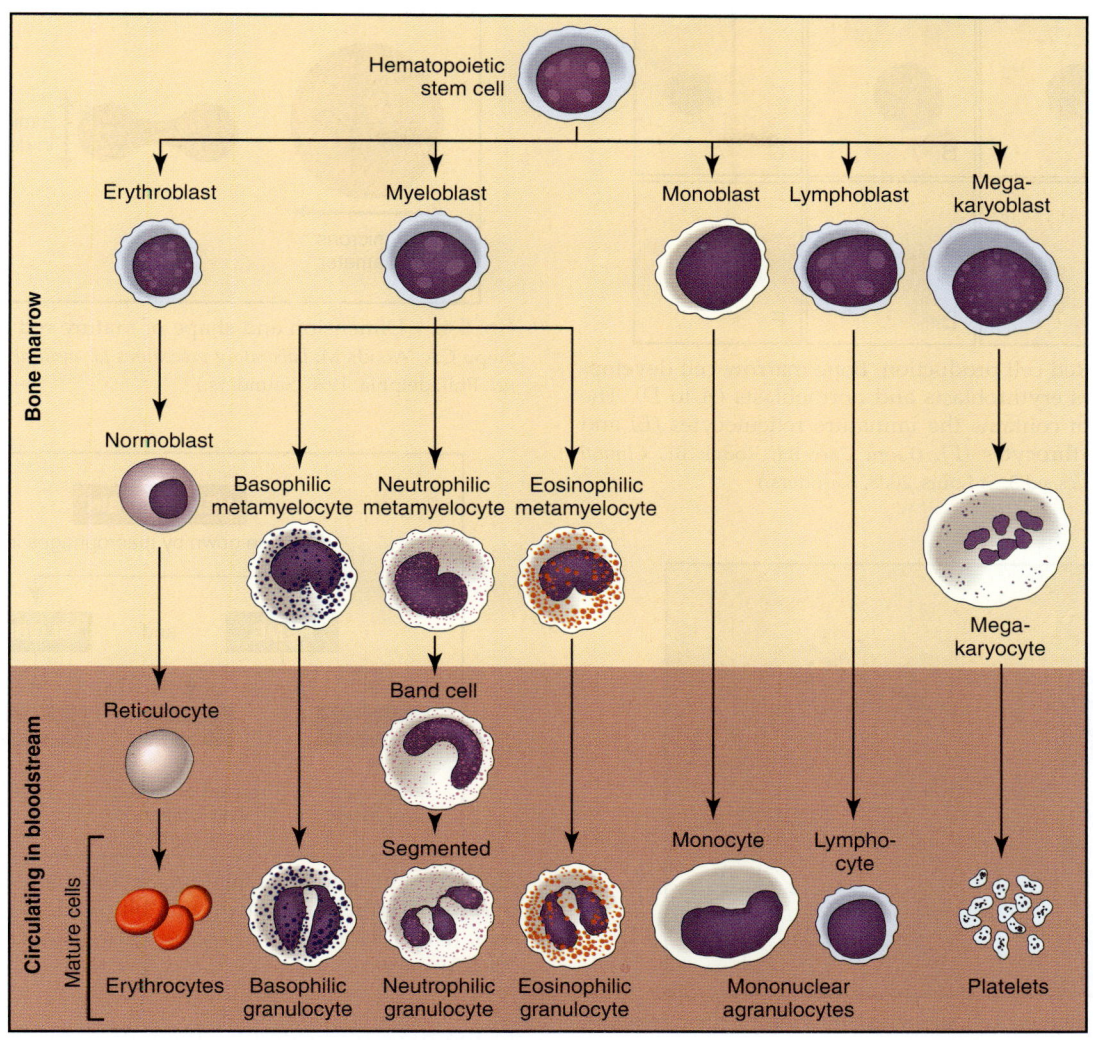

Fig. 5-3. Hematopoiesis. Note the stem cell's differentiation in the bone marrow *(top)* and immature and mature cellular elements in the peripheral bloodstream *(bottom)*. (From Chabner D: *The language of medicine,* ed 8, St Louis, 2007, Saunders.)

(immature RBCs), also called *rubriblasts,* become **normocytes** that shed their nuclei before entering the bloodstream. In the bloodstream the young RBCs, which still contain some nuclear deoxyribonucleic acid (DNA), are called **reticulocytes** (Fig. 5-5). The average amount of reticulocytes found in peripheral blood is approximately 1%. A percentage higher than 3% indicates that the individual is actively producing new red cells because of a loss of RBCs, such as when hemorrhaging occurs. As the reticulocytes continue to mature, they shed their remaining intracellular nuclear material while retaining millions of **hemoglobin (Hgb)** molecules (reddish pigment capable of carrying oxygen).

Mature red cells are biconcave disks filled with a reddish pigment called *hemoglobin* (Fig. 5-6). Hgb consists of an iron (heme) and a protein (globin) molecule. Hgb has a strong affinity for oxygen that it picks up and carries from the lungs to the cells of the body. This oxygen-carrying capacity of RBCs is critical to sustaining life energy throughout the body. Because of their critical role, RBCs account for almost half of the blood volume. After 80 to 120 days, RBCs disintegrate, releasing the iron (heme) portion, which goes back to the bone marrow to make new RBCs (Fig. 5-7). The remaining elements convert to bilirubin, which is further processed through various stages in the liver, intestines, and kidneys (Fig. 5-8).

White Blood Cells

WBCs fall into two general categories: granulocytes, consisting of neutrophils, basophils, and eosinophils; and nongranulocytes, consisting of lymphocytes and monocytes.

Granulocytes
Myeloblasts are the stem cells in the bone marrow that become myelocytes (see Fig. 5-3). The myelocytes develop into the three kinds of granulocytes:

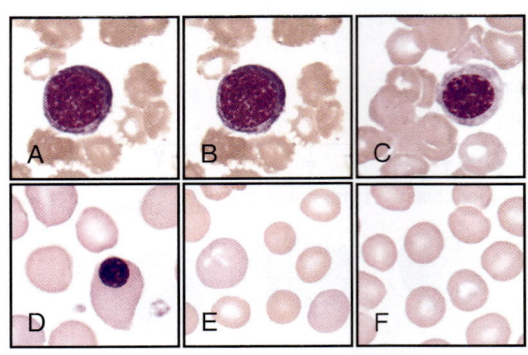

Fig. 5-4. Red cell production. Bone marrow cell development shows erythroblasts and normoblasts *(A to D)*. The bloodstream contains the immature reticulocytes *(E)* and mature erythrocytes *(F)*. (From Carr JH, Rodak BF: *Clinical hematology atlas,* ed 3, St Louis, 2008, Saunders.)

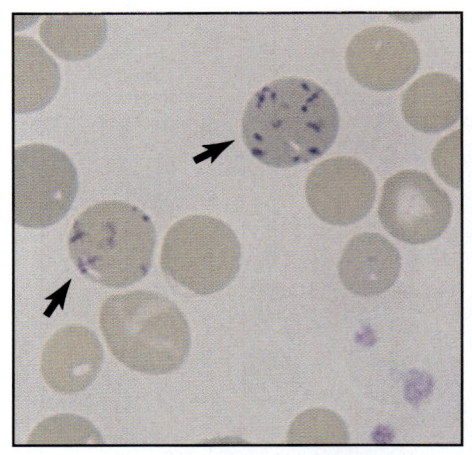

Fig. 5-5. Stained reticulocytes showing nuclear remains. (From Rodak BF: *Hematology: clinical principles and applications,* ed 3, St Louis, 2007, Saunders.)

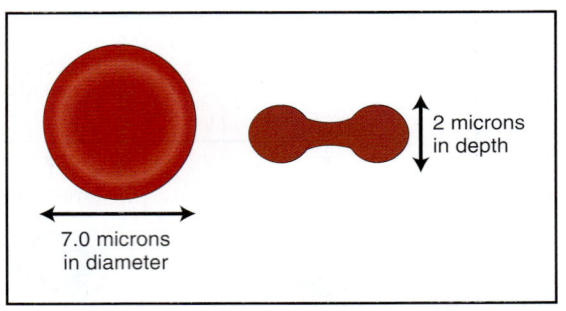

Fig. 5-6. Dimension and shape of mature red cells. (From Stepp CA, Woods M: *Laboratory procedures for medical office personnel,* Philadelphia, 1998, Saunders.)

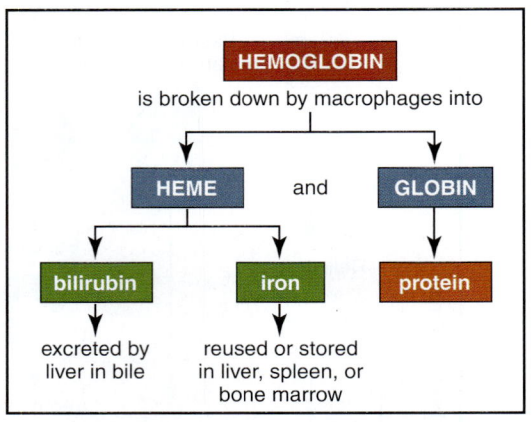

Fig. 5-7. Breakdown of hemoglobin into heme and globin and their further breakdown into bilirubin, iron, and protein. (From Chabner D: *The language of medicine,* ed 8, St Louis, 2007, Saunders.)

neutrophils, eosinophils, and basophils. Fig. 5-9 illustrates a myeloblast becoming a myelocyte and metamyelocyte within the bone marrow. The granulocyte enters the bloodstream with its **nucleus** (the central controlling structure in the cell) in an elongated "band" shape. The maturing nuclei of the eosinophils and basophils become segmented into two lobes. The mature neutrophil's multisegmented nucleus is referred to as *polymorphonuclear (PMN)* or as a *seg* (Fig. 5-10).

The three mature **granulocytes** in the bloodstream are distinguished from one another by the staining characteristics of the granules located in their **cytoplasm** (fluid within cells between the nucleus and the outer cell membrane). When a drop of whole blood is smeared onto a slide and then stained, the three different granulocytic WBCs show an affinity, or attraction, to either the *red* acid dye **(eosino)**, the *blue* alkaline dye **(baso)**, or *both* colors **(neutro)**. The WBCs are named on the basis of their *attraction* to the dyes (indicated by the suffix -**phil**) and have distinct purposes in aiding the body during infection and inflammation.

Neutrophils. Neutrophils have small granules that stain lavender/pink {Leave the / in rather than "or"}. They are usually the most numerous WBCs in the blood because of their ability to engulf and digest foreign matter, especially pathogenic bacteria.

Eosinophils. Eosinophils have large granules that stain red. They increase in number during allergic reactions and parasitic infestations.

Basophils. Basophils have large granules that stain dark blue. They are the rarest WBCs in the blood and are involved in preventing blood from excessive clotting by producing the anticoagulant heparin. They also mediate the inflammatory response.

Nongranulocytes (Agranulocytes). Bone marrow also produces the following two **nongranulocytes,** or **agranulocytes,** which may have a few or no granules in their gray and sky-blue cytoplasm:

Fundamental Concepts

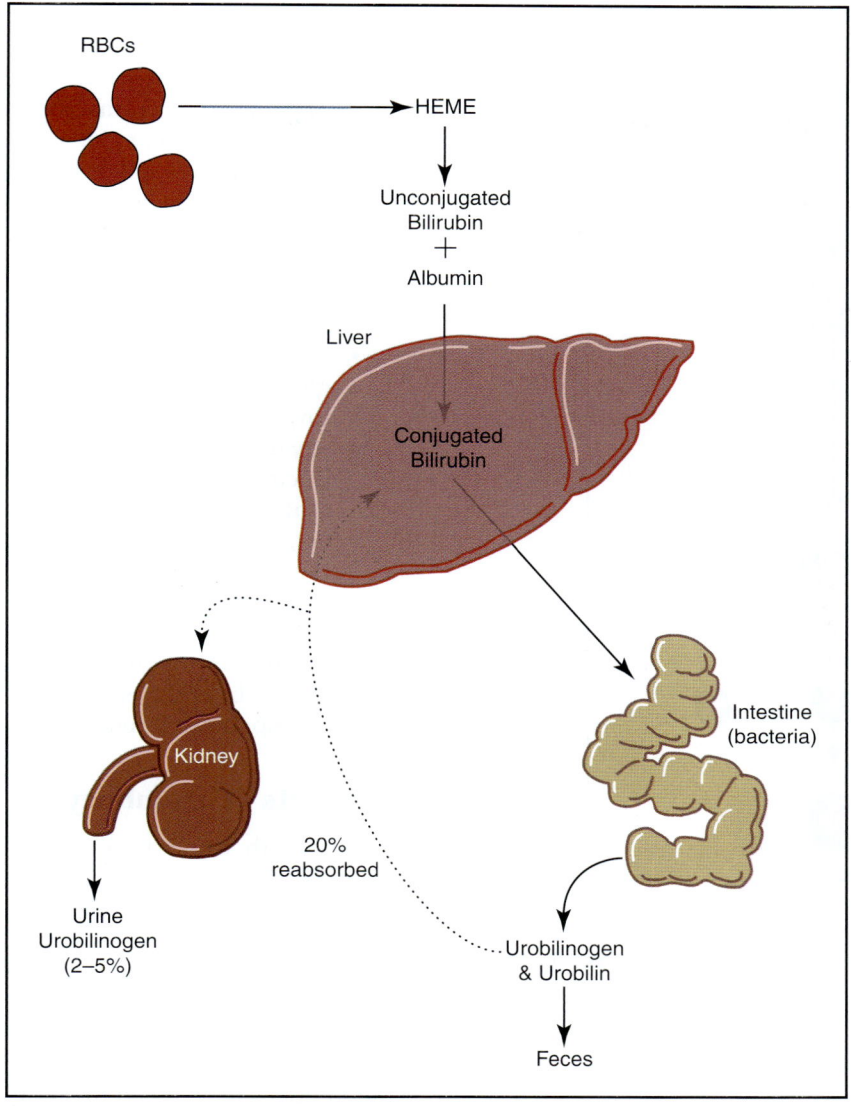

Fig. 5-8. Bilirubin metabolism in the liver, intestines, and kidney. (From Rodak BF: *Hematology: clinical principles and applications,* ed 3, St Louis, 2007, Saunders.)

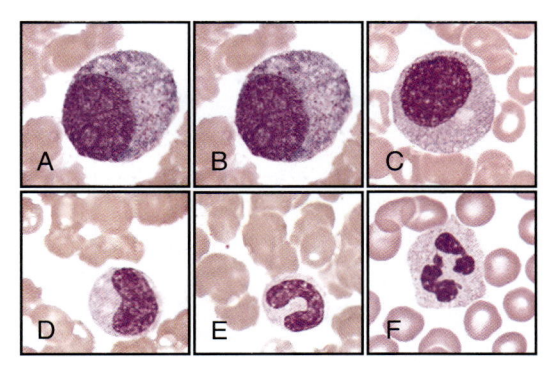

Fig. 5-9. Granulocytic white blood cell production. Bone marrow cell development shows myeloblasts becoming myelocytes (**A** to **D**). The bloodstream contains the immature band (**E**) and the mature polymorphonuclear neutrophil (**F**), also referred to as *seg*. (From Carr JH, Rodak BF: *Clinical hematology atlas,* ed 3, St Louis, 2008, Saunders.)

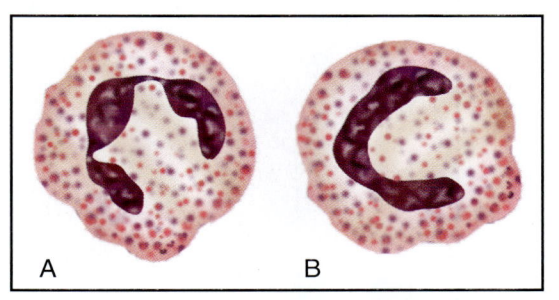

Fig. 5-10. Compare the multilobed mature nucleus in the seg (**A**) with the immature nucleus in the band neutrophil (**B**). (From Stepp CA, Woods M: *Laboratory procedures for medical office personnel,* Philadelphia, 1998, Saunders.)

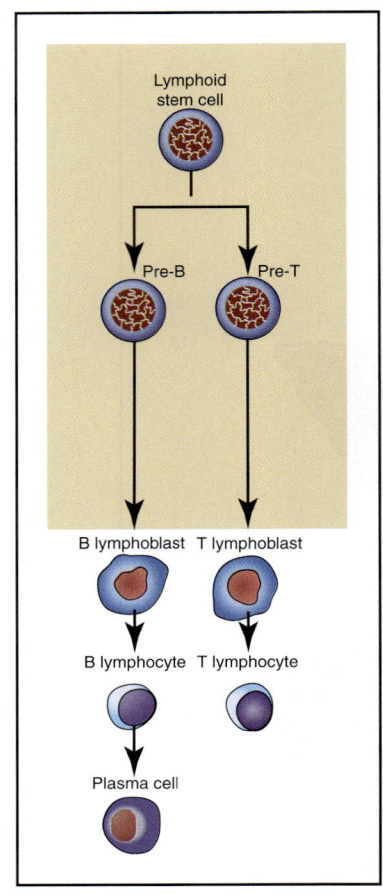

Fig. 5-11. Lymphocytic flow chart showing the lymphoblast differentiating into B and T lymphoblasts and cells. The B cells become plasma cells when they leave the bloodstream and enter body tissues. (From Carr JH, Rodak BF: *Clinical hematology atlas*, ed 3, St Louis, 2008, Saunders.)

1. **Monocytes** in the blood originate as monoblasts (immature monocytes) in the bone marrow. They are the largest WBCs and can leave the bloodstream to enter the tissues as **macrophages** (large, engulfing cells). Their numbers increase during the recovery stage of infection and during the healing of traumatized tissue when debris needs to be cleaned up.
2. **Lymphocytes** are the smallest, nongranular WBCs that develop from lymphoblasts (immature lymphocytes) in the bone marrow. They further differentiate into B and T cells (Fig. 5-11).
   - *T lymphocytes* are stimulated by the thymus gland to develop a variety of immune responses toward invaders.
   - *B lymphocytes* become plasma cells capable of producing specific antibodies (**immunoglobulins**) that destroy or render harmless foreign invaders, especially viruses. (The immune response involving T and B lymphocytes is covered in Chapter 7.)

   Lymphocytes are the smallest WBCs in the bloodstream. They move freely among the blood vessels, lymph vessels, and tissues as they constantly survey for and respond to foreign invaders.

Platelets (Thrombocytes)

The seventh formed element also comes from the stem cell (hemocytoblast) after it differentiates into a megakaryoblast and then into a **megakaryocyte** (large nuclear cell) in the bone marrow (Fig. 5-12). This very large cell releases fragments of its cytoplasm into the bloodstream, which are seen as small **thrombocytes,** or platelets.

Platelets gather around the site of a damaged blood vessel in an effort to "plug" the leak (Fig. 5-13).

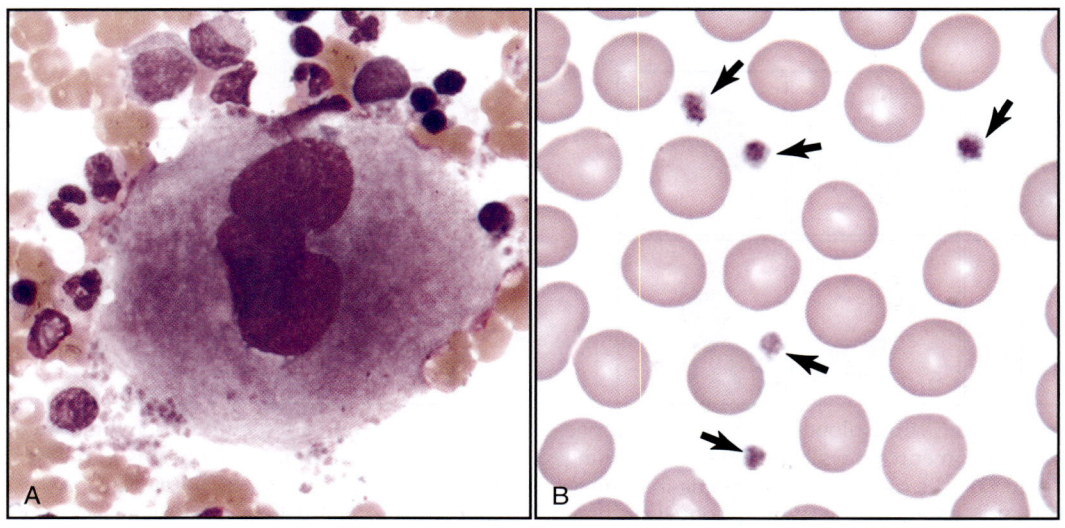

Fig. 5-12. Megakaryocyte in the bone marrow (**A**) and cytoplasmic platelets in the bloodstream (**B**). (From Carr JH, Rodak BF: *Clinical hematology atlas*, ed 3, St Louis, 2008, Saunders.)

Fundamental Concepts

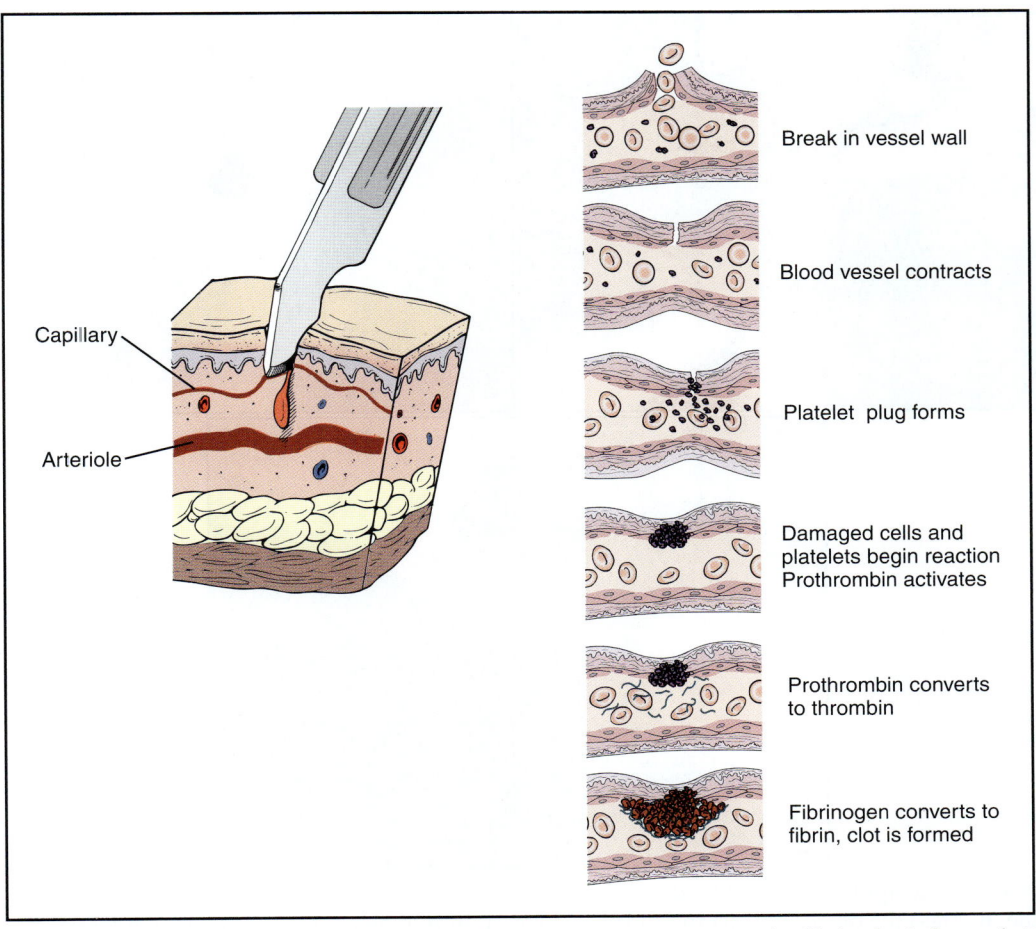

Fig. 5-13. Hemostasis. The damaged blood vessel constricts, platelets congregate, and a fibrin clot is formed. (From Stepp CA, Woods M: *Laboratory procedures for medical office personnel,* Philadelphia, 1998, Saunders.)

They also release clotting chemicals that activate the formation of sticky fibrin strands that entangle the blood cells and form a clot (Fig. 5-14).

Preparing a Blood Smear for Observation by Physician or Laboratory Technician

A blood smear can be made by using fresh blood from a gently mixed lavender-topped EDTA Vacutainer tube (Becton Dickinson, Franklin Lakes, N.J.) or from a fresh capillary puncture. A drop of blood is placed on the end of a clean slide with a Diff safety device (Becton Dickinson) inserted into the lavender EDTA tube. This device is a convenient and safe way to obtain a drop of blood from the Vacutainer tube without removing the sealed top of the tube. Push the white device into the top of the EDTA lavender tube, then invert the tube and press the device against the slide (Fig. 5-15). The pressure on the slide causes a drop of blood to flow onto the

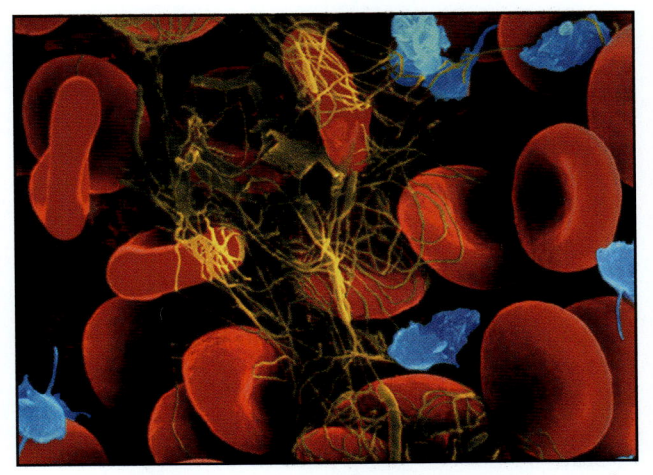

Fig. 5-14. Fibrin strands enmesh the cells and form a clot that plugs the bleeding vessel. (From Chabner D: *The language of medicine,* ed 8, St Louis, 2007, Saunders. Originally from Page J et al: *Blood: the river of life,* Washington, DC, 1981, New Books.)

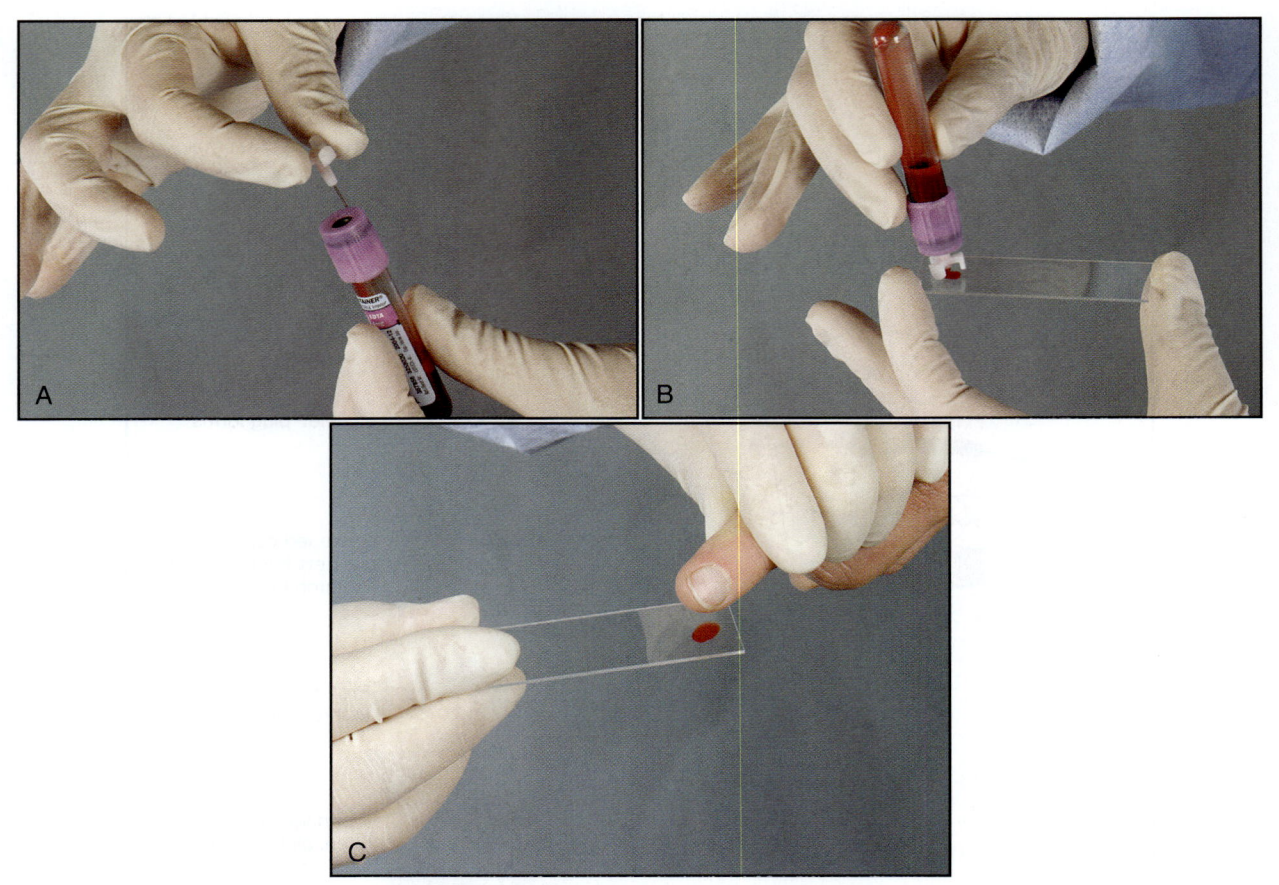

Fig 5-15. **A,** One way to apply a drop of blood to a slide for smearing is to push a Safety Diff device into a lavender-topped Vacutainer tube. **B,** Press the device against the slide to deliver a drop of blood. **C,** Another method is to apply the drop of blood directly from a finger stick.

slide. A drop of blood can also be obtained from a finger capillary puncture. Next, the drop of blood is spread across the slide by bringing a clean "pusher" slide back into the drop at a 30- to 35-degree angle. As soon as the blood spreads approximately three fourths along the edge, quickly move the pusher slide forward (Fig. 5-16). Allow the slide to air dry. A properly performed smear will look like the one in Fig. 5-17. Improper, unacceptable smears resemble those in Fig. 5-18.

Evaluate the smear to see if the following are present:
1. A feathered edge
2. A well-distributed "body" with margins on each side
3. Smooth, thick-to-thin spreading of the smear with no ridges or tails

The smeared blood slide is then stained with either Wright's stain or a Quick Diff (Becton Dickinson) stain. Both of these staining methods use three ingredients: a methanol fixative, a red acid dye, and a blue alkaline dye. The Wright's stain also uses a buffer solution to change the pH. Refer to the material safety data sheets in the workbook and the labels on the bottles when working with stains, and take appropriate precautions. The simple Quick Diff staining procedure used in ambulatory settings is provided in the workbook and is demonstrated in Procedure 5-1 at the end of this section.

Stained blood smears must be observed by the physician, a trained hematologist, or a laboratory technician.

White Blood Cell Identification and Differential

The hematologist scans stained blood smears to identify the distribution of the five types of leukocytes on the basis of their staining characteristics, shapes, and sizes. This procedure is called a **differential count.** See the WBC atlas on pp. 140-141, which lists and shows the distinguishing characteristics that are observed for each of the leukocytes.

Fundamental Concepts

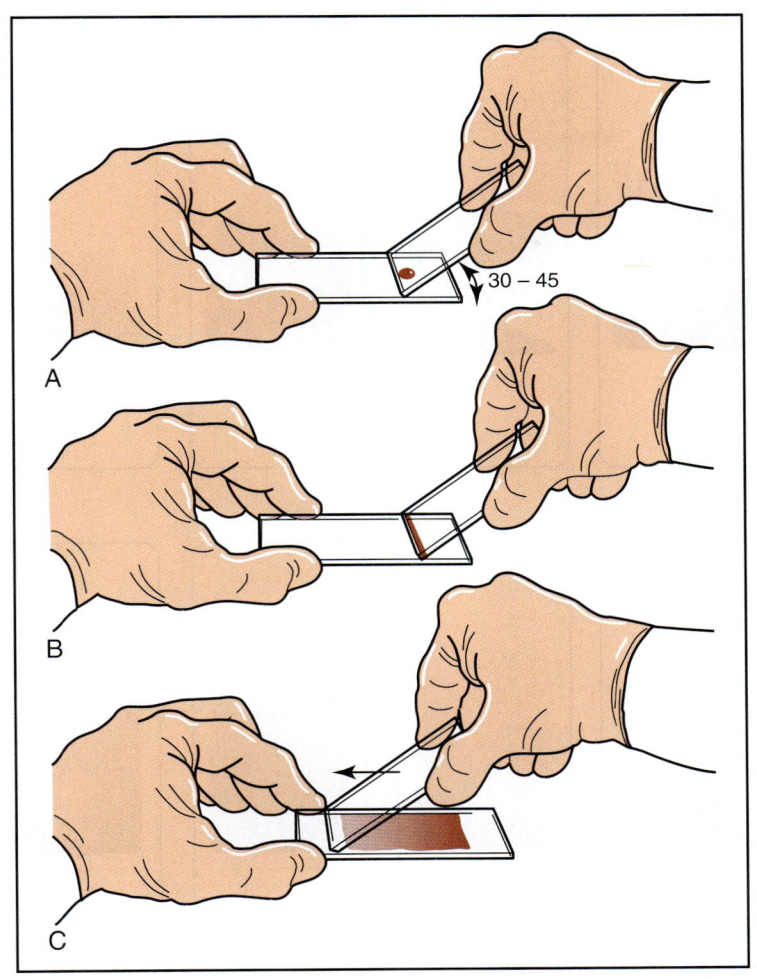

Fig. 5-16. Proper blood smear technique. **A,** Pull upper slide back into the drop of blood. **B,** Allow blood to spread along the edge of the slide. **C,** Then, with downward pressure, quickly push the slide to the other end until stopped by the fingers. (From Rodak BF: *Hematology: clinical principles and applications,* ed 3, St Louis, 2007, Saunders.)

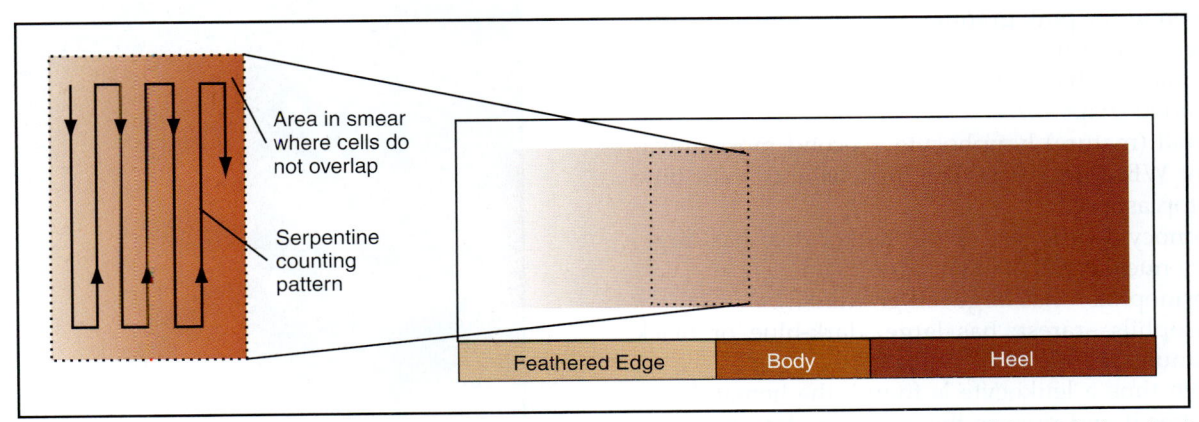

Fig. 5-17. Ideal smear, showing the thinning out of the feathered edge on the left with the body of the slide for viewing the cells. The "heel" is the thick area of blood cells that were pulled from the drop of blood. Note the serpentine pattern of moving the slide up and over and down and over the body of the smear to observe many different fields without duplicating an area. (From Stepp CA, Woods M: *Laboratory procedures for medical office personnel,* Philadelphia, 1998, Saunders.)

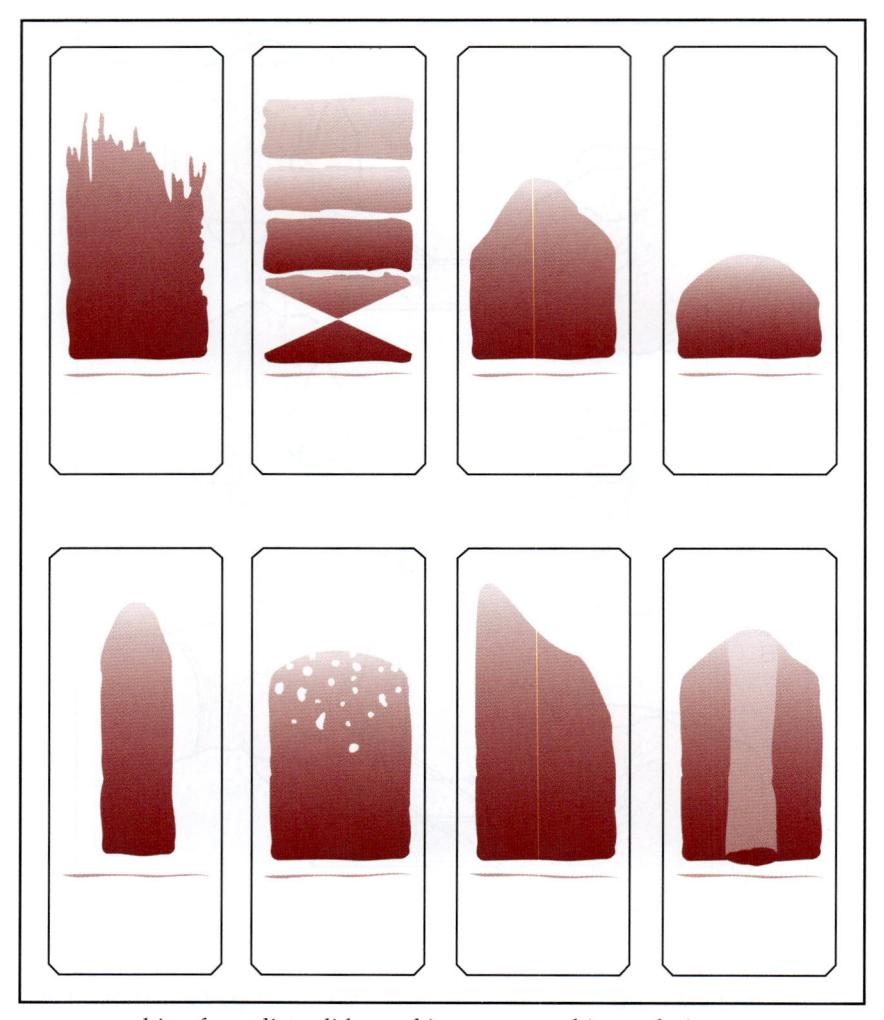

Fig. 5-18. Improper smears resulting from dirty slides and improper pushing techniques. (From Rodak BF: *Hematology: clinical principles and applications,* ed 3, St Louis, 2007, Saunders.)

Note the following facts found in the atlas for each of the following:
- Segmented neutrophil—most prevalent WBC; fine lavender or pink granules in the cytoplasm and a segmented nucleus *(A)*
- Immature banded neutrophil; nucleus has a banded shape *(B)*
- Small (mature) lymphocyte—second most prevalent WBC: dense circular nucleus and scant blue cytoplasm *(C)*
- Monocytes—largest of the leukocytes; has large, lacy nucleus *(D)*
- Eosinophils—has large red granules *(E)*
- Basophils—rarest; has large, dark-blue or black granules *(F)*

Each time a leukocyte is found, the hematologist identifies it and presses the corresponding key on a differential counter (Fig. 5-19). After identifying 100 leukocytes, the counter sounds a bell. Each of the five leukocytes is then displayed as a percentage of the total 100 cells identified.

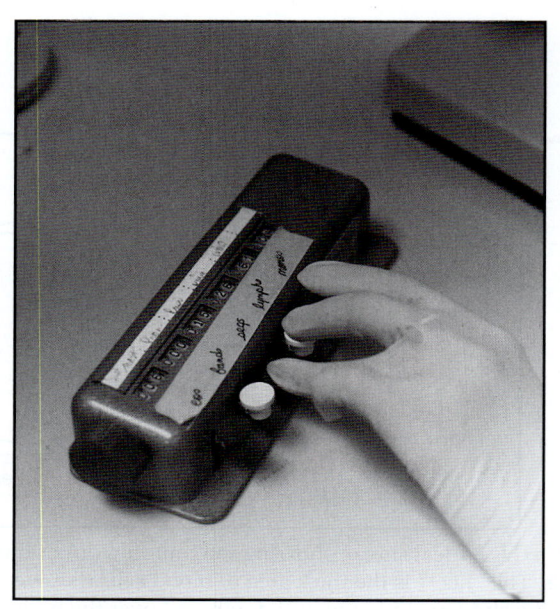

Fig. 5-19. Differential counter. (From Rodak BF: *Hematology: clinical principles and applications,* ed 3, St Louis, 2007, Saunders. Courtesy Beckman Coulter.)

Red Blood Cell Identification and Description

Next, the hematologist observes and reports the appearance of the RBCs. Normal RBC appearance and distribution are shown in the Fig. 5-20). In a diseased state, the RBCs may become altered in appearance. The three columns in flow chart *(A) in the RBC Atlas* show how RBCs can vary in size **(anisocytosis)**, shape **(poikilocytosis)**, and color **(polychromia, hypochromia,** and **hyperchromia)**. The hematologist reports the degree of these variances by using +1, +2, and so on. The following abnormal RBC sizes, colors, and shapes are shown in the RBC Atlas on pp. 142-143:

- Macrocyte (large cell) *(B)*
- Microcyte and hypochromic RBCs (small cell and faded color cells) *(C)*
- Polychromatic RBCs (multicolored cells) *(D)*
- Dacryocytes (tear-shaped cells) *(E)*
- Ovalocytes (elliptical-shaped cells) *(F)*
- Spherocytes (ball-shaped round cells) *(G)*
- Sickle cells (collapsed, C-shaped cells) *(H)*

Platelet Description

Platelets (thrombocytes) are also assessed while scanning the slide (Fig. 5-21). Their quantity is approximated by the hematologist while observing various fields under oil immersion.

Theory of Hemostasis

The cardiovascular system is equipped with a remarkable mechanism that swiftly stops blood from escaping out of a damaged blood vessel. First the blood vessel constricts, slowing down the blood flow. Then platelets concentrate around the damaged site and initiate a clot made of a sticky fibrin mesh (see Figs. 5-13 and 5-14). The fibrin strands are the result of a complex chain reaction of 13 clotting factors, including the two plasma proteins, **fibrinogen (factor I),** and **prothrombin (factor II)** (Table 5-1). The formation of the sticky fibrin can be simplified into four steps, as illustrated in Fig. 5-22.

Once the clot is formed and has fulfilled its purpose, the body stops the reaction to prevent excessive clotting. The body produces a natural anticoagulant, heparin, to keep the clotting mechanism in balance. The anticoagulant will prevent the blood from forming an unwanted stationary clot, or **thrombus,** or releasing a traveling clot, or **embolus.**

Coagulation and Testing

Most coagulation tests are performed at the hospital or reference laboratory to help determine why a patient is bleeding, bruising, or forming clots abnormally. Table 5-2 lists reference values for selected coagulation tests.

A patient who is prone to **thrombosis** (an abnormal condition of clotting) may need to take anticoagulant drugs such as warfarin or coumarin. Patients receiving anticoagulant therapy must be monitored on a predetermined schedule, sometimes weekly moving to monthly over time. They are tested to see the amount of time a sample of their blood takes to coagulate. If their blood coagulates too rapidly, they may have an underdosage of their anticoagulant, which may lead to a life-threatening blood clot. If, on the other hand, the blood coagulates too slowly, it may indicate an overdosage of their anticoagulant, which may cause a fatal hemorrhage.

The CLIA-waived testing method for monitoring these patients' coagulation times is called the prothrombin time, or **protime test.** The result of the test is expressed in seconds as well as in an international normalized ratio **(INR)** that can be compared with recommended therapeutic values regardless of different methods. The INR facilitates the comparison of results of different methods of prothrombin tests. The therapeutic goal is to keep the patient's protime within a range of approximately 9 to 18 seconds (depending on the test method) or at a standardized 2 to 2.5 INR (occasionally higher). A therapeutic protime at this level prolongs the clotting time enough to prevent unwanted clotting but not so long that the patient is in danger of abnormal bleeding.

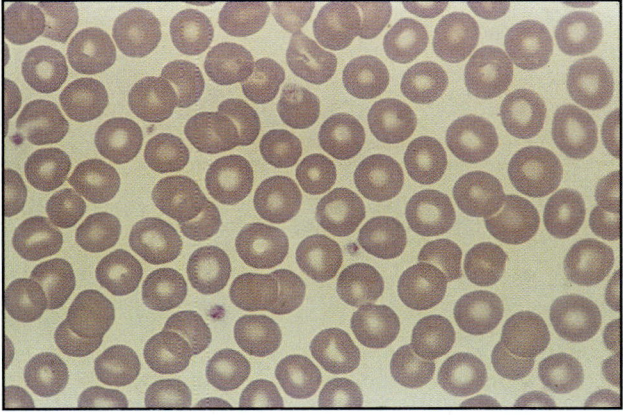

Fig. 5-20. Normal red blood cell appearance and distribution in the body of the smeared slide. This slide contains predominantly red blood cells with a few platelets. (From Rodak BF: *Hematology: clinical principles and applications,* ed 3, St Louis, 2007, Saunders.)

White Blood Cell

	Cell Type	Cell Size (μm)	Nucleus	Chromatin in Nucleus	Cytoplasm
A	Polymorphonuclear neutrophil (poly, PMN), segmented neutrophil (seg)	10-15	Two to five lobes connected by thin filaments	Coarsely clumped	Pale blue to pink
B	Band neutrophil (band)	10-15	C or S shaped, constricted but no thread-like filaments	Coarsely clumped	Pale blue to pink
C	Lymphocyte (lymph)	7-18*	Round to oval; may be slightly indented; occasional nucleoli	Condensed to deeply condensed	Scant to moderate; sky blue; vacuoles may be present
D	Monocyte (mono)	12-20	Variable; may be round, horse-shoe, or kidney shaped; often has folds producing "brainlike" convolutions	Lacy	Blue-gray; may have pseudopods; vacuoles may be absent or numerous
E	Eosinophil (eos)	12-17	Two to three lobes connected by filaments	Coarsely clumped	Pink; may have irregular borders
F	Basophil (baso)	10-14	Usually two lobes connected by thin filaments	Coarsely clumped	Lavender to colorless

*The difference in size from small to large lymphocyte is primarily caused by a larger amount of cytoplasm.
A, Segmented neutrophils, the most prevalent white blood cell, have fine lavender/pink granules throughout the cytoplasm.
B, Banded neutrophils show immature nonsegmented nucleus.
C, Lymphocytes are typically the second most frequently seen white blood cell. Note dense nucleus with scanty cytoplasm.
D, The large monocytes contain a convoluted nucleus and abundant cytoplasm.
E, The eosinophils have large red granules.
F, The basophils have large, dark-blue granules.
Illustrations modified from Carr JH, Rodak BF: Clinical hematology atlas, ed 3, St Louis, 2008, Saunders.

Granules	Reference Range	Microscopic View
Abundant lavender/ pink granules	50%-70%	A
Abundant lavender/ pink granules	0%-5%	B
±Few	20%-40%	C
Many fine granules frequently giving the appearance of ground glass	3%-11%	D
Granules are large red to orange, round	0%-7%	E
Large dark blue/ black; variable in number with uneven distribution	0%-1%	F

Red Blood Cells

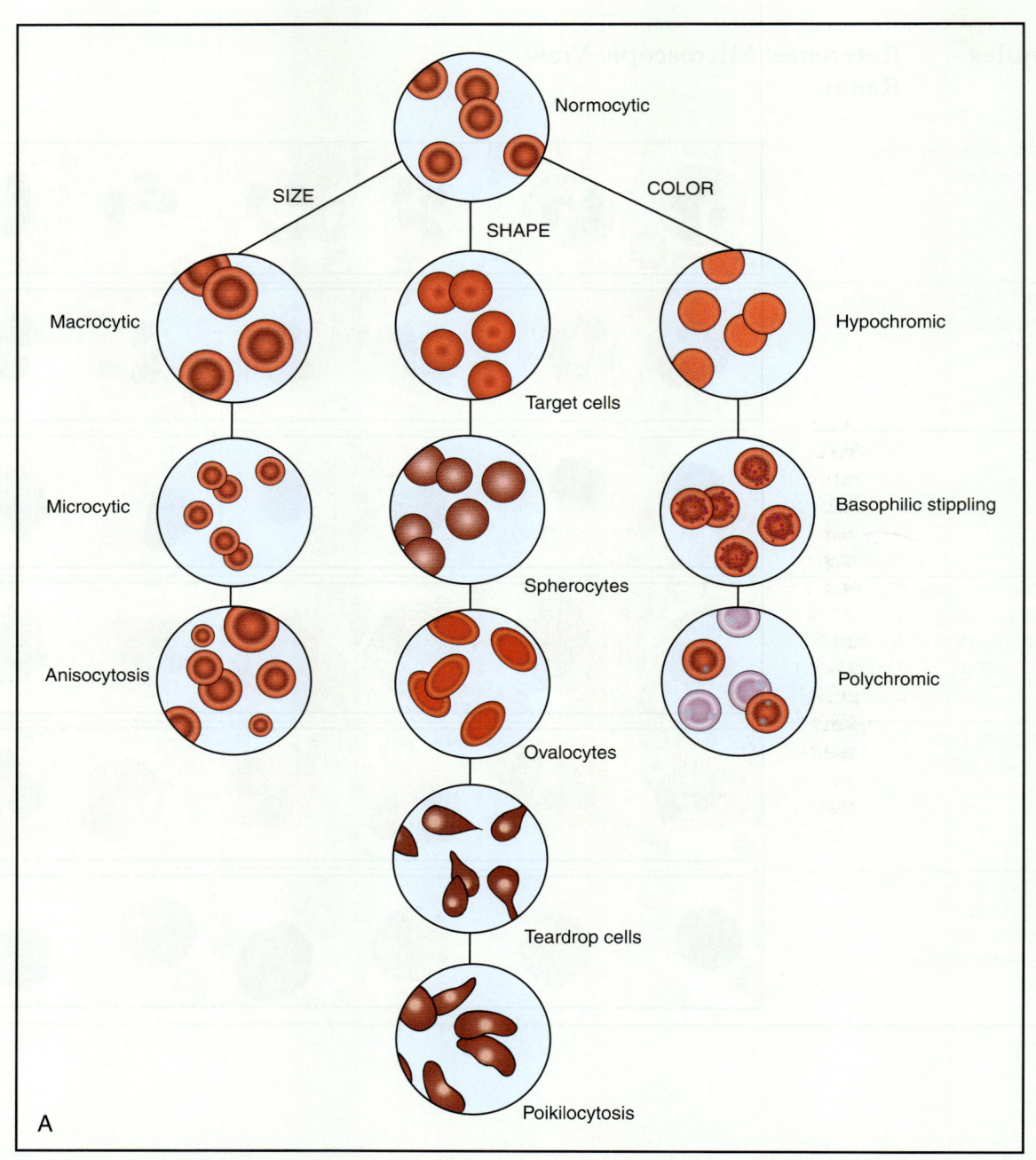

A, Flow chart with the terms relating to variations in red blood cell size *(left)*, shape *(middle)*, and color *(right)*. (From Stepp CA, Woods M: *Laboratory procedures for medical office personnel*, Philadelphia, 1998, Saunders.)

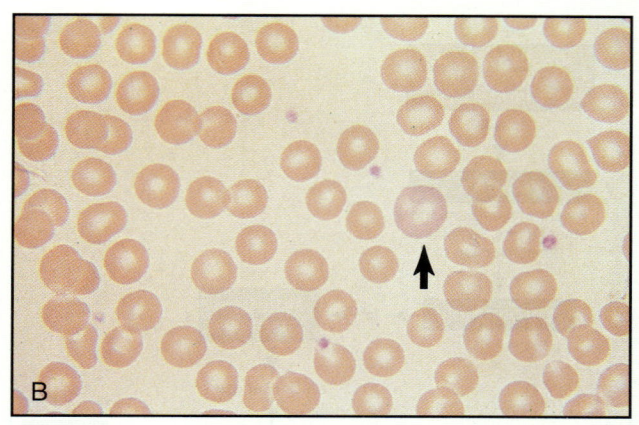

B, Macrocytic red blood cell. (From Rodak BF: *Hematology: clinical principles and applications,* ed 3, St Louis, 2007, Saunders.)

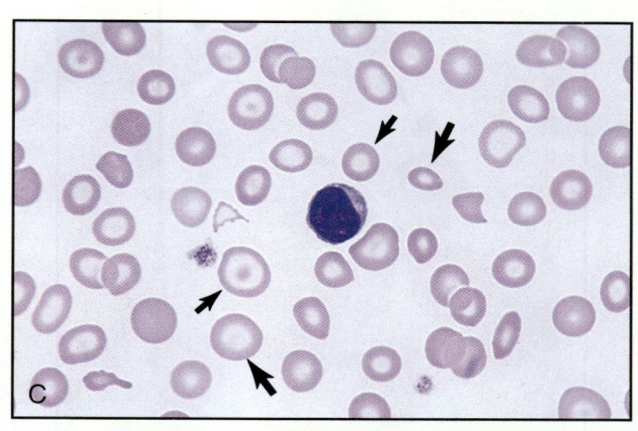

C, Microcytes; hypochromic red blood cells. (From Rodak BF: *Hematology: clinical principles and applications,* ed 3, St Louis, 2007, Saunders.)

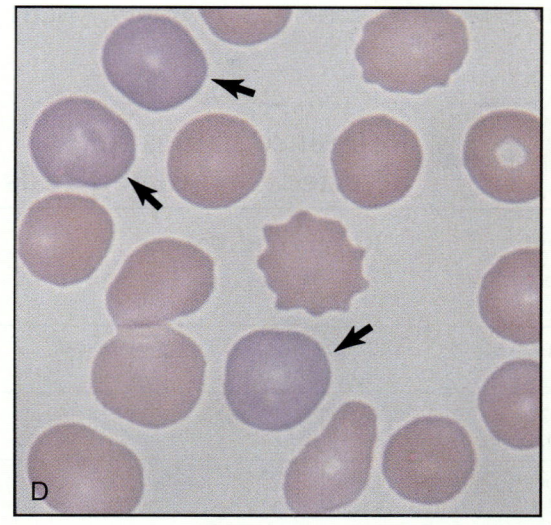

D, Polychromatic red blood cells. (From Carr JH, Rodak BF: *Clinical hematology atlas,* ed 3, St Louis, 2008, Saunders.)

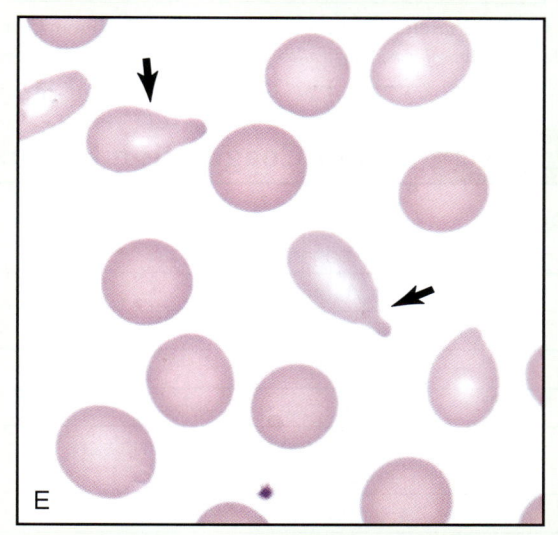

E, Tear drop (dacryocytes). (From Carr JH, Rodak BF: *Clinical hematology atlas,* ed 3, St Louis, 2008, Saunders.)

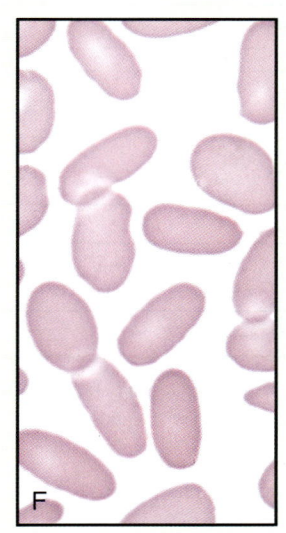

F, Ovalocytes. (From Carr JH, Rodak BF: *Clinical hematology atlas,* ed 3, St Louis, 2008, Saunders.)

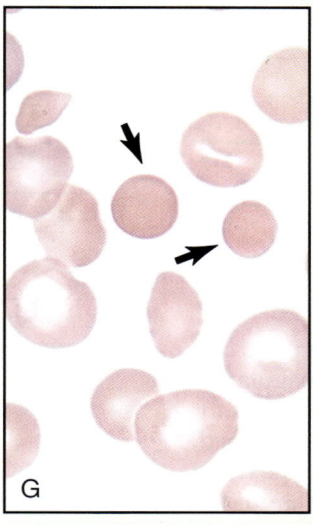

G, Spherocytes. (From Rodak BF: *Hematology: clinical principles and applications,* ed 3, St Louis, 2007, Saunders.)

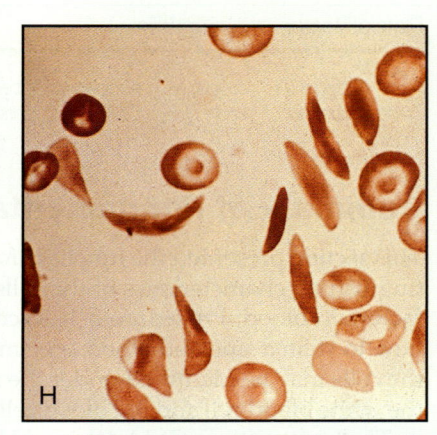

H, Sickle cells. (From Rodak BF: *Hematology: clinical principles and applications,* ed 3, St Louis, 2007, Saunders.)

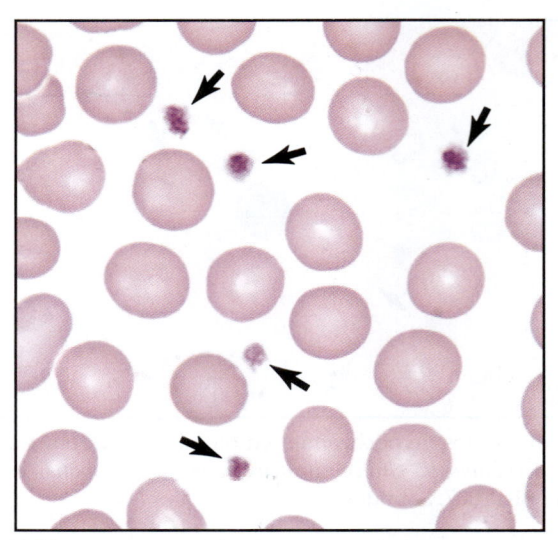

Fig. 5-21. Platelets among the red blood cells. (From Carr JH, Rodak BF: *Clinical hematology atlas*, ed 3, St Louis, 2008, Saunders.)

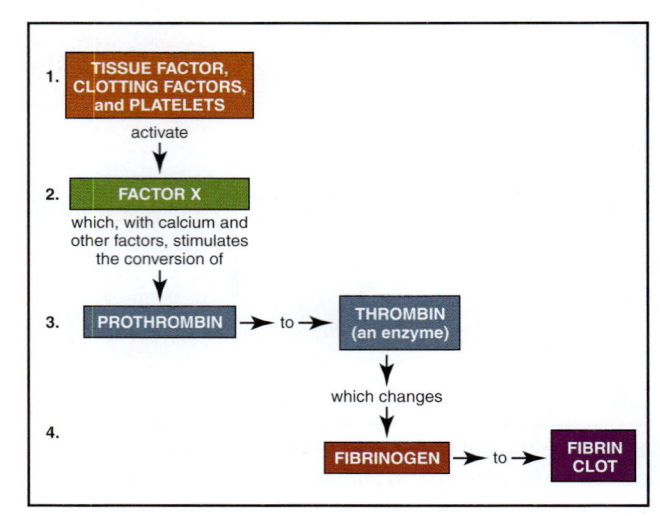

Fig. 5-22. Four steps of the formation of fibrin. (From Chabner D: *The language of medicine*, ed 8, St Louis, 2007, Saunders.)

TABLE 5-1 List of Coagulation Factors

Factor	Name
I	Fibrinogen
II	Prothrombin
III	Tissue factor; thromboplastin
IV	Calcium
V	Labile factor; proaccelerin
VII	Serum prothrombin conversion accelerator; proconvertin
VIII	Antihemophilic factor
IX	Plasma thromboplastin component
X	Stuart–Prower factor
XI	Plasma thromboplastin antecedent
XII	Hageman factor
XIII	Fibrin stabilizing factor
Platelet factor	Cephalin

From Stepp CA, Woods M: *Laboratory procedures for medical office personnel*, Philadelphia, 1998, Saunders.

Summary of Fundamental Concepts

This section presented the function, formation, and distinguishing characteristics of the cells and coagulation factors in blood. Procedure 5-1 describes the steps for how to stain a smeared blood specimen. Once stained, the cells may be identified under the microscope using the white blood cell and red blood cell atlases as guides.

The next section, CLIA-Waived Hematology Tests, describes the most common hematology tests performed in physician office laboratories (POLs).

TABLE 5-2 Reference Values for Selected Coagulated Tests

Test	Reference Values
Bleeding time (Ivy)	1-8.5 min (average, 3-6 min)
Platelet count	150,000-400,000/mm^3 (average, 250,000/mm^3)
Platelet aggregation	Aggregation visible within <5 min
Capillary fragility	Normal: <10 petechiae/2 in circle Grade 1: 0-10 petechiae/2 in circle Grade 2: 11-20 petechiae/2 in circle Grade 3: 21-50 petechiae/2 in circle Grade 4+: >50 petechiae/2 in circle
Activated clotting time	70-120 sec
Partial thromboplastin time	30-45 sec
Prothrombin time	11.0-13.0 sec
Thrombin time	7.0-12.0 sec
Fibrinogen assay	200-400 mg/dL or 2.0-4.0 g/L
Clot retraction	50% in 2 hr; 90% in 4 hr

Modified from Stepp CA, Woods M: *Laboratory procedures for medical office personnel*, Philadelphia, 1998, Saunders.

Fundamental Concepts

PROCEDURE 5-1 Diff Staining Procedure

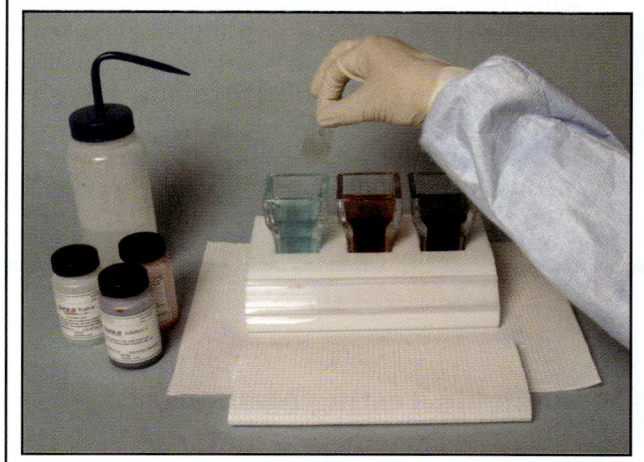

A. Slide is dipped in fixative three times and allowed to dry completely.

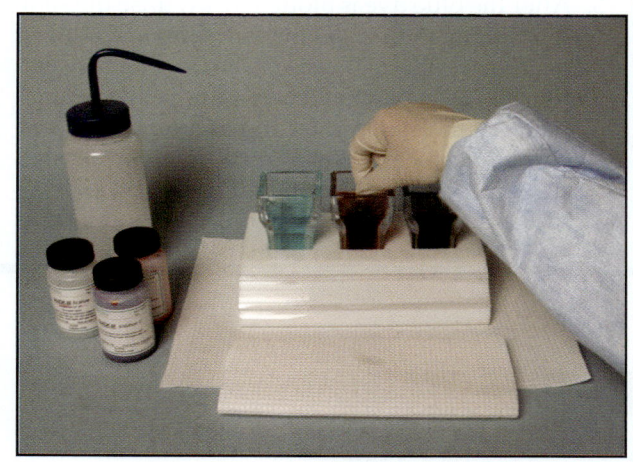

B. Slide is dipped into the red eosin dye three to five times.

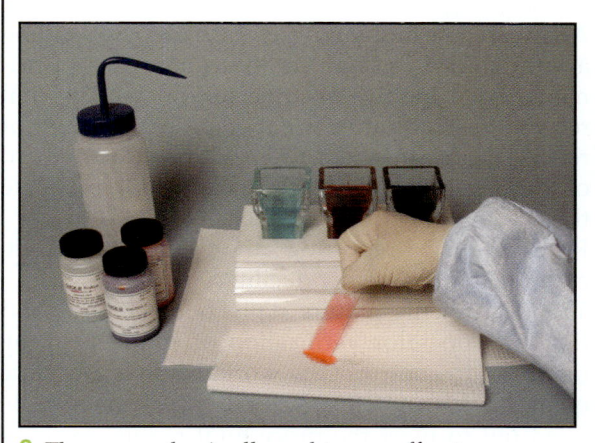

C. The excess dye is allowed to run off onto an absorbent paper.

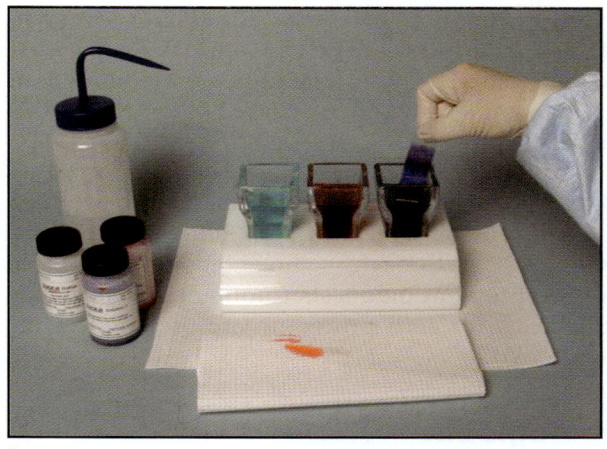

D. The slide is dipped into the blue baso dye three to five times.

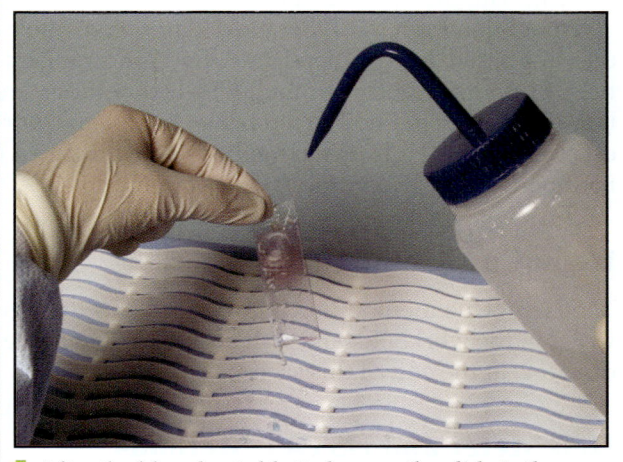

E. After the blue dye is blotted away, the slide is thoroughly rinsed with water on both sides and dried, then brought to the microscope for viewing under the oil immersion lens.

Equipment and Supplies

Quick Diff stain: fixative, red eosin dye, blue baso dye; staining rack; water source (bottled or running water); bibulous paper

Procedure

1. Dip the slide in fixative three times, and allow it to dry completely (Fig. A).
2. Dip the slide into the red eosin dye three to five times (Fig. B).
3. Let the excess dye run off and blot the rest away with absorbent paper (Fig. C).
4. Dip the slide into the blue baso dye three to five times (Fig. D).

(continued)

> **PROCEDURE 5-1** **Diff Staining Procedure—cont'd**
>
> 5. After the blue dye is blotted away, rinse the slide thoroughly with water on both sides and allow it to air dry (Fig. E). It can also be pressed between two bibulous papers to help remove the water.
> 6. Observe the slide under the oil immersion lens of the microscope. Refer to the microscope skill sheet in Chapter 2 for the proper steps to bring the slide into focus under the oil immersion lens. The cells and platelets will be enlarged 1000 times (100× oil objective times the 10× ocular lens). The slide will show predominantly RBCs with some small platelet clumps throughout. The challenge is to find the WBCs. The two most commonly found WBCs are segmented neutrophils and small lymphocytes. See Table 5-1 for assistance in identifying the WBCs.

CLIA-WAIVED HEMATOLOGY TESTS

The most common procedure associated with hematology is the CBC. A CBC generally consists of the following seven laboratory tests: RBC, WBC, platelet counts, Hgb, hematocrit (HCT), differential, and RBC indices. The Hgb and HCT are CLIA-waived tests. The other five tests are moderately or highly complex and are discussed at the end of this chapter.

Four hematology tests have been approved as CLIA-waived hematology tests and can be performed in certificate of waiver (CoW) offices: Hgb tests, HCT tests, erythrocyte sedimentation rates (ESR), and prothrombin time tests (protime). (Competency skill sheets for each procedure are provided in the workbook.)

Hemoglobin

The Hgb within the RBCs is measured by **hemolyzing** (destroying the RBCs) and measuring the amount of released Hgb present. The value is expressed as grams per deciliter **(g/dL)**, which represents the weight of the Hgb (g) per the volume of blood (dL). The result is compared with the reference range. Expected Hgb values are as follows:

Adult men	13 to 18 g/dL
Adult women	11 to 16 g/dL
Children	10 to 14 g/dL (increases with age)
Newborns	16 to 23 g/dL

Notice that the Hgb ranges in women are lower than in men because women lose blood during menstruation each month during their reproductive years. Newborns are born with high Hgb levels that fall during early childhood and then build up to the adult levels. When any of the patient results fall below their reference range, it is referred to as *anemia*.

Hemoglobin Testing Methods

Common procedural steps in all Hgb tests include the following:
1. Collecting blood into an appropriate testing device
2. Hemolyzing the RBCs to release their Hgb
3. Analyzing the amount of released Hgb by sending a light source through the specimen. The instruments have highly sensitive optical readers that receive the light after it either passes through or reflects off the specimen; the resulting measurement of the light then allows the instrument to calculate the amount of Hgb within the specimen.
4. Reading and reporting the digital readout, expressed in grams per deciliter
5. The instruments require daily optics checks and first-time operator verification of competency by using liquid controls. The workbook has a generic quantitative competency check sheet that may be filled out to meet the procedural requirements of these test methods. All the control results and patient results must be logged and evaluated by comparing them with their provided reference ranges.

Three common CLIA-waived Hgb test methods approved by the Food and Drug Administration (FDA) and used in ambulatory care settings are the HemoCue method (HemoCue Inc., Lake Forest, Calif.), the Hgb meter method, and the i-STAT method (Abbott Laboratories, Abbott Park, Ill.).

HemoCue Method

The HemoCue method procedure check sheet is provided in the workbook and is demonstrated in Procedure 5-2, at the end of this section.

Hgb Meter and i-STAT Methods

The Hgb meter and the i-STAT are handheld point-of-care instruments that can be brought to the patient for a rapid assessment of Hgb and other blood test results (Fig. 5-23).

CLIA-Waived Hematology Tests

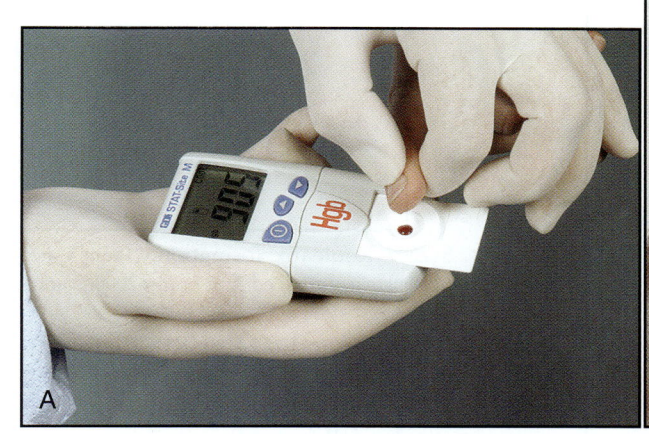

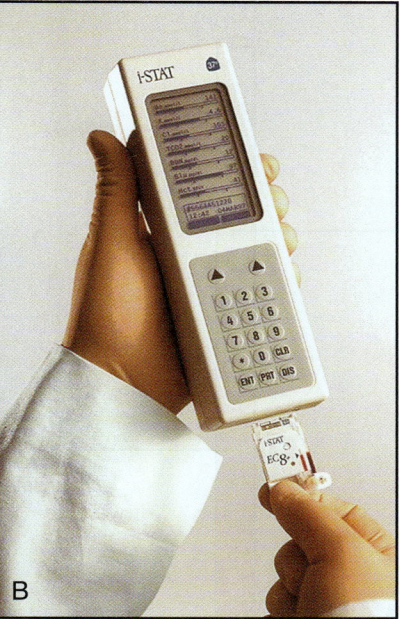

Fig. 5-23. **A,** Hemoglobin meter. **B,** i-STAT Point-of-Care blood analyzer. (**B,** From Rodak BF: *Hematology: clinical principles and applications,* ed 3, St Louis, 2007, Saunders. Courtesy i-STAT Corporation, East Windsor, NJ.)

Hematocrit

Hematocrit (HCT) measures the percentage of packed RBCs that result after centrifuging a specimen and comparing the volume of the packed cells with the total volume of the measured specimen (Fig. 5-24). The packed RBCs are expressed as a percentage of whole blood. HCT expected values are the following:

Adult men	42% to 52%
Adult women	36% to 48%
Children	34% to 42% (increases with age)
Infants	32% to 38%
Newborns	51% to 60%

Notice that the RBCs occupy almost 50% of the total volume of blood. Also notice that the numeric values of Hgb are approximately one third the numeric values of the HCT. If a patient falls below the expected HCT range, this is considered anemia. A patient with an abnormally high HCT level is referred to as polycythemic.

General Spun Microhematocrit Procedures

Steps common to all microhematocrit procedures include the following:
- Collecting blood into two appropriate capillary tubes containing an anticoagulant to prevent clotting of the specimens (NOTE: OSHA safety precautions recommend using plastic capillary tubes, not glass, to prevent possible breakage and blood exposure incidents.)
- Sealing the capillary tubes with clay or a stopper at one end
- Centrifuging the specimens in a HCT centrifuge with the sealed end against the outer rubber gasket or down in the sleeved plastic holder for 5 minutes
- Observing the centrifuged layers: plasma, buffy coat, red cell layer, and sealant (see Fig. 5-24).
- Determining the percent of RBC volume compared with the total blood volume by using a built-in scale or a variable volume scale

The results of the two capillary tubes should be within 2% of agreement, and the final result is recorded as the average of the two tubes. If the results of the two tubes are not within 2%, the test should be repeated. Also take note if the appearance of the plasma is red, indicating hemolysis; white, indicating lipemia (fat in the blood); or dark yellow–brown, indicating jaundice.

Procedure 5-3, presented at the end of this section, describes the general HCT procedure, and its corresponding check sheet is provided in the workbook.

HemataSTAT Procedure

Procedure 5-4 describes an alternate method for measuring blood HCTs in which plastic-covered tubes are rapidly spun in a centrifuge for only 1 minute. The centrifuge has a built-in reading tray that provides a digital readout. A proficiency check sheet is provided in the workbook.

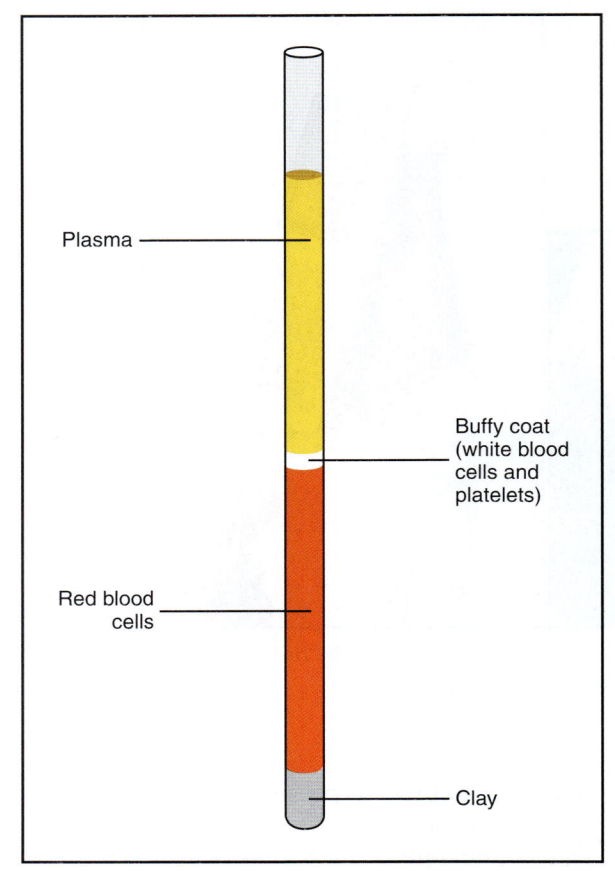

Fig. 5-24. HCT tube layers: plasma, buffy coat, red blood cell layer, sealant.

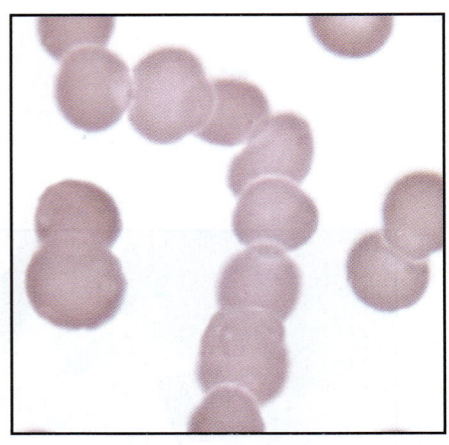

Fig. 5-25. Rouleaux formation. (From Carr JH, Rodak BF: *Clinical hematology atlas*, ed 3, St Louis, 2008, Saunders.)

Erythrocyte Sedimentation Rate

The **erythrocyte sedimentation rate (ESR)** is the rate at which RBCs settle out of an anticoagulated blood specimen after 60 minutes. The result is reported in millimeters per hour. ESR expected values are as follows:

Adult men <50 years	0 to 15 mm/hr
Adult men >50 years	0 to 20 mm/hr
Adult women <50 years	0 to 20 mm/hr
Adult women >50 years	0 to 30 mm/hr

The ESR is a nonspecific screening test to help confirm and monitor changes in inflammatory diseases, autoimmune diseases, carcinomas, and certain forms of leukemia. Patients with these diseases will show sedimentation rates greater than the expected values in the preceding list depending on the amount of inflammation occurring when blood is drawn.

The principle of the ESR is based on the effect of plasma proteins (especially globulins and fibrinogen) produced during inflammatory conditions. These proteins cause the RBCs to become sticky and stack together in a **rouleaux formation** (resembling stacked chips) (Fig. 5-25). The stacked RBCs fall (sediment) at an increased rate that is directly proportional to the increased amount of proteins that were produced during inflammation.

The shape and size of RBCs also affect ESR. For example, spherocytes fall and create an increased rate, whereas sickle cells fall at a slower rate, and macrocytes fall faster than microcytes.

Other technical factors, such as the following, can also interfere with obtaining accurate sedimentation rate results:

False Increased Rates

- Tilting the test tubes results in an erroneous increase in sedimentation.
- Vibrations falsely increase sedimentation.
- Extreme hot room temperatures falsely increase the sediment rate.
- Timing is critical; the results must be read at exactly 60 minutes because taking a reading after the specified time gives a result that is too high.

False Decreased Rates

- Extreme cold room temperatures falsely decrease the sediment rate.
- Taking a reading before the specified time gives a result that is too low.

Other Interferences

- Air bubbles in the tube interfere with sedimentation by breaking up the specimen and causing an erroneous lower value.
- The blood must be fresh, tested within 2 hours of collection or within 6 hours if the specimen has been refrigerated.

SEDIPLAST System

The SEDIPLAST (Polymedco Inc., Courtlandt Manor, N.Y.) ESR method uses a safe, disposable, calibrated plastic pipette that is inserted into a vial containing a mixture of transferred EDTA blood and a premeasured citrate solution. This closed-system test provides a sedimentation rate after allowing the pipette to stand in a vertical rack for 1 hour. The SEDIPLAST procedure check sheet is provided in the workbook and is demonstrated in Procedure 5-4, at the end of this section.

Prothrombin Time

Prothrombin time **(PT)** is a commonly performed CLIA-waived test that measures the amount of time the blood takes to form a fibrin clot. The PT test uses thromboplastin as the active reagent to initiate the coagulation process (see Fig. 5-22).

The PT test is used as a *screening* test for patients who lack clotting factors, have a liver disease, or are deficient in **vitamin K** (a critical element in the production of prothrombin). The PT of these patients will be prolonged, indicating they will be prone to bleeding. The PT test is also widely used to *monitor* patients who have been placed on anticoagulant therapy. These patients are taking anticoagulant drugs (warfarin, coumarin) because they have had a tendency to produce internal clots, which could lead to strokes and heart attacks. The anticoagulant drugs suppress the liver from synthesizing prothrombin. The PT test measures both normal and therapeutic PTs in fresh whole blood. Results are displayed in plasma equivalent seconds and INR. The reference range varies depending on the method of testing but is usually approximately 11 to 13 seconds. The rate can also be expressed as an INR, which is the patient's PT divided by the time of the normal control supplied by the manufacturer for each lot of thromboplastin. The INR rate is the coagulation value that can be more accurately compared against other PT test methods. The therapeutic goal is to keep the patient's PT at approximately 12 to 18 seconds (depending on the method used), or 2 to 2.5 INR (occasionally higher depending on therapeutic need).

Procedure 5-6, at the end of this section, presents the PT/INR method, and a proficiency check sheet is provided in the workbook. The PT/INR method uses a highly sensitive instrument that runs its optics check before each test and runs the high and low controls alongside the patient's blood specimen. It will not give a patient's result unless all controls are accurate and precise (i.e., reliable).

Becoming Proficient at CLIA-Waived Hematology Tests

Now that you have learned about the significance of Hgb, HCT, ESR, and PT tests, take time to complete the following:
1. Answer the questions at the end of this chapter and the CLIA-waived portion in Chapter 5 of the workbook using your structured notes and text.
2. View the videos on-line to see Hgb and HCT performed.
3. Perform the Chapter 5 exercises on-line, which were designed to reinforce your knowledge of terminology and CLIA-waived test procedures.
4. Study Procedures 5-2 through 5-6 before your lab.

PROCEDURE 5-2 Hemoglobin: HemoCue Method

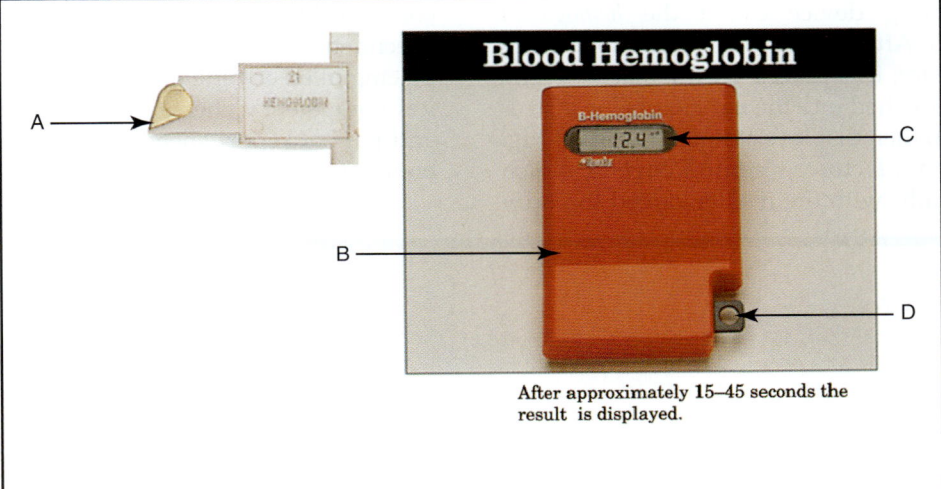

After approximately 15–45 seconds the result is displayed.

A. HemoCue equipment and procedure. *a*, Hgb microcuvette; *b*, HemoCue instrument; *c*, digital readout; *d*, cuvette holder. (From Zakus SM: *Clinical skills for medical assistants*, ed 4, St Louis, 2001, Mosby.)

(continued)

PROCEDURE 5-2 Hemoglobin: HemoCue Method—cont'd

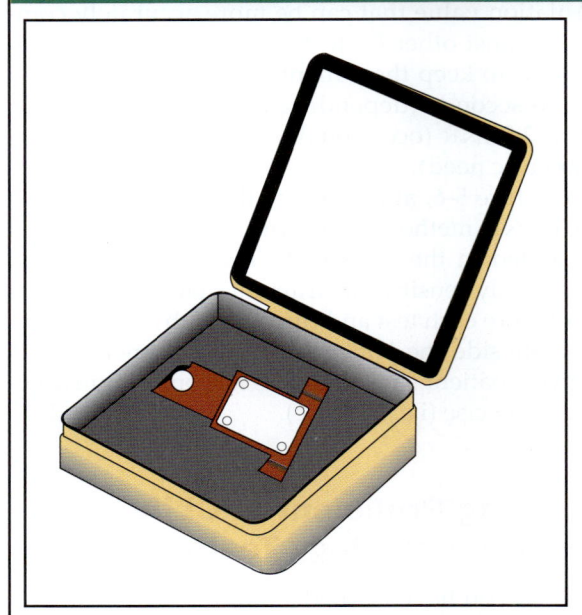

B. HemoCue calibration with red control cuvette.

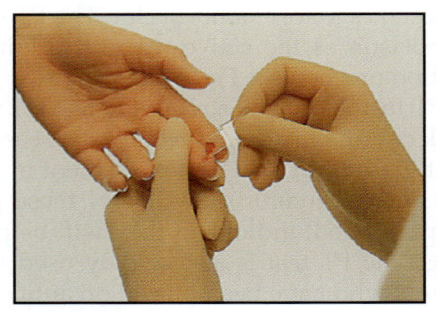

C. Fill the cuvette in one continuous process. It should never be topped up after the first filling.

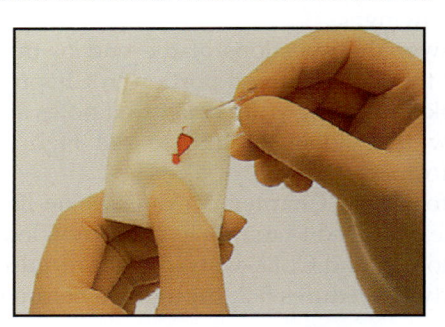

D. Wipe off the excess blood on the outside of the cuvette tip. Make sure that no blood is drawn out of the cuvette in this procedure.

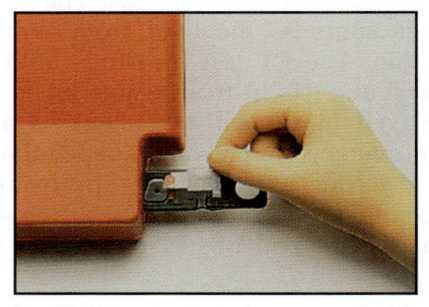

E. Place the filled cuvette into the cuvette holder immediately, and push it into measuring position.

Fig. A shows the HemoCue system, which uses a blood-collecting device called the *hemoglobin microcuvette (a)*. After it has filled with blood from a finger puncture, it is placed on the black cuvette holder *(d)* and pushed into the red HemoCue instrument *(b)*, which then displays a digital result *(c)*. Fig. B shows the manufacturer's control cuvette, which must be run daily, with the results logged to verify that the instrument's optical system is working correctly. Figs. C to E show the steps for obtaining specimen (C), wiping away excess blood (D), and placing filled cuvette into instrument (E). An analytical competency check-off sheet, control log sheet, and patient report sheet are included in the workbook for documenting each of these steps.

CLIA-Waived Hematology Tests

PROCEDURE 5-3 — Hematocrit: General Procedure

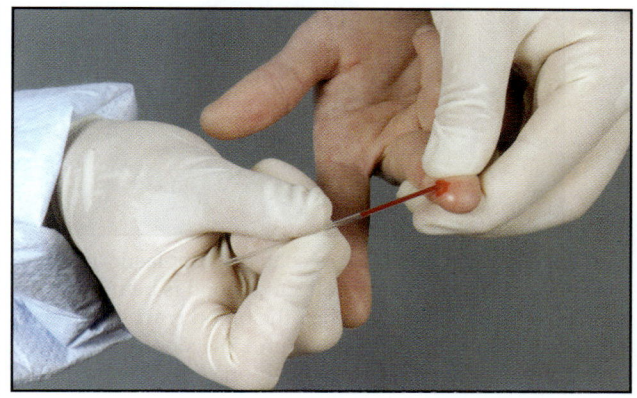

A. Hold capillary in a horizontal position or slightly tipped down to allow capillary action to pull blood into the tube.

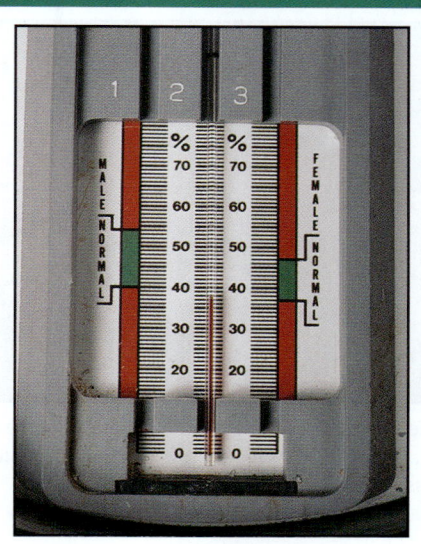

B. When using a built-in hematocrit scale as seen above, the capillary tube must be filled to the designated line on the capillary tube. (From Bonewit-West K: *Clinical procedures for medical assistants,* ed 7, St Louis, 2008.)

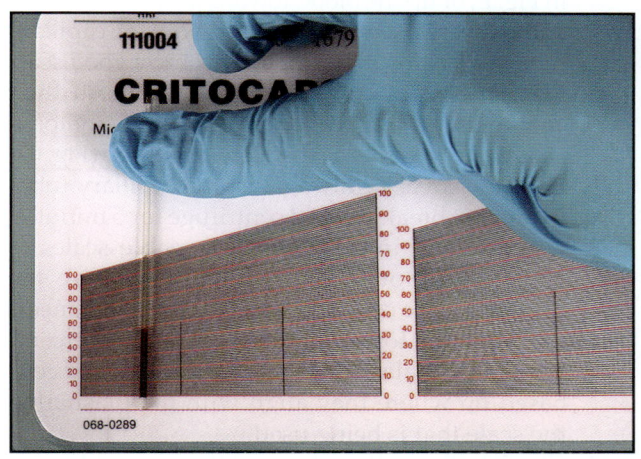

C. The blood sample is being read on a variable reader to determine the percentage of total blood occupied by the red blood cells.

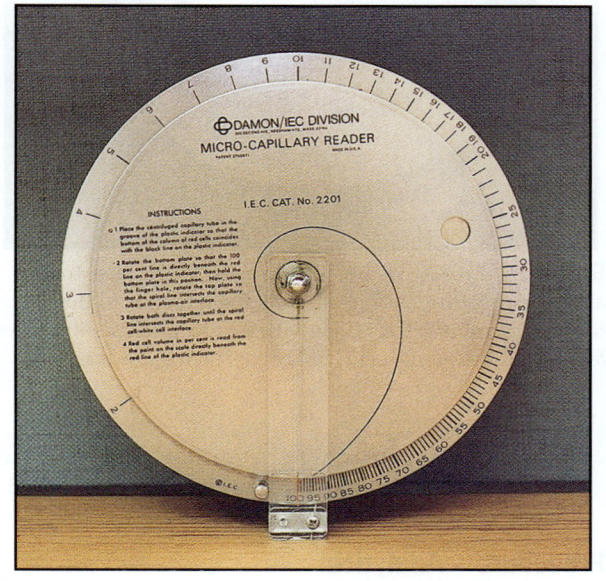

D. This Micro-capillary reader is also able to adjust and read various volumes of blood collected and spun during the hematocrit test. (From Rodak BF: *Hematology: clinical principles and applications,* ed 3, St Louis, 2007, Saunders.)

Equipment and Supplies

- Hematocrit centrifuge with locking cover for safety when spinning the specimens
- Plastic capillary tubes and sealing clay (or self-sealing plastic protected capillary tubes)
- Two liquid controls to check accuracy of high and low hematocrit readings
- Blood specimens used in test—either venous blood collected in **lavender EDTA tube** or **capillary blood** from finger using a lancet, alcohol, and sterile gauze

Preparation—Preanalytical

1. Sanitize the hands and put on fluid-impermeable gown, and gloves.
2. Check the expiration date and storage requirements of all supplies and controls.
3. All first-time operators should run and log results of the controls to check that their technique produces accurate results. Controls

(continued)

PROCEDURE 5-3 Hematocrit: General Procedure—cont'd

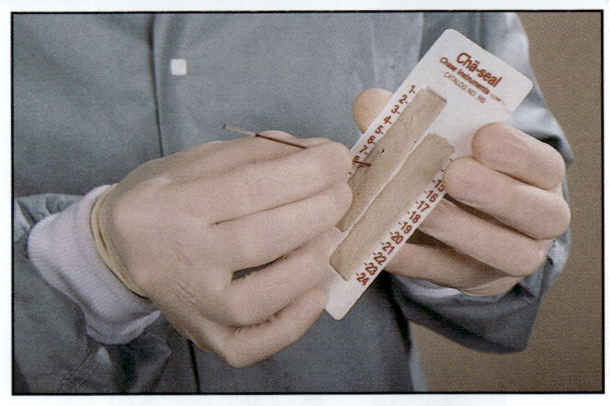

E. Seal the clean end of the tube with clay before centrifuging. (From Bonewit-West K: *Clinical procedures for medical assistants*, ed 7, St Louis, 2008.)

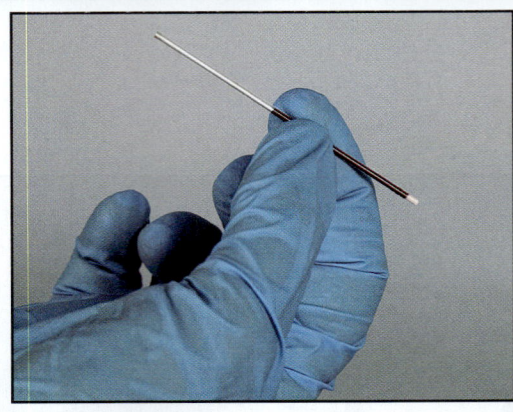

F. This is a safety tube that is coated with plastic and able to self-seal. The capillary collected blood is being tilted toward the sealing clay. When the blood reaches the clay, it automatically seals itself within 15 seconds of contact while holding it in a vertical position.

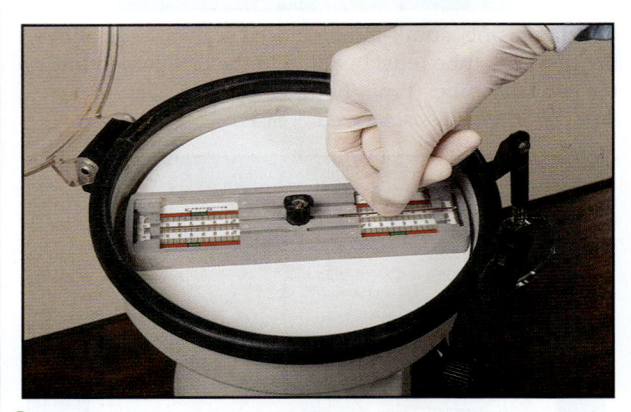

G. The filled tubes are placed opposite each other to balance the centrifuge while it spins the red cells to the bottom of the tube. (From Bonewit-West K: *Clinical procedures for medical assistants*, ed 7, St Louis, 2008, Saunders.)

should also be run whenever new supplies are used and on days when patients will be tested.

Procedure—Analytical

4. Collect two heparin anticoagulated capillary tubes with blood from a finger or an EDTA tube of blood.
   - Hold the capillary tube in a horizontal position or slightly tilted down to allow capillary action to pull the blood into the tube, as shown in Fig. A.
   - Avoid allowing bubbles into your specimen, and fill exactly to the line if using a built-in centrifuge scale, as seen in Fig. B.
   - If a variable scale reader that can adapt to any volume of blood is being used (Fig. C or Fig. D), the tubes may be filled approximately ½ to ¾ full.

5. Seal the clean end of both tubes with clay, as seen in Fig. E, or tip the blood toward the presealed end of the tubes as seen in Fig. F and hold the capillary tube vertical for 15 seconds to ensure a good seal.
6. Place the tubes opposite each other with their clay ends toward the outside of the hematocrit centrifuge to create a balanced centrifuge (Fig. G).
7. Lock the cover firmly against the capillary tubes to prevent breaking, and centrifuge for 5 minutes.
8. Use the built-in scale or the variable scales to adjust your total volume (starting where the clay meets the cells and where the plasma meets the air at the top). Then determine the percentage of the total volume occupied by the red cells based on where they align with the plasma on the scale that is being used.
9. Check both readings to see if they are within 2% of each other, and then record the average of the two tubes. (NOTE: See the two readings in Fig. C: Do their results fall within 2% of each other?)

Follow-up—Postanalytical

10. Results of control and patient should be logged, and the patient results should be charted in the patient record.
11. Properly dispose of the lancets and capillary tubes in the biohazard sharps container and any other blood-contaminated supplies in the biohazard waste container. Disinfect the work area.
12. Remove personal protective equipment, and sanitize the hands.

Figs. C and F courtesy Zack Bent.

CLIA-Waived Hematology Tests

PROCEDURE 5-4 Hematocrit: HemataSTAT Method

The HemataSTAT (Separation Technology, Inc., Altamonte Springs, Fla.) is a rapid portable microhematocrit system that uses replaceable plastic holders and plastic capillary tubes for increased operator safety. It has a built-in reading system that supplies a digital readout.

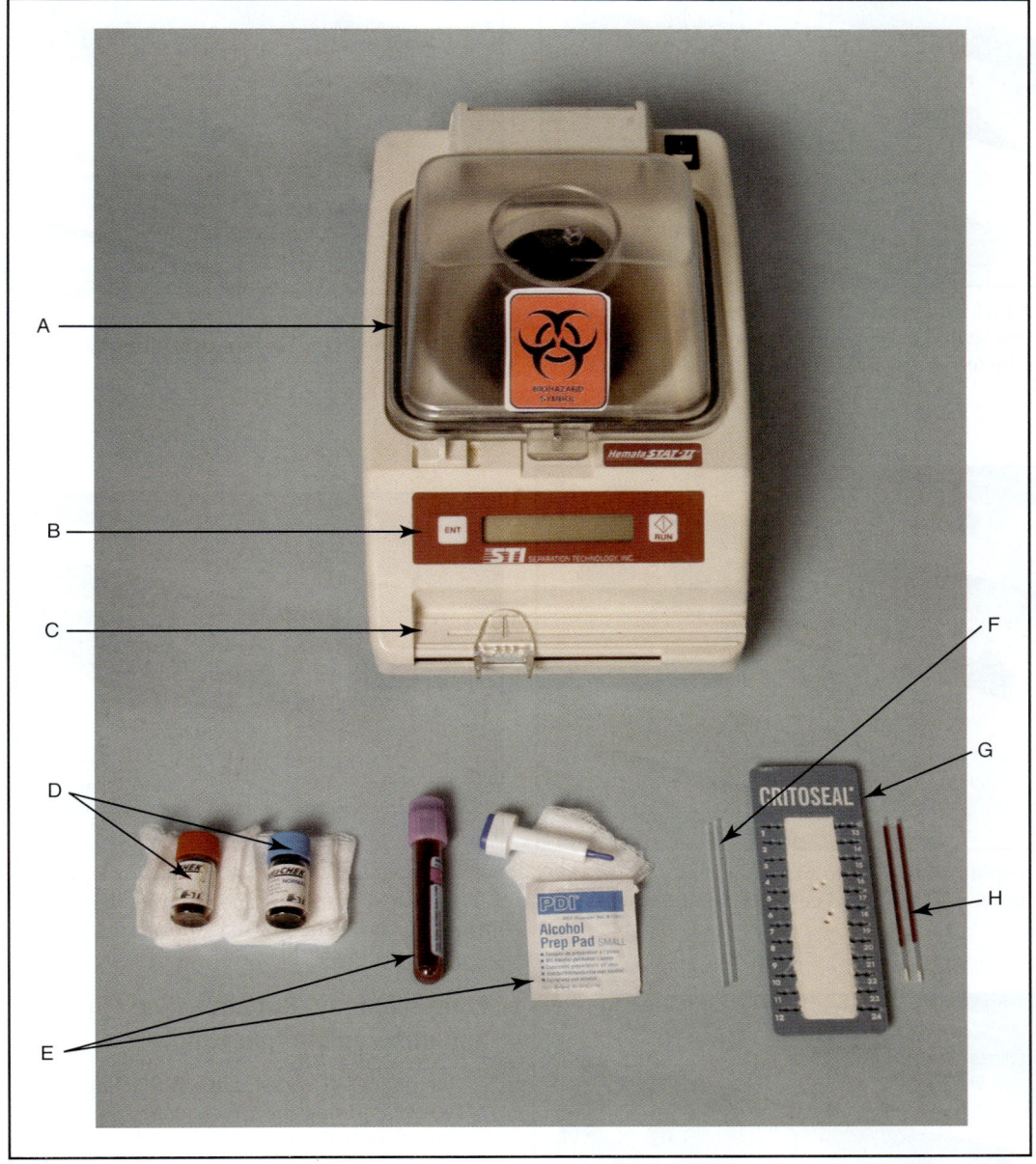

A. HemataSTAT instrument and supplies. *a*, HemataSTAT centrifuge area; *b*, HemataSTAT input controls; *c*, capillary tube reading tray with plastic slider; *d*, two liquid controls; *e*, blood specimens used in test; *f*, two plastic capillary tubes; *g*, Critoseal plastic sealant; *h*, two capillary tubes filled with blood and sealed before centrifuging.

(continued)

PROCEDURE 5-4 Hematocrit: HemataSTAT Method—cont'd

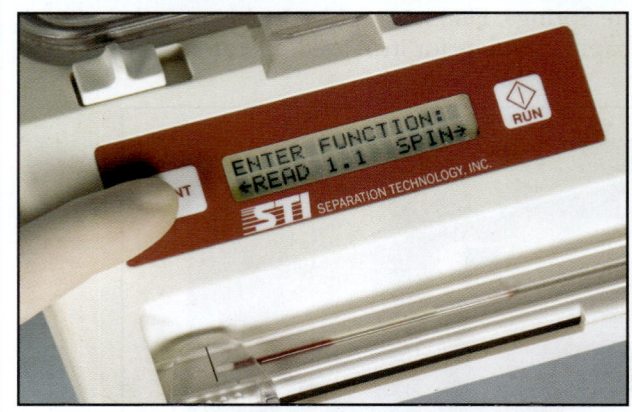

B. HemataSTAT tube reading procedure. With both the capillary tube sealed end and the movable slider all the way to the left, press ENT to "read" according to the display.

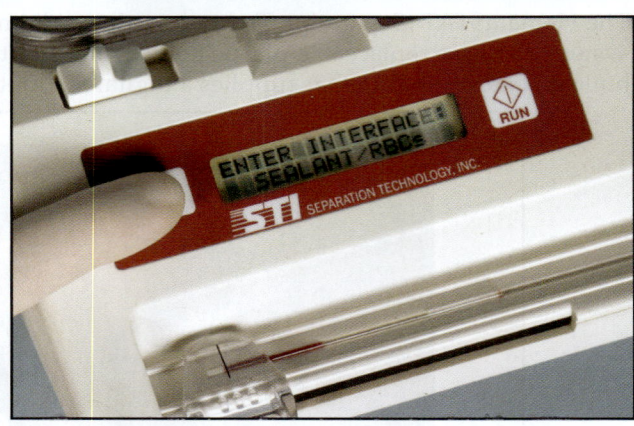

C. Follow display command to move the slider so the line is directly above the sealant/RBC interface, and press ENT.

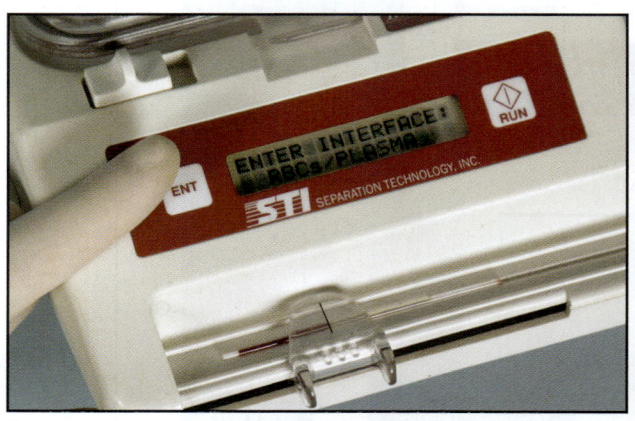

D. Follow display command to move the slider so the line is directly above the red blood cell–plasma interface, and press ENT.

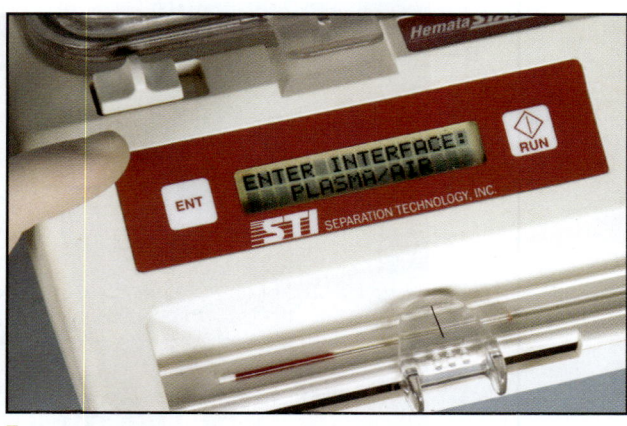

E. Follow display command to move the slider so the line is directly above the plasma–air interface, and press ENT.

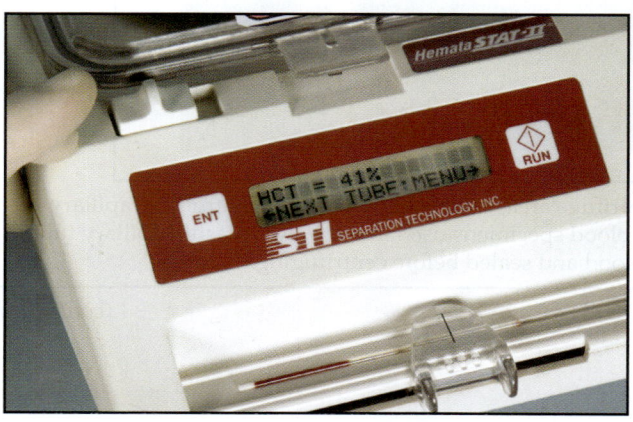

F. Read the final result on the display, record, and press ENT for the next tube.

Equipment and Supplies (See Fig. A, and observe the following)

a) HemataSTAT centrifuge with locking cover for safety when spinning the specimens
b) input controls on each side of the digital screen
c) Capillary tube reading tray with plastic slider
d) Two liquid controls to check accuracy of high and low HCTs
e) Blood specimens used in test—either venous blood collected in lavender EDTA tube or capillary
f) Blood from finger using the lancet, alcohol, and sterile gauze
g) Two plastic capillary tubes
h) Critoseal plastic sealant for sealing one end of each capillary tube after collecting the blood specimen
i) Two capillary tubes that have been filled with blood and sealed before centrifuging

PROCEDURE 5-4 Hematocrit: HemataSTAT Method—cont'd

Preparation—Preanalytical

1. Sanitize the hands, and put on fluid-impermeable gown, gloves.
2. Check the expiration date and storage requirements of all supplies and controls.
3. All first-time operators should run and log results of the controls to check that their technique produces accurate results. Controls should then be run and logged periodically and whenever new supplies are used.

Procedure—Analytical

4. Collect two capillary tubes of anticoagulated blood, then seal and centrifuge them as directed
5. Read the two tubes in the HemataSTAT instrument by following the digital screen instructions:
   - With the tube and slider all the way to the left, press ENT to "Read" (Fig. B).
   - Move the slider so the line is directly above the sealant–RBC interface, and press ENT (Fig. C).
   - Move the slider so the line is directly above the RBC–plasma interface, and press ENT (Fig. D).
   - Move the slider so the line is directly above the plasma–air interface, and press ENT (Fig. E).
   - Observe the final digital result, record, and press ENT to set the instrument for the next tube (Fig. F).
6. Repeat the preceding procedure with the second tube. Check both readings to see if they are within 2% of each other, then record the average of the two tubes.

Follow-up—Postanalytical

7. Log and chart all results
8. Properly dispose of biohazard waste materials, and disinfect the work area.
9. Remove personal protective equipment, and sanitize the hands.

PROCEDURE 5-5 ESR: SEDIPLAST System Procedure

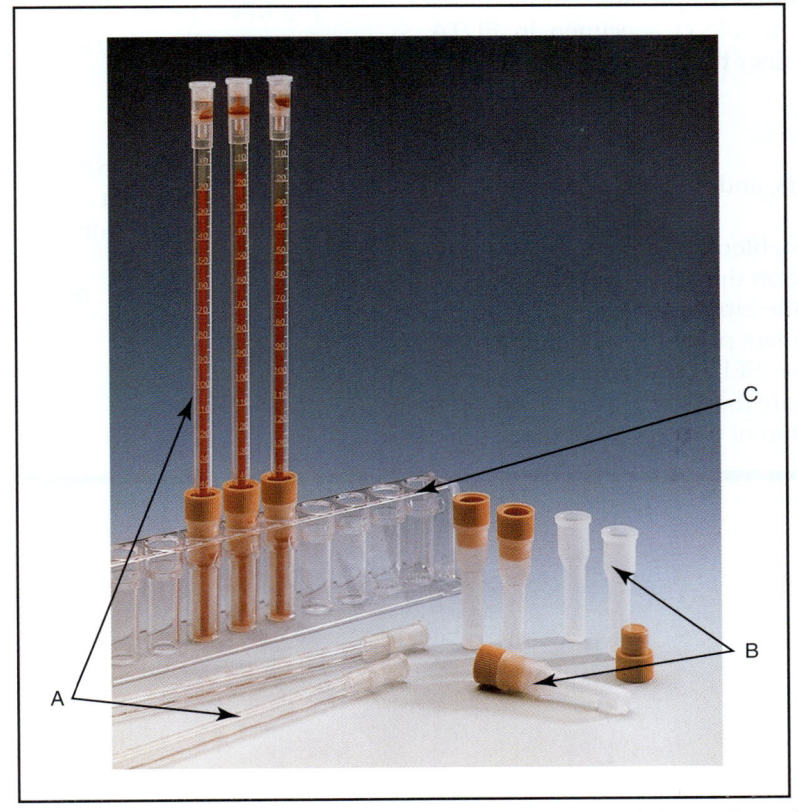

A. SEDIPLAST system. *a*, 200-mm scaled pipette; *b*, citrate tubes; *c*, rack. (From Rodak BF: *Hematology: clinical principles and applications*, ed 3, St Louis, 2007, Saunders. Courtesy Polymedco, Cortlandt Manor, NY.)

(continued)

PROCEDURE 5-5 ESR: SEDIPLAST System Procedure—cont'd

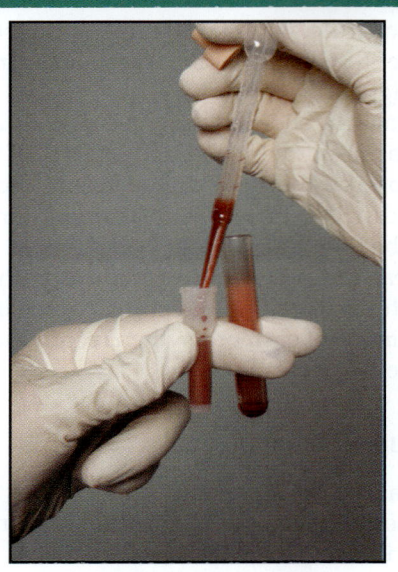

B. Transfer whole blood from the EDTA Vacutainer tube to the indicated line on the citrate tube.

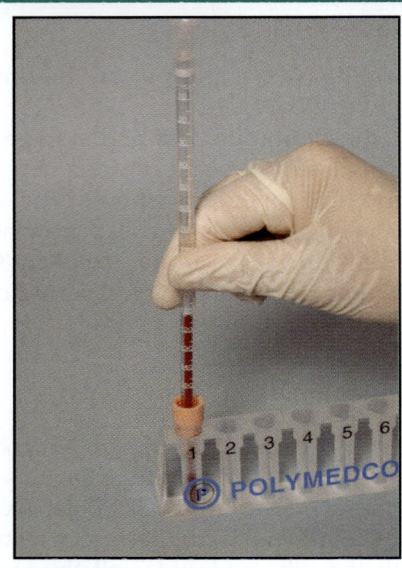

C. After replacing the citrate tube's pink top and mixing, place it in rack. Press the pipette down fully into the citrate tube so that the blood rises up and over the top of the pipette. After 1 hour measure the red blood cell sedimentation (note the three readings in Fig. A).

Equipment and Supplies (Fig. A)

200-mm scaled SEDIPLAST pipette; citrate tubes and rack; fresh venous blood specimen in EDTA (lavender top) Vacutainer tube

Procedure

1. Sanitize the hands, and don personal protective equipment.
2. Transfer the whole blood from the EDTA tube to the indicated line on the citrate tube (Fig. B).
3. After replacing the citrate tube's pink top and mixing the specimen, place the tube in the rack.
4. Slowly press the SEDIPLAST pipette down fully into the citrate tube so that the blood rises up and over the top of the pipette (Fig. C).
5. After 1 hour, measure the number of millimeters the RBC fell in the pipette. This number is the RBC sedimentation rate (note the three different readings in Fig. A).

Follow-up

6. After recording the results as millimeters per hour in the patient chart, dispose of the biohazardous pipettes properly and disinfect the work area.
7. Remove personal protective equipment, and sanitize hands.

CLIA-Waived Hematology Tests

PROCEDURE 5-6 Prothrombin Time INRatio (HemoSense) Method

INRatio is a portable, precalibrated, battery-operated instrument that has its own built-in quality control testing method.

Intended for use in quantitative prothrombin time (PT) testing in fresh capillary whole blood with the INRatio system. The INRatio system is intended for use by health care professionals or properly trained patients to monitor oral anticoagulation therapy.

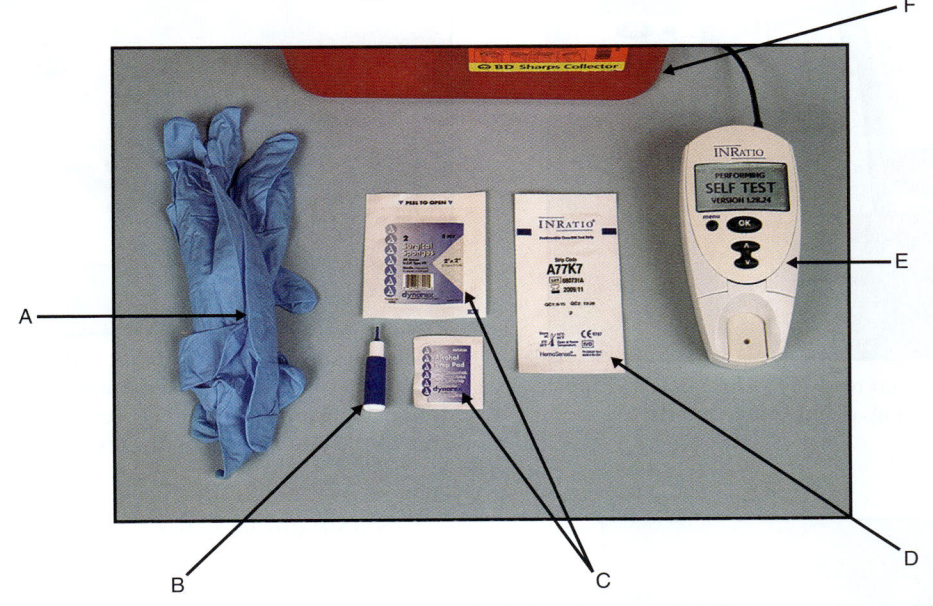

A. INRatio—equipment and supplies. *a*, Gloves; *b*, lancet; *c*, alcohol and gauze; *d*, INRatio test strips; *e*, INRatio meter; *f*, biohazard sharps container.

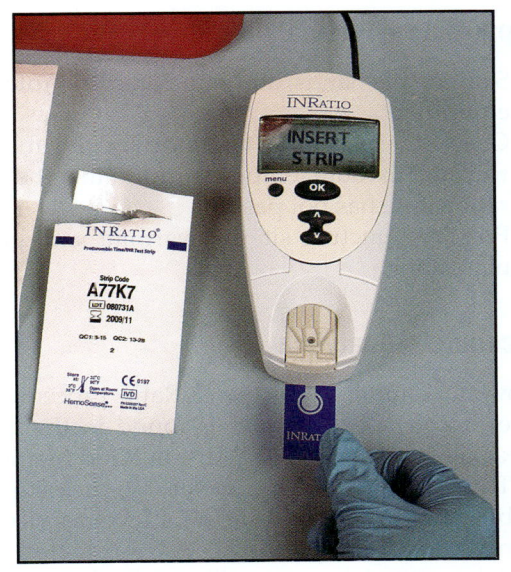

B. Insert the strip into the meter with "INRatio" readable at the bottom of the test strip.

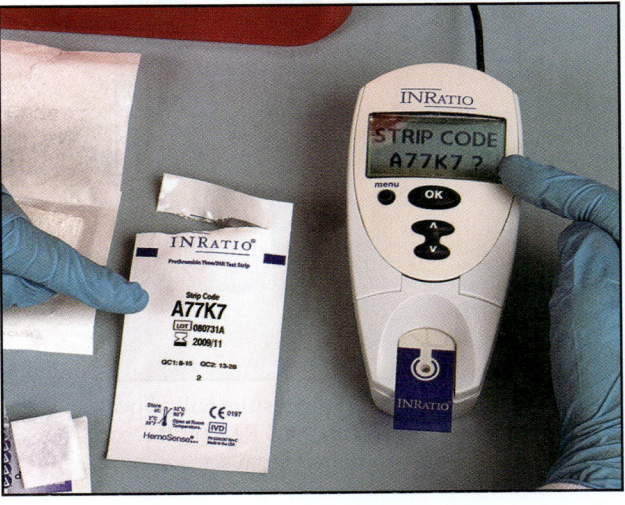

C. Check that the strip code on the meter matches the one on the test strip pouch when "STRIP CODE ####" appears in the display. If it does, press the OK key.

(continued)

PROCEDURE 5-6   Prothrombin Time INRatio (HemoSense) Method—cont'd

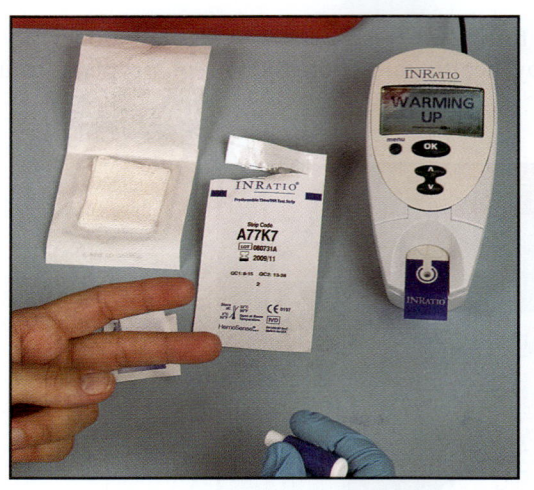

D. The meter will then read "WARMING UP." Prepare the finger by warming, disinfecting, and drying thoroughly.

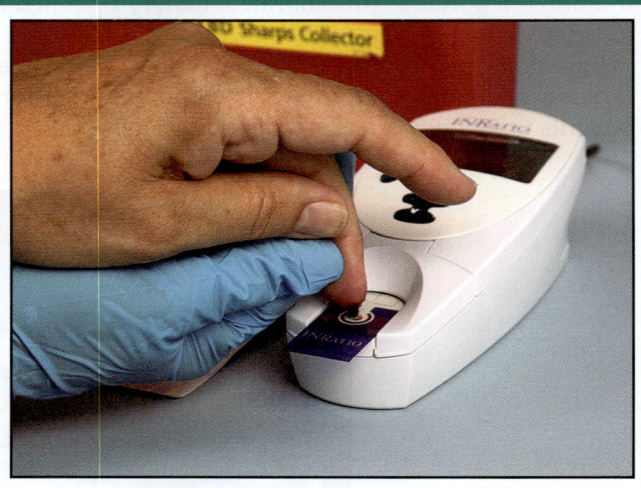

E. After the beep and the prompt "APPLY SAMPLE," incise the finger with the lancet and form a large hanging drop using gentle continuous pressure. Apply the hanging drop to the sample well on the test strip.

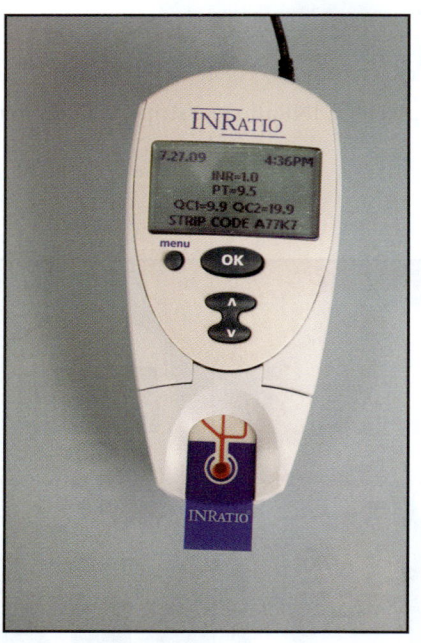

F. The meter will beep, and the results will appear on the display when the test is complete. Read and record the INR and PT seconds from the digital screen.

Equipment and Supplies (Fig. A)

- Gloves (a)
- Lancet with 21 gauge (b)
- Alcohol, gauze, and bandage for capillary puncture site care (c)
- INRatio test strips (d) (at room temperature and sealed in foil container until within 10 minutes of testing)
- INRatio meter (e) with digital readout screen that guides the operator through the procedure
- Biohazard sharps container (f)

Preparation—Preanalytical

1. Sanitize the hands, and don personal protective equipment.
2. Check to see if the test strip in the foil has warmed to room temperature and that the expiration date has not passed.
3. Prepare puncture site by warming and gently massaging.

Procedure—Analytical

Below is a summary of the INRatio procedure. A more thorough explanation is found in the workbook skill sheet for PRO-TIME—INRatio Method.

4. Turn on the INRatio meter by pressing any button. Meter should be on a level service. Do not move during testing.
5. After self-test the meter will read "INSERT STRIP."
6. Open a test strip foil pouch, and remove the test strip. Insert the strip into the meter with "INRatio" readable at the bottom of the test strip (Fig. B).

Advanced Concepts

PROCEDURE 5-6 Prothrombin Time INRatio (HemoSense) Method—cont'd

7. Check that the strip code matches the one on the test strip pouch when "STRIP CODE ####" appears in the display (Fig. C). If it does, press the OK key. If it does not, press the UP/DOWN button to change the first digit. Press OK to enter the new digit. Repeat for each new digit until the instrument and the strip codes match, then press OK to finalize the code. The meter will then read "WARMING UP" (Fig. D).
8. Prepare the finger by warming, disinfecting, and drying thoroughly. Then wait for the beep and the prompt "APPLY SAMPLE." The green sample light will also appear through the test strip sample well.
9. Incise the finger with the lancet. Wipe away the first drop, and form a large hanging drop using gentle continuous pressure.
10. Apply the hanging drop to the sample well on the test strip (Fig. E).
11. Wait while the meter performs the test and calculates the results. The message "TESTING SAMPLE" will display. The blood sample is traveling down the three channels. The center channel is the patient, and the outside channels are the controls.
12. The meter will beep, and the results will appear on the display when the test is complete. If an error message occurs, see the INRatio User's Guide for proper action.
13. Read and record the INR and PT seconds from the digital screen (Fig. F).

	INR	PT Seconds (NOTE: Ranges Vary Depending on Method)
Normal Range	0.8 to 1.2	6.5 to 11.9 seconds
Therapeutic Ranges		NOTE: Physician must determine therapeutic range for each patient
Low Anticoagulation	1.5 to 2.0	19.6 to 26.1 seconds
Moderate Anticoagulation	2.0 to 3.0	26.1 to 39.2 seconds
High anticoagulation	2.5 to 4.0	32.6 to 52.2 seconds

Follow-up—Postanalytical

14. Discard the strip and any biohazard materials appropriately. The meter will turn off automatically after 10 minutes. Identify any critical values, and take appropriate steps to notify the physician.
15. Dispose of waste in the appropriate biohazard containers, and disinfect the work area.
16. Remove personal protective equipment, and sanitize the hands.

Figs. A through F courtesy Zack Bent.

ADVANCED CONCEPTS

Complete Blood Count

Many physicians order a CBC because they want a more complete picture of the internal status of the blood cells. The CBC specimen usually requires a lavender-topped Vacutainer tube with EDTA. EDTA acts as a preservative that maintains the integrity of the blood cells and also works as an anticoagulant. Because the CBC consists of some moderately to highly complex tests, the blood specimen is usually sent to a reference laboratory to be tested with highly sophisticated instruments. A sample laboratory requisition form for ordering the CBC is shown in Fig. 5-26. The subsequent laboratory report form with the results of the CBC is seen in Fig. 5-27.

A CBC generally consists of seven or more laboratory tests that reflect the total count, analysis, and microscopic descriptions of the various cellular elements: RBCs, WBCs, and platelets.

1. RBCs are counted and reported in millions per cubic millimeter or as a whole number times 10 to the ninth power per liter (International Units [SI]). Totals are then compared with reference ranges established for neonates (newborns), infants, children, men, and women (Table 5-3).
2. HCT measures the percentage of packed RBCs compared with the total blood volume.
3. The Hgb within the RBCs is measured. The value is expressed as grams per deciliter and is compared with the reference range.
4. The **RBC indices** are mathematic ratios of the three aforementioned tests (Hgb, HCT, RBC count). These RBC tests are valuable for identifying various forms of **anemia** (a condition in which the RBC or Hgb levels are below normal) and **polycythemia** (abnormal condition of increased RBCs).

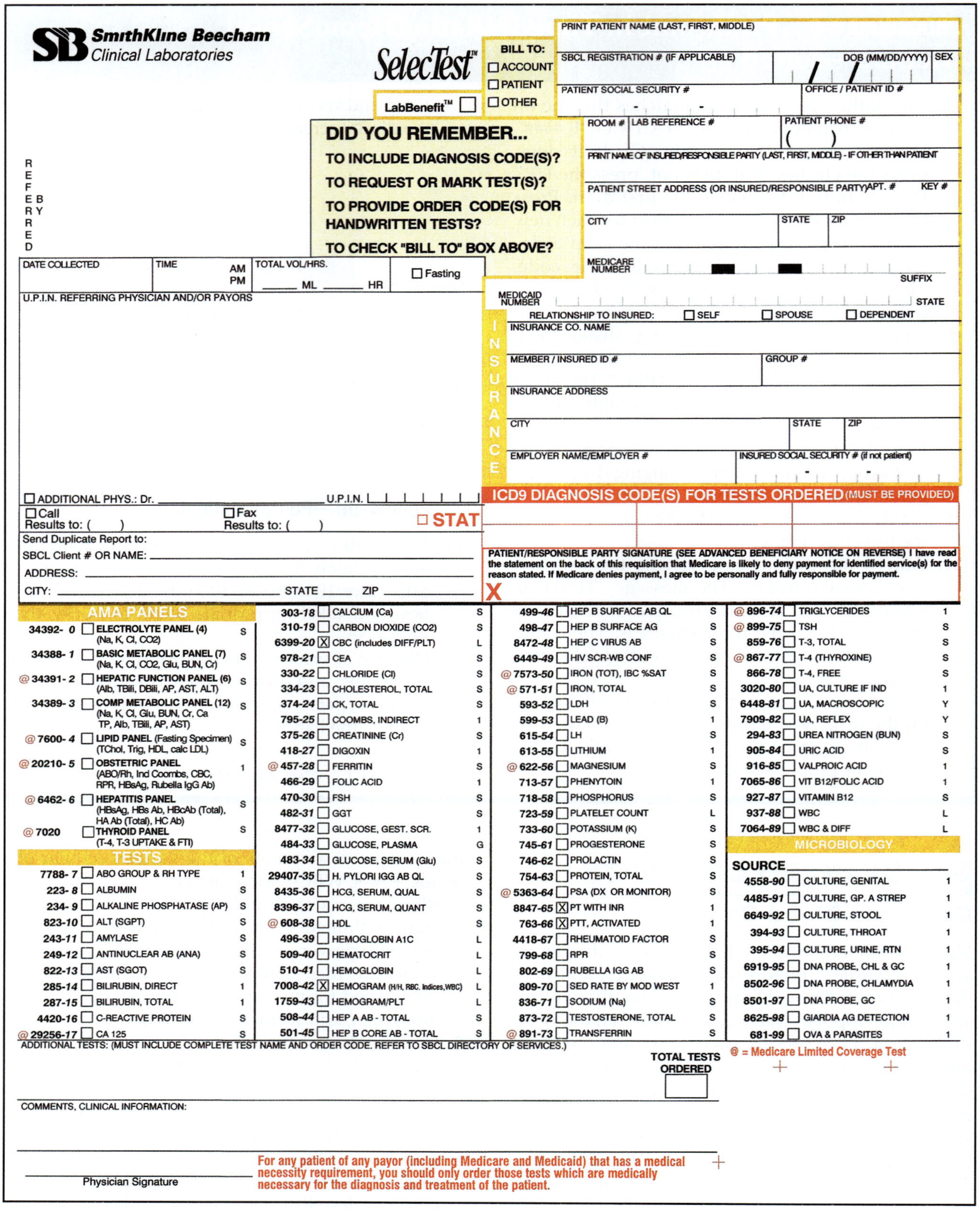

SmithKline Beecham Clinical Laboratories

SelecTest™

LabBenefit™ ☐

BILL TO: ☐ ACCOUNT ☐ PATIENT ☐ OTHER

PRINT PATIENT NAME (LAST, FIRST, MIDDLE)

SBCL REGISTRATION # (IF APPLICABLE) | DOB (MM/DD/YYYY) | SEX

PATIENT SOCIAL SECURITY # | OFFICE / PATIENT ID #

ROOM # | LAB REFERENCE # | PATIENT PHONE #

PRINT NAME OF INSURED/RESPONSIBLE PARTY (LAST, FIRST, MIDDLE) - IF OTHER THAN PATIENT

PATIENT STREET ADDRESS (OR INSURED/RESPONSIBLE PARTY) APT. # | KEY #

CITY | STATE | ZIP

MEDICARE NUMBER | SUFFIX

MEDICAID NUMBER | STATE

RELATIONSHIP TO INSURED: ☐ SELF ☐ SPOUSE ☐ DEPENDENT

INSURANCE

INSURANCE CO. NAME

MEMBER / INSURED ID # | GROUP #

INSURANCE ADDRESS

CITY | STATE | ZIP

EMPLOYER NAME/EMPLOYER # | INSURED SOCIAL SECURITY # (if not patient)

DID YOU REMEMBER...

TO INCLUDE DIAGNOSIS CODE(S)?

TO REQUEST OR MARK TEST(S)?

TO PROVIDE ORDER CODE(S) FOR HANDWRITTEN TESTS?

TO CHECK "BILL TO" BOX ABOVE?

REFERRED BY

DATE COLLECTED | TIME AM PM | TOTAL VOL/HRS. ______ ML ______ HR | ☐ Fasting

U.P.I.N. REFERRING PHYSICIAN AND/OR PAYORS

☐ ADDITIONAL PHYS.: Dr. ______ U.P.I.N.

☐ Call Results to: ( ) ☐ Fax Results to: ( ) ☐ STAT

Send Duplicate Report to:

SBCL Client # OR NAME: ______

ADDRESS: ______

CITY: ______ STATE ____ ZIP ______

ICD9 DIAGNOSIS CODE(S) FOR TESTS ORDERED (MUST BE PROVIDED)

PATIENT/RESPONSIBLE PARTY SIGNATURE (SEE ADVANCED BENEFICIARY NOTICE ON REVERSE) I have read the statement on the back of this requisition that Medicare is likely to deny payment for identified service(s) for the reason stated. If Medicare denies payment, I agree to be personally and fully responsible for payment.

X

AMA PANELS

- 34392-0 ☐ ELECTROLYTE PANEL (4) (Na, K, Cl, CO2) S
- 34388-1 ☐ BASIC METABOLIC PANEL (7) (Na, K, Cl, CO2, Glu, BUN, Cr) S
- @ 34391-2 ☐ HEPATIC FUNCTION PANEL (6) (Alb, TBili, DBili, AP, AST, ALT) S
- 34389-3 ☐ COMP METABOLIC PANEL (12) (Na, K, Cl, Glu, BUN, Cr, Ca TP, Alb, TBili, AP, AST) S
- @ 7600-4 ☐ LIPID PANEL (Fasting Specimen) (TChol, Trig, HDL, calc LDL) S
- @ 20210-5 ☐ OBSTETRIC PANEL (ABO/Rh, Ind Coombs, CBC, RPR, HBsAg, Rubella IgG Ab) 1
- @ 6462-6 ☐ HEPATITIS PANEL (HBsAg, HBs Ab, HBcAb (Total), HA Ab (Total), HC Ab) S
- @ 7020 ☐ THYROID PANEL (T-4, T-3 UPTAKE & FTI) S

TESTS

- 7788-7 ☐ ABO GROUP & RH TYPE 1
- 223-8 ☐ ALBUMIN S
- 234-9 ☐ ALKALINE PHOSPHATASE (AP) S
- 823-10 ☐ ALT (SGPT) S
- 243-11 ☐ AMYLASE S
- 249-12 ☐ ANTINUCLEAR AB (ANA) S
- 822-13 ☐ AST (SGOT) S
- 285-14 ☐ BILIRUBIN, DIRECT 1
- 287-15 ☐ BILIRUBIN, TOTAL 1
- 4420-16 ☐ C-REACTIVE PROTEIN S
- @ 29256-17 ☐ CA 125 S
- 303-18 ☐ CALCIUM (Ca) S
- 310-19 ☐ CARBON DIOXIDE (CO2) S
- 6399-20 ☒ CBC (includes DIFF/PLT) L
- 978-21 ☐ CEA S
- 330-22 ☐ CHLORIDE (Cl) S
- 334-23 ☐ CHOLESTEROL, TOTAL S
- 374-24 ☐ CK, TOTAL S
- 795-25 ☐ COOMBS, INDIRECT 1
- 375-26 ☐ CREATININE (Cr) S
- 418-27 ☐ DIGOXIN 1
- @ 457-28 ☐ FERRITIN S
- 466-29 ☐ FOLIC ACID 1
- 470-30 ☐ FSH S
- 482-31 ☐ GGT S
- 8477-32 ☐ GLUCOSE, GEST. SCR. 1
- 484-33 ☐ GLUCOSE, PLASMA G
- 483-34 ☐ GLUCOSE, SERUM (Glu) S
- 29407-35 ☐ H. PYLORI IGG AB QL S
- 8435-36 ☐ HCG, SERUM, QUAL S
- 8396-37 ☐ HCG, SERUM, QUANT S
- @ 608-38 ☐ HDL S
- 496-39 ☐ HEMOGLOBIN A1C L
- 509-40 ☐ HEMATOCRIT L
- 510-41 ☐ HEMOGLOBIN L
- 7008-42 ☒ HEMOGRAM (H/H, RBC, Indices, WBC) L
- 1759-43 ☐ HEMOGRAM/PLT L
- 508-44 ☐ HEP A AB - TOTAL S
- 501-45 ☐ HEP B CORE AB - TOTAL S
- 499-46 ☐ HEP B SURFACE AB QL S
- 498-47 ☐ HEP B SURFACE AG S
- 8472-48 ☐ HEP C VIRUS AB S
- 6449-49 ☐ HIV SCR-WB CONF S
- @ 7573-50 ☐ IRON (TOT), IBC %SAT S
- @ 571-51 ☐ IRON, TOTAL S
- 593-52 ☐ LDH S
- 599-53 ☐ LEAD (B) 1
- 615-54 ☐ LH S
- 613-55 ☐ LITHIUM 1
- @ 622-56 ☐ MAGNESIUM S
- 713-57 ☐ PHENYTOIN 1
- 718-58 ☐ PHOSPHORUS S
- 723-59 ☐ PLATELET COUNT L
- 733-60 ☐ POTASSIUM (K) S
- 745-61 ☐ PROGESTERONE S
- 746-62 ☐ PROLACTIN S
- 754-63 ☐ PROTEIN, TOTAL S
- @ 5363-64 ☐ PSA (DX OR MONITOR) S
- 8847-65 ☒ PT WITH INR 1
- 763-66 ☒ PTT, ACTIVATED 1
- 4418-67 ☐ RHEUMATOID FACTOR S
- 799-68 ☐ RPR S
- 802-69 ☐ RUBELLA IGG AB S
- 809-70 ☐ SED RATE BY MOD WEST 1
- 836-71 ☐ SODIUM (Na) S
- 873-72 ☐ TESTOSTERONE, TOTAL S
- @ 891-73 ☐ TRANSFERRIN S
- @ 896-74 ☐ TRIGLYCERIDES 1
- @ 899-75 ☐ TSH S
- 859-76 ☐ T-3, TOTAL S
- @ 867-77 ☐ T-4 (THYROXINE) S
- 866-78 ☐ T-4, FREE S
- 3020-80 ☐ UA, CULTURE IF IND 1
- 6448-81 ☐ UA, MACROSCOPIC Y
- 7909-82 ☐ UA, REFLEX Y
- 294-83 ☐ UREA NITROGEN (BUN) S
- 905-84 ☐ URIC ACID S
- 916-85 ☐ VALPROIC ACID 1
- 7065-86 ☐ VIT B12/FOLIC ACID 1
- 927-87 ☐ VITAMIN B12 S
- 937-88 ☐ WBC L
- 7064-89 ☐ WBC & DIFF L

MICROBIOLOGY

SOURCE ______

- 4558-90 ☐ CULTURE, GENITAL 1
- 4485-91 ☐ CULTURE, GP. A STREP 1
- 6649-92 ☐ CULTURE, STOOL 1
- 394-93 ☐ CULTURE, THROAT 1
- 395-94 ☐ CULTURE, URINE, RTN 1
- 6919-95 ☐ DNA PROBE, CHL & GC 1
- 8502-96 ☐ DNA PROBE, CHLAMYDIA 1
- 8501-97 ☐ DNA PROBE, GC 1
- 8625-98 ☐ GIARDIA AG DETECTION 1
- 681-99 ☐ OVA & PARASITES 1

ADDITIONAL TESTS: (MUST INCLUDE COMPLETE TEST NAME AND ORDER CODE. REFER TO SBCL DIRECTORY OF SERVICES.)

TOTAL TESTS ORDERED

@ = Medicare Limited Coverage Test

COMMENTS, CLINICAL INFORMATION:

Physician Signature

For any patient of any payor (including Medicare and Medicaid) that has a medical necessity requirement, you should only order those tests which are medically necessary for the diagnosis and treatment of the patient.

Fig. 5-26. Requisition (note the checked-off hematology tests). (From Zakus SM: *Clinical skills for medical assistants,* ed 4, St Louis, 2001, Mosby.)

Advanced Concepts

		DATE & TIME RECEIVED	ACCESSION NUMBER
		10/20/2010 20:45	
		LOCATION	DATE REPORTED
			10/21/2000

PHYSICIAN	PATIENT INFORMATION

TEST		RESULTS	REFERENCE RANGE	UNITS
HEMOGRAM	LO	2.9	4.5-10.5	CU. MM.
WHITE BLOOD COUNT	LO	2.39	4.40-5.90	CU. MM.
RED BLOOD COUNT	LO	7.4	14.0-18.0	GM/100 ML
HEMOGLOBIN	LO	22.3	40.0-52.0	%
MEAN CORPUSCULAR VOLUME		93	80-100	fL
MEAN CORPUSCULAR HGB		31.0	27.0-32.0	PG
MEAN CORPUSCULAR HGB CONC		33.2	31.0-36.0	%
DIFFERENTIAL, WBC				
SEGMENTED NEUTROPHILS		57	38-80	%
LYMPHOCYTE		29	15-45	%
MONOCYTES		7	1-10	%
EOSINOPHILS		1	0-4	%
BAND NEUTROPHILS	HI	6	0-5	%
ANISOCYTOSIS	ABN	SLIGHT		
HYPOCHROMIA	ABN	SLIGHT		
PLATELET ESTIMATE	ABN	DECREASED		
PARTIAL THROMBOPLASTIN TIME				
PARTIAL THROMBOPLASTIN TIME		31.7	20.0-40.0	SECONDS
CONTROL PTT		30.4	20.0-40.0	SECONDS
PROTHROMBIN TIME				
PROTHROMBIN TIME		12.2	10.0-13.5	SECONDS
CONTROL PT		12.0	11.0-13.0	SECONDS
FINAL Report		(Summary)		

Fig. 5-27. Laboratory report (note the values outside the reference range). (Modified from Zakus SM: *Clinical skills for medical assistants*, ed 4, St Louis, 2001, Mosby.)

- The mean (average) cell Hgb concentration (**MCHC**) is determined by the following formula:

  $MCHC = Hgb \times 100 / HCT = gm/dL$ or %

- This ratio is commonly calculated in the ambulatory care setting because Hgb and HCT are both CLIA-waived tests. The reference ranges for MCHC in Table 5-3 show a 1:3 relation of Hgb to HCT, which is approximately 33%. If the patient's values fall below the reference range, the RBCs contain less Hgb than normal. This is often the case in iron-deficiency anemia, chronic blood loss anemia, macrocytic anemia, and hypochromic anemia. All these conditions can be confirmed during the microscopic examination of a stained blood smear.

- The mean cell volume (**MCV**) and mean cell Hgb (**MCH**) indices compare the HCT volume and the Hgb value to the total RBC count, respectively. The formulas are as follows:

  $MCV = HCT \times 1000 / RBC\ count$
  $= \mu m$ or fL (femtoliters)

  $MCH = Hgb \times 10 / RBC\ count = pg$ (picograms)

- By comparing the patient's MCV to the reference range, the general size of the RBCs can be determined. If the MCV is less than 80, for example, the RBCs are microcytic (small); if the MCV is greater than 100, the RBCs are macrocytic (large). The MCH indicates the concentration of Hgb compared with the average size of the RBCs.

5. WBCs are counted and reported in thousands per cubic millimeter or as a whole number multiplied by 10 to the ninth power per liter in SI units. The total WBC count is compared with reference ranges, such as those in Table 5-3.

6. A differential count that uses the stained blood smear is performed, and the five types of leukocytes are reported with the percentage of each type compared with reference values, as in Table 5-3. The hematologist uses a manual differential counter to determine the differential (see Fig. 5-19). The appearance of the RBCs and platelets is also observed and described in the report. The WBC tests are valuable in identifying **leukocytosis** (an abnormal increase in WBCs), forms of **leukemia** (various cancers of the WBCs), and **leukopenia** (an abnormal decrease in WBCs).

7. Platelets are counted by approximation on the stained slide or by an automated instrument and are expressed in hundreds of thousands per cubic millimeter, or in SI units as a decimal fraction multiplied by 10 to the twelfth power per liter. The patient's results are compared with a reference range, such as that in Table 5-3. This information is useful in diagnosing various bleeding and clotting disorders.

Abnormal Complete Blood Count Findings

The CBC gives a complete picture of the RBCs, WBCs, and platelets. High-quality medical care requires that laboratory values always be correlated with the clinical state. For example, if a patient exhibits signs and symptoms of fatigue and **hypoxemia** (lack of oxygen in the blood), the physician may suspect that a form of anemia is present. By ordering a CBC and observing all the RBC test results (RBC count, Hgb, HCT, and indices), the physician can then make a differential diagnosis.

Anemias

Table 5-4 shows the effect of various forms of anemia on CBC test results. This information is confirmed by observing the stained blood smear during the differential. Fig. 5-28 illustrates the way RBCs appear in the following forms of anemia:

- Folate (folic acid)-deficiency anemia: The macrocytic (enlarged) RBCs are caused by the poor formation of the RBCs in the bone marrow.
- Iron-deficiency anemia: The **hypochromic** (less than normal color) and microcytic (small) RBCs result from the inability to build healthy Hgb. This is the most common type of anemia and is caused by blood loss or inadequate iron in the diet.
- Hereditary spherocytosis: Because of a genetic abnormality, the RBCs have a spherical shape rather than the normal disk shape.
- Aplastic anemia: All the blood cell elements show a decrease in aplastic anemia as a result of the inability to produce cells in the bone marrow (see Table 5-4). Enlarged ovalocytes are the result of trauma to the stem cells in the bone marrow.
- Pernicious anemia: The cells appear enlarged, fragile, and abnormally shaped because the diet is deficient in vitamin B_{12} or because intrinsic factor (a chemical that allows B_{12} to be absorbed into the blood from the digestive tract) is lacking.
- Sickle cell disease: The RBCs collapse into a sickle shape under certain circumstances. This condition is caused by an inherited Hgb-S molecule.
- Thalassemia and hemolytic anemia: The increase of reticulocytes in the peripheral blood is associated with RBC destruction from inherited thalassemia or other hemolytic causes.

TABLE 5-3 Reference Ranges for Complete Blood Count

Test	Neonates	Infants (6 mo)	Children	Adults Men	Adults Women
Red blood cells	4.8-7.1 million/mm³	3.8-5.5 million/mm³	4.5-4.8 million/mm³	4.5-6.0 million/mm³	4.0-5.5 million/mm³
Hematocrit	44%-64%	30%-40%	35%-41%	42%-52%	36%-45%
Hemoglobin	17-21 g/dL	10-15 g/dL	11-16 g/dL	15-18 g/dL	12-16 g/dL
Red blood cell indices					
MCV	96-108 μm	—	—	82-98 μm	
MCH	32-34 pg	—	—	26-34 pg	
MCHC	31-33 g/dL	—	—	31-37 g/dL	
White blood cells	9000-30,000/mm³	6000-16,000/mm³	5000-13,000/mm³	4000-11,000/mm³	
Differential white blood cell count					
Neutrophils	≥45% by 1 week of age	32%	60% of children 2 years and older	50%-65%	
Bands	—	—	—	0%-7%	
Eosinophils	—	—	0%-3%	1%-3%	
Basophils	—	—	1%-3%	0%-1%	
Monocytes	—	—	4%-9%	3%-9%	
Lymphocytes	≥41% by 1 week of age	61%	59% for children 2 years or older	25%-40%	
Platelets	140,000-300,000/mm³	200,000-473,000/mm³	150,000-450,000/mm³	150,000-400,000/mm³	

MCV, Mean cell volume; *MCH*, mean cell hemoglobin; *MCHC*, mean (average) cell hemoglobin concentration.
From Stepp CA, Woods M: *Laboratory procedures for medical office personnel*, Philadelphia, 1998, Saunders.

White Blood Cell Disorders

The WBC count and differential can also be correlated to the patient's clinical state. For example, if a patient has an infection, the total WBC count may rise as the body fights the infection (leukocytosis). The type of infection can be determined by observing the percentage of each type of WBC in the differential. For example, a rise in neutrophils would indicate a bacterial infection as opposed to a rise in lymphocytes, which would indicate a viral infection. Also, the viral infection referred to as *mononucleosis* is known for the presence of atypical lymphocytes that appear larger than normal (Fig. 5-29). An abnormally low WBC count (leukocytopenia) may be a sign of malnutrition.

An extremely high abnormal WBC count with a decrease in the RBC and platelet count may indicate leukemia. Again, the stained blood smear will shed more light on what is happening. As previously stated, all the blood cells come from one stem cell or hemocytoblast. If the differentiation phase of the myeloblasts goes out of control, the bone marrow myelocytes increase and begin to appear in the peripheral blood in increasingly greater numbers, to the detriment of RBCs and platelets. The patient would be diagnosed with acute myelocytic leukemia (**AML**) if this condition developed suddenly, or with chronic myelocytic leukemia (**CML**) if it is a long-term condition. If, on the other hand, the formation of the lymphocytes goes out of control, then immature lymphoblasts will appear in the peripheral blood. This form of leukemia can also be classified as acute (acute lymphocytic leukemia [**ALL**]) or chronic (chronic lymphocytic leukemia [**CLL**]). Monocytic leukemia, consisting of the overgrowth of monoblasts, is rare but can be either acute or chronic in nature.

TABLE 5-4 Complete Blood Count and Forms of Anemia

	RBC (per mm³)	Hgb (g/dL)	Hct (%)	MCV (per μm³)	MCH (pg)	MCHC (g/dL)	WBC (per mm³)	Reticulocyte Count (per mm³)	Platelet Count (per mm³)
Normal	Male, 4.7-6.1; female, 4.2-5.4	Male, 14-18; female, 12-16	Male, 42-52; female, 37-47	80-90	27-31	32-36	5000-10,000	0.5-2	150,000-400,000
Acute hemorrhagic anemia	Initial increase, latent decrease	Initial decrease, latent decrease	Normal initially, latent decrease	Increase	Decrease	Normal	Increase	Increase	Decrease
Chronic hemorrhagic anemia	Decrease	Decrease	Decrease	Slight decrease	Slight decrease	Slight decrease	Normal	Decrease	Normal
Iron-deficiency anemia	Decrease	Decrease	Decrease	Decrease	Decrease	Decrease	Normal	Decrease	Normal to increase
Aplastic anemia	Gross decrease	Gross decrease	Gross decrease	Moderate decrease	Gross decrease	Gross decrease	Gross decrease	Decrease	Gross decrease
Pernicious anemia	Decrease	Gross decrease	Gross decrease	Increase	Increase	Increase	Slight decrease	Decrease	Slight decrease
Folate-deficiency anemia	Decrease	Gross decrease	Gross decrease	Increase	Increase	Increase	Slight decrease	Decrease	Slight decrease
Sickle-cell anemia	Decrease	Decrease	Decrease	Decrease	Normal	Normal	Increase	Increase	Normal
Hemolytic anemia	Decrease	Decrease	Decrease	Increase	Slight decrease	Normal	Normal	Increase	Normal to increase

From Frazier MS, Drzymkowski J: *Essentials of human disease and condition*, ed 3, Philadelphia, 2004, Saunders.
RBC, Red blood cell; *Hgb*, hemoglobin; *HCT*, hematocrit; *MCV*, mean cell volume; *MCH*, mean cell hemoglobin; *MCHC*, mean (average) cell hemoglobin concentration; *WBC*, white blood cell.

Advanced Concepts

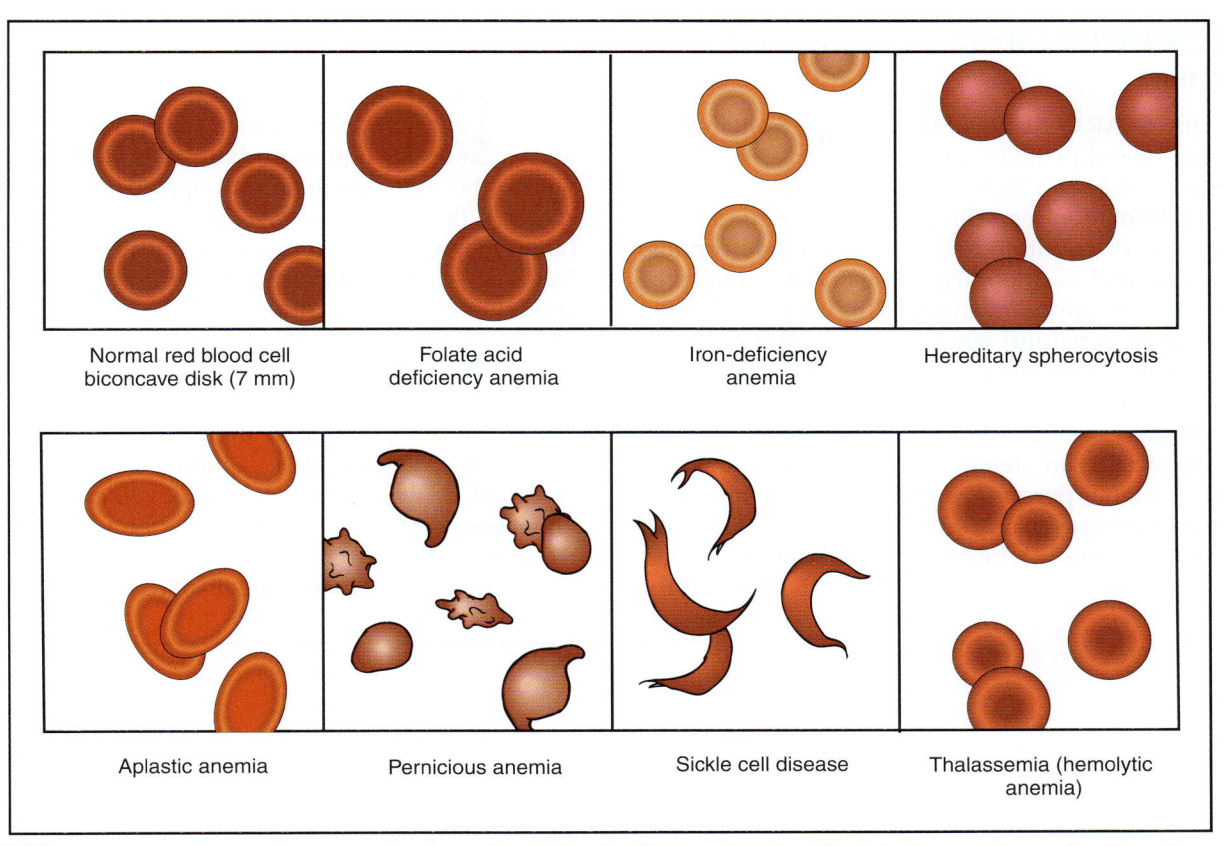

Fig. 5-28. Distinctive sizes, shapes, and colors of red blood cells associated with eight forms of anemia. (From Stepp CA, Woods M: *Laboratory procedures for medical office personnel*, Philadelphia, 1998, Saunders.)

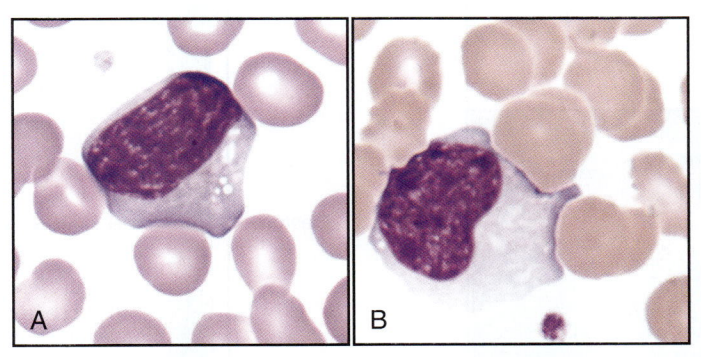

Fig. 5-29. Atypical reactive lymphocytes seen in mononucleosis. (From Carr JH, Rodak BF: *Clinical hematology atlas*, ed 3, St Louis, 2008, Saunders.)

CLIA-Nonwaived (Moderately Complex) Automated Hematology Systems

For offices that require more hematological information than just the waived Hgb and HCT, semi-automated hematology instruments that are CLIA approved as moderately complex may be appropriate. When performing this level of diagnostic testing, the laboratory professional will need to go through the registration, accreditation, and certification process with the Centers for Medicare and Medicaid Services (CMS) and comply with more rigorous quality control and assurance standards, including the documented training of operators and additional quality assurance standards, to include documentation of the following:

- Daily instrument calibrations and standards
- Two levels of controls run routinely
- Maintenance checks of the instrument, temperature, and supplies
- Proficiency testing

To pass the required proficiency testing, the office must run a sample from an outside proficiency laboratory twice a year and submit its results to see if they are within the acceptable range established by the accreditation agency. If the results are not in the acceptable range, the office must take the appropriate steps to correct the problem.

QBC STAR Centrifugal Hematology System

The QBC STAR Centrifugal Hematology System (Becton Dickinson) provides the ambulatory care setting with more than just Hgb and HCT values. It also provides information regarding the WBC count, platelet count, and distribution of granulocytes (neutrophils, basophils, and eosinophils) versus nongranulocytes (lymphocytes and monocytes). This additional WBC information is helpful when dealing with infections. Neutrophils predominantly fight bacterial infections, whereas lymphocytes fight viral infections. If the patient shows a high total WBC count (leukocytosis), the physician can determine which WBC demonstrates a higher percentage and act accordingly. This information is especially valuable to the pediatrician who needs to know whether a child should be placed on antibiotics for a bacterial infection. Laboratory values must always be correlated with the clinical state.

The QBC system spins down a capillary sample of blood into its various layers (red cells, buffy coat, and plasma). A fluorescent dye and a miniature float within the tube can stain and spread out the buffy coat of WBCs and platelets into three additional layers (granulocytes, nongranulocytes, and platelets). Fig. 5-30 shows the relative size of the centrifuged capillary specimen and the distribution of the centrifuged cell layers. A laser beam or a tungsten–halogen light beam is then directed at the separated layers of blood cells in the capillary tube to analyze each layer. The light beam strikes the cell layers at an angle, allowing sensors to detect the amount of light scattered and the amount absorbed by the cells. Each type of cell creates a different angle of scatter based on its volume, shape, and refractive index. After all the blood cell layers have been analyzed, the results are displayed and printed.

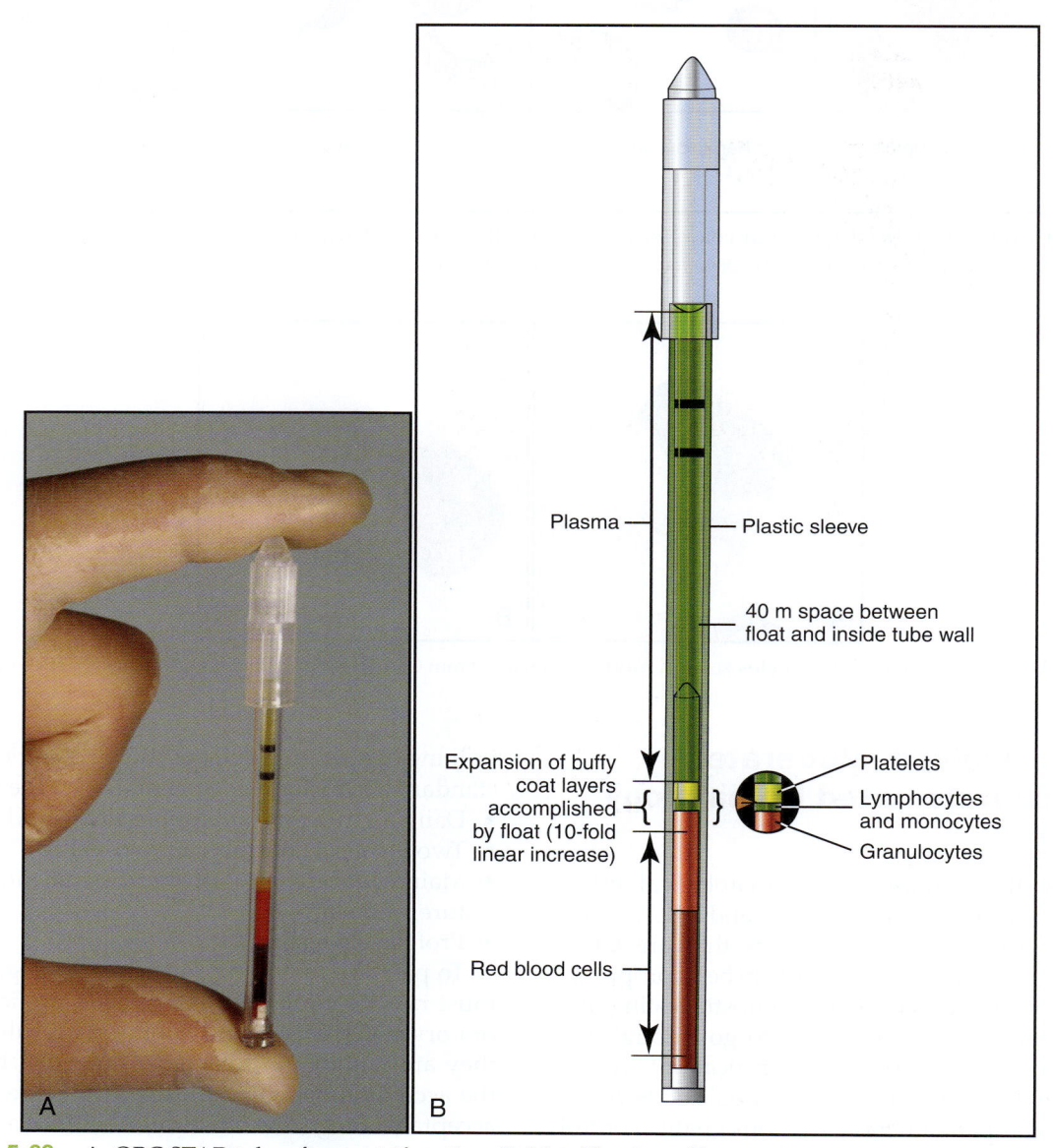

Fig. 5-30. **A,** QBC STAR tube after centrifugation. **B,** Identification of layers. (**B,** Courtesy of Becton Dickinson.)

Advanced Concepts

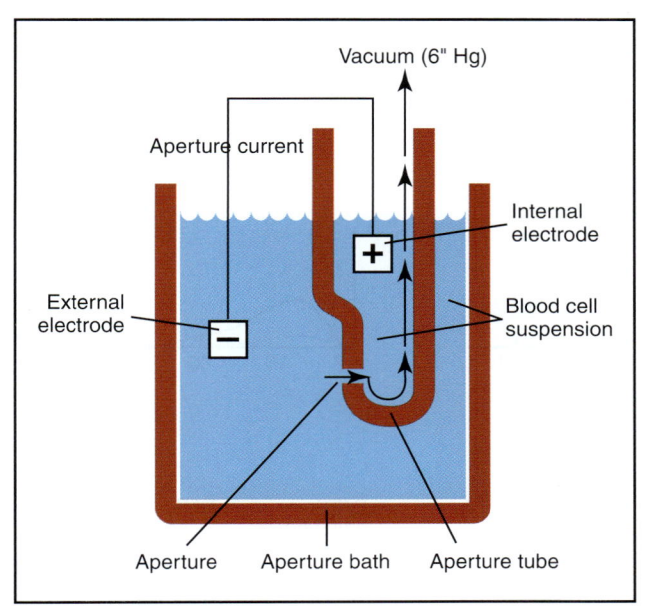

Fig. 5-31. The Coulter Counter system, which uses electrical impedance technology. (From Rodak BF: *Hematology: clinical principles and applications,* ed 3, St Louis, 2007, Saunders. Courtesy Beckman Coulter.)

Quality Assurance

The QBC is a moderately complex instrument that requires regular monitoring with the high and low liquid controls. The control test results must be logged and plotted to pick up any shifts, trends, or signs of inaccuracy. Proficiency testing with a specimen from an outside laboratory must also be done twice a year.

Coulter Counter System

The Coulter Counter (Beckman Coulter, Fullerton, Calif.) is a highly sophisticated hematology analyzer that performs an automated CBC. The test uses blood cells diluted with an electrolyte solution capable of conducting electricity. When the blood cells, which are poor conductors of electricity, pass through an opening (aperture) in the instrument, they cause a pulse or interruption (impedance) of the electrical circuit (Fig. 5-31). The pulses are counted, analyzed, and calculated by the instrument, which produces a readout. Compare the normal and abnormal reports in Fig. 5-32.

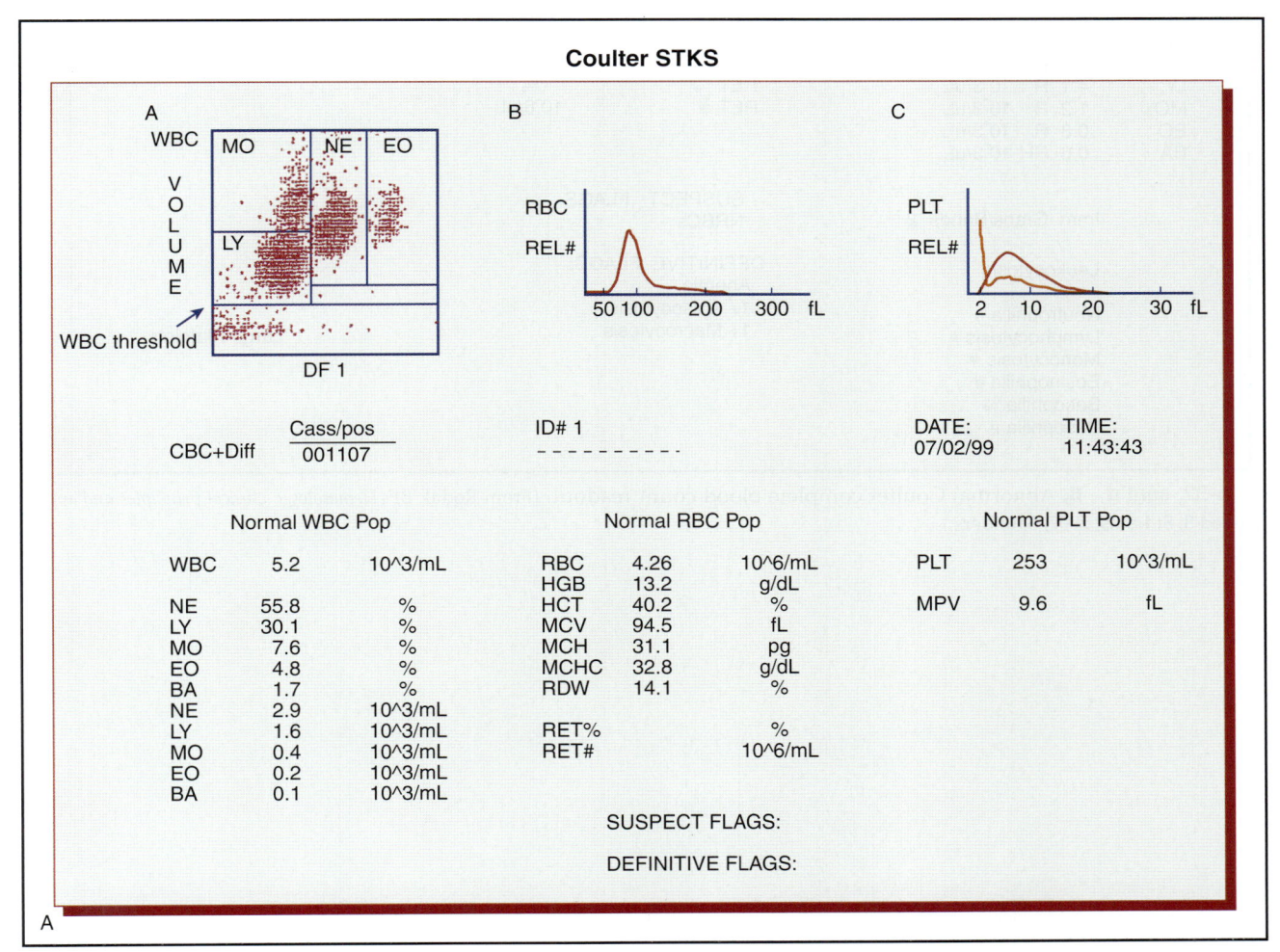

Fig. 5-32. **A,** Normal Coulter complete blood count readout.

Coulter STKS

A WBC VOLUME / DF 1

B RBC REL# (50 100 200 300 fL)

C PLT REL# (2 10 20 30 fL)

CBC+Diff   Cass/pos 001104

ID 1

DATE: 07/02/99   TIME: 11:41:03

Abnormal WBC Pop

WBC	18.0*RH	10^3/uL
NE	63.0	%
LY	22.6	%
MO	6.9	%
EO	4.3	%
BA	3.2	%
NE	11.3 RH	10^3/uL
LY	4.1 R	10^3/uL
MO	1.2 R	10^3/uL
EO	0.8 R	10^3/uL
BA	0.6 RH	10^3/uL

Imm Grans/Bands 2

Leukocytosis

Neutrophilia #
Lymphocytosis #
Monocytosis #
Eosinophilia #
Basophilia %
Basophilia #

Abnormal RBC Pop

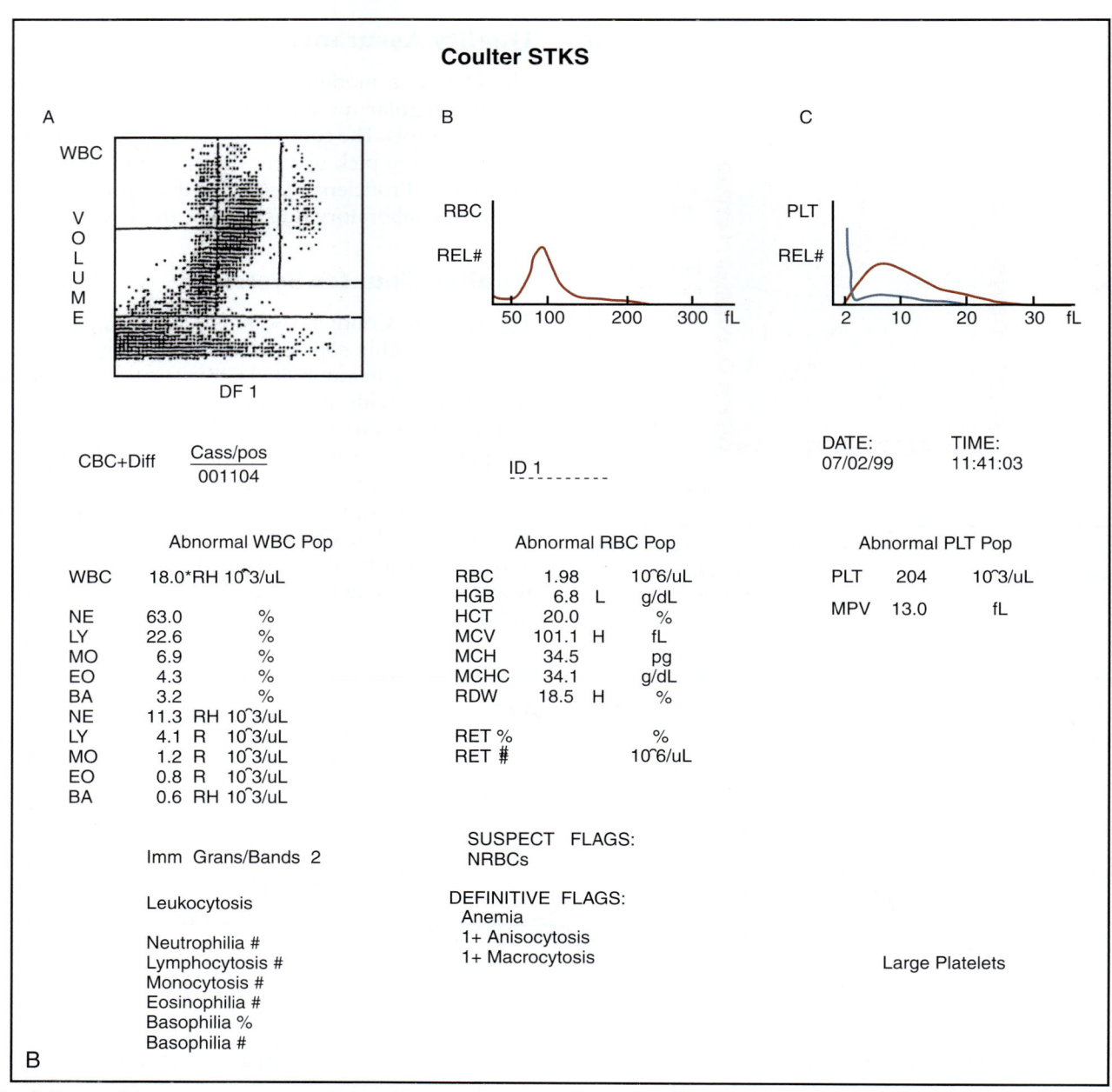

RBC	1.98	10^6/uL
HGB	6.8 L	g/dL
HCT	20.0	%
MCV	101.1 H	fL
MCH	34.5	pg
MCHC	34.1	g/dL
RDW	18.5 H	%
RET %		%
RET #		10^6/uL

SUSPECT FLAGS:
NRBCs

DEFINITIVE FLAGS:
Anemia
1+ Anisocytosis
1+ Macrocytosis

Abnormal PLT Pop

PLT	204	10^3/uL
MPV	13.0	fL

Large Platelets

Fig. 5-32, cont'd **B,** Abnormal Coulter complete blood count readout. (From Rodak BF: *Hematology: clinical principles and applications*, ed 3, St Louis, 2007, Saunders.)

Review Questions

1. Which of the following is not a formed element in the blood?
   a. Platelets
   b. Prothrombin
   c. RBCs
   d. WBCs

2. Match the following terms with their description: granulocytes anticoagulant erythrocytes megakaryocyte plasma platelet EDTA
   _____ complex liquid in which blood cells are suspended
   _____ most numerous blood cells (occupying almost 50% of the blood)
   _____ WBC group made up of neutrophils, eosinophils, and basophils
   _____ agent that prevents clotting of whole blood
   _____ cellular element important in hemostasis
   _____ most common anticoagulant used in routine hematology procedures
   _____ large bone marrow cell from which platelets are derived

3. Match the following terms with their definitions:
   ___ red cell   a. immature neutrophil
   ___ neutrophil   b. has coarse orange-red granules
   ___ eosinophil   c. smallest WBC
   ___ basophil   d. largest WBC
   ___ lymphocyte   e. has blue-black granules
   ___ monocyte   f. made of fragments of cytoplasm
   ___ platelet   g. biconcave disk
   ___ band cell   h. nucleus has two to five segments, and cytoplasm is pink/lavender with granules

4. Provide the missing terms found in the final steps of the common pathway of coagulation:
   _____ → Thrombin
   Fibrinogen → _____

5. Prothrombin (factor II) is a plasma protein dependent on vitamin ____.

6. Match each testing method with its appropriate test:
   ___ HemoCue   a. CBC
   ___ QBC   b. sedimentation rate
   ___ Westergren   c. coagulation test
   ___ HemataSTAT   d. Hgb
   ___ Protime   e. HCT

7. Match each RBC index with its ratio elements:
   ___ MCV   a. Hgb/RBC
   ___ MCHC   b. HCT/RBC
   ___ MCH   c. Hgb/HCT

8. Match each anemia with its cause:
   ___ iron-deficiency anemia   a. destruction of circulating RBCs
   ___ hemolytic anemia   b. seen with blood loss (menses, ulcers, hemorrhaging)
   ___ aplastic anemia   c. inherited abnormal Hgb-S molecule
   ___ sickle-cell anemia   d. destruction of stem cells in bone marrow from toxins
   ___ pernicious anemia   e. caused by decreased vitamin B_{12}

9. Match these leukocyte disorders with their descriptions:
   ___ leukocytopenia   a. presence of atypical "reactive" lymphocytes
   ___ ALL   b. increase in WBCs (usually from infection)
   ___ mononucleosis   c. long-term cancer of granulocytes in bone marrow
   ___ CML   d. sudden cancer of a nongranulocyte
   ___ leukocytosis   e. abnormal decrease of WBCs

Review Question Answers

1. b
2. plasma, erythrocytes, granulocytes, anticoagulant, platelet, EDTA, megakaryocyte
3. g, h, b, e, c, d, f, a
4. prothrombin, fibrin
5. K
6. d, a, b, e, c
7. b, c, a
8. b, a, d, c, e
9. e, d, a, c, b

Websites

American Society of Hematology's image bank of slides of normal and abnormal blood cells:
www.ashimagebank.org/contents.asp

Dr. Joseph F. Smith Medical Library site offers information on ESRs:
www.chclibrary.org/micromed/00047230.html

Manufacturer information on INRatio (HemoSense):
http://www.hemosense.com/support/productlit.shtml

CHAPTER 6

Chemistry

Objectives
After completing this chapter you should be able to:

Fundamental Concepts
1. Identify the plasma components in peripheral blood, and describe their function and significance.
2. Describe the proper specimen collection for various chemistry tests.
3. Explain the basic principles of glucose and fat metabolism.

CLIA-Waived Chemistry Tests
1. Follow the most current OSHA safety guidelines when performing chemistry tests.
2. Perform FDA-approved glucose, hemoglobin A1c, lipid panel, and fecal occult blood CLIA-waived tests according to the stated task, conditions, and standards listed on the Learning Outcome Evaluation found in the student workbook.
3. Describe the Beer–Lambert law and the principle supporting the way in which chemical analytes are measured by photometry.
4. Explain the importance of performing instrument calibrations, optics checks, quality controls, and Westgard's rules of quality control monitoring.

Advanced Concepts
1. List eight critical chemistry tests performed during medical emergencies.
2. Match chemistry panels with the tests performed.
3. Identify and inform the physician when laboratory reports show chemistry values out of the expected range by comparing patient results with the laboratory's reference range.
4. Using the chart of basic blood chemistry tests, identify a possible disease condition related to high or low patient test results.
5. Perform and/or discuss the use of the hand-held i-STAT analyzer for point-of-care testing blood electrolytes, anion gap, blood gases, BUN, and creatinine.

Key Terms

absorbance photometry indirect measurement of the amount of light that a solution absorbs
anion negatively charged ion
atherosclerosis formation of plaque along the inside walls of blood vessels
Beer–Lambert Law law stating that intensity of color change is directly proportional to the concentration of an analyte in a solution
carbohydrates sugars and starches
catalysts chemicals that produce specific changes in other substances without being changed themselves
cation positively charged ion
clinical diagnosis diagnosis based on the patient's initial signs and symptoms
clot activator chemical additive that speeds up the clotting of a blood specimen
definitive diagnosis final, confirmed diagnosis based on clinical signs and symptoms and the results of diagnostic tests
dyslipidemia abnormal amounts of fat and lipoproteins in the blood
endogenous cholesterol cholesterol manufactured in the liver
exogenous cholesterol cholesterol derived from the diet

galvanometer instrument capable of measuring the intensity of light
glucagon hormone produced by the pancreas to raise blood glucose by converting glycogen into glucose and noncarbohydrates into glucose
glycogen stored form of glucose found especially in muscles and the liver
glycosylated hemoglobin hemoglobin A molecule within red blood cells that becomes permanently bound to glucose
gout form of arthritis caused by accumulation of uric acid crystals in the synovial fluid
hyperglycemia elevated blood sugar
hyperinsulinemia excessively high blood insulin levels
hyperlipidemia excessive fat in blood, which gives plasma a milky appearance
hypoglycemia low blood sugar
insulin hormone produced by the pancreas to lower blood glucose level by moving it into body cells and converting glucose into glycogen for future use
insulin resistance condition in which insulin is not effective at moving the glucose from the blood into the cells (seen in type 2 diabetes)

Key Terms—cont'd

ions electrolytes consisting of positively or negatively charged particles
ketoacidosis acidosis caused by an accumulation of ketones in the body, a result of the excessive breakdown of fats; occurs primarily as a complication of type 1 diabetes mellitus
lipoproteins protein-linked lipids
myoglobin iron-containing, oxygen-binding protein found in muscles
occult hidden or not visible to the naked eye
panels groups of tests that focus on blood cells, particular organs, or metabolic functions
reflectance photometry indirect measurement of the light that reflects off a solution
trans fats synthetic hydrogenated fats
transmittance photometry measurement of the amount of light passing through a solution
troponin I and T heart-specific indicators of a recent myocardial infarction

Abbreviations

2 hr PP	2-hour postprandial (after eating)	IDDM	insulin-dependent diabetes mellitus (type 1)
A1c	hemoglobin A1c, glycosylated hemoglobin, or glycated hemoglobin	Ig	immunoglobulins (antibodies)
ALP or AP	alkaline phosphatase (also abbreviated as alk phos)	IGT	impaired glucose tolerance
		K^+	potassium ion
ALT	alanine aminotransferase	LD	lactic dehydrogenase
AST	aspartate aminotransferase	LDL	low-density lipoproteins, or "lousy" cholesterol
BUN	blood urea nitrogen		
Ca	calcium	Na^+	sodium ion
Cl^-	chloride ion	NIDDM	non–insulin-dependent diabetes mellitus (type 2)
CK	creatine kinase		
DM	diabetes mellitus	OGTT	oral glucose tolerance test
FBG	fasting blood glucose	SST	serum separator tube
FPG	fasting plasma glucose	T_3	triiodothyronine
GGT	gamma-glutamyltransferase	T_4	thyroxine
GTT	glucose tolerance test	TC/HDL ratio	total cholesterol compared with high-density lipoprotein
HCO_3^-	bicarbonate ion	TSH	thyroid-stimulating hormone
HDL	high-density lipoproteins, or "healthy" cholesterol	VLDL	very-low-density lipoprotein (e.g., protein and triglyceride)

FUNDAMENTAL CONCEPTS

Clinical chemistry is the testing of the chemical analytes found in various liquid body specimens, such as urine, whole blood, serum, plasma, **synovial fluid** (from joints), pleural fluid (from the chest cavity), pericardial fluid (from the sac surrounding the heart), peritoneal fluid (from the abdominal cavity), and cerebrospinal fluid. The specimens most commonly tested in the ambulatory setting are urine and blood.

Chapter 5 detailed the various cellular elements found in blood (red blood cells [RBCs], white blood cells, and platelets) and the blood coagulation process. This chapter deals with the *liquid* portion of blood: plasma.

Blood Plasma

Plasma is a pale yellow, sweet-smelling, sticky fluid occupying slightly more than 50% of the total blood volume. For a complete understanding of the numerous blood chemistry tests and their significance, the composition of plasma must be reviewed. Refer to the numbered flow chart (Fig. 6-1) while reading about each component.

Approximately 90% of plasma (1) is water (2), with hundreds of dissolved substances and gases, including the following:

- *Salts* (3)—electrolytes consisting of positively and negatively charged particles **(ions)** that maintain acid/base balance (e.g., sodium, chloride, potassium, and bicarbonate)
- *Nutrients* (4)—derived from the gastrointestinal tract after it digests and absorbs **carbohydrates** (sugars and starches) into glucose, fats into fatty acids, and proteins into amino acids, along with the essential vitamins and minerals
- *Waste products* (5)—from cellular and molecular metabolism; carried in the plasma and excreted by the urinary system (e.g., urea, creatinine, uric acid)
- *Hormones* (6)—from various endocrine glands (e.g., thyroid, pancreas)
- *Enzymes* (7)—**catalysts** produced by living cells that produce specific changes in other substances without being changed themselves
- *Proteins* (8)—a major portion of plasma that can be divided into three categories: albumin, globulin, and clotting proteins

Fundamental Concepts

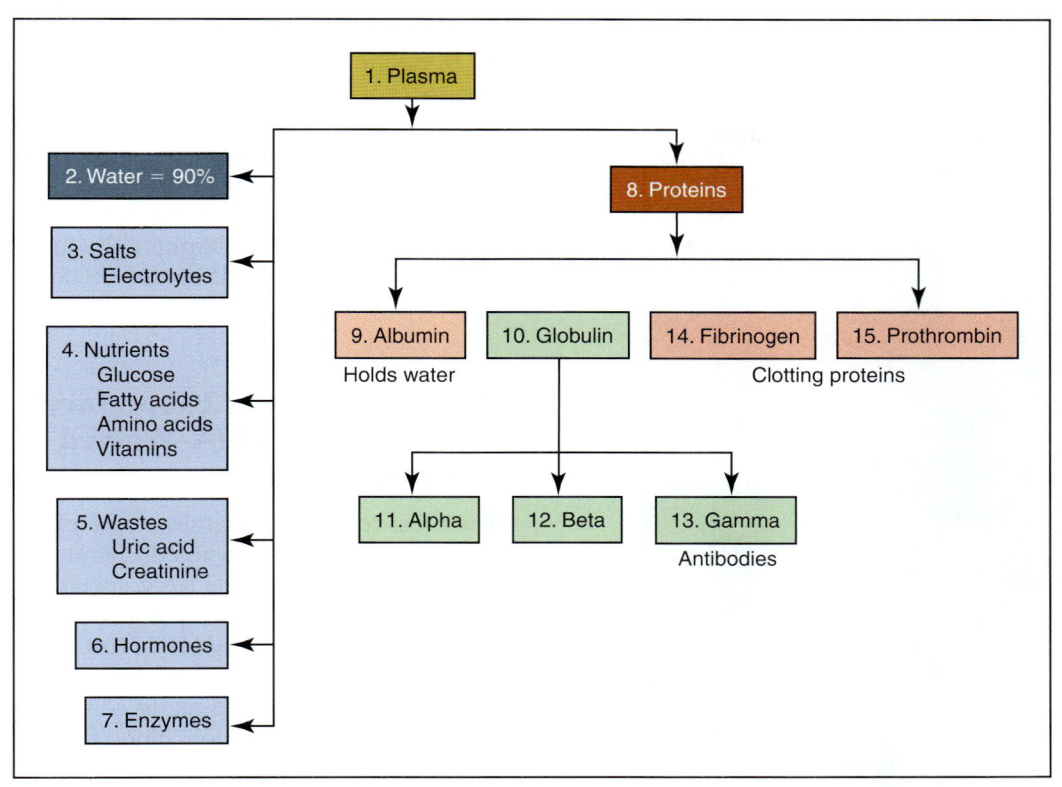

173

Fig. 6-1. Plasma flow chart.

- *Albumins* (9)—hold the water within the blood vessels
- *Globulins* (10)—simple proteins further classified into *alpha* (11), *beta* (12), and *gamma* (13); gamma globulins are also called immunoglobulins (**Igs** or antibodies)
- *Fibrinogen* (14) and *prothrombin* (15)—clotting proteins produced by the liver (when these clotting factors have been removed from plasma during the clotting process, the remaining fluid is referred to as *serum*)

Blood plasma is a dynamic, ever-changing liquid that reflects the inner workings of internal organs and tissues. In good health, each organ is constantly producing or removing its various chemical products within the plasma to maintain homeostasis. When disease strikes a particular organ or body system, homeostasis is interrupted and a change is seen in the blood chemistry. The measured change in blood chemistry allows a physician to detect or confirm the **clinical diagnosis** (diagnosis made on the basis of the patient's initial signs and symptoms). Follow-up chemistry tests allow the physician and patient to monitor the progress of the disease.

Blood Chemistry Specimens

The required blood specimens for chemistry testing differ depending on what analyte is being tested and what testing method is used at the reference laboratory or ambulatory setting.

Reference Laboratory Specimens for Blood Chemistry Testing

Blood chemistry tests derived from a reference laboratory generally require a *serum specimen*, which is obtained from a coagulated (clotted) blood specimen. The vacuum tube of choice for serum specimens is usually the gold serum separator tube **(SST)** containing a gel and a **clot activator** (a chemical additive that speeds up the clotting of the blood specimen). The SST containing the blood specimen must sit for 30 minutes after drawing to form a dense clot. The clotted specimen is then centrifuged for 10 to 15 minutes. The centrifugation forces the clotted cells to the bottom of the tube. Also during centrifugation, the gel migrates up over the cells, separating the serum from the clot. Fig. 6-2 shows the SST specimen (gold-topped tube) before and after centrifugation and the serum from a centrifuged red-topped "clot" tube.

Some chemical analytes may be affected by the clot activator or gel in the SST tube, so the laboratory may request that the serum specimen be collected in a plain red-topped tube that allows the blood to clot with no additives. Be sure to check the reference laboratory requisition (or the laboratory reference manual) to confirm the correct tube to draw for the ordered analyte(s). In the sample laboratory requisition in Fig. 6-3, note the routine chemistry tests and the required tube for each of the following:

- G for gold or gel found in the SSTs —yields a serum specimen that is separated from the clot tests that give results on either the blood cells (such as complete blood count [CBC] panels), particular organs (e.g., hepatic panel), or metabolic functions (e.g., Met. panels). A panel of tests can usually be run on one analyzer with one serum specimen at a much lower cost than a series of individual tests. (The various panels of tests run in reference laboratories are discussed later in this chapter.) The individual blood and urine tests are listed in alphabetical order on the requisition.

Physician's Office Laboratory Specimens for CLIA-Waived Chemistry Tests

The most common specimen in the physician's office laboratory (POL) for waived chemistry tests is the capillary puncture *whole blood* specimen. The blood is usually collected in a capillary tube containing an anticoagulant or directly into a testing device within a specified time frame. Testing devices may test the whole blood specimen directly, or they may separate the plasma from the whole blood before testing. The manufacturer's instructions must be read for each procedure to determine the exact type of specimen that should be used for each waived test.

Some waived tests may also use a venous anticoagulated whole blood specimen in place of the capillary blood specimen. Once again, only tubes designated by the manufacturer should be used. The following are examples of CLIA-waived specimens:

- **Glucose testing** may be run with the whole blood from a capillary puncture or venous blood collected in a **gray-topped tube.** The gray tube contains an antiglycosylating additive that prevents the glucose from being metabolized by RBCs. NOTE: Some glucose monitors will not work with the gray-topped blood specimens.
- The test for **glycosylated hemoglobin** (hemoglobin A1c molecule within RBCs that becomes permanently bound to glucose) can be performed with a capillary puncture specimen or a venous blood specimen collected in a **lavender-topped hematology tube.**
- **Cholestech** (Cholestech Corporation, Hayward, Calif.) lipid tests must be run with whole blood from either a capillary puncture or venous blood collected in a **green-topped vacuum tube** containing the anticoagulant *lithium* **heparin.** (NOTE: Green-topped *sodium* heparin tubes should *not* be used because they will interfere with the Cholestech testing method.)
- The basic metabolic chemistry tests run on an **I-Stat instrument** use whole blood from a finger stick collected in a capillary tube or venous blood collected in a **syringe or green heparin tube.**

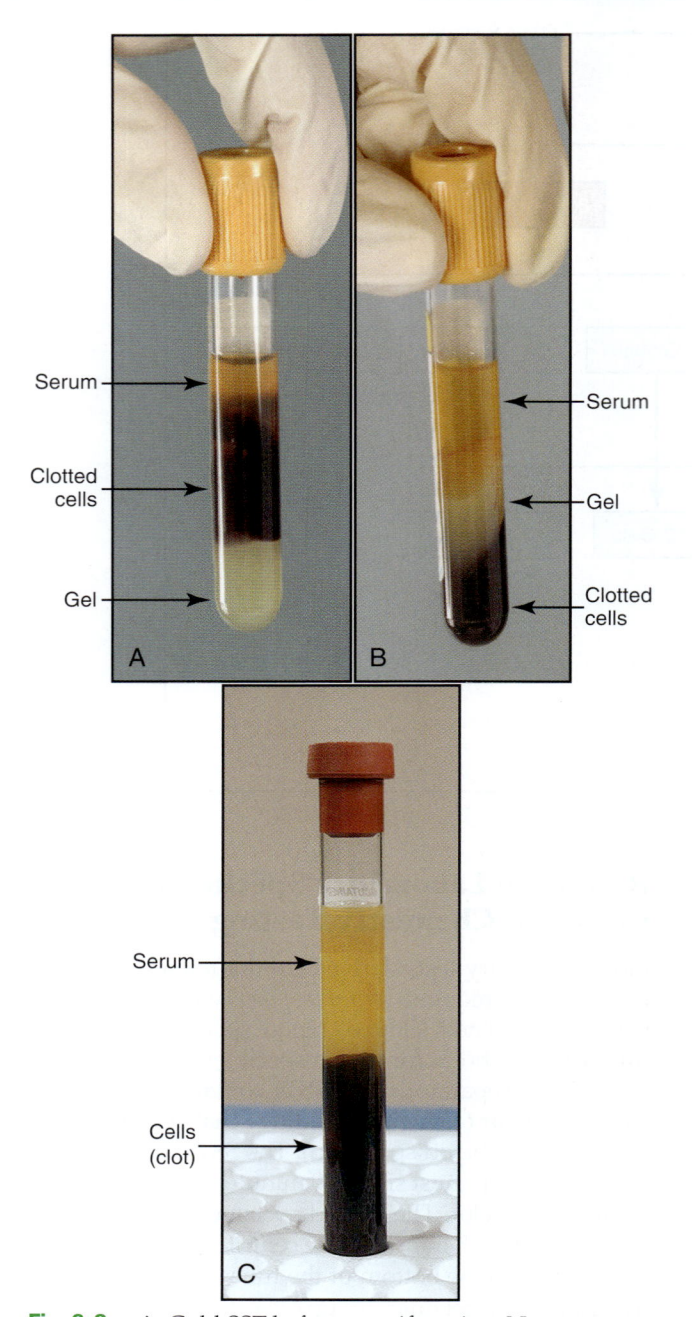

Fig. 6-2. A, Gold SST before centrifugation. Note position of the gel on the bottom. **B,** Gold SST after centrifugation. Note that the gel now separates the serum from the clotted cells. **C,** Centrifuged red-topped "clot" tube with no gel or clotting additive. (Modified from Bonewit-West K: *Clinical procedures for medical assistants,* ed 7, St Louis, 2008, Saunders.)

- R for red-topped "clot" tubes—yields a serum specimen with no clot activators or gel
- P for purple ethylenediamine tetraacetic acid (EDTA) anticoagulant tubes—for hematology testing
- Lt. Blue for sodium citrate anticoagulant—for coagulation testing

Also, notice the list of *panels* on the sample reference laboratory requisition. **Panels** are groups of

Fundamental Concepts

Patient Name: _____ DOB: _____ SS#: _____
Ordering Physician Signature: _____ Date: _____
Routine: _____ Standing Order: _____ Fasting: _____ Nonfasting: _____
Diagnosis Code: 1. _____ 3. _____
                2. _____ 4. _____
Copy to: _____

Panels
_____ CBC w/Diff	P	
_____ CBC without Diff	P	
_____ Electrolyte Panel	G	
_____ Hepatic Panel	G	
_____ Hgb and Hct	P	
_____ Lipid Panel	G	
_____ Met. Panel, Basic	G	
_____ Met. Panel, CMP	G	
_____ Renal Function Panel	G	

Urine Testing
_____ U/A w/Micro
_____ Urinalysis-dip only

Individual Chemistry
_____ Alk Phos (ALP)	G
_____ BUN	G
_____ Calcium, Serum	G
_____ Cholesterol	G
_____ CK, Creat. Kinase Tot.	G
_____ FSH	G
_____ Glucose	G
_____ Hemoglobin, A1c	P
_____ H. Pylori	G
_____ Iron	G
_____ Iron Panel, inc binding	G
_____ K (potassium)	G
_____ Magnesium	G
_____ Na (sodium)	G
_____ Phosphorus	G
_____ Prothrombin Time	Lt. Blue
_____ Rheumatoid Factor	G
_____ RA Titer	G
_____ Sed Rate	P
_____ SGOT (ALT)	G
_____ SGPT (AST)	G
_____ Uric Acid	G

Prostate Testing
_____ PSA Diag	G
_____ PSA M-Screening	G

Thyroid Specific Testing
_____ TSH	G
_____ T4 (Thyroxine)	G
_____ T3 Uptake	G
_____ Thyroid Panel w/TSH	G

Testing by Alpha
_____ 2 hr GTT	G
_____ 3 hr GTT	G
_____ 5 hr GTT	G
_____ Albumin	G
_____ Amylase	G
_____ APTT	Lt. Blue
_____ Bilirubin-Dorest	G
_____ Bilirubin-Total	G
_____ Chloride	G
_____ CO_2	G
_____ Digoxin	R
_____ HDL Cholesterol	G
_____ LD Lactate Dehyd.	G
_____ Mono Test	R
_____ Phenytoin	R
_____ Platelet Count	P
_____ Preg. Test	G
_____ RPR	G
_____ Protein, Total	G
_____ Tegretol	G
_____ TIBC	G
_____ Triglycerides	G
_____ Valproic Acid	R

G = Gold gel (SST tube)
R = Red (clot tube)
P = Purple (EDTA tube)
Lt. Blue = (sodium citrate)

Fig. 6-3. Sample requisition.

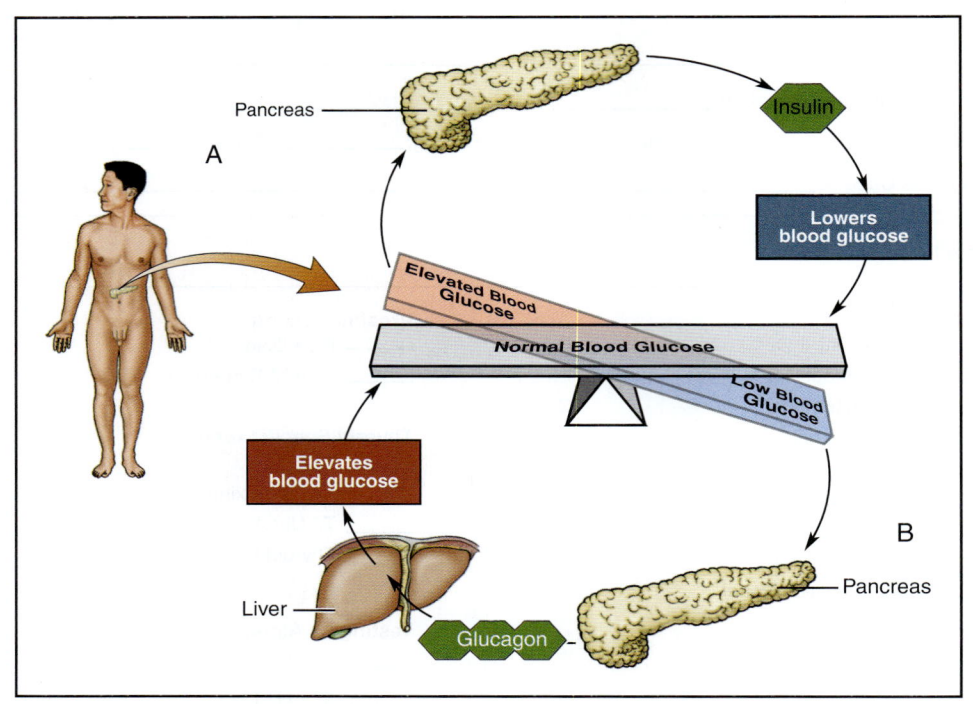

Fig. 6-4. Homeostatic balancing of glucose levels. **A,** When glucose level is too high, insulin lowers it to normal. **B,** When glucose level is too low, glucagon raises it to normal. (From Herlihy M: *The human body in health and illness,* ed 3, St Louis, 2006, Saunders.)

Glucose Metabolism and Testing

In the ambulatory care setting, the most common CLIA-waived chemistry tests are designed to screen and monitor glucose and lipid metabolism. These in-office tests allow the physician to receive results immediately and counsel the patients while they are still in the office. The physician may then order additional diagnostic tests from the reference laboratory to reach a **definitive diagnosis** (the final, confirmed diagnosis based on the initial clinical signs and symptoms of the patient compared with the results of the tests from the reference laboratory).

Glucose Metabolism

Glucose is a simple six-carbon sugar that all cells and tissues require for life-giving energy. Glucose enters the blood after the digestion of carbohydrates. Once glucose is in the blood, it is distributed, metabolized, and processed in the following cells, tissues, and organs:
- Body cells—all take in blood glucose for energy
- Muscles—store and convert excess glucose into **glycogen** (stored form of glucose found especially in the muscles and liver) for future needs
- Adipose tissues (fat)—take in fatty acids and glucose to produce triglycerides
- Liver—converts excess glucose into glycogen or combines glucose with fatty acids to produce triglycerides

Glucose levels in the blood must be maintained within a homeostatic range of 70 to 110 mg/dL. The monitoring and control of glucose levels within this range are controlled by two hormones: **insulin** and its antagonist, **glucagon** (Fig. 6-4). Both hormones are produced by the islets of Langerhans within the pancreas.

When glucose levels rise, as seen after eating, the hormone insulin is secreted from the beta cells within the islets of Langerhans. Insulin *reduces* the level of plasma glucose by (1) promoting movement of glucose from the blood into body cells, (2) stimulating the conversion of glucose to glycogen in the liver and muscles, and (3) stimulating the conversion of glucose and fatty acids into triglycerides within the liver and adipose tissues.

When blood glucose levels decrease, as during fasting, the hormone glucagon is secreted from alpha cells within the islets of Langerhans. Glucagon *increases* plasma glucose by stimulating the conversion of the stored glycogen in the liver and muscles back into glucose and then releasing the glucose into the blood.

Diabetes Mellitus

Diabetes mellitus **(DM)** is a disorder of carbohydrate metabolism characterized by **hyperglycemia** (elevated blood sugar) and glycosuria (sugar in the urine) resulting from the inadequate production or use of insulin. DM occurs when the pancreas is unable to produce enough effective insulin to move the glucose from the blood into the body cells. There are several types of diabetes.

Insulin-Dependent Diabetes Mellitus (Type 1)
Insulin-dependent diabetes mellitus (**IDDM**) occurs in 5% to 10% of the diabetic population. It is the result of an autoimmune destruction of the pancreatic beta cells, which are then unable to produce insulin. Without insulin the body cannot move glucose out of the blood and into the tissues. Consequently, patients with IDDM must constantly monitor their blood sugar levels and inject the appropriate amount of insulin to prevent the harmful effects of hyperglycemia. If glucose levels remain high for long periods, the following severe complications may occur:
- *Microvascular problems*, caused by the abundance of sugar blocking the small blood vessels, may lead to kidney disease and renal failure; retinopathy and blindness; and poor circulation in the extremities (e.g., the feet), resulting in recurring infections that may lead to gangrene and amputation.
- *Cardiovascular problems* caused by the subsequent formation of fatty plaque on the arteries may lead to atherosclerotic heart disease, hypertension, and stroke.
- *Ketoacidosis*, a dangerous blood condition, may lead to diabetic coma. Ketoacidosis occurs in IDDM when insulin is not present and the cells do not receive their glucose. It is the result of the body's effort to obtain its energy from fat rather than glucose. The by-products of the fat breakdown are ketones, which eventually make the blood dangerously acidic. When blood acidity and glucose levels are excessive, the patient becomes comatose.

By frequently monitoring glucose levels, the diabetic patient must administer insulin to keep any rising glucose levels down, thus preventing the harmful effects of hyperglycemia and ketoacidosis. The insulin-dependent diabetic patient can also keep glucose levels in control by following a low-carbohydrate diet and exercising.

Non–Insulin-Dependent Diabetes Mellitus (Type 2)
Non–insulin-dependent, or type 2, diabetes (**NIDDM**) accounts for 90% to 95% of the diabetic population. It has become epidemic in the United States because of the increasing numbers of obese, sedentary individuals. These individuals generally produce insulin, but it cannot effectively move the glucose from the blood into the cells, a condition known as **insulin resistance**. This resistance creates high blood glucose levels (hyperglycemia). Scientific research has found that the beta cells of the pancreas become sluggish and cannot release the right amount of insulin at the right time, causing fluctuating periods of hypoglycemia (low blood sugar) and hyperglycemia. The ineffectiveness of insulin's response to glucose is referred to as *impaired glucose tolerance* (**IGT**). IGT may then lead to **hyperinsulinemia** (excessive blood insulin levels). Hyperinsulinemia causes abnormal amounts of fat levels in the blood (**dyslipidemia**) that lead to **atherosclerosis** (the formation of plaque along the inside walls of blood vessels) and hypertension. The cascade effect of NIDDM that begins with insulin resistance and hyperinsulinemia, which then leads to high blood pressure and heart disease, has been described as *metabolic syndrome* (Fig. 6-5).

If individuals with NIDDM do not bring their high glucose levels under control, they incur the same microvascular and cardiovascular complications as out-of-control insulin-dependent diabetics. Research has shown that if individuals with NIDDM are diagnosed early, they can begin diet management, exercise, and the use of oral hypoglycemic medication to bring their sugar levels down. They may then avoid developing any of the negative complications caused by abnormally high blood sugar.

Table 6-1 summarizes the differences between type 1 and type 2 diabetes.

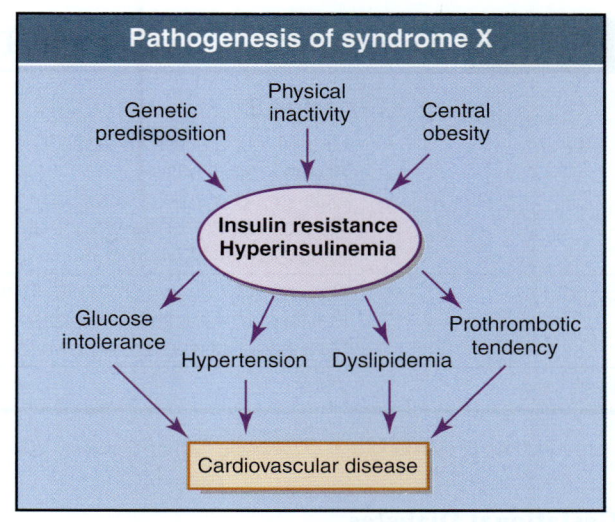

Fig. 6-5. Pathogenesis of syndrome X, also known as *metabolic syndrome*. (From Belchetz P, Hammond P: *Mosby's color atlas and text of diabetes and endocrinology,* St Louis, 2003, Mosby.)

Prediabetes
Prediabetes is the state that occurs when blood glucose levels are higher than normal but not high enough for a diagnosis of diabetes. Studies have shown that type 2 diabetes develops in most people with prediabetes within 10 years. Studies have also shown that people with prediabetes can prevent or delay the development of type 2 diabetes by up to 58% through changes in lifestyle that include modest weight loss with diets containing fewer refined carbohydrates (sugars and processed flour) and regular exercise.

TABLE 6-1 Comparison of Type 1 and Type 2 Diabetes Mellitus

	Type 1	Type 2
Features	Usually occurs before age 30 Abrupt, rapid onset Little or no insulin production Thin or normal body weight at onset Ketoacidosis often occurs	Usually occurs after age 30 Gradual onset; asymptomatic Insulin usually present 85% are obese Ketoacidosis seldom occurs
Symptoms	Polyuria (glycosuria promotes loss of water) Polydipsia (dehydration causes thirst) Polyphagia (tissue breakdown causes hunger)	Polyuria sometimes seen Polydipsia sometimes seen Polyphagia sometimes seen
Treatment	Insulin	Diet; oral hypoglycemic or insulin

From Chabner D: *The language of medicine*, ed 8, St Louis, 2007, Saunders.

Gestational Diabetes

Gestational diabetes occurs during pregnancy. The mother's IGT usually subsides after delivery of the baby. Signs and symptoms of gestational diabetes include glucosuria, hyperglycemia, excessive weight gain in the mother, and a baby weighing 9 pounds or more. Women who have gestational diabetes are also prone to developing type 2 diabetes later in life.

Transient Diabetes

Individuals may have diabetes during acute illness or steroid therapy. This form of diabetes usually lasts as long as the condition or treatment continues, then subsides.

Blood Glucose Screening and Monitoring Tests

The American Diabetes Association recommends two tests to identify diabetes and prediabetes in the early stages: the fasting plasma glucose test **(FPG)** and the oral glucose tolerance test **(OGTT)**. The blood glucose levels measured from these tests determine whether an individual has prediabetes or diabetes. The POL may perform CLIA-waived whole blood glucose tests that act as a screening test for potential diabetics. If the results of the screening tests are high, they must be confirmed by the plasma test or serum test methods that are usually performed by moderately complex reference laboratories.

Fasting Blood Glucose

For a fasting blood glucose test **(FBG),** a patient's fasting sample is usually taken in the morning after a fast of 10 to 14 hours. Patients cannot have any food from 10 PM until the test the next morning. Usually, they may drink only water, but check your institutional protocol for fasting preparations regarding proper timing and dietary restrictions. If the FBG is between 100 mg/dL and 126 mg/dL on two different days, the patient is considered prediabetic. If the FBG is greater than 126 mg/dL, the patient is considered diabetic (based on American Diabetes Association criteria). CLIA-waived glucose tests are for screening only and should be followed up with the more complex plasma tests for blood glucose. A definitive diagnosis is usually made with a venous specimen that has been collected in a gray-topped tube.

Oral Glucose Tolerance Test or 2-Hour Postprandial Blood Sugar

Another method of screening for diabetes mellitus is the OGTT, also called a 2-hour postprandial blood sugar **(2 hr PP)**. The OGTT begins with the measurement of FBG. If the results are within an acceptable range after the initial test, the patient is given a glucose-rich drink or meal and retested after 2 hours. Normal blood glucose levels should be brought down to less than 140 mg/dL 2 hours after the drink. If the glucose level does not fall below 140 mg/dL but is not greater than 200 mg/dL, the patient is considered prediabetic. If the glucose level is greater than 200 mg/dL after 2 hours, the patient is considered diabetic.

Random Glucose Test

A blood specimen can also be collected at any time to see if the glucose level is within the normal range of less than 140 mg/dL. A random blood specimen greater than 200 mg/dL is indicative of diabetes.

Glucose Tolerance Test

A more thorough test for measuring an individual's glucose metabolism is the full glucose tolerance test **(GTT),** in which blood glucose levels are measured at fasting and then at 1-hour intervals for 2 to 6 hours. The test generally takes place at a reference laboratory or hospital outpatient laboratory.

The GTT begins the same way the OGTT does, in that the patient comes in fasting and is initially tested for blood glucose level. If the results of the fasting

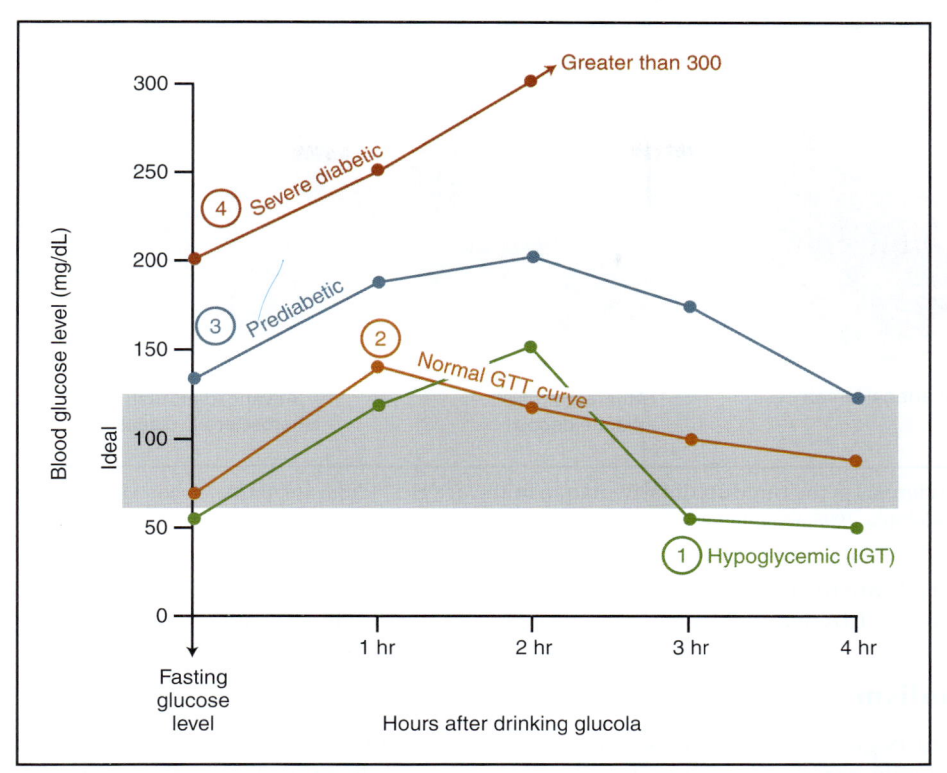

Fig. 6-6. Comparative patterns of GTT results. Compare the blood glucose levels for each condition during the initial fasting test, then the subsequent levels for each hourly test after consumption of the glucose drink.

test show a high glucose level (above 126), no further testing is done. If the results are within an acceptable range, the patient is given a 100-g dose of glucose to drink. Blood and urine specimens are collected and tested for glucose levels after the first half hour and then every hour for a specified period of time. The urine is tested to see if and when the blood glucose levels exceed the renal threshold for glucose of 160 to 180 mg/dL. When the renal threshold is exceeded, glucose is present in the urine.

During this test the patient should be monitored for signs of fainting or nausea. If these occur, or if the blood glucose levels exceed 300 mg/dL, the test should be terminated. If the doctor suspects hyperglycemia (diabetes), it is typically a 3-hour GTT. If the doctor suspects hypoglycemia, the test may continue for 5 or 6 hours. Fig. 6-6 shows the patterns of faulty glucose metabolism during a GTT.

Glycosylated Hemoglobin/Glycated Hemoglobin (Hgb A1c)

When hemoglobin A in the RBCs is exposed to high levels of glucose, the hemoglobin molecule is permanently glycosylated and changes into hemoglobin A1c **(Hgb A1c)**. Because the life span of an RBC is 80 to 120 days, the percentage of glycosylated hemoglobin molecules will be proportional to the overall concentration of glucose levels in the blood over the average life span of the RBCs (approximately 2 to 3 months). A normal percentage range of glycosylated hemoglobin in a whole blood specimen from adults is 2.2% to 4.8%.

The Hgb A1c test result is especially valuable to the person who is diagnosed with diabetes (or prediabetes) because it provides an accurate long-term index of the patient's average blood glucose level. Also, Hgb A1c test results are not subject to the daily fluctuations that occur in plasma glucose monitoring. Therefore the American Diabetes Association recommends the Hgb A1c as the best test to determine whether a patient's blood sugar has been under control during the previous 2 to 3 months. For example, if an Hgb A1c test result rises above the recommended 6% to 8%, the patient is at risk of developing the microvascular and cardiovascular complications previously discussed. This information can be used to encourage the patient to better understand and follow the treatment plan to prevent those complications.

Lipid Metabolism and Testing

Lipids, or fats, are essential to the body. They are an alternate source of energy when blood glucose levels are down and are critical to cellular health. Research has shown that poor lipid metabolism and cardiovascular disease are directly linked. In an effort to help correct the growing problems of obesity and heart disease in the United States, annual lipid screening

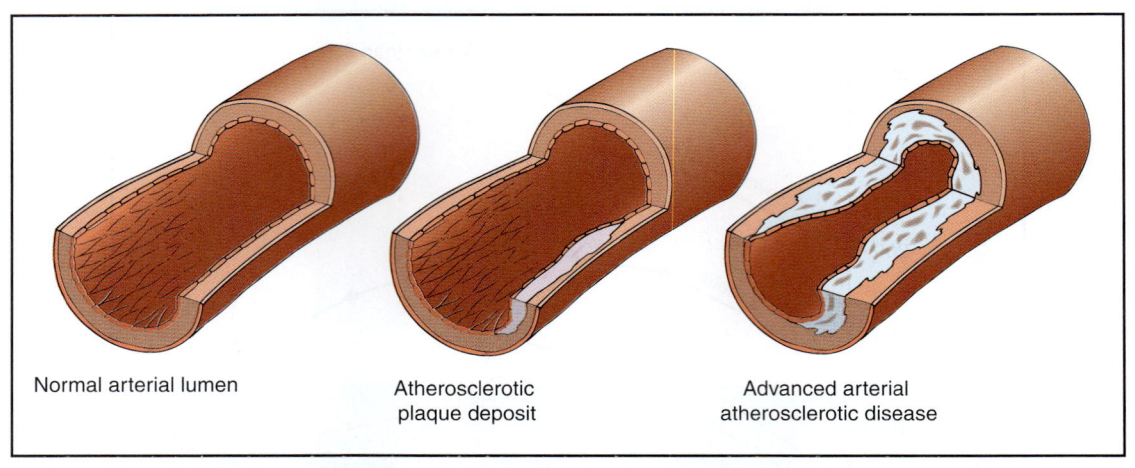

Fig. 6-7. Atherosclerosis is the buildup of fatty plaque in the arteries. (From Stepp CA, Woods M: *Laboratory procedures for medical office personnel*, Philadelphia, 1998, Saunders.)

and monitoring tests are recommended. Lipid screening is approved as a CLIA-waived test.

Lipid Metabolism

Lipid metabolism begins with the ingestion of fats. Dietary fats and oils are digested into fatty acids, which are transported to the liver to be reassembled into lipids. These lipids, like glucose, are then transported by the blood to all the body tissues. The lipids are used in critical cellular metabolism or stored as body fat. Some of the essential functions and uses of lipids are the following:
- Production of steroidal hormones
- Transportation of fat-soluble vitamins (vitamins A, D, and E)
- Insulation against extreme temperatures
- Maintenance of healthy skin
- Protection of vital organs and nerves
- Potential source of energy when glucose is not available
- Satisfies the feeling of hunger

The two plasma lipids most routinely tested are cholesterol and triglycerides. These two lipids can be further categorized and tested according to the three ways they are transported in the blood in the form of **lipoproteins** (protein-linked lipids): high-density lipoproteins **(HDL)**, low-density lipoproteins **(LDL)**, and very-low-density lipoproteins **(VLDL)**. Cholesterol, triglyceride, and lipoprotein levels are frequently ordered together in a lipid panel.

Cholesterol

Cholesterol is essential for the production of cell membranes, bile, myelin sheaths on nerves, and steroid hormones. Cholesterol is also required in the absorption of vitamin D. Cholesterol is found in the blood, bile, liver, brain, kidneys, and adrenal glands. Most of the cholesterol found in the blood is manufactured in the liver and is called **endogenous cholesterol.** In fact, the liver is able to produce all the cholesterol the body needs.

Another source of cholesterol, **exogenous cholesterol,** comes from what we eat. Foods high in saturated fats and **trans fats** tend to raise the blood level of cholesterol. Trans fats are synthetic hydrogenated fats found in partially hydrogenated margarines and oils used in cooking and baking. Saturated fats are found in meat, egg yolks, milk, and other dairy products that are usually hard or semisolid at room temperature. Both trans fats and saturated fats are known to elevate cholesterol levels, causing atherosclerosis (Fig. 6-7).

Not all dietary fats have the adverse effects of saturated fats and trans fats. Research has found that mono*unsaturated* fats and poly*unsaturated* fats, which are naturally liquid at room temperature, actually lower the blood level of cholesterol. These fats can also reverse plaque buildup on blood vessel walls. Examples of "good" monounsaturated fats are canola oil, olive oil, and omega-3 oil from fish. Examples of good polyunsaturated fats are soybean, safflower, corn, and cottonseed oils.

Lipoproteins

Cholesterol and triglycerides are lipids that do not mix with the water in plasma. Consequently, the liver attaches a protein to these lipids, which then become lipoproteins. The following three types of lipoproteins are manufactured in the liver and are classified on the basis of their density:
- HDL (high-density lipoprotein) is referred to as the "healthy" cholesterol because it has the lowest fat content and appears to protect against the accumulation of fatty deposits on blood vessels. In fact, HDL is capable of removing excess cholesterol from the walls of the blood vessels and carrying it back to the liver to be excreted.

- LDL (low-density lipoprotein) is referred to as the "lousy" cholesterol because it forms plaque on the walls of the blood vessels (atherosclerosis) because of its higher fat content. LDL becomes elevated in the blood after saturated fats and trans fats are ingested. Some individuals are also genetically predisposed to producing LDL endogenously within the liver.
- VLDL (very-low-density lipoprotein) is made predominantly of proteins linked to triglycerides. VLDL is also directly linked to the formation of plaque and atherosclerosis.

Total Cholesterol/High-Density Lipoprotein Ratio

The total blood cholesterol level (TC) is compared with the HDL level in the form of a ratio. This ratio provides an important index for determining the cardiac risk a patient faces because of atherosclerosis. The **TC/HDL ratio** is more valuable than TC alone because it takes into account whether a high level of TC is made up of the HDL "healthy" cholesterol or the undesirable LDL cholesterol. A ratio above 4.5 indicates that the person either is not producing enough good HDL or is producing too much bad LDL. In either case, the individual will need to do the following to lower cardiovascular risk:

- Exercise routinely, which will cause the HDL level to rise and the triglyceride level to go down.
- Change eating habits in favor of foods that are low in refined carbohydrates and high in fiber (e.g., whole grains, vegetables, fruits), which will lower glucose and triglyceride levels.
- Lower the dietary intake of trans fats and saturated fats found in baked goods, dairy, and fatty meats. This will lower the LDL levels.
- Change to a diet containing natural monounsaturated fats and polyunsaturated fats found in olive, canola, soybean, safflower, and other oils. This will raise HDL levels.
- Begin cholesterol-lowering medications (e.g., statins) as prescribed by the physician.

Triglycerides

Triglycerides are a direct result of diets rich in carbohydrates. Triglycerides account for 95% of the fat stored in adipose tissue. High levels of triglycerides are also associated with atherosclerotic risk. Like cholesterol, triglycerides are transported in the plasma bound to proteins as either LDL (15%) or VLDL (85%). When elevated, triglycerides produce a milky-white appearance in the plasma, a condition called **hyperlipidemia**. Triglyceride levels rise significantly in the blood after sweets or alcohol are ingested and when blood insulin levels are high (hyperinsulinemia). Therefore, when testing for triglyceride levels in the blood, most laboratories require the patient to fast 12 to 14 hours before testing and to refrain from alcohol 2 days before testing. Triglyceride levels can be lowered by exercising and decreasing dietary intake of sweets and alcohol.

The Lipid Panel

The lipid panel of tests consists of TC, HDL, LDL, VLDL, triglycerides, and the TC/HDL ratio. Medical research has established a direct link between blood lipid levels and coronary artery disease that may lead to subsequent myocardial infarcts (heart attacks). Myocardial infarction is the leading cause of death in the United States. An individual's cardiovascular risk can be determined by comparing the results of the tests in the lipid panel with the individual's age, weight, height, blood pressure, and smoking habits. Early detection of an at-risk individual can reduce the risk of cardiovascular disease and heart attack if the individual is placed on an appropriate preventive treatment plan consisting of exercise, diet, and medication therapy.

CLIA-WAIVED CHEMISTRY TESTS

Most of the CLIA-waived blood chemistry tests that are performed or observed in ambulatory settings are *quantitative* analyses. The numeric blood levels of glucose, lipids, glycosylated hemoglobin, electrolytes, BUN, and creatinine are all quantified by electronic photometers. The CLIA-waived fecal **occult** blood (hidden or not visible to the naked eye) test is a *qualitative* analysis that simply detects the presence or absence of blood in a fecal specimen.

Principle of Photometers and Spectrophotometers

Each blood chemistry testing method in this section involves collecting a capillary puncture whole blood specimen into a testing device containing premeasured reagents that react with the analyte being tested. The reagents change color as they react to the analyte in question (similarly to the color changes occurring in urine dipsticks). The testing devices are inserted into an electronic analyzer that sends a spectrum of light through the specimen. A photometer located within the analyzer measures the amount of light that passed through the specimen or reflected off the specimen. The intensity of the color changed by the specimen is directly proportional to the concentration of the analyte within the specimen. This equation is known as the **Beer–Lambert law**.

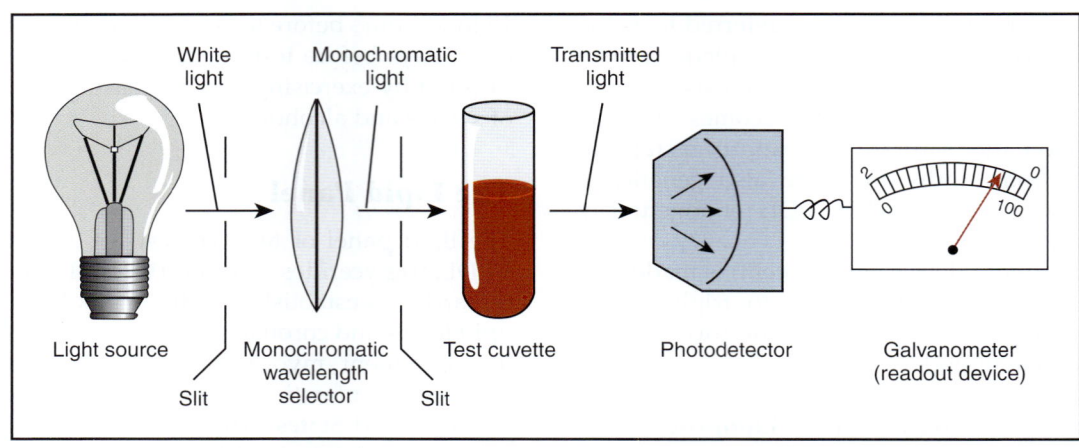

Fig. 6-8. Principles of photometry: A spectrum of light passes through the specimen and strikes a photodetector. The intensity of light received by photodetector is then sent to a readout device that is able to convert the light intensity to a quantitative concentration of the analyte being tested. The intensity of the color changed by the specimen is directly proportional to the concentration of the analyte within the specimen based on the Beer–Lambert law. (From Stepp CA, Woods M: *Laboratory procedures for medical office personnel,* Philadelphia, 1998, Saunders.)

The chemical analyzers used in blood chemistry testing are highly sensitive photometers and spectrophotometers that directly measure the amount of light passing through the solution **(transmittance photometry)**, indirectly measure the amount of light that the solution absorbs **(absorbance photometry)**, or indirectly measure the amount of light the solution reflects **(reflectance photometry)**. Once the light passes through the solution (or reflects off the specimen), it activates a photodetector that activates a **galvanometer** (an instrument capable of measuring the intensity of light). The galvanometer sends the information to an electronic program that converts the information into a quantitative digital readout (Fig. 6-8).

Quality Assurance When Using Optical Instruments

Optical tests depend on all the elements in the light path functioning correctly to receive accurate and reliable results. To accomplish this, each analyzer provides an "optics check" or calibration device or setting that ensures the instrument's optics are working correctly.

Be sure to observe and document all the quality assurance and quality control steps in the instruction manuals for the various chemical analyzers. The skill check sheets and corresponding logs for the tests covered in this text are located in the workbook. They all have the following preanalytical requirements:

- Instruments must be calibrated *daily*, and the calibration results must be logged in the calibration log. Newer analyzers may self-calibrate with each specimen and will not require logging.
- Run liquid controls for each test method according to the manufacturer's recommendations to check the technique and accuracy of the various testing devices, such as the glucose strip, the Hgb A1c cartridge, and the Cholestech cassette. Log the results of the controls. If they do not fall within the manufacturer's acceptable range, check the following:
  1. Was the control specimen processed poorly, or was the testing technique poor?
  2. Were the reagents or liquid controls stored at the wrong temperature? Had they expired?
  3. Was the instrument dirty or faulty?
- Always check the expiration date of the testing device, and do not run the test if the expiration date has passed.
- Because the testing device kits for each test must be stored and tested within a specific temperature range, record and monitor the daily room temperature and refrigerator temperature on a log sheet, as found in the workbook. Also pay strict attention to the length of time it is necessary to wait for a testing device that has been stored in the refrigerator to come to room temperature.
- Always retain the most current package inserts that come with the liquid controls and the testing kits and attach them to the procedure sheets for each test method.

Westgard's Rules for Monitoring Quality Control Results

In Chapter 2 the weekly logging of the liquid control results were placed onto a Levy–Jennings graph and analyzed for excessive scatter, trends, and shifts (see Figs. 2-4 through 2-7). The control's mean (average) value and its reference range (+/- 2 standard deviations) were compared with a target that would show if the daily results were consistently accurate and precise (see Fig. 2-8). In this chapter each of the chemical analyzers require the periodic running of one to three liquid controls to determine whether the testing procedure is able to consistently detect both the normal values and the abnormal values of the chemicals being measured.

Westgard has set up four additional rules to help evaluate the reliability of a test method when the controls have been run over time. By plotting the monthly logged control results onto a Levy–Jennings graph, one can see if any of the following rules have been broken, which indicates a faulty testing system. Do not run patient tests, and contact the manufacturer if any of the following patterns show up on the Levy–Jennings chart:

1. Both levels of control results are outside the manufacturer's reference range.
2. The same control level falls outside of the reference range in two successive runs.
3. One of the controls falls outside of the plus or minus one standard deviation in four successive runs.
4. One of the controls consistently falls above the mean value or consistently falls below the mean value for 10 consecutive runs.

A monthly Levy–Jennings graph and exercise are provided in the workbook. Also, when running the tests in the lab class, plot the results of the controls for all the students and analyze their accuracy and precision to see if the plotted results pass the criteria for reliability.

CLIA-Waived Glucose Tests

Present blood glucose levels can be readily screened and monitored with simple handheld glucometers. Blood glucose levels over time can also be monitored by testing the percentage of glycosylated hemoglobin (A1c) in a whole blood specimen.

Glucose Monitoring Devices

Numerous brands of glucose meters have been approved for home use and for point-of-care monitoring and screening. Technology continues to make it easier to obtain blood specimens and obtain the glucose results in seconds. For example, multiple-site lancets can now be used to collect a very small amount of blood from sites other than the finger, such as the forearm. NOTE: Although forearm testing can give sensitive fingertips a break from testing, forearm testing is not recommended whenever the blood sugar levels may be running low, such as before meals, after exercising, and after administering insulin. It has been proved that fingerstick blood samples will show hypoglycemia more quickly than forearm testing, thus alerting the patient to possible insulin shock.

Noninvasive infrared absorption technology has also made it possible to measure the blood glucose levels with no stick at all.

Glucose meters are also becoming more and more sophisticated, with computerized readouts that graph the patient's glucose readings throughout each day of the week. The computerized visual data help the patient and physician see exactly when glucose levels become out of control during the week. The patient may then take the appropriate steps to prevent those problems. The Contour (Bayer, Pittsburgh, Penn.) procedure check sheet is provided in the workbook and is demonstrated in Procedure 6-1, located at the end of this section. This monitor is similar to the One-Touch Ultra (LifeScan, Milpitas, Calif.). Both devices can be viewed on the Internet (along with many other glucose monitoring methods) by going to the various manufacturers' websites. (NOTE: Never run the supplies or controls from one manufacturer on a different manufacturer's analyzer.)

Glycosylated Hemoglobin A1c

The Hgb A1c test is generally used for monitoring diagnosed diabetics or prediabetics at 3- and 6-month intervals to make sure they are keeping their long-term glucose levels under control. Several brands of analyzers measure Hgb A1c. The Bayer A1c NOW+ procedure check sheet is provided in the workbook and is demonstrated in Procedure 6-2, located at the end of this section. It uses a dedicated testing meter that is packaged with 20 test cartridges and 20 sampling packets that all share the same code as the meter. When the 20 tests are completed, the meter is deactivated. Another kit with a new dedicated meter and its 20 coded cartridges and sampling packets is then purchased for the next 20 A1c tests.

Cholesterol and Lipid Profiles with the Cholestech LDX

Total blood cholesterol testing and lipid profiles have become standard screening tests in POLs. The Cholestech LDX is a popular analyzer capable of measuring either single blood cholesterol levels or the full panel of lipids plus glucose. Its procedure check sheet is provided in the workbook and demonstrated in Procedure 6-3, located at the end of this section.

The Cholestech is also approved for CLIA-waived testing for the two liver enzymes alanine aminotransferase **(ALT)** and aspartate aminotransferase **(AST)**. These enzymes may become elevated if a person who is taking statin drugs (i.e., cholesterol-lowering drugs such as Zocor or Lipitor) is experiencing liver damage. If enzyme results are elevated, the physician may consider a different therapeutic drug. NOTE: Because these enzymes are also elevated during muscle damage, the physician must interpret the significance of the results on the basis of an entire clinical evaluation of the patient.

Fecal Occult Blood Testing with the Guaiac Method

Fecal occult blood testing is a simple, inexpensive test to detect blood that may be hidden or not visible to the naked eye (occult) on or in a stool specimen. It is a useful aid in the diagnosis of a number of gastrointestinal disorders and is typically part of a routine physical examination or a mass screening clinic of the population for colorectal cancer.

The presence of blood in fecal matter may be the result of bleeding from hemorrhoids, polyps, diverticulitis, dysentery, parasites, fissures, colitis, or colorectal cancer. If a positive result is obtained, additional follow-up diagnostic tests are performed, such as proctosigmoidoscopy, colonoscopy, or barium enema x-ray studies to determine the cause of the bleeding.

Cancer of the colon is one of the leading causes of death in the United States. The early stages of colon cancer are usually painless and asymptomatic. By the time an individual becomes aware of the condition, the cancer is typically at the metastasizing phase. Therefore early detection is especially critical while it is still localized and curable. The American Cancer Society recommends that a fecal occult blood test be a routine part of the physical examination of adults.

The principle of the test is to apply samples from various fecal specimens to paper slides coated with guaiac (a wood resin that reacts with blood). The paper slides are contained within cardboard testing devices that are then mailed or returned to the testing site. If blood is present, the hemoglobin will react with the guaiac and turn blue when a developing solution is applied. The developing solution consists of hydrogen peroxide. False-positive test results can occur if the patient's diet is high in red meat, turnips, horseradish, or bananas. Certain therapeutic drugs, such as nonsteroidal antiinflammatory drugs, aspirin, iron preparations, and anticoagulants, may also cause positive findings because of their effects on the gastrointestinal tract. The procedure for fecal occult blood check sheet is provided in the workbook and is demonstrated in Procedure 6-4, located at the end of this section.

An alternative patient-friendly method of testing for occult blood consists of simply floating a test pad in the toilet after a bowel movement. The pad is checked for a change in color caused by the presence of blood in the toilet water. See the second part of Procedure 6-4 for this ColoCARE method of testing for fecal occult blood. Another highly sensitive method for testing fecal occult blood is found in Chapter 7. It is referred to as the iFOB test, which is the acronym for immunoassay fecal occult blood.

Summary of CLIA-Waived Tests

All the CLIA-waived tests covered in the preceding sections are *screening* tests to detect possible risks to a patient's health. The glucose test detects possible diabetes, the lipid profile detects possible cardiovascular disease, and the occult blood test detects possible colon cancer.

Diabetes and cardiovascular diseases have become so prevalent in the United States that in 2005 the Center for Medicare and Medicaid Services approved coverage of glucose screening and preventive cardiovascular screening for all Medicare beneficiaries. The new coverage went into effect as part of the larger Medicare Prescription Drug, Improvement, and Modernization Act of 2003. The approved cardiovascular screening includes three tests to detect early risk for cardiovascular disease: TC, HDL, and triglycerides. The TC/HDL ratio can also be determined by these tests, which can be ordered individually or as part of a lipid panel.

Becoming Proficient at CLIA-Waived Chemistry Testing

Now that you have learned about the significance of glucose, hemoglobin A1c, lipid panels, and occult blood tests, take time to complete the following:
1. Answer the CLIA-waived portion in Chapter 6 of the workbook using your structured notes and text.
2. View the videos on-line to see glucose quality controls and fecal occult instructions and testing.
3. Perform the Chapter 6 on-line exercises, which are designed to reinforce your terminology and CLIA-waived test knowledge.
4. Study Procedures 6-1 through 6-4 at the end of this section before your lab.

CLIA-Waived Chemistry Tests

PROCEDURE 6-1 Glucometer Procedure

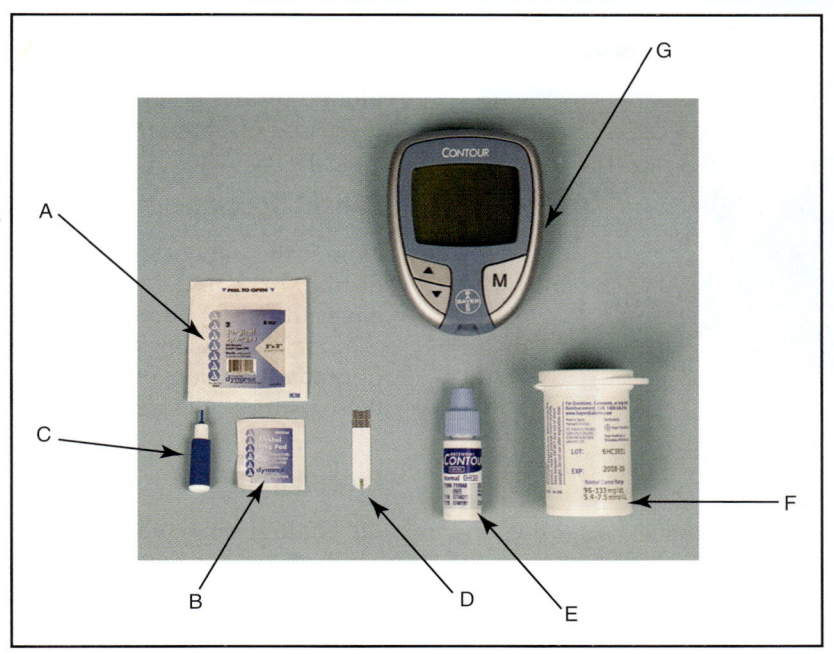

A. Equipment and supplies. *a,* Gauze; *b,* alcohol; *c,* lancet; *d,* test strip; *e,* liquid control; *f,* test strip container with control reference range; *g,* contour glucometer.

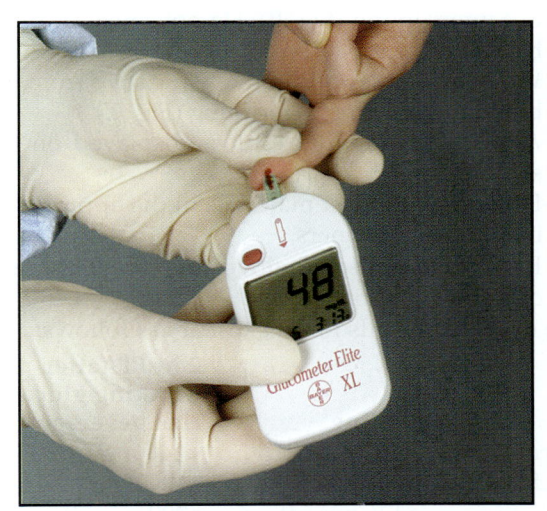

B. Glucometer (Ascensia) procedure. Collecting the specimen into the tip of the strip.

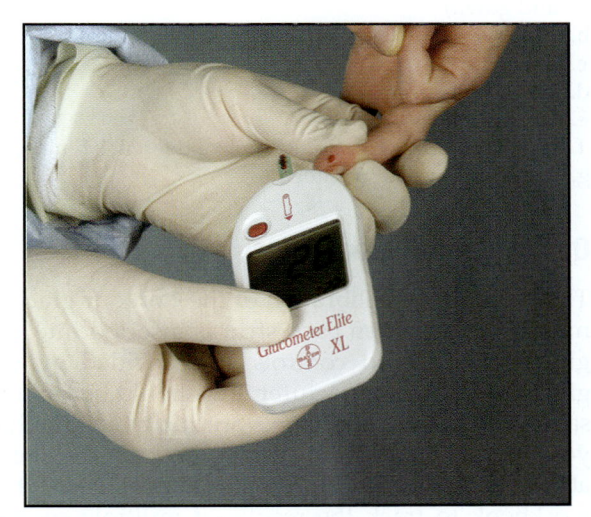

C. When a beep sounds, remove the strip from the drop of blood.

(Continued)

PROCEDURE 6-1 Glucometer Procedure—cont'd

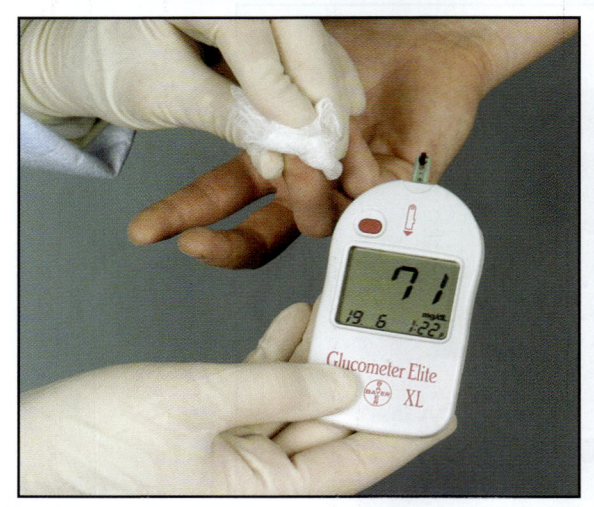

D. After 30 seconds the glucometer will display the glucose result.

Equipment and Supplies (Fig. A)

a. Gauze and personal protective equipment (gloves and gown)
b. Alcohol
c. Lancet
d. Test strips
e. Liquid control
f. Strip container with liquid control reference range
g. Contour glucose monitor

Quality Control Procedures

The "coding" or calibration of the Contour glucose monitor is set when each strip is inserted into the glucometer. Liquid controls are provided by the glucose meter manufacturer and should be run the same way patient specimens are run to ensure that your technique and the system are providing reliable results. A control log has been provided in the workbook to track the results of multiple control readings. The results can then be plotted on a graph as seen in Chapter 1 in order to pick up trends, shifts, randomized errors, and so forth. A control log and control graph are provided in the workbook to plot the results of multiple control readings. Check the plotted control graph for signs of trends or drifts, as discussed in Chapter 1.

Patient Specimen

Note if the patient's capillary specimen is random, fasting, or 2 hr PP. Each of these specimens will have a different reference range.

NOTE: The Contour pictured in Fig. A is an upgraded version of the Elite glucometer seen in these pictures; the procedure steps remain the same.

Procedure

1. Sanitize the hands, and don gloves.
2. Turn on the meter by inserting the end of the strip that contains the metallic contact bars.
3. Perform a capillary puncture, and wipe away the first drop. Then touch the exposed end of the strip to the base of the second drop of blood, allowing the blood to "sip" into the strip without interruption (Fig. B). Do not smear or place blood on the top or bottom of the strip.
4. When a beep sounds, remove the strip from the blood to keep from overfilling (Fig. C).
5. After 5 seconds the result is displayed on the screen (Fig. D).
6. Discard all the test materials in the appropriate biohazard containers.
7. Remove and discard gloves into the biohazard container. Sanitize hands.

The expected results for this test are as follows:

	Fasting	2 hr PP (after drinking glucose-rich beverage)
Normal	<100 mg/dL	<140 mg/dL
Prediabetes	100-125 mg/dL	140-199 mg/dL
Diabetes	≥126 mg/dL or above	≥200 mg/dL

Fig. A courtesy Zack Bent.

CLIA-Waived Chemistry Tests

PROCEDURE 6-2 A1c NOW+ Glycosylated Hemoglobin Procedure

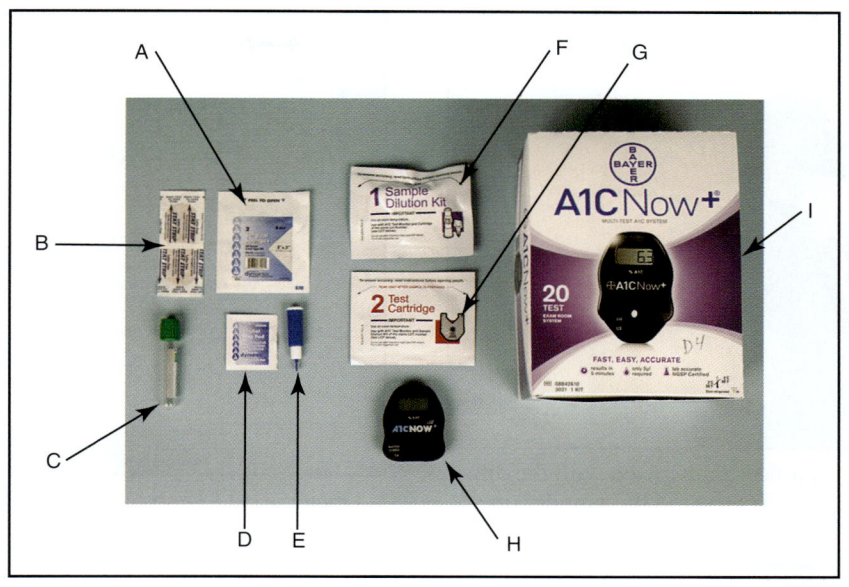

A. Supplies and equipment for the Test Kit Method for A1c.

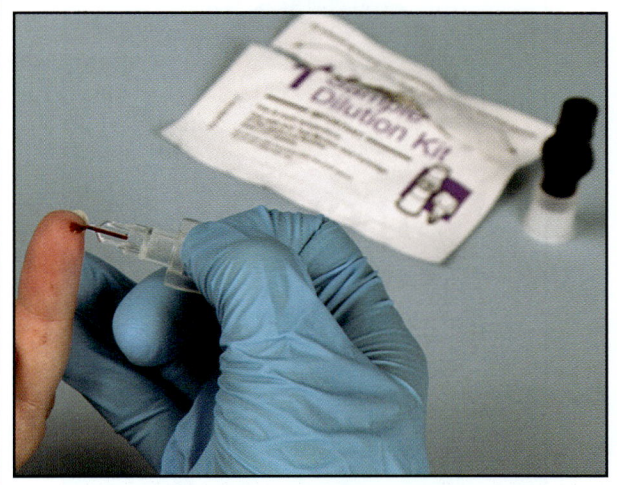

B. After lancing the finger and wiping away the first drop, gently touch the blood drop and fill the capillary blood collector from the #1 packet, as seen above.

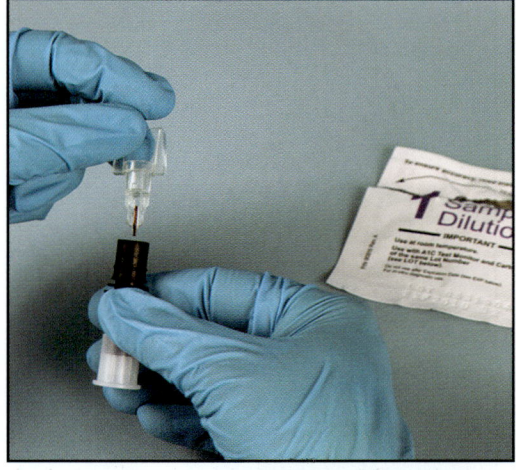

C. After wiping any blood from the outside of the capillary tube, firmly insert the blood collector into the top of the dilution sampler body, as seen above.

Equipment and Supplies for the Test Kit Method for A1c (Fig. A)

a. Gauze
b. Bandage,
c. Heparin tube for venous blood sample
d. Alcohol swab,
e. Lancet for capillary blood sample
f. Sample dilution kit containing capillary tube collector and sampler body
g. Test cartridge
h. A1c monitor programmed to work only with the 20 cartridges in the kit
i. Box containing one monitor and 20 sample dilution kits and 20 cartridges

Patient Specimen

Use only **fresh capillary blood** or venous whole blood collected in a **green heparin tube.** Venous blood can be used only if the tube is less than 1 week old and has been under refrigeration during that time. The blood being tested should fill the small glass capillary tube located on the capillary holder provided in the kit. Do not allow blood to touch the holder. If using the venous tube of blood, dispense the well-mixed blood onto a slide, and obtain the blood by dipping the capillary tube into the drop at a 45-degree angle. Once the glass capillary tube

(Continued)

PROCEDURE 6-2 A1c NOW+ Glycosylated Hemoglobin Procedure—cont'd

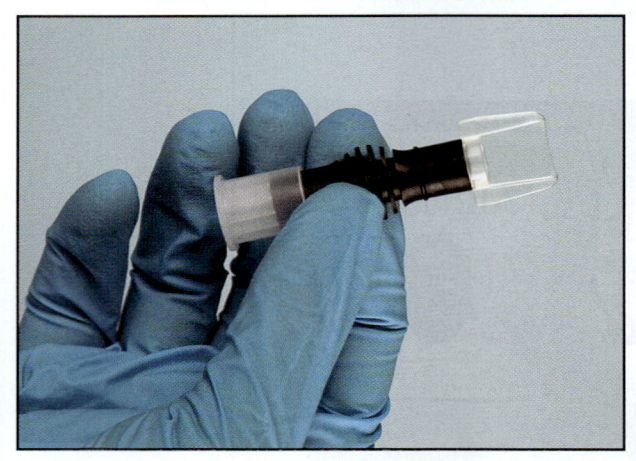

D. The fully inserted sample is then mixed with the dilution by tilting 6 to 8 times. Then stand the sampler on the table.

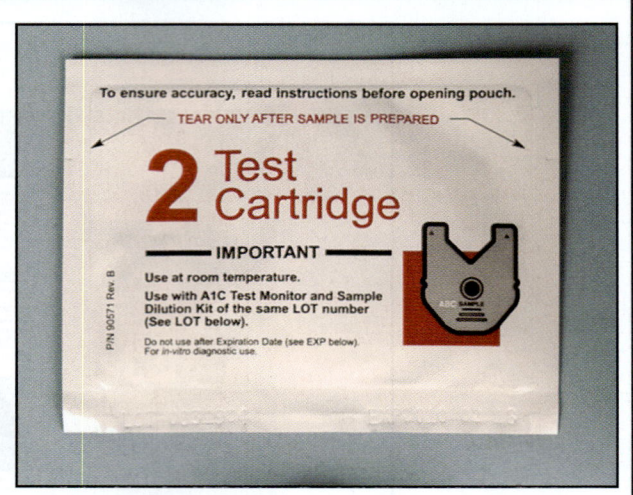

E. Open packet #2 and use within 2 minutes. Click the cartridge into the monitor from the same kit.

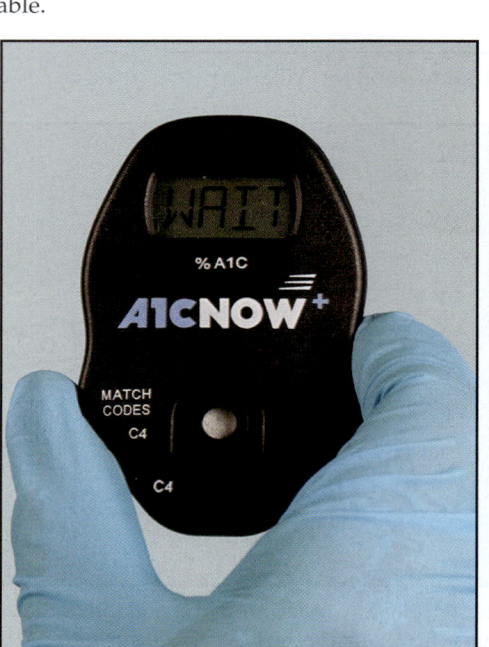

F. The inserted cartridge will start the monitor, which indicates a "WAIT" message.

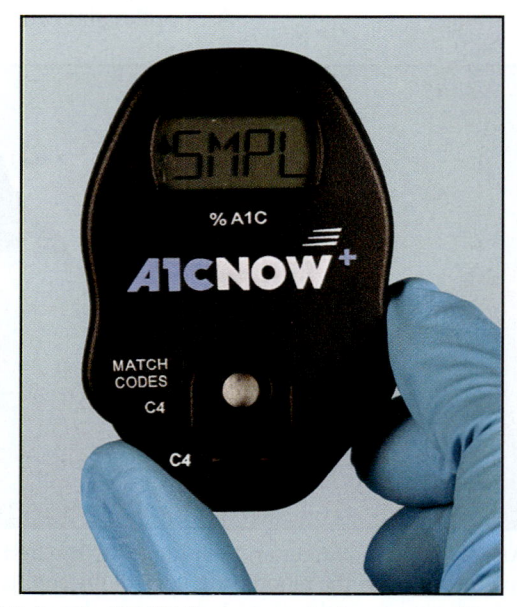

G. Wait for the "SMPL" to appear before proceeding with the next step.

has been filled with the specimen, the analysis must begin within 5 minutes.

Procedure

1. Sanitize the hands, and don personal protective equipment (gown and gloves).
2. Remove the blood collector from the foil #1 sampler dilution kit. Touch the tip of the capillary tube that is attached to the holder into the small drop of blood from the finger stick or the venous blood drop on the slide until the capillary is filled (Fig. B).
3. Wipe the sides of the capillary tube with tissue.
4. Insert the capillary holder into the sampler body that also came from the #1 sampler dilution kit (Fig. C). Push together and twist until the holder and sampler body snap into place.
5. The fully inserted sample is then mixed with the dilution by tilting 6 to 8 times (Fig. D). Then, stand the sampler on the table

PROCEDURE 6-2   A1c NOW+ Glycosylated Hemoglobin Procedure—cont'd

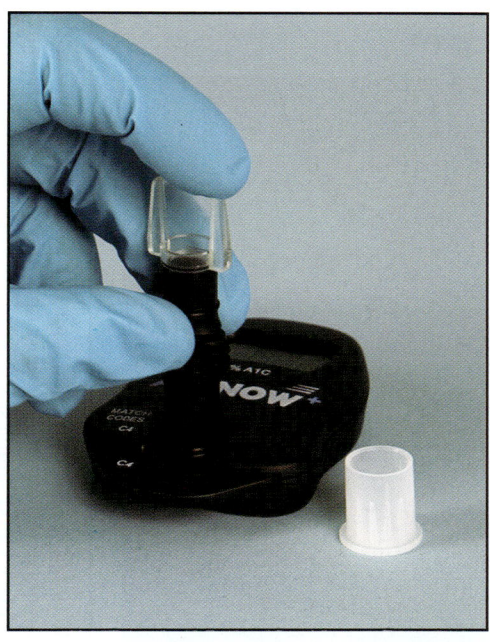

H. Remove the sampler from its base, and push it down onto the white well of the cartridge. The monitor must be on a level surface and cannot be moved until the test is complete.

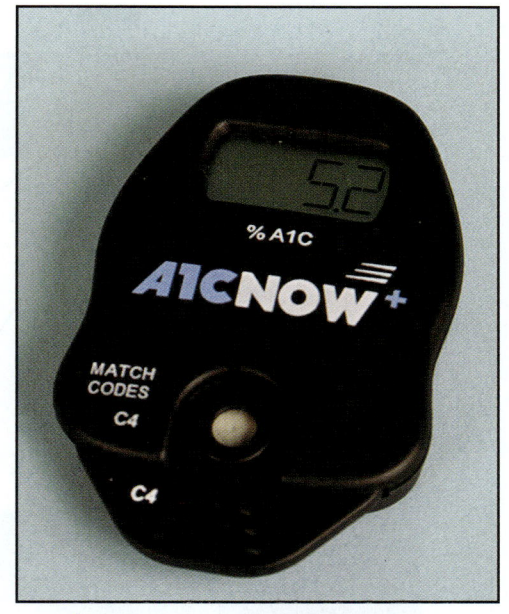

I. Next, the A1C result will appear.

6. Open the #2 test cartridge (Fig. E) foil package, and perform the following within 2 minutes:
   - Click the cartridge into the monitor that came in the same kit box. Check code numbers, which must match.
   - While the monitor indicates "WAIT" (Fig. F), prepare the sample by removing the base.
   - Do not add the sample until the monitor indicates "SMPL" (Fig. G).
   - Push sampler down onto the white well of the cartridge (Fig. H). The monitor must be on a level surface and cannot be moved until the test is complete.
7. After several minutes, the monitor will indicate "QCOK" followed by the test result (Fig. I shows a result of 5.2) followed by the number of tests left in the kit.
8. Record the results from the display, and report to the physician.
9. Properly dispose of all biohazard supplies, disinfect the area, remove gloves, and sanitize the hands.

The expected results of an A1c test are the following:

Nondiabetics	3%-6%
Controlled diabetics	6%-8%
Poorly controlled diabetics	As much as 20% or higher

NOTE: Because A1c is also affected by the hemoglobin concentration, normal ranges should be determined by each laboratory to conform to the population being tested.

Quality Control Procedures

The liquid controls must be run with each new shipment of test cartridges (foil package #2) and their accompanying monitor and the sample dilution kits (foil package #1). Use the capillary holder from one of the sampler dilution kits to collect the control specimens. Insert the filled capillary holder into the sampler body as for a patient specimen. Patient samples cannot be run if the controls do not check out. If the controls are run again and they still do not check out, there are three areas to investigate: (1) the *technique* used to process the specimen and run the test, (2) the liquid control and *reagent* expiration dates and their temperature and time requirements, and (3) the *analyzer's* optics and maintenance requirements. If all these areas check out and a new set of controls still does not work, call the manufacturer.

Figs. A through I courtesy Zack Bent.

PROCEDURE 6-3 Cholestech Method of Measuring Lipids and Glucose

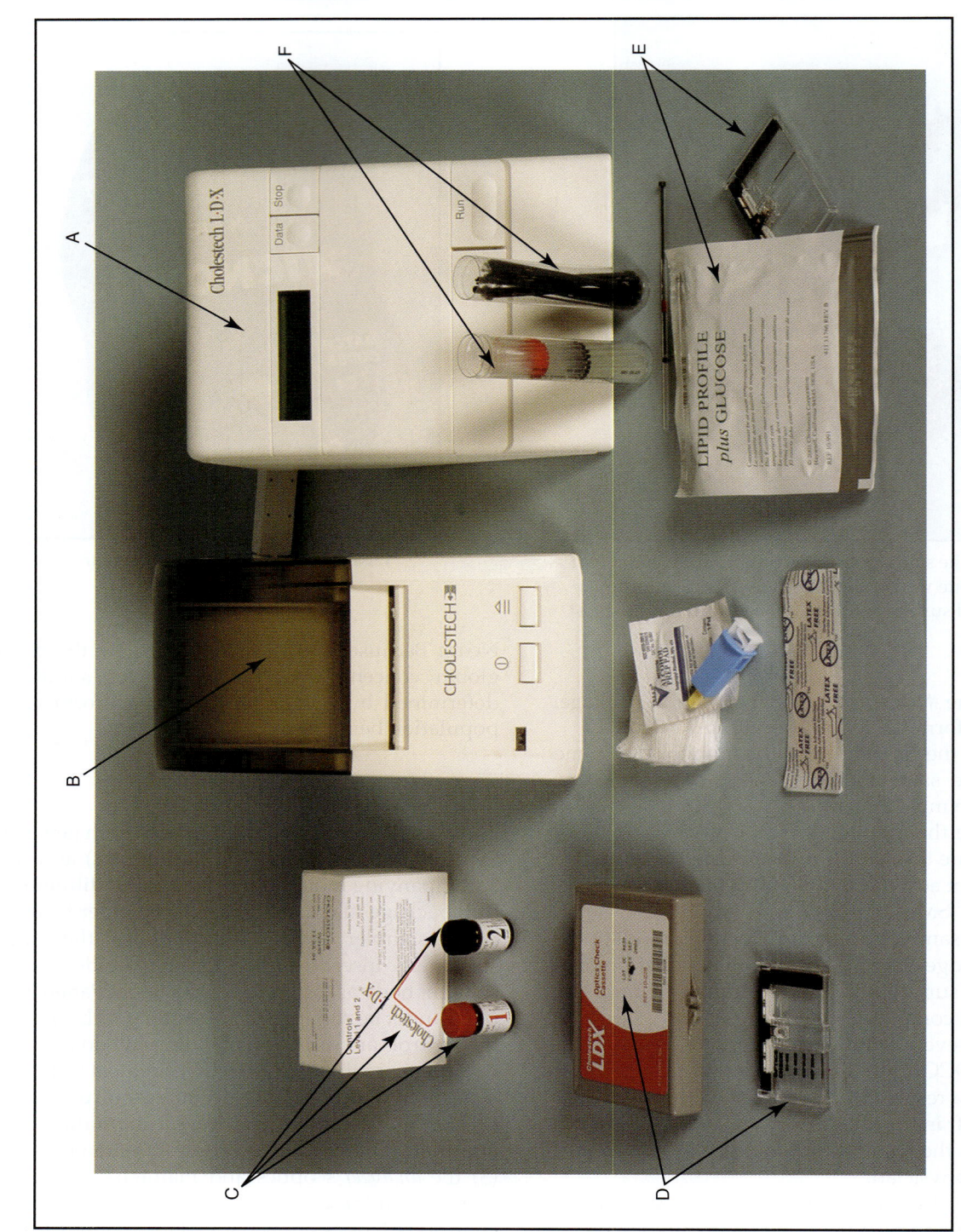

A. Cholestech analyzer and supplies. *a*, Cholestech LDX analyzer; *b*, printer with self-adhesive individual reports; *c*, liquid control box with insert reference sheet of values for level 1 and level 2 controls; *d*, optics check container and cassette for daily optics checks; *e*, foil wrap and testing cassette; *f*, capillary tubes and plungers for collecting and dispensing capillary blood samples.

PROCEDURE 6-3 Cholestech Method of Measuring Lipids and Glucose—cont'd

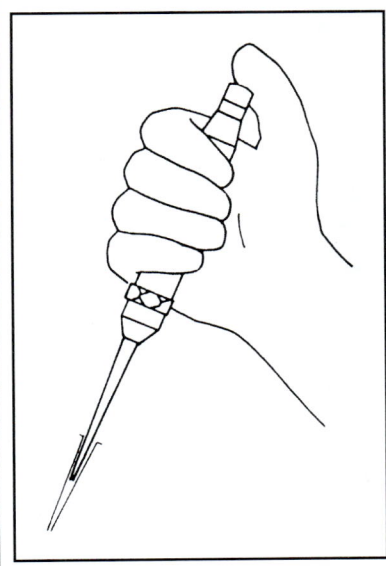

B. Micropipetter for obtaining and dispensing liquid controls and venous blood collected in a green lithium heparin tube. (1) Press thumb down before entering sample. (2) Release thumb while in sample, causing the pipette to fill. (3) Clean outside of pipette with gauze. (4) Press thumb down again to deliver the sample into the cassette, and then remove the pipetter from the device before releasing thumb to avoid pulling the specimen back into the pipetter. (From Young A, Kennedy D: *The medical assistant: an applied learning approach,* ed 10, St Louis, 2007, Saunders.)

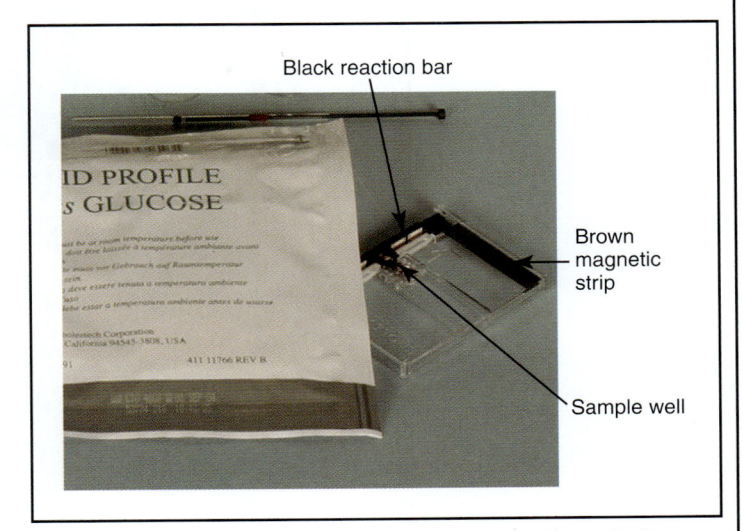

C. Remove the cassette from the foil without touching the brown magnetic strip or black reaction bar. Also, observe the position of the sample well.

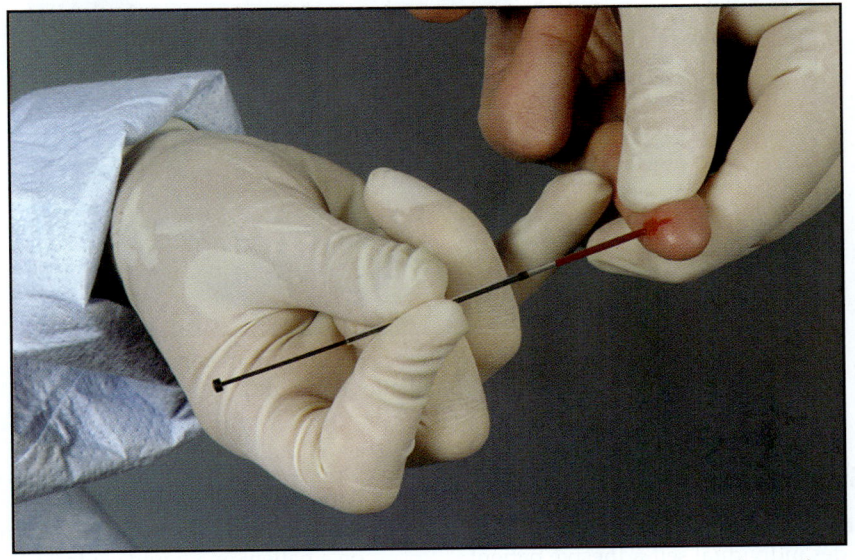

D. Collect blood into the capillary tube with the black plunger inserted into the red end of the capillary tube. Collection should be completed within 10 seconds.

(Continued)

PROCEDURE 6-3 Cholestech Method of Measuring Lipids and Glucose—cont'd

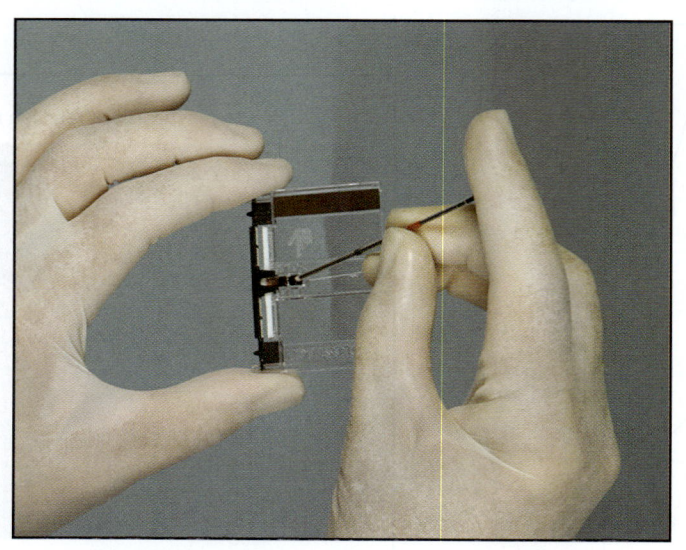

E. Transfer the blood into the cassette test well within the next 5 minutes using the plunger (this avoids clotting of the specimen).

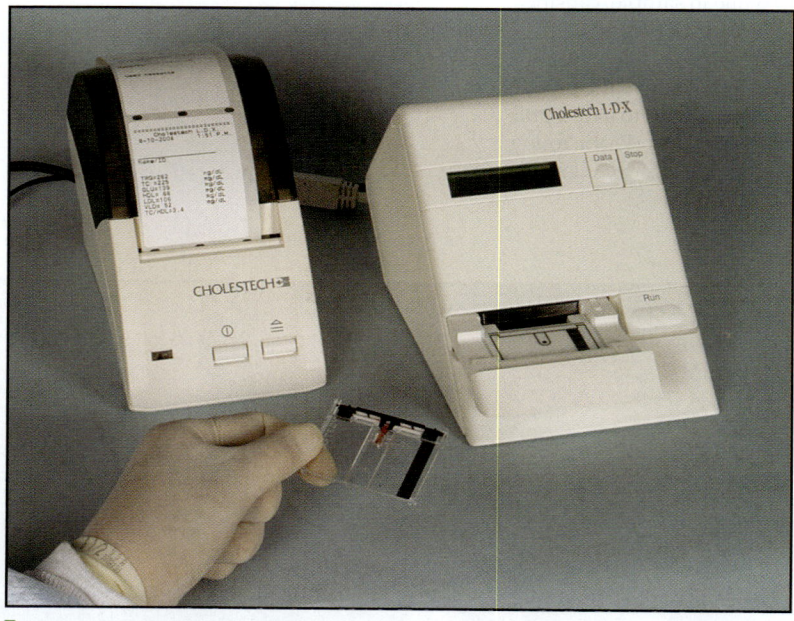

F. Immediately place the cassette with the specimen in the opened drawer, and press RUN. Results will be printed after 5 minutes.

Equipment and Supplies (Fig. A)

a. Cholestech LDX analyzer
b. Printer that provides individual self-adhesive patient readouts
c. Control box with level 1 and level 2 liquid controls (stored in refrigerator)
d. Optics check container and optics check cassette (stored at room temperature)
e. Individual foil wrap and test cassette for running a test on a patient or a liquid control (stored in refrigerator)
f. Cholestech capillary tubes and black plungers for collecting and transferring capillary blood samples (stored at room temperature)

PROCEDURE 6-3 Cholestech Method of Measuring Lipids and Glucose—cont'd

Patient Sample

If a lipid panel including triglycerides is ordered, the patient should not drink alcohol for 48 hours before testing and should have fasted for 10 to 12 hours. The test can be run with whole blood from a finger stick that is collected in the appropriate capillary tube with its black plunger inserted. Whole blood from a green-topped lithium heparin vacuum tube can also be used. (NOTE: Green-topped sodium heparin tubes are not acceptable.) Cholestech provides an automatic micropipetter that consists of a disposable plastic-tipped pipette placed on the end of a plunger (Fig. B). The plunger is pushed in before entering the tube of blood. Once in the blood the plunger is released, causing the correct amount of blood to flow into the plastic tip. The blood can then be transferred to the Cholestech testing device by pushing down on the plunger.

Procedure

1. Allow the refrigerated cassette to come to room temperature (at least 10 minutes before opening).
2. Make sure the analyzer is plugged in and warmed up.
3. Remove the cassette from its foil pouch, and place it on flat surface. Do not touch the black bar or the brown magnetic strip (Fig. C). Hold the cassette by the short sides only.
4. Press RUN. The analyzer will perform a self-test, and the screen will display "Self-Test Running," then "Self-Test OK."
5. The cassette drawer will open, and the screen will display "Load Cassette and Press Run." The drawer will remain open for 4 minutes, after which it will close with the message "System timeout. Run to continue." If the RUN button is not pushed within 15 seconds of the message, the drawer will close and the screen will go blank. If this happens, simply press RUN and allow the analyzer to go through the self-test again, then proceed.
6. Collect a blood sample from a finger stick into the Cholestech LDX capillary tube with its plunger in place (Fig. D). (Or use the Mini-Pet pipette provided by Cholestech to collect the Vacutainer blood and the control samples.)
7. The blood or control sample must then be plunged into the cassette well within 5 minutes after collection, or the blood may clot (Fig. E).
8. Immediately place the filled cassette into the drawer of the analyzer (Fig. F).
   - Keep the cassette level after the sample is applied.
   - The black reaction bar faces toward the analyzer.
   - The brown magnetic strip is on the right.
9. Press RUN. The drawer will close and the screen will display "(Test names) Running."
10. When the test is complete, the analyzer will beep and the screen will display results. At the same time, the printer will provide the results. (NOTE: Pressing the DATA button will display the calculated results of all tests on the screen if you are running a panel of tests. The DATA button will also display questions that must be answered to determine the cardiac risk factor.)

The interpretation of the lipid panel as it relates to cardiovascular risk is as followed (based on American Heart Association recommendations):

Total Cholesterol Levels	What It Means
Less than 200 mg/dL	Desirable
200-239 mg/dL	Borderline high risk for heart disease
240 mg/dL and above	High risk for heart disease

LDL Cholesterol Levels	What It Means
Less than 100 mg/dL	Optimal
100-129 mg/dL	Near optimal
130-159 mg/dL	Borderline high
160-189 mg/dL	High
190 mg/dL and above	Very high

HDL Cholesterol Levels	What It Means
Less than 40 mg/dL	High risk for heart disease
40-59 mg/dL	Less risk for heart disease
60 mg/dL	Desirable

TC/HDL ratio ≤ 4.5 or less is desirable

Triglycerides	What It Means
<150 mg/dL	Desirable
150-199 mg/dL	Borderline high
200-499 mg/dL	High
500 mg/dL	Very high

A normal ALT range is 10-40 U/L (units per liter).
A normal AST range is 10-30 U/L.

(Continued)

PROCEDURE 6-3 Cholestech Method of Measuring Lipids and Glucose—cont'd

ALT and AST are enzymes that are measured to help assess liver damage. ALT and AST levels are monitored in patients who are taking certain medications to lower cholesterol, control diabetes, or treat other diseases.

Quality Control Procedures

The calibration "optics check" cassette should be run daily. It does not require any specimen in its well. Simply place the cassette in the drawer of the Cholestech. The results of the optical reading in all four testing areas will be displayed and printed. Log and compare the numbers with the required range designated on the cassette. If any number falls out of range, patient tests cannot be run until the cause is determined and corrected.

The two levels of liquid controls should be run at least monthly, or whenever a new set of cassettes is opened. Use the Mini-Pet to transfer the control solution into the cassette well, and run the control as you would a patient sample. Log the results and compare them with the control package insert. If the results do not fall in the required range, patient samples cannot be run until the cause is determined and corrected.

PROCEDURE 6-4 Occult Blood: ColoScreen III Method and ColoCARE Method

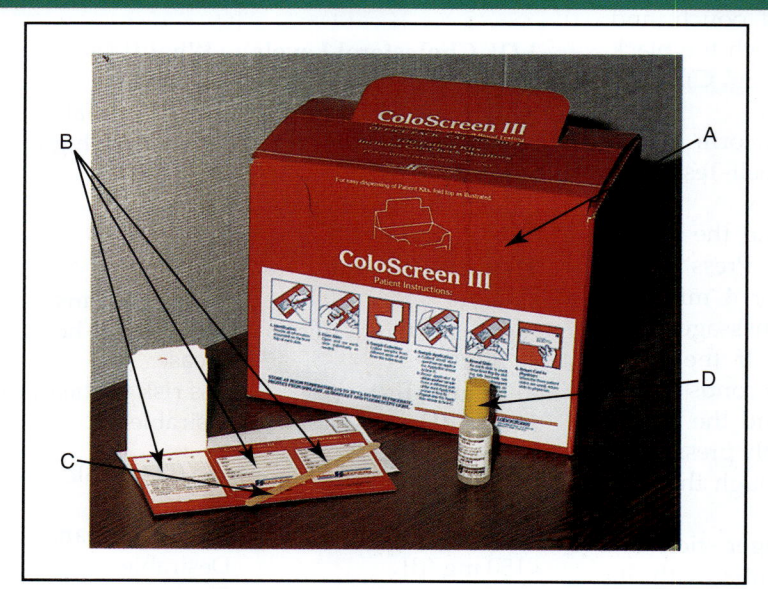

A. Fecal occult blood kit and supplies. *a*, ColoScreen III box with supplies and directions; *b*, three specimen slides; *c*, three wooden applicators; *d*, hydrogen peroxide developer.

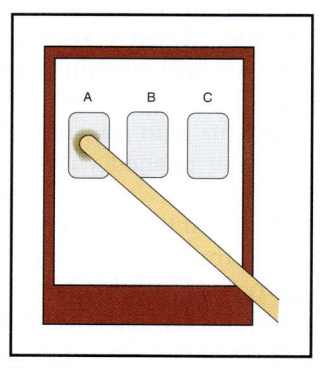

B. The patient applies a thin fecal smear to each box after lifting the *front flap* of the specimen slide. (From Stepp CA, Woods M: *Laboratory procedures for medical office personnel,* Philadelphia, 1998, Saunders.)

CLIA-Waived Chemistry Tests

PROCEDURE 6-4 Occult Blood: ColoScreen III Method and ColoCARE Method—cont'd

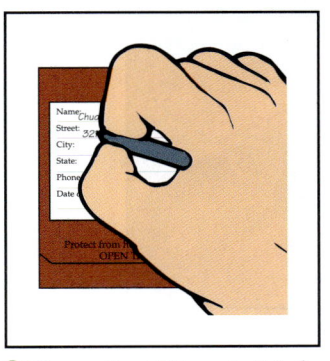

C. The patient fills out all information on the front flap of each slide *after* the application of the three different specimens. The specimens are mailed or carried to the laboratory. (From Stepp CA, Woods M: *Laboratory procedures for medical office personnel*, Philadelphia, 1998, Saunders.)

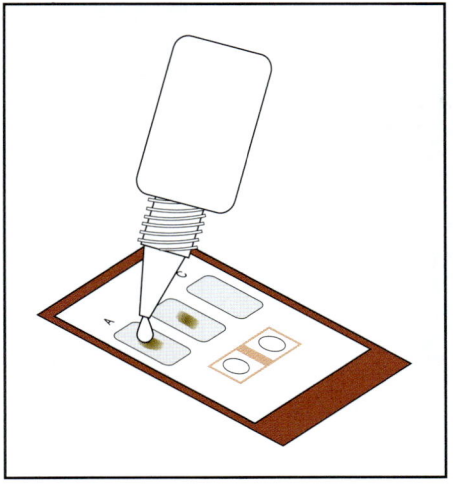

D. Two drops of developer are applied to each test area after lifting the *flap on the back* of the specimen slide. (From Stepp CA, Woods M: *Laboratory procedures for medical office personnel*, Philadelphia, 1998, Saunders.)

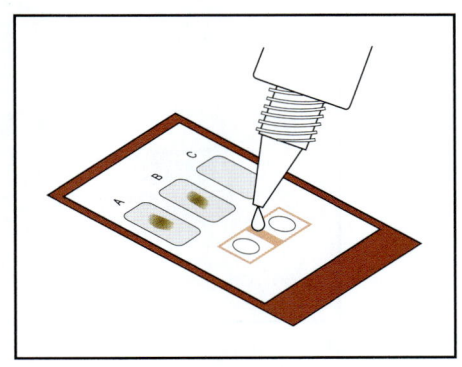

E. Apply developer to the monitoring section of the slide to confirm that the positive turns blue and the negative does not. (From Stepp CA, Woods M: *Laboratory procedures for medical office personnel*, Philadelphia, 1998, Saunders.)

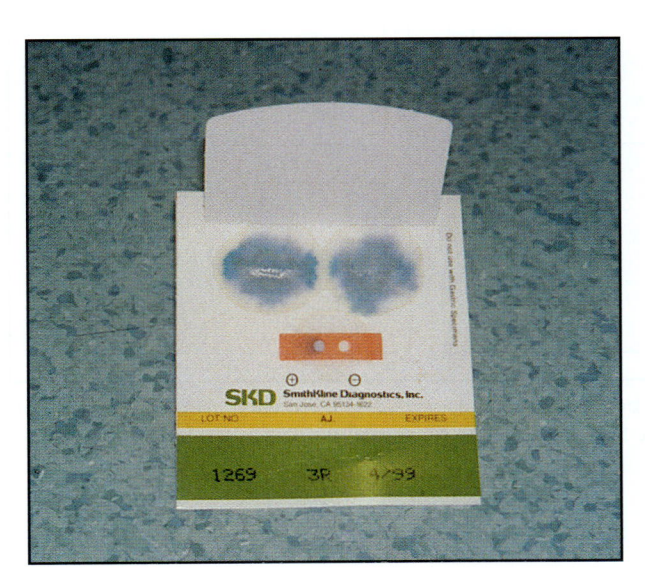

F. Observe the positive occult blood test results in the upper areas of the slide and confirm the control results at the bottom: positive *(left)* and negative *(right)*. (From Stepp CA, Woods M: *Laboratory procedures for medical office personnel*, Philadelphia, 1998, Saunders.)

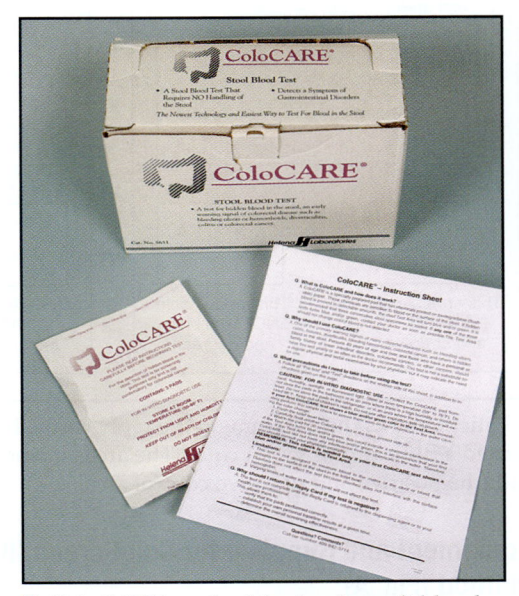

G. ColoCARE method for fecal occult blood. Patient receives foil packet with three test pads, a reply card, and an instruction sheet.

(Continued)

PROCEDURE 6-4 Occult Blood: ColoScreen III Method and ColoCARE Method—cont'd

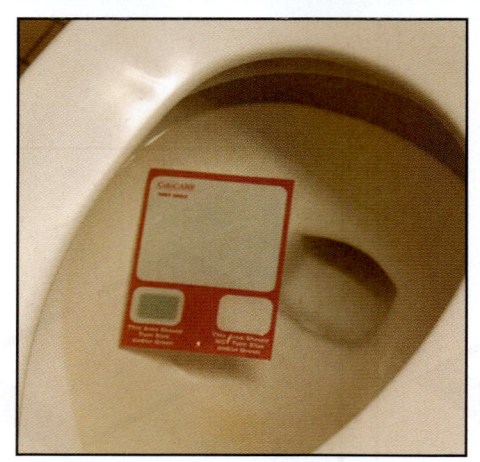

H. Negative occult blood test result with no color in the large test box. The controls show blue in the positive left lower corner and no color in the negative control box in the lower right corner.

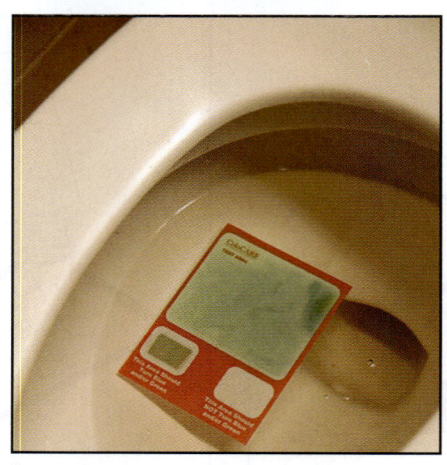

I. Positive occult blood test showing blue color in the large test box. The controls once again show blue in the positive left lower corner and no color in the negative control box in the lower right corner.

First Bowel Movement	Second Bowel Movement	Third Bowel Movement
Date _____	Date _____	Date _____
ColoCARE Test area	ColoCARE Test area	ColoCARE Test area
This area should turn blue and/or green / This area should NOT turn blue and/or green	This area should turn blue and/or green / This area should NOT turn blue and/or green	This area should turn blue and/or green / This area should NOT turn blue and/or green

J. Patient marks the diagram on the reply card labeled "first bowel movement" with an **"x" in each area of the pad that turned a blue and/or green color.** The areas include the large test area and the two smaller areas at the bottom of the pad (the positive and negative control areas).

Equipment and Supplies for ColoScreen III Method (Fig. A)

a. ColoScreen III
b. Three specimen slides
c. Three wooden applicators
d. Hydrogen peroxide developer

Check for proper storage (e.g., temperature, light). Check the expiration date. Locate the package insert and patient instructions.

PROCEDURE 6-4 Occult Blood: ColoScreen III Method and ColoCARE Method—cont'd

Patient Preparation and Pretest Instruction

Two days before the test and during the specimen-collecting day, the patient should eat a high-fiber diet, including well-cooked poultry or fish, cooked fruits and vegetables, bran cereals, raw lettuce, carrots, and celery, and moderate amounts of peanuts and popcorn. The patient should refrain from ingesting the following items, which may interfere with the test results: red and partially cooked meats, turnips, cauliflower, broccoli, parsnips, melons (especially cantaloupe), alcohol, aspirin, and vitamin C.

When collecting specimens, the patient should use the slides, applicators, and the take-home instructions as follows:

1. After a bowel movement, use the wooden applicator to collect a small sample by scraping the surface of the feces and spread a thin layer in box A of the slide (Fig. B). Using the same applicator, collect a second sample from a different part of the feces and spread it in box B.
2. Discard the wooden applicator, reseal the cover of the slide, and complete the information requested on the outside of the cover (Fig. C).
3. Repeat the preceding steps with the next two consecutive bowel movements and the two remaining slides.

Test Procedure

4. Apply gloves, and observe universal precautions. Confirm that all necessary information was written on slide covers.
5. Open the back sides of all three slides, and place two drops of developer on each specimen (Fig. D). If a blue reaction occurs anywhere in the specimen area, this indicates a positive result. A positive result may be read in as early as 30 seconds to 2 minutes, but do not record a negative (no blue) until at less 2 minutes have passed.
6. Perform the monitor test (internal control) by placing one or two drops between the monitor boxes and waiting 30 seconds to 2 minutes to read the results and confirm that the positive turned blue and the negative did not (Fig. E).
7. Observe the positive blue specimen reactions and the results of the control monitors showing blue on the positive dot and nothing on the negative dot (Fig. F).

Equipment and Supplies for ColoCARE Method

Patient receives foil packet containing three test pads and a reply card, along with an instruction sheet (Fig. G).

Patient Preparation and Pretest Instruction

Two days before the test and during the specimen-collecting day, the patient should eat a high-fiber diet, including well-cooked poultry or fish, cooked fruits and vegetables, bran cereals, raw lettuce, carrots, celery, and moderate amounts of peanuts and popcorn. The patient should refrain from ingesting the following items, which may interfere with the test results: red and partially cooked meats, turnips, cauliflower, broccoli, parsnips, melons (especially cantaloupe), alcohol, aspirin, and vitamin C.

At-Home Test Procedure

1. After a bowel movement, do not flush or put toilet paper in the toilet. **Perform the following steps within 5 minutes after bowel movement.**
2. Open foil pouch by tearing along the dotted line at the bottom of the pouch, being careful not to tear the pad inside and remove one ColoCARE pad from the pouch. Tape the pouch closed to protect the remaining pads from light and moisture.
3. Hold the ColoCARE pad with the printed side up. Carefully release the pad, allowing it to float on the water in the center of the toilet bowl.
4. Observe the ColoCARE pad for 30 seconds, and note any blue or green appearance on the pad (see Figs. H and I below for possible negative and positive results).
5. After testing the first bowel movement, mark the diagram on the reply card (Fig. J) labeled "First Bowel Movement" with an **"X" in each area of the pad that turned a blue or green color**. The areas include the large TEST AREA and the two smaller areas at the bottom of the pad (the positive and negative control areas). After recording the results on the reply card, flush the floating test pad down the toilet.

(Continued)

PROCEDURE 6-4 Occult Blood: ColoScreen III Method and ColoCARE Method—cont'd

6. Repeat step 5 for the next two consecutive bowel movements, and mark the second and third diagrams on the reply card according to the same instructions.

7. Fill out all the information required on the reply card, and send it to the office or bring the card back to the office for interpretation.

Figs. G, H, and I courtesy Zack Bent.

TABLE 6-2 Normal and Critical Blood Chemistry Results (on i-STAT Analyzer)

Reference Ranges

	Arterial	Venous	Critical Ranges
pH	7.35-7.45	7.32-7.42	<7.200 or >7.55
PCO_2	35-45 mmHg	41-51 mmHg	<20 or >65 mmHg
PO_2	80-100 mmHg		<50 mmHg
Sodium	136-146 mmol/L		<120 or >160
Potassium	3.5-5.0 mmol/L		<2.5 or >6.0
Chloride	101-114 mmol/L		<80 or >130
Glucose	Fasting: 73-115 mg/dL		Adult: <40 or >500 Newborn (0-3 mos): <40 or >200
BUN (UN)	Adults (≥12 yrs): 8-20		
Hct	Male subjects: 42%-52% Female subjects: 37T-47%		<15%

ADVANCED CONCEPTS

i-STAT

Additional CLIA-waived point-of-care chemistry tests, such as the i-STAT, have been approved for POLs. Originally, this handheld i-STAT device was designed for critical care situations in which blood chemistry test results were needed immediately (STAT). The technology was designed to ensure that a non–laboratory-trained health professional could run the chemistry tests at the patient's bedside and obtain reliable results. Table 6-2 shows the critical test values that are typically monitored during a patient's "crisis" situation. The reasons that these values are needed are discussed in the following paragraphs.

Almost all metabolic processes in the body are dependent on or affected by pH, blood gas, and electrolyte levels. The pH is critical for maintaining proper physiological molecular structure and chemical reactions. The electrolytes (Na, K, Cl, and ionized Ca) are involved with pH regulation, water distribution, proper muscle and nerve function, oxidation-reduction reactions, and enzymatic reactions. Blood gases (oxygen and carbon dioxide) are also critical for maintaining proper tissue oxygenation and pH balance.

Glucose determinations help in evaluating disorders of carbohydrate metabolism; evaluating acidosis and ketoacidosis; evaluating dehydration, coma, hypoglycemia, and neuroglycopenia; and establishing a diagnosis of diabetes.

Blood urea nitrogen (BUN) and creatinine are commonly used to evaluate renal function. An abnormally high level of urea nitrogen in the blood is an indication of kidney function, impairment, or failure. Other causes of increased values for urea nitrogen include gastrointestinal bleeding and a high-protein diet. Causes of decreased urea values include pregnancy, severe liver insufficiency, overhydration, and malnutrition.

The whole blood hematocrit and hemoglobin measurements are useful for determining if RBC quantity is sufficient to maintain a proper oxygen level during a surgical procedure. It is a key indicator of the body's state of hydration, anemia, or severe blood loss, as well as the blood's ability to transport oxygen.

The i-STAT system consists of a handheld analyzer and single-use disposable cartridges.

The analyzer automatically controls all functions of the testing cycle including fluid movement within the cartridge, calibration, and continuous quality monitoring (NOTE: A pictorial Procedure 6-5 i-STAT has been placed at the end of this chapter and

Advanced Concepts

a complete procedure skill sheet is provided in the workbook.)

The CLIA-waived i-STAT CHEM8+ cartridge can be used to test all the following blood chemistries and print out the results in minutes:
- Sodium (Na)
- Potassium (K)
- Chloride (Cl)
- Ionized calcium (Ca)
- TCO_2
- Glucose (Glu)
- Blood urea nitrogen (BUN)
- Creatinine (Crea)
- Hematocrit (Hct)
- Hemoglobin (Hgb)

Piccolo

Demands for improved patient care and greater cost control are driving profound changes in the structure of health care delivery. Within and outside of traditional hospital environments, evolving technology is permitting some types of diagnostic testing and patient monitoring to move from the clinical laboratory to the near-patient environment. Many health care professionals whose roles have traditionally involved hands-on patient care are now being asked to take a role in clinical chemistry testing as well.

Laboratorians, with their training and experience, know that rigorous quality control (QC) is an absolute necessity for accurate test results on which treatment decisions can confidently be based. The Piccolo Xpress Point-of-Care Chemistry Analyzer incorporates a process called iQC ("intelligent Quality Control") that meets established QC standards independently of the operator's skill level. iQC is a series of sophisticated automatic checks that verify the chemistry, optics, and electronic functions of the analyzer during each run and ensures that operators in a wide range of environments report only accurate and reliable results.

The Piccolo Xpress Point-of-Care Chemistry Analyzer is a lightweight portable instrument that processes whole blood, serum, or plasma samples in self-contained, single-use reagent discs. Transparent to the operator, iQC checks the analyzer, the reagent disc, and the sample during each run to verify correct electronic and chemistry performance. If it detects uncharacteristic performance, iQC automatically suppresses a single chemistry or the entire panel and immediately alerts the operator to any problems. From the self-test at power-up to the recording and printing of patient results, the Piccolo Xpress conducts multiple QC checks automatically with each run; iQC ensures that the operator reports only accurate and reliable results.

Metabolic Panels: Basic and Comprehensive

Not all offices can afford the previously described chemistry analyzers. When physicians need to know blood chemistry values to arrive at a definitive diagnosis, either they will have the medical assistant or phlebotomist draw a blood sample (usually a gold SST) and send it to a reference laboratory for testing, or they will send the patient to the reference laboratory. Depending on what the physician needs to know, a metabolic panel, which typically consists of 6 to 12 or more chemistry tests, will be ordered. The panels are usually ordered as part of an annual physical exam or when a patient is being prepared for surgery. Metabolic panels provide the physician with a comprehensive picture of the patient's carbohydrate and lipid metabolism. They also provide information regarding the liver, kidney, heart, and thyroid functions. Typical tests in a metabolic panel include electrolytes, lipids, glucose, BUN, bilirubin, enzymes, and hormones. The report in Fig. 6-9 shows each analyte's result along with its reference range. Note that when an analyte is out of range, it is noted to the left of its value. The physician must interpret these chemistry results along with the rest of the patient's examination to make a definitive diagnosis.

Renal Panel

The renal, or kidney, panel consists of tests that portray how the kidney is functioning. The kidney is responsible for excreting the following chemical wastes: urea, creatinine, and uric acid. By observing increases in **BUN**, blood creatinine, and uric acid, the physician can see when the kidney has become impaired and to what degree. This panel of tests is helpful in monitoring the diabetic who is at risk for kidney failure. Elevated uric acid levels alone are associated with **gout** (a form of arthritis caused by the accumulation of uric acid crystals in the synovial fluid of joints). The kidneys and lungs maintain the body's water and pH balance by releasing or retaining charged electrolyte ions—chloride (**Cl^-**), potassium (**K^+**), sodium (**Na^+**), and bicarbonate (**HCO_3^-**). Therefore testing the levels of these electrolytes may also be included in the renal panel.

Electrolyte Panel

Electrolyte panels give a picture of the patient's water–salt balance and the ability to maintain proper pH. The most common electrolytes measured in the serum are the following:
- K^+ and Na^+, two positively charged ions, or **cations**
- Cl^- and HCO_3^-, two negatively charged ions, or **anions**

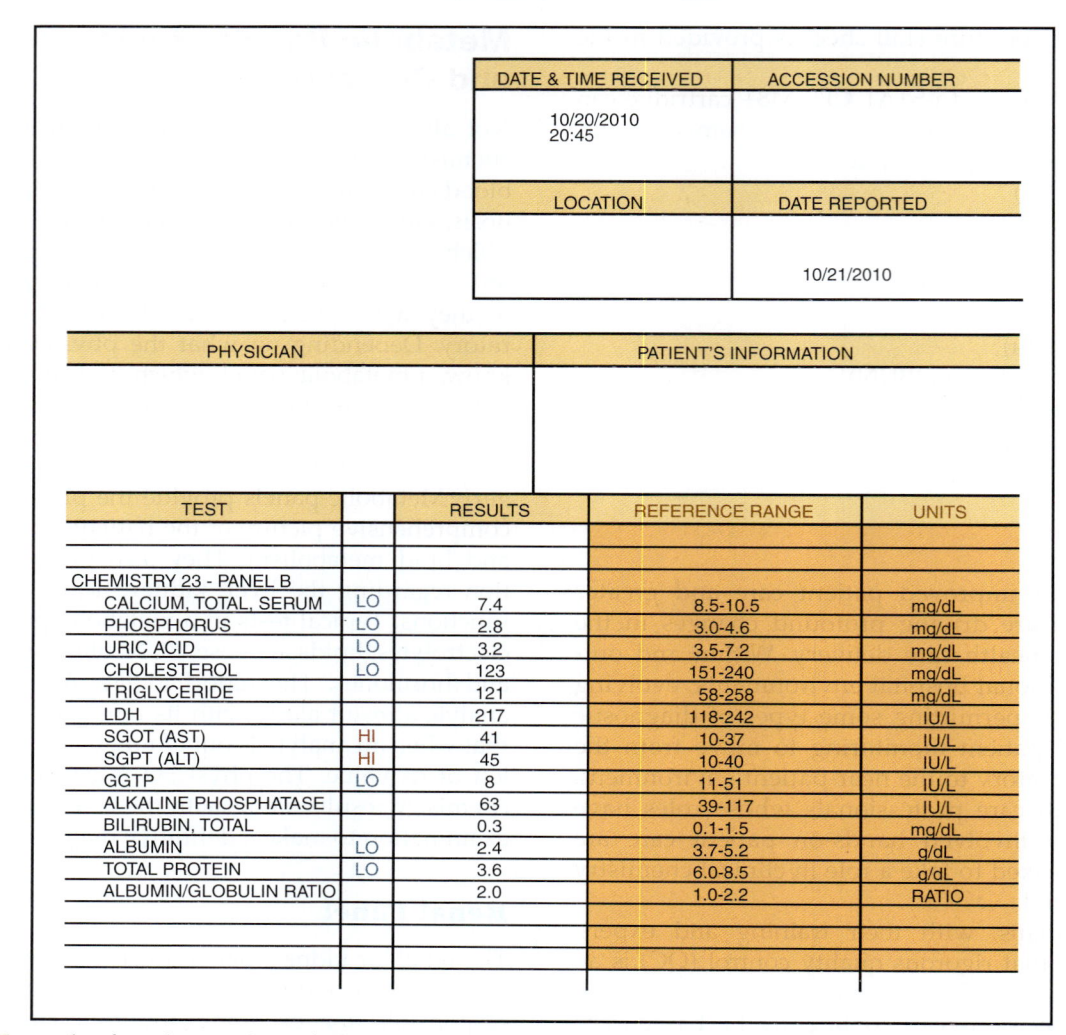

TEST		RESULTS	REFERENCE RANGE	UNITS
CHEMISTRY 23 - PANEL B				
CALCIUM, TOTAL, SERUM	LO	7.4	8.5-10.5	mg/dL
PHOSPHORUS	LO	2.8	3.0-4.6	mg/dL
URIC ACID	LO	3.2	3.5-7.2	mg/dL
CHOLESTEROL	LO	123	151-240	mg/dL
TRIGLYCERIDE		121	58-258	mg/dL
LDH		217	118-242	IU/L
SGOT (AST)	HI	41	10-37	IU/L
SGPT (ALT)	HI	45	10-40	IU/L
GGTP	LO	8	11-51	IU/L
ALKALINE PHOSPHATASE		63	39-117	IU/L
BILIRUBIN, TOTAL		0.3	0.1-1.5	mg/dL
ALBUMIN	LO	2.4	3.7-5.2	g/dL
TOTAL PROTEIN	LO	3.6	6.0-8.5	g/dL
ALBUMIN/GLOBULIN RATIO		2.0	1.0-2.2	RATIO

Fig. 6-9. Example of an abnormal metabolic panel report. (From Zakus SM: *Mosby's clinical skills for medical assistants*, ed 4, St Louis, 2001, Mosby.)

Hepatic Panel

The hepatic panel is a series of tests to determine liver function and damage. The liver is involved in the following metabolic functions:
- It metabolizes glucose from the gastrointestinal tract into stored glycogen.
- It metabolizes amino acids from the gastrointestinal tract into plasma proteins—albumin, some globulins, and the clotting proteins (fibrinogen and prothrombin).
- It metabolizes fatty acids from the gastrointestinal tract into the various blood lipids.
- It processes bilirubin, a waste product from the breakdown of hemoglobin, and excretes it in the bile.
- When the liver is impaired, the blood chemistry will reflect *increases* in bilirubin levels and *decreased* levels of albumins and clotting proteins owing to the impairment of protein production. However, significant impaired liver function must be present for these analytes to show abnormality. Therefore a liver panel will also include a series of enzyme tests to help determine whether the liver is damaged.
- Enzymes are usually located within the cells of organs and tissues. Enzymes are catalysts that assist in the particular metabolic changes required of the cells. An enzyme's name always ends with the suffix *–ase*. The word root preceding the *–ase* explains the chemical reaction the enzyme is involved in. When a tissue or organ is damaged, it releases its specific enzymes into the blood. Because the liver is involved in so many intracellular metabolic reactions, levels of all the following enzymes may become elevated in the blood when it is damaged:
- Alkaline phosphatase (alk phos, **ALP**, or **AP**)
- Gamma-glutamyltransferase **(GGT)**
- Aspartate aminotransferase **(AST)**
- Alanine aminotransferase **(ALT)**
- Lactic dehydrogenase **(LD)**

Advanced Concepts

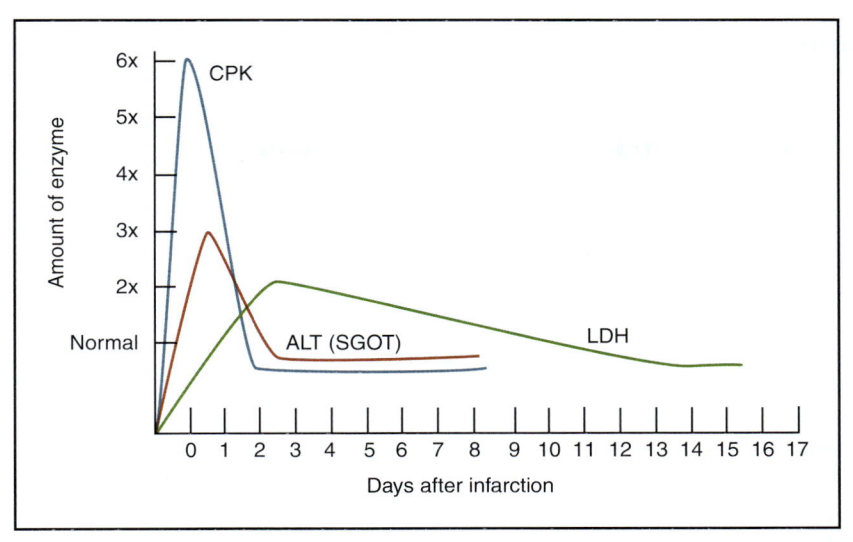

Fig. 6-10. Myocardial infarction enzyme patterns during the 9 days after a heart attack. (From Stepp CA, Woods M: *Laboratory procedures for medical office personnel,* Philadelphia, 1998, Saunders.)

Patients who are taking medications (e.g., statin drugs that lower blood cholesterol) may have their ALT or AST levels tested to see if the liver is being damaged by the medication. Other damaged organs may release some of these enzymes as well. Once again, the physician must interpret the chemical results along with the complete clinical picture of the patient before making a definitive diagnosis.

Cardiac Panel

When the heart is injured, as in a myocardial infarction, it releases the following into the blood:
- **Troponin I and T**—muscle proteins that, when elevated, are excellent heart-specific indicators of a recent myocardial infarction.
- Creatine kinase **(CK or CPK)**—an enzyme found in muscle and brain tissue that is elevated soon after the heart is damaged. Two other enzymes, LD (LDH) and ALT (SGOT), are also elevated. Fig. 6-10 illustrates the cardiac enzyme pattern typical of patients with myocardial infarction.
- **Myoglobin** is an iron-containing, oxygen-binding protein found in muscles (similar to hemoglobin in RBCs) that is also elevated in blood after a myocardial infarction.

Thyroid Panel

The thyroid gland plays a critical role in body metabolism by producing two hormones: thyroxine **(T_4)** and triiodothyronine **(T_3)**. Their production is regulated by the pituitary gland, which sends out thyroid-stimulating hormone **(TSH).** A panel of these analytes—TSH, T_4, and T_3 uptake—would be ordered to help in the diagnosis of an overactive or underactive thyroid gland. The T_3 uptake is a test that measures the amount of iodine that is "taken up" to synthesize the T_3 hormone.

Individual Analytes and Their Disease Associations

The laboratory requisition seen in Fig. 6-3, at the beginning of the chapter, listed many individual tests that can be ordered, as well as the panels of tests. Individual tests are preferred over panels once the diagnosis is made and the condition requires frequent monitoring. Table 6-3 lists the most common chemistry tests categorically, their expected ranges, and the possible disease associations if the test results are high or low.

Summary

Because blood chemistry is so crucial to diagnosis and patient care, technology will continue to provide POLs with new and improved, user-friendly chemical testing analyzers. Be sure to stay informed through local diagnostic test suppliers and the Internet for the latest in chemistry testing. The websites for each of the CLIA-waived testing methods presented in this chapter are listed below. Review the latest news at each site, as well as their educational departments and their demonstration videos.

TABLE 6-3 Common Chemistry Panels and Possible Disease Associations

Test	Expected Range*	Possible Disease Associations — High Levels	Possible Disease Associations — Low Levels
Renal Panel			
BUN (blood urea nitrogen)	8-26 mg/dL	Impaired kidney function Acute renal failure Cardiovascular failure Obstruction of urine flow	No clinical significance
BUN/creatinine ratio	10-20	Prerenal impairment Dehydration Congestive heart failure Gastrointestinal bleed	Renal tubular necrosis
Creatinine	0.7-1.4 mg/dL	Impaired kidney function Acute glomerulonephritis Obstruction of urine flow	No clinical significance
Uric acid	3.6-8 mg/dL (male subjects) 2.5-6.78 mg/dL (female subjects)	Gout Decreased renal function Emotional stress Total fasting	Use of some drugs
Electrolytes			
Chloride	98-108 mmol/L	Congestive heart failure Dehydration Cushing's disease Diabetes insipidus Severe hyperaldosteronism	Nephritis Diuretic administration Starvation Severe vomiting Severe hypoaldosteronism
Potassium	3.5-5.3 mmol/L	Urinary obstruction Renal failure Ketoacidosis Hypoaldosteronism	Diarrhea Diuretic administration Starvation Hyperaldosteronism Renal tubular defects
Sodium	135-146 mmol/L	Severe dehydration Brain injuries Diabetic coma Cushing's disease Hyperaldosteronism Lack of ADH Renal failure	Metabolic acidosis Diarrhea Renal tubular disease Polyuria Addison's disease Overhydration Hypoaldosteronism Renal SIADH
Hepatic			
Bilirubin	0.1-1.2 mg/dL	Massive hemolysis Obstructive jaundice Cirrhosis Carcinoma Renal calculi	No clinical significance
A/G ratio (albumin/globulin ratio)	1.1-2.5	No clinical significance	Viral hepatitis Ulcerative colitis Burns Multiple myeloma Sarcoidosis Metastatic carcinoma Nephrotic syndrome Diabetic ketosis Congestive heart failure

Advanced Concepts

TABLE 6-3   Common Chemistry Panels and Possible Disease Associations—cont'd

		POSSIBLE DISEASE ASSOCIATIONS	
Test	Expected Range*	High Levels	Low Levels
Albumin	3.5-5.0 g/dL	Dehydration	Impaired synthesis (cirrhosis, hepatitis) Hemorrhage Acute nephritis Protein-losing gastro-enteropathies Inadequate protein intake Excessive protein breakdown Burns
Globulin	1.7-3.5 g/dL	Chronic active hepatitis Multiple myeloma Hodgkin's disease Collagen disease Tuberculosis Brucellosis Sarcoidosis	No clinical significance
Protein	6-8.5 g/dL	Multiple myeloma Dehydration Vomiting Diarrhea	Impaired kidney function

Blood Enzymes

Test	Expected Range*	High Levels	Low Levels
ALP (alkaline phosphatase)	117-390 u/L (child) 39-117 u/L (adult)	Obstructive jaundice Paget's disease Rickets Osteomalacia Hepatocellular disease Biliary obstruction Cirrhosis	Scurvy
ALT or SGOT (alanine aminotransferase)	0-37 u/L (male) 0-31 u/L (female)	Myocardial function Acute hepatitis Cirrhosis Mononucleosis	No clinical significance
AST or SGPT (aspartate aminotransferase)	0-40 u/L (male) 0-31 u/L (female)	Viral hepatitis Biliary obstruction	No clinical significance
CK (creatine kinase)	10-90 u/L (depending on method of testing)	Myocardial infarction Duchenne's muscular dystrophy	No clinical significance
GGT (gamma-glutamyl-transferase)	11-50 u/L (male) 7-32 u/L (female)	Cirrhosis Congestive heart failure Alcoholism Obstructive jaundice Hepatocellular disease	No clinical significance
LD or LDH (lactic dehydrogenase)	118-242 u/L (male) 122-220 u/L (female)	Myocardial infarction Hemolytic anemia Acute leukemia Hepatic disease Pulmonary infarction	No clinical significance

(Continued)

TABLE 6-3 Common Chemistry Panels and Possible Disease Associations—cont'd

Test	Expected Range*	POSSIBLE DISEASE ASSOCIATIONS High Levels	Low Levels
Minerals			
Calcium	8.5-10.5 mg/dL	Dehydration Myeloma Hyperparathyroidism Sarcoidosis Bone metastases Leukemia Lymphoma Paget's disease Acute renal failure Hypervitaminosis D Addison's disease	Regional enteritis Ulcerative colitis Diarrhea Hypoparathyroidism Cushing's disease Pancreatitis Malabsorption Malnutrition Rickets Tetany (neonates) Vitamin D deficiency Some renal and intestinal disorders
Phosphorous	2.5-4.5 mg/dL	Addison's disease Hypervitaminosis D Acromegaly Hypoparathyroidism Chronic renal failure	Hyperparathyroidism Vitamin D deficiency Rickets Malabsorption IDDM
Iron	40-160 µg/dL	Hemolytic anemia Hemochromatosis Increased release from body stores Decreased use of iron (e.g., lead poisoning) Sideroblastic anemia	Iron-deficiency anemia Pregnancy Insufficient dietary intake of iron
Blood Gases			
Carbon dioxide	Dependent on method and if blood is arterial or venous	Aldosteronism Respiratory acidosis Metabolic alkalosis	Diarrhea Metabolic acidosis Respiratory alkalosis
Metabolism			
Cholesterol	140-240 mg/dL LDL <100 mg/dL HDL >50 mg/dL	Atherosclerotic disease Alcoholism Defects in lipoprotein metabolism Hypothyroidism Diabetes mellitus	Malnutrition
Glucose	65-110 mg/dL	Diabetes mellitus (hyperglycemia) Cushing's disease	Hypoglycemia Addison's disease
Triglycerides	30-150 mg/dL	Atherosclerotic disease Alcoholism Hyperlipidemia Hypothyroidism Pancreatic disorders Diabetes mellitus (poorly controlled)	Malnutrition

*Ranges vary depending on test method, regional populations, and so forth.
ADH, Antidiuretic hormone; *SIADH*, syndrome of inappropriate secretion of antidiuretic hormone; *IDDM*, insulin-dependent diabetes mellitus.

Advanced Concepts

PROCEDURE 6-5 i-STAT Chemistry Analyzer Procedure

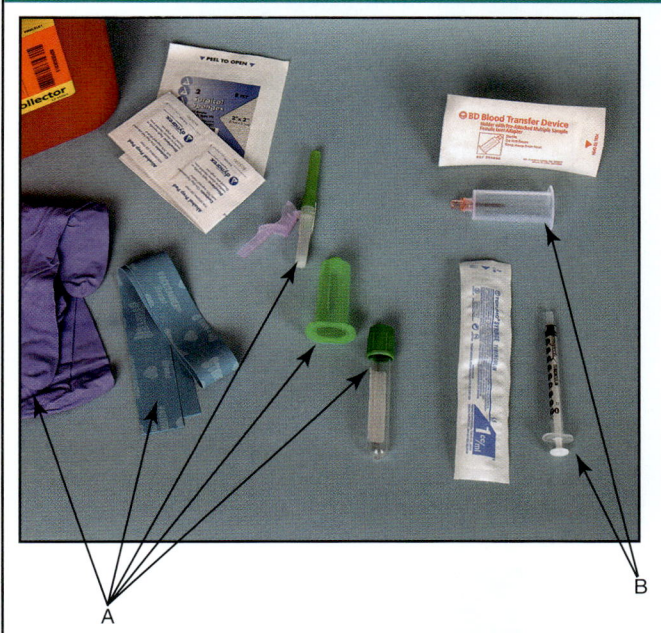

Preanalytical supplies: Venipuncture items using a 4-cc lithium heparin tube (a), and the safety transfer device that will be used with the 1-cc syringe (b).

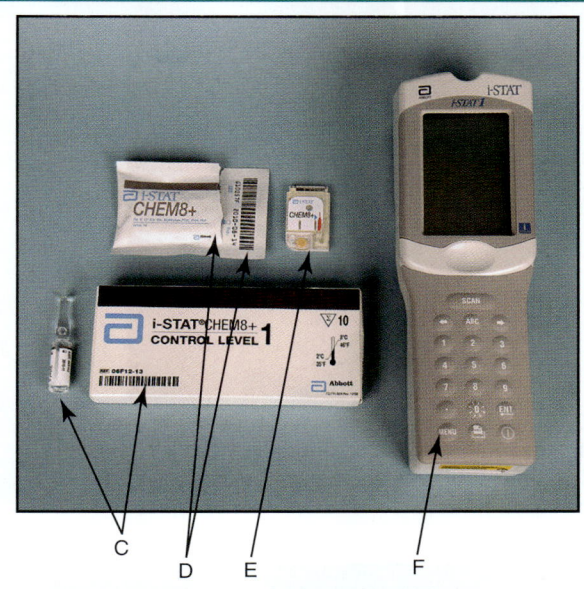

Analytical supplies and analyzer: Liquid control ampule and package (c), foil cartridge package with barcode (d), cartridge (e), and the hand-held analyzer (f).

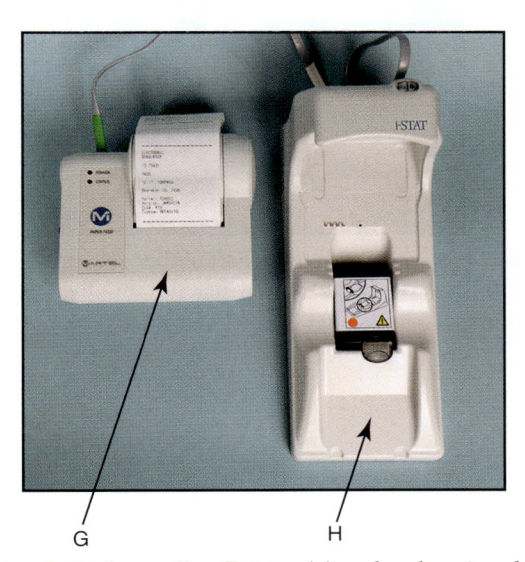

Postanalytical supplies: Printer (g) and recharging dock for analyzer (h).

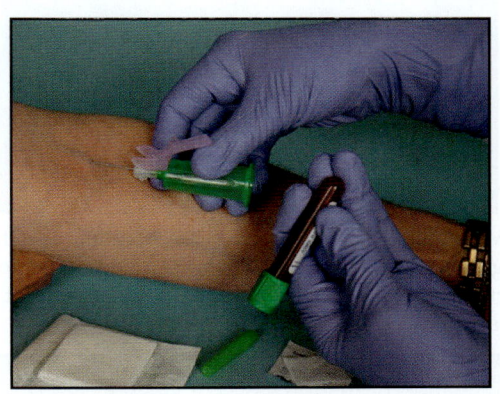

A. Collect blood, making sure the 4-cc heparin tube fills completely and that the blood is mixed by tilting 10 times. The specimen should be tested within 10 minutes. NOTE: During this time, key in operator and patient information followed by scanning the cartridge bar code.

(Continued)

PROCEDURE 6-5 i-STAT Chemistry Analyzer Procedure—cont'd

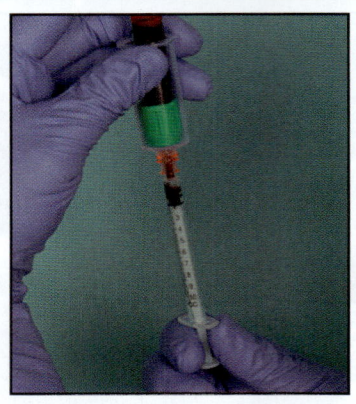

B. Using safety transfer device, pull well-mixed blood from the tube into about half of a 1-cc syringe. If air enters the syringe, do not push it back into the blood tube.

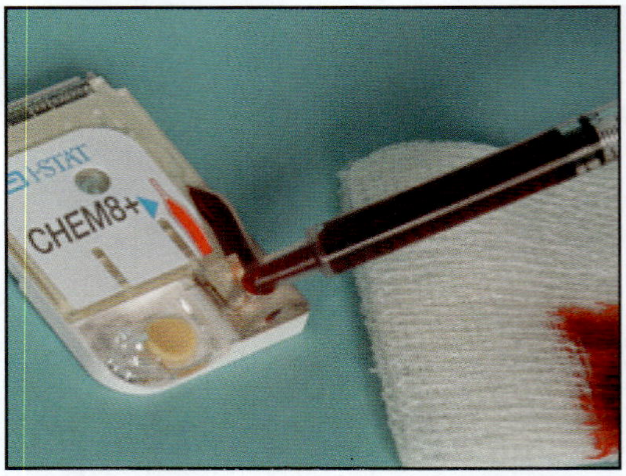

C. Remove any air at the tip of the syringe along with three drops of blood. Then carefully push the blood into the cartridge well until the blood reaches the arrow and there is still blood remaining in the well but not overflowing.

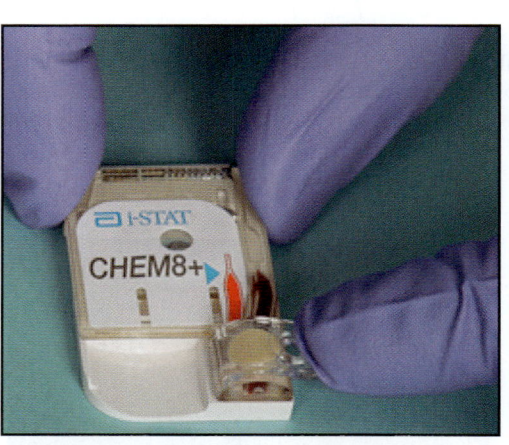

D. Swing the cover tab over the well from left to right using one finger. Do not press on the beige circle area directly over the well. Push down on the tab until it snaps into place.

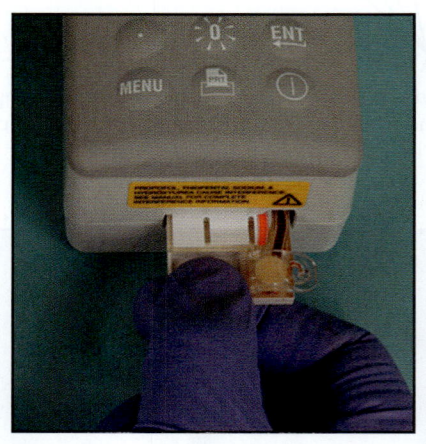

E. Use the grooved area to the left of the well, or the sides of the cartridge, to slowly insert it into the analyzer.

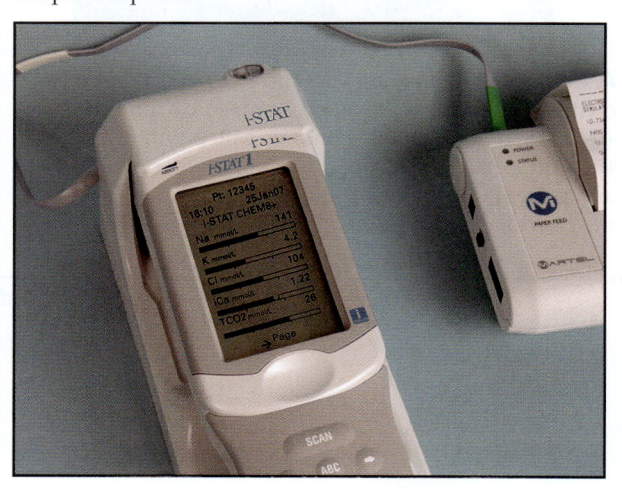

F. After 2 to 3 minutes the results will appear on the screen. Note "→ Page" command on bottom of the screen indicating more results will appear on a second screen. Press the print button to send the results to the printer via wireless transmission or via the docking device USB connection.

Figures courtesy Zack Bent.

Review Questions

1. What type of specimen is required for most blood chemistry tests in the POL (hint: think of the waived tests)?
   _____

   When collecting blood for a reference laboratory?
   _____

2. When plasma glucose is high, what hormone is secreted?
   _____

3. What percentage of diabetes mellitus cases in the United States are type 2, or non–insulin dependent?
   _____

4. The presence of sugar in the urine is called
   _____

5. A type of blood glucose test that requires no special fasting or other preparation is the
   a. GsTT
   b. fasting glucose
   c. 2-hour postprandial glucose
   d. random glucose test

6. Explain the reason for testing Hgb A1c.
   _____
   _____.

7. Match the following:
   _____ LDL   a. an abnormal increase in the glucose level in the blood
   _____ HDL   b. a complex molecule consisting of protein and a fat such as cholesterol
   _____ glycogen   c. the form in which carbohydrate is stored in the body
   _____ hypoglycemia d. a lipoprotein consisting of protein and cholesterol that removes excess cholesterol from blood vessel walls
   _____ hyperglycemia e. an abnormally low level of glucose in the blood
   _____ lipoprotein   f. a lipoprotein consisting of protein and cholesterol that adheres to blood vessel walls, forming plaque

8. List the two main sources of cholesterol in the blood.
   1. _____
   2. _____

9. Why is LDL cholesterol referred to as "lousy" cholesterol and HDL referred to as "healthy" cholesterol?
   _____

10. What is the purpose of calibrating a blood chemistry analyzer?
    _____
    _____

11. List three reasons that a control would not fall within its designated range.
    1. _____
    2. _____
    3. _____

12. List the ranges for each of the following total cholesterol categories:
    a. desirable cholesterol level:
    _____
    b. low-risk cholesterol level:
    _____
    c. high cholesterol level:
    _____

13. What is the main reason for performing the fecal occult blood test?
    _____
    _____

14. Match the blood chemistry profiles for the various body organs or diseases with their corresponding chemistry tests.
    ___ renal profile   a. uric acid
    ___ liver profile   b. BUN, creatinine, uric acid, electrolytes
    ___ cardiac profile c. CK, LD, AST, and lipids
    ___ lipid profile   d. bilirubin, alkaline phosphatase, albumin, globulin
    ___ gout   e. cholesterol, LDL, HDL, triglycerides

Review Question Answers

1. whole blood from a finger stick; serum from a red clot tube or gold SST
2. insulin
3. 90% to 95%
4. glucosuria
5. d
6. It provides a picture of average glucose levels over a 3-month period and helps determine whether the patient is keeping glucose levels under control.
7. f, d, c, e, a, b
8. from the diet (exogenous); from the liver (endogenous)
9. LDL adheres to the arteries, causing plaque, whereas HDL removes the plaque.
10. To check the instrument's optical performance
11. poor specimen processing or technique; reagents stored at wrong temperature or expired; instrument dirty or faulty
12. less than 200 mg/dL; 200 to 240 mg/dL; higher than 240 mg/dL
13. To determine if bleeding is present within the colon, which might indicate possible carcinoma
14. b, d, c, e, a

Websites

American Diabetes Association home page:
www.diabetes.org/home.jsp

"How to Tell If You Have Pre-Diabetes" from the American Diabetes Association:
www.diabetes.org/pre-diabetes/pre-diabetes-symptoms.jsp

Bayer Contour information:
http://www.bayerdiabetes.com/sections/ourproducts/meters/contour.aspx

Information and demonstration video on how to use the Bayer computer monitoring systems for adults and children:
http://www.bayerdiabetes.com/sections/ourproducts/software.aspx
http://www.bayerdidget.co.uk/about-didget/Product-Demo

Demonstration video on how to use the LifeScan OneTouch Ultra glucose monitor from Johnson & Johnson:
www.lifescan.com

Training video on how to run the Cholestech LDX:
http://www.cholestech.com/support/ldx_training.htm

i-STAT information:
http://www.abbottpointofcare.com/istat/www/products/Cartridge_Brochure.pdf
www.codemap.com/abbott

Piccolo Express information:
http://www.abaxis.com/medical/

Excellent physician office resource for lab equipment and supplies:
http://www.physiciansofficeresource.com/physicians/physician-office-lab.asp

CHAPTER 7

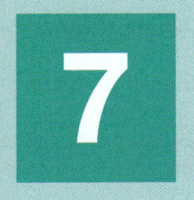

Immunology

Objectives
After completing this chapter you should be able to:

Fundamental Concepts
1. Explain the immune process.
2. Differentiate between cell-mediated immunity and humoral immunity.
3. List and match the classes of immunoglobulins (antibodies) with their locations and/or functions.
4. List the four ways to acquire adaptive immunity.
5. Discuss the principles of in vivo and in vitro immunology tests as they relate to allergy testing.

CLIA-Waived Immunology Tests
1. Give examples of direct and indirect immunology tests based on the detection of antigens or antibodies.
2. Perform a CLIA-waived pregnancy test, infectious mononucleosis test, and *Helicobacter pylori* test according to the stated task, conditions, and standards listed in the Learning Outcome Evaluation in the student workbook.
3. Describe mononucleosis, and explain how it is diagnosed.
4. Discuss HIV and CLIA-waived testing for HIV.
5. Discuss and/or perform the highly sensitive iFOB test using the lateral flow immunoassay method to detect fecal occult blood.

Advanced Concepts
1. Discuss advanced immunological techniques such as agglutination, enzyme-linked immunosorbent assay, and chromatographic immunoassay.
2. Observe a slide test for ABO blood typing for the presence or absence of immunological agglutination to determine blood type.
3. Observe a slide test for Rh blood typing, and explain how Rh incompatibility can cause erythroblastosis fetalis.
4. Explain how titers are used by physicians in the diagnosis and prognosis of disease conditions.
5. Identify common immunology tests within three categories: bacterial infections, viral infections, and detection of other antigens such as hormones and cancer-related substances.

Key Terms

active immunity long-term protection against future infections resulting from the production of antibodies that were formed naturally during an infection or artificially by vaccination

agglutination clumping together of blood cells or latex beads caused by antibodies adhering to their antigens

allergen an antigen that causes an allergic reaction

antibodies immunoglobulins produced specifically to destroy foreign invaders

antigens substances that are perceived as foreign to the body and elicit an antibody response

autoimmune diseases destructive tissue diseases caused by antibody/self-antigen reactions

cell-mediated immunity T lymphocytic cell response to antigens

chromatographic pertaining to a visual color change that appears when an enzyme-linked antibody/antigen reaction takes place

complement proteins proteins that stimulate phagocytosis and inflammation and are capable of destroying bacteria

erythroblastosis fetalis a hemolytic anemia in newborns resulting from maternal–fetal blood group incompatibility

helper T cells (TH4 or CD4) antigen-activated lymphocytes that stimulate other T cells and help B cells produce their antibodies

heterophile antibody antibody that appears during an Epstein–Barr viral infection (mononucleosis) that has an unusual affinity to antigens on sheep red cells

histamine compound released by injured cells that causes the dilation of blood vessels

humoral immunity B lymphocytic cell response to antigens resulting in the production of specific antibodies to destroy a foreign invader; also called antibody-mediated immunity

iFOB immunoassayed fecal occult blood

immunosorbent pertaining to the attachment of an antigen or antibody to a solid surface such as latex beads, wells in plastic dishes, or plastic cartridges

Key Terms—cont'd

inflammation overall reaction of the body to tissue injury or invasion by an infectious agent, characterized by redness, heat, swelling, and pain

interferons proteins secreted by infected cells to prevent the further replication and spread of an infection into neighboring cells

in vitro within a laboratory apparatus

in vivo within a host or living organism

killer T cells antigen-activated lymphocytes that attack foreign antigens directly and destroy cells that bear the antigens; also called *cytotoxic cells*

memory B cells antigen-activated B lymphocytes that remember an identified antigen for future encounters

memory T cells antigen-activated T lymphocytes that remember an antigen for future encounters

mucous membrane thin sheets of tissue that line the internal cavities and canals of the body and serve as a barrier against the entry of pathogens into the body

natural killer cells special type of lymphocyte that attacks and destroys infected cells and cancer cells in a nonspecific way

normal flora nonpathogenic microorganisms that normally inhabit the skin and mucous membranes

passive immunity short-term acquired immunity created by antibodies received naturally through the placenta (or the colostrum to an infant) or artificially by injection

phagocytes cells capable of engulfing and ingesting microorganisms and cellular debris

phagocytosis process of engulfing and digesting microorganisms and cellular debris

plasma cells a subgroup of B lymphocytes that produce the antibodies that travel through the blood specifically targeting and reacting with antigens

self-antigens substances within the body that induce the production of antibodies that attack an individual's own body tissues; also called *autoantigens*

serology branch of laboratory medicine that performs antibody/antigen testing with serum

suppressor T cells antigen-activated lymphocytes that inhibit T and B cells after a sufficient number of cells have been activated

titer a quantitative test that measures the amount of antibody that reacts with a specific antigen

vaccination process of injecting harmless or killed microorganisms into the body to induce immunity against a potential pathogen (also called *immunization*)

wheal raised induration

FUNDAMENTAL CONCEPTS

Overview of Immunology

The immune system is a remarkable defense system that protects the human body against invading pathogens, toxins, allergens, and cancer cells. When the body is under attack by any of these invaders, it has a full arsenal of defenses to destroy the invader, as well as protect itself from future attacks. A key ingredient in this defense mechanism is the body's production of **antibodies** (immunoglobulins produced specifically to destroy foreign invaders). These antibodies are produced after the body detects the presence of specific **antigens** (substances that are perceived as foreign to the body). Once antibodies are produced, they attack the antigens, forming an antibody/antigen complex that destroys or renders the invader harmless.

Biotechnology research has made it possible to detect and measure specific antibodies and their specific antigens in blood and body fluids. Antibody/antigen testing is a rapidly expanding laboratory science called *immunology*. Because antibodies are usually found in serum, the laboratory department performing antibody/antigen testing may also be referred to as the *serology* department.

The science of immunology dates to the 1500s, when it was recorded that China had developed a technique of exposing individuals to a powder made from smallpox scabs to produce protection against the disease. The thought was that if children or young adults were exposed in a healthy state, the disease would not be as devastating; unfortunately, that did not always occur. In the late 1700s, Edward Jenner, an English country doctor, found that injecting individuals with material from cowpox provided effective protection against smallpox. This preventive process of injecting harmless or killed microorganisms into the body to induce immunity against a potential pathogen was known as **vaccination** or immunization.

The field of immunology has benefited from a tremendous amount of new research and subsequent knowledge over the past 100 years. In fact, the cells responsible for the body's immune response were not discovered until the 1960s. Another recent finding is that the body may respond to **self-antigens** (substances within the body that induce the production of antibodies that attack an individual's own body tissues; also called *autoantigens*). Antibody/self-antigen reactions cause a variety of destructive tissue diseases referred to as **autoimmune diseases.**

The Immune Process

The overall immune process that occurs as the body protects itself against foreign invaders can be viewed as three lines (or battlefields) of defensive mechanisms. Fig. 7-1 is a simplified picture of these

Fundamental Concepts

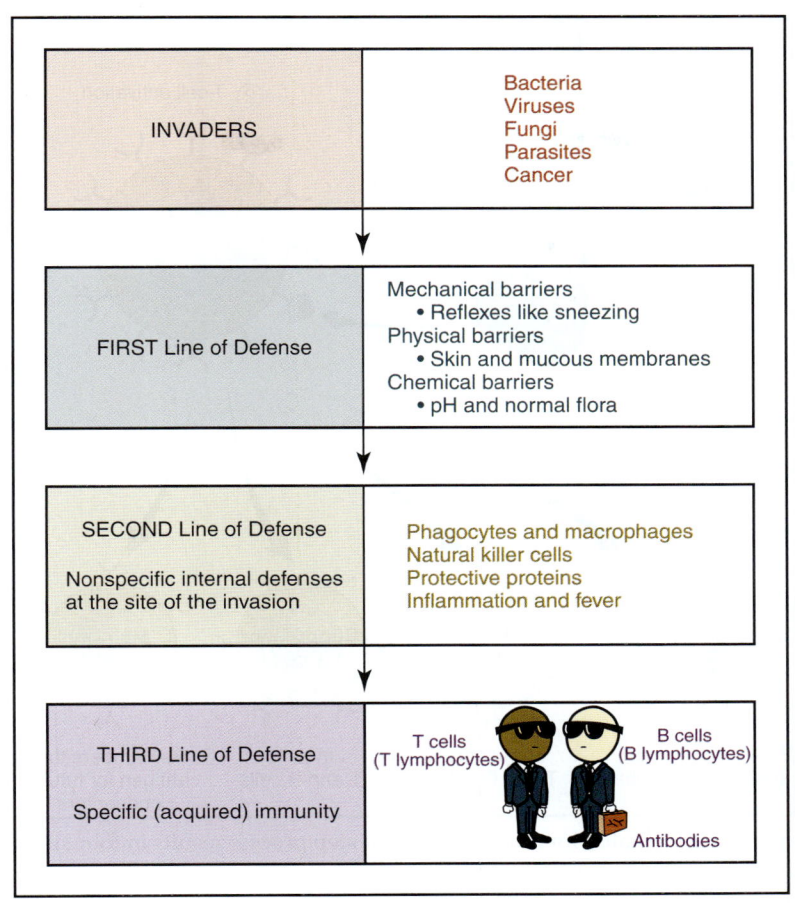

Fig. 7-1. Three lines of defense against harmful invaders. Nonspecific immunity defenses are external barriers, then internal responses to the invaders. Specific immunity (the third line of defense) involves "intelligent" T cells, B cells, and the production of antibodies. (Modified from Herlihy M: *The human body in health and illness,* ed 3, St Louis, 2006, Saunders.)

lines of defense. The foreign invaders are portrayed at the top of the flowchart. Their goal is to enter the body and cause destruction. The first two lines of defense are considered "nonspecific immunity"—nonspecific because they fight all invaders in the same way. The third line of defense, at the bottom of the illustration, is referred to as "specific immunity" because it intelligently identifies each invader on the basis of its specific antigens. The B cells are then able to produce a specific antibody capable of destroying the invader.

First Line of Defense: Natural Barriers
The first line of defense stops invaders from entering or growing on the body. The skin and **mucous membrane** (thin sheets of tissue lining the internal cavities and canals) serve as anatomical barriers that prevent the entry of pathogens into the body. They also secrete chemicals that discourage the growth of pathogenic bacteria. These secretions maintain a skin pH of 5.6, which allows the growth of **normal flora** (nonpathogenic microorganisms that normally inhabit the skin and mucous membranes) while inhibiting the growth of pathogens. In the respiratory tract the mucous membranes contain mucus, which entraps foreign organisms. Coughing and sneezing help move foreign organisms out of the body.

Second Line of Defense: Nonspecific Internal Response
The second line of defense is the internal nonspecific response to all invaders that have passed the natural barriers and entered the body. When invaders break through the barriers, the body quickly responds by sending **phagocytes** (cells capable of engulfing and ingesting pathogens and cellular debris) to the site of invasion. White blood cells, neutrophils, and monocytes (which become macrophages in the tissue) engulf and ingest the invaders by the process of **phagocytosis**.

Natural killer cells are a special type of lymphocyte sent to the scene of invasion to attack and destroy the body's infected cells and cancer cells in a nonspecific way. Protective proteins such as interferons and complement proteins also play an important role at the site of invasion. **Interferons** are proteins secreted by infected cells to prevent the further replication and spread of the infection into neighboring cells. **Complement proteins** are proteins that further stimulate phagocytosis and **inflammation** (reaction of the body

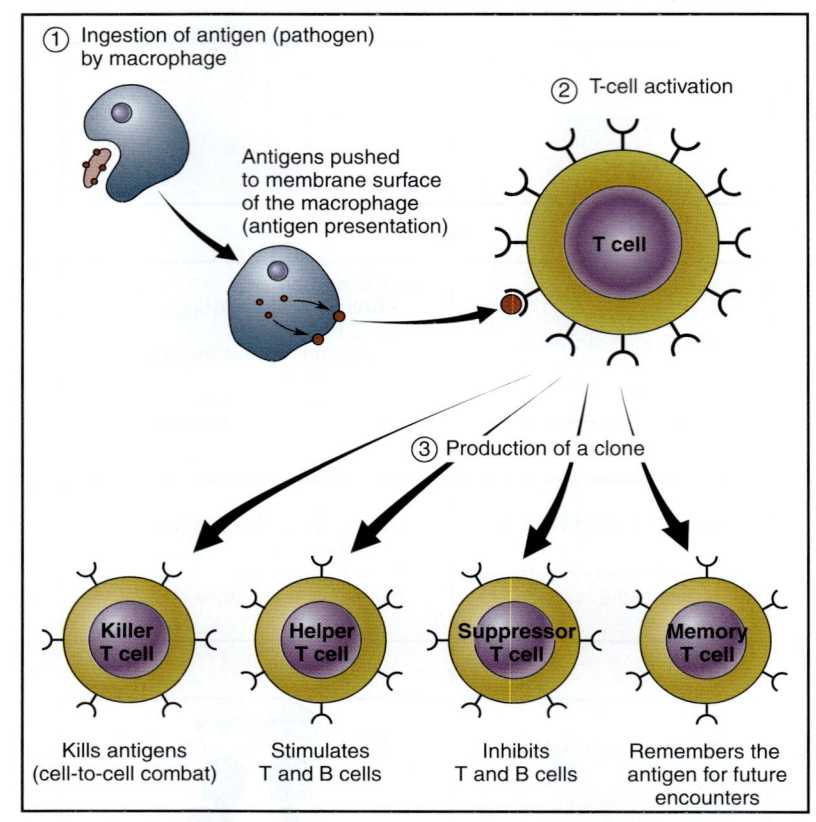

Fig. 7-2. T-cell activation and cell-mediated immunity. The three-step process results in four subsets of T cells. (From Herlihy M: *The human body in health and illness*, ed 3, St Louis, 2006, Saunders.)

to tissue injury or invasion by an infectious agent) and are capable of destroying bacteria. Complement proteins swarm over a bacterium and punch holes in its membrane, causing it to fill with fluid and explode.

At the same time that these defenders are doing their jobs to destroy the invader, the injured tissues are initiating a nonspecific *inflammatory* response. The clinical signs of inflammation are heat, redness, swelling, and pain. Inflammation begins when **histamine** is released by the injured cells, causing the dilation of blood vessels. The increased blood flow to the affected areas results in redness and heat. Fluids in the plasma leak into the tissue because of the increased permeability of the vessels, causing the swelling and pain.

The second line of defense is generally seen within the first 12 hours of an infection. For example, the first signs and symptoms of influenza start with swollen glands, sore throat, chills, and fever. These symptoms are the result of an active nonspecific battle against the invaders consisting of the phagocytes, natural killer cells, protective proteins, and the subsequent inflammatory response.

Third Line of Defense: Adaptive or Acquired Immunity

The third line of defense goes into action when the first two lines have failed to bring the invasion under control. It is the "intelligent" identification of the invader based on its antigenic properties. The T cells and B cells work together to produce the specific antibodies that will destroy the invader or render it harmless once and for all. This adaptive process takes 6 to 10 days to accomplish. The T and B cells are also capable of developing immunological memory so that a second encounter with the same organism will induce a heightened immune reaction.

Both these intelligent lymphocytes provide different immunological functions, as described in the following sections.

Cell-Mediated Immunity. T cells, small lymphocytes associated with the thymus gland, are involved in **cell-mediated immunity.** They become involved at the site of the invasion, where they become activated after they receive an antigen presentation from the macrophages (Fig. 7-2).

Once activated, T cells rapidly duplicate themselves into clones that differentiate into the following four subgroups:
1. **Killer T cells,** or cytotoxic cells (TC), are antigen-activated lymphocytes that attack foreign antigens directly and destroy cells that bear the antigens.
2. **Helper T cells** (TH4 or CD4) stimulate other T cells and help B cells produce their antibodies. (These are the cells infected by the human immunodeficiency virus [HIV].)

Fundamental Concepts

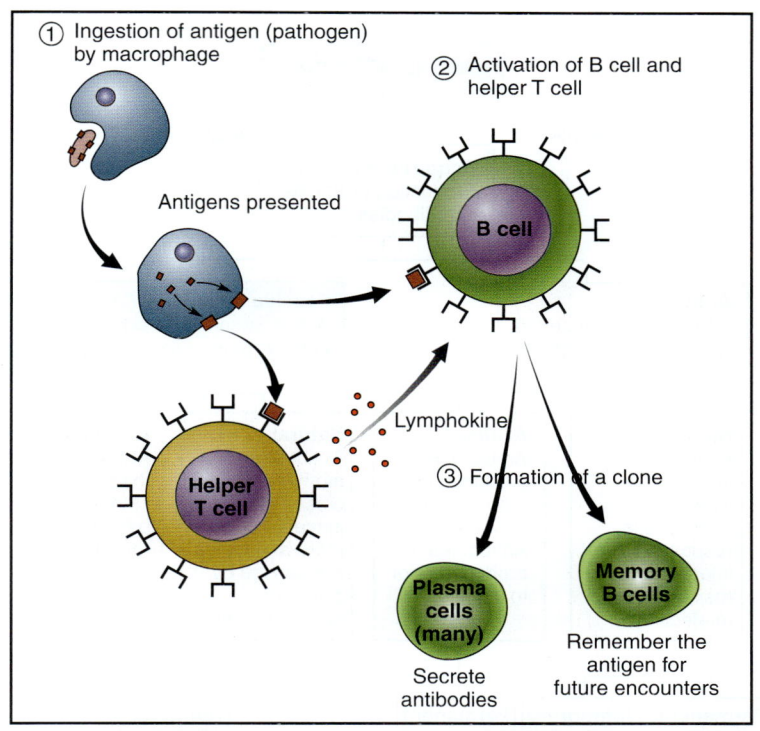

Fig. 7-3. B-cell activation and humoral (antibody) immunity. The three-step process results in the production of antibodies by the plasma cells. (From Herlihy M: *The human body in health and illness*, ed 3, St Louis, 2006, Saunders.)

3. **Suppressor T cells** (TS) inhibit the T and B cells after a sufficient number of cells have been activated.
4. **Memory T cells** remember the antigen for future encounters. They are ready to respond to subsequent exposure to the specific antigens with increased speed and intensity.

Of the lymphocytes circulating in the blood, 70% to 80% are T cells.

Humoral Immunity (Antibody-Mediated Immunity). B cells are involved in **humoral immunity**. Humoral immunity begins with the interaction of a B cell with a specific antigen and the lymphokine (chemicals) from the T helper cell (Fig. 7-3). Once it is activated, it rapidly duplicates into a clone and differentiates into the following two subgroups:
1. **Plasma cells** produce the antibodies (immunoglobulins) that travel through the blood specifically targeting and reacting with the antigens, resulting in the destruction of the invader.
2. **Memory B cells** remember the antigen for future encounters. They also are ready to respond to subsequent exposure to the specific antigens with increased speed and intensity.

Classes of Antibodies (Immunoglobulins). Biomedical researchers have found that antibodies are part of the globulin group of proteins that circulate in the blood. Because of their globulin properties, antibodies are referred to as *immunoglobulins (Igs)*. The researchers have classified immunoglobulins into the following groups, based on their shapes, locations, and functions:
- IgE are the immunoglobulins involved in acute allergic reactions.
- IgM are the primary responders in the first encounter with an invading antigen.
- IgG respond to the antigens and allergens in subsequent invading or allergic encounters.
- IgA protect mucous membranes from bacterial and viral infections.
- IgD are involved in lymphocyte activation and suppression.

Ways to Acquire Specific Immunity. Once a specific antibody is present in the blood, the individual is said to be immune to its particular disease, pathogen, or antigen. There are four ways to acquire specific immunity: (1) active immunity acquired naturally, (2) active immunity acquired artificially, (3) passive immunity acquired naturally, and (4) passive immunity acquired artificially (Fig. 7-4).

Active immunity is long-term protection against future infections that results from the production of antibodies that were formed naturally during an infection or artificially by vaccination. In both cases the antibody is remembered in the memory B cells, making the individual immune to future encounters with the pathogen.

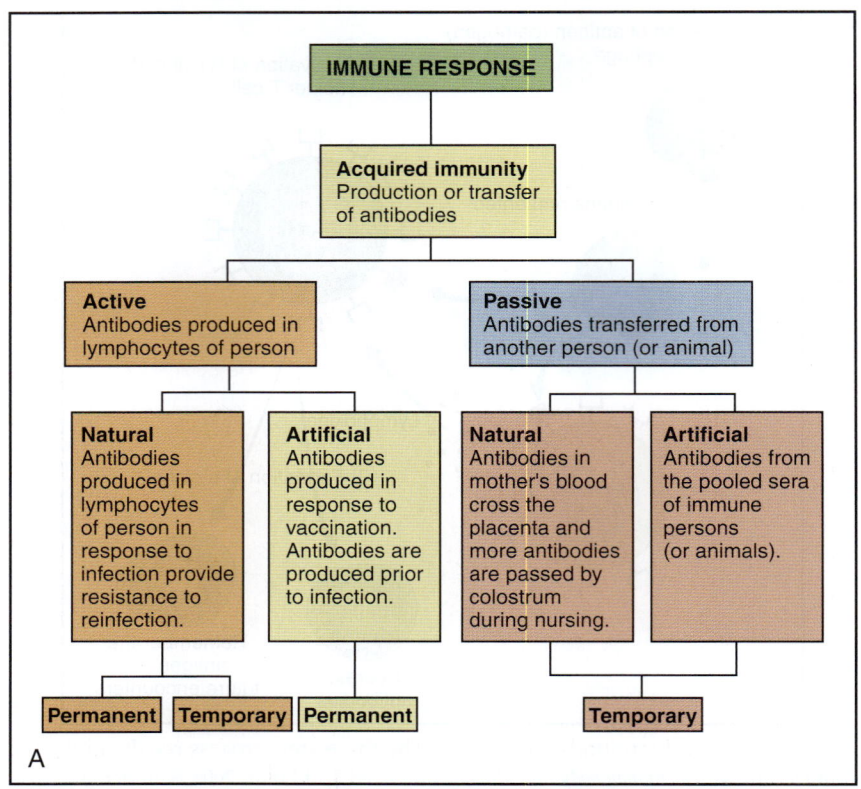

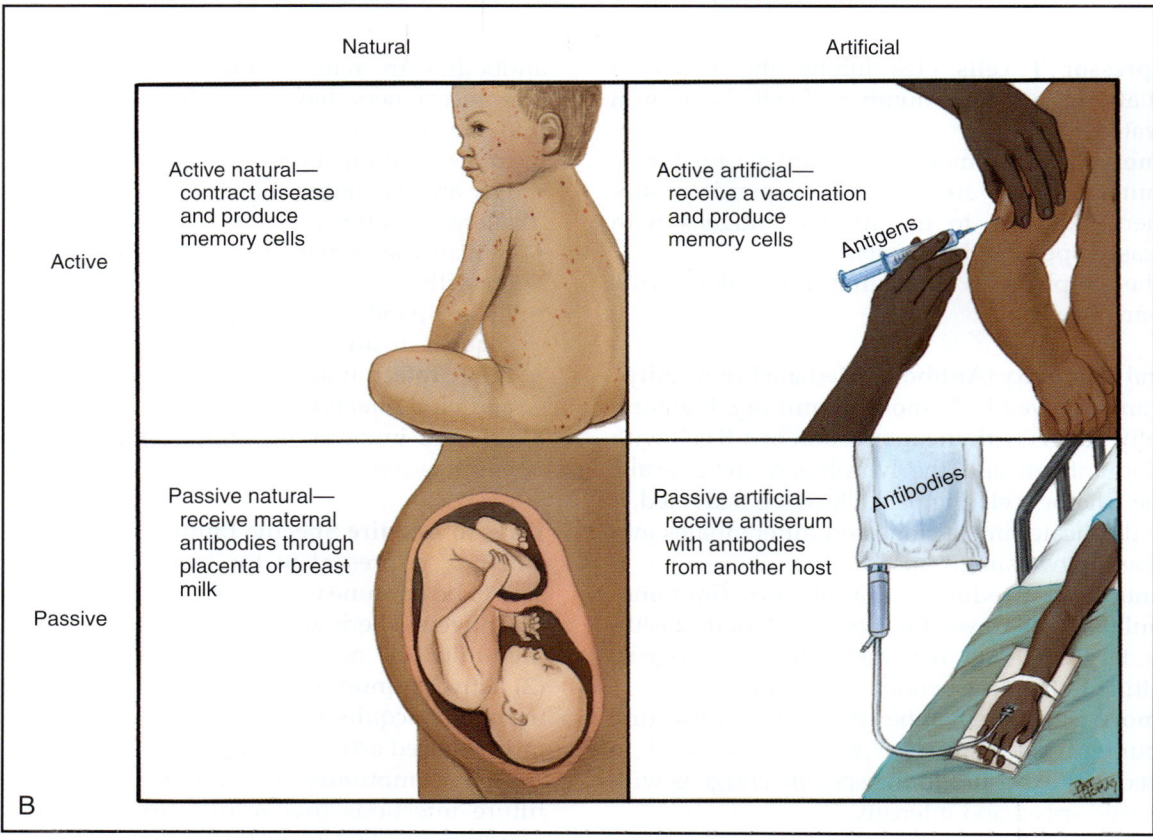

Fig. 7-4. A, Forms of acquired humoral (antibody) immunity and their ability to provide permanent or temporary immunity. **B,** Examples of the four combinations of active/passive immunity and natural/artificial immunity. (**A,** From Stepp CA, Woods M: *Laboratory procedures for medical office personnel,* Philadelphia, 1998, Saunders; and **B,** From Applegate EJ: *The anatomy and physiology learning system,* ed 3, St Louis, 2006, Saunders.)

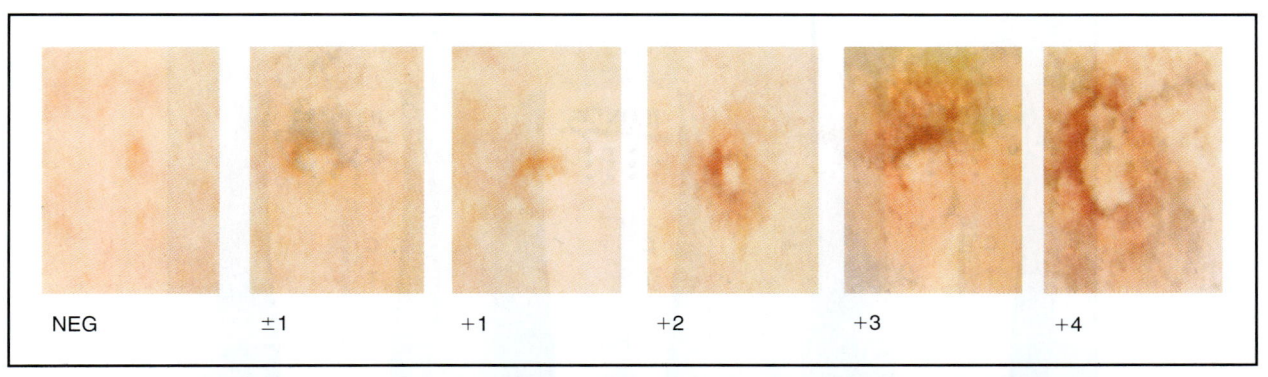

Fig. 7-5. In vivo antibody/antigen test, with negative and positive skin reactions to an antigen. If the patient has the specific antibodies that react with the injected antigen, a wheal forms. (From Bonewit-West K: *Clinical procedures for medical assistants*, ed 7, St Louis, 2008, Saunders.)

Passive immunity is short-term protection against infections created by antibodies received naturally through the placenta (or the colostrum to an infant) or artificially by the injection of antiserum or gamma globulins. Passive immunity is only temporary.

Two Types of Allergy Testing

In Vivo Testing

The body is capable of overreacting to antigens by producing too many antibodies (immunoglobulins), resulting in allergic or autoimmune conditions such as asthma, hives, breathing difficulties, and gastrointestinal inflammation. Allergy tests have been performed to visualize the specific reaction between an **allergen** (an antigen that causes an allergic reaction) and its specific antibody. Tests are done **in vivo** (within a host or living organism) by injecting or pricking an antigen into the skin and seeing whether a **wheal** (raised induration) forms in response to the antibody/antigen reaction. Fig. 7-5 shows a negative reaction and various positive reactions to skin tests. Tuberculosis screening tests and allergy skin tests are examples of in vivo immunology tests.

In Vitro Testing

Laboratory immunology tests (also referred to as *serology tests*) are now being performed **in vitro** (within the laboratory test tube) outside of the body. It is now available to test the antigen/antibody reaction using only the serum from a tube of blood. Through this testing method, a multiwell plate is coated with various food proteins and/or inhalants that are possible allergens capable of causing allergic reactions. The patient's serum is then added to each well. If the patient's serum contains IgE or IgG antibodies to any of the specific food or inhalant proteins, a binding reaction occurs. The degree of antibody–antigen binding depends on the concentration of antibodies present in the patient's serum. The reaction is then detected through a color change and assessed spectrophotometrically. The wells showing a strong reaction and high level of IgG immunoglobulins will indicate an allergic response to the items in the wells. A typical serological food panel test will indicate possible allergies in the following food groups: dairy, meat/fowl, fruits, fish/crustacea/mollusk, grains, vegetables, spices, herbs.

CLIA-WAIVED IMMUNOLOGY TESTS

CLIA-Waived Enzyme-Linked Immunoassays

Manufacturers produce a variety of immunology testing devices. In most of these rapid screening tests, a liquid specimen is absorbed and travels across a testing area that enzymatically changes color if an antibody/antigen reaction takes place. The tests typically include an internal control that must also change color to prove the testing device is working. The control area is usually located just beyond the test area to make sure the solution has traveled all the way through the test area. This method is often referred to as a *lateral flow immunochromatographic assay*. Fig. 7-6 shows the before and after reactions of a positive and negative urine pregnancy test.

The presence of specific antibodies or antigens associated with a specific disease can be detected in the blood or other body specimens by mixing them with their specific antigen or antibody and checking for a reaction. The tests usually provide a visual reaction when the antibody/antigen complex is formed. Biotechnology has made available numerous CLIA waived test kits designed to detect rapidly the presence of an antigen (direct test) or an antibody (indirect test) associated with a particular disease or infection. These screening tests are usually

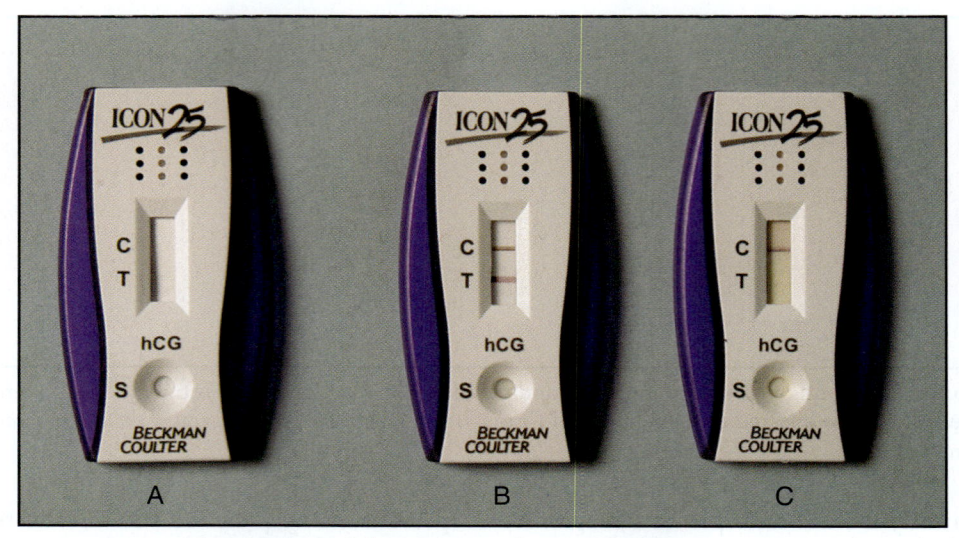

Fig. 7-6. In vitro pregnancy test showing lateral flow immunochromatographic assay. **A,** Test device before adding specimen (S: specimen is placed in well; T: specimen travels through test area; C: control must turn color to prove device is working). **B,** Positive reactions in test area and control area (two pink bands). **C,** Negative reaction in test area and positive reaction in control area.

displayed and interpreted **chromatographically** (pertaining to a visual color change that appears when an enzyme-linked antibody/antigen reaction takes place).

Table 7-1 lists the common CLIA-waived tests that use the lateral flow method to detect the presence of an antigen or antibody associated with a specific disease or condition. Some test kits provide the antibody and test for its antigen in the specimen (direct tests). Other test kits provide the antigen and test for its specific antibody within the specimen (indirect tests). In both cases a color reaction occurs if both antibody and antigen are present, and the results are recorded as positive. If the color reaction does not occur in the test area, the result is recorded as negative.

A variety of test kits are available for CLIA-waived screening tests for pregnancy, mononucleosis, *Helicobacter pylori* infections, HIV, and a new immunological method for testing fecal occult blood. NOTE: This text provides directions that apply to the specific kits portrayed in the procedures. Never assume that the instructions from a new kit or a kit from another manufacturer are the same. The instructions packaged with each particular kit should be followed.

Pregnancy Testing

Pregnancy testing is based on the detection of a hormone called *human chorionic gonadotropin (HCG)*, which is found in urine or blood. HCG levels in blood and urine may detect pregnancy 1 to 5 days after conception. HCG is produced by the chorionic villi of the developing placenta, with levels peaking between the fiftieth and eightieth days of pregnancy. After this time the levels decline and remain at a lower level, then disappear a few days after the birth.

The CLIA-waived immunoassay provides a qualitative detection of HCG. The test takes approximately 5 minutes to perform and is easy to read. The following points are important to remember:
- The urine specimen container must be free of detergents; a clean, disposable urine container is best for collection.
- A first morning urine specimen is recommended because it will contain the highest concentration of HCG. Specific gravity testing should be performed to determine if the urine specific gravity is more than 1.010. An overly diluted specimen below 1.010 could cause a false-negative result.
- The urine should be refrigerated if testing cannot be performed within an hour. The urine must be brought back to room temperature before testing.
- Follow the manufacturer's recommendations for storage of the kit. If the kit is refrigerated, it also must be brought to room temperature before testing.
- Do not use expired kits.
- Do not use the supplies or reagents from one kit with another kit.
- Test results will show "negative" or "positive," but be sure to chart "negative for pregnancy" or "positive for pregnancy."
- Observe Health Insurance Portability and Accountability Act (HIPAA) guidelines regarding patient confidentiality.
- Observe Occupational Safety and Health Administration (OSHA) guidelines when dealing with specimens.

CLIA-Waived Immunology Tests

TABLE 7-1 Common CLIA-Waived Tests That Use the Lateral Flow Method

When Both Antigen and Antibody Are Present → Positive Result

Screening Tests	Antigens (When testing for antigen in specimen = DIRECT TEST)	Antibodies (When testing for antibody in specimen = INDIRECT TEST)
Pregnancy	HCG from mother's placenta in urine specimen (DIRECT)	Anti-HCG antibodies in test kit
Bladder tumor–associated antigen (BTA)	BTA from bladder cancer in urine specimen (DIRECT)	Monoclonal antibodies in test kit react with BTA.
Mononucleosis	Heterophile antigens in test kit	IgM heterophile antibody produced against EBV found in blood specimen (INDIRECT)
Helicobacter pylori	*H. pylori* antigens in test kit	IgG antibodies specific against *H. pylori* found in blood specimen (INDIRECT)
HIV	HIV-1 antigens in test kit	Antibodies against HIV-1 found in blood or cheek cells (INDIRECT)
Fecal occult blood	Blood from fecal matter (DIRECT)	Immunochemical color reaction occurs if positive.
Influenza A and B*	Viral antigens from nasal swab specimen (DIRECT)	Antiviral antibodies in test kit
Streptococcus A infection*	Streptococcal antigen extracted from throat swab (DIRECT)	Antistreptococcal antibodies in test kit
Drug testing in urine†	Drug will inhibit immune reaction	Reaction does not appear in test area if positive.

HCG, human chorionic gonadotropin; *EBV*, Epstein–Barr virus; *HIV*, human immunodeficiency virus.
*The antigenic direct testing for the presence of influenza A and B infection and streptococcus A infection are covered in Chapter 8.
†Drug testing in urine is covered in Chapter 9.

The **SureStep Pregnancy Test** procedure check sheet is provided in the workbook and is demonstrated in Procedure 7-1, located at the end of this section.

Mononucleosis Testing

The causative agent of mononucleosis is the Epstein–Barr virus (EBV). The infection is often called the "kissing disease" because it is transmitted by direct oral contact through saliva. Mononucleosis is an acute infectious disease most frequently seen in children and young adults. *Clinical signs* and symptoms are mental and physical fatigue, severe weakness, headache, fever, sore throat, and swollen lymph nodes. *Hematological findings* may show an increase in reactive lymphocytes. *Immunologically*, the antibody that is produced during EBV infection is called a **heterophile antibody.** This heterophile antibody has an unusual affinity for antigens on the red blood cells (RBCs) of sheep. The heterophile antibody is produced by patients infected with mononucleosis usually by the fifth to eighth day after infection. Within 3 weeks of infection, 80% of the patients have a detectable level of heterophile antibodies. In the 20% of patients who do not produce the antibody, the diagnosis depends solely on the clinical and hematological findings. In the outpatient laboratory, rapid mononucleosis tests that detect heterophile antibodies are easy to perform and provide reliable results.

The QuickVue+ Mononucleosis Test Procedure check sheet is provided in the workbook and is demonstrated in Procedure 7-2 at the end of this section.

Helicobacter pylori Testing

H. pylori are spiral-shaped bacteria believed to be the cause of most peptic ulcers (90% of duodenal and 80% of gastric ulcers). This organism weakens the mucous lining of the stomach and duodenum. Stomach acids and bacteria are able to penetrate the sensitive lining beneath the mucous layer and cause an ulcer. Symptoms of an ulcer include a gnawing pain in the abdominal area a few hours after eating and during the night. These symptoms are relieved by eating and taking antacids. Ulcers are now being treated with antibiotic drugs that kill the *H. pylori* bacteria along with drugs that reduce stomach acid.

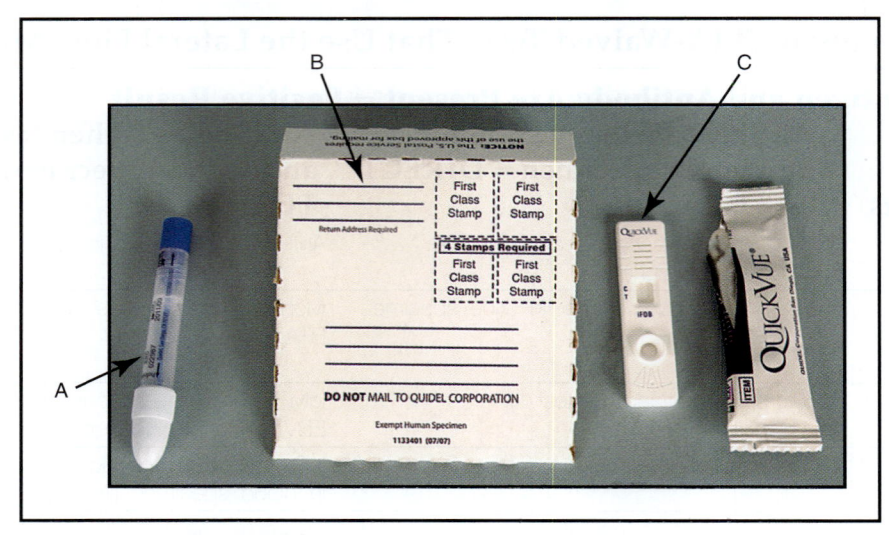

Fig. 7-7. Latest iFOB (immuno-Fecal Occult Blood test) showing (a) patient at-home collection tube, (b) mailer, and (c) in-office test kit. (Courtesy Zack Bent.)

The **QuickVue *Helicobacter pylori* gII Test** procedure check sheet is provided in the workbook and is demonstrated in Procedure 7-3, located at the end of this section.

Human Immunodeficiency Virus

HIV attacks and destroys the T helper (CD4) lymphocytes. As previously stated, the T helper cells play a critical role in protecting the body against infection by cell-mediated immunity. They also help B cells produce their specific antibodies during humoral immunity. As more and more T helper cells are destroyed by the HIV infection, the body becomes less able to fight off infections and becomes more susceptible to opportunistic infections. Acquired immune deficiency syndrome (AIDS) is the condition that eventually occurs and is characterized by the presence of life-threatening infections and cancers. Transmission is primarily through sexual contact and the sharing of drug injection needles with infected persons. Health care workers should adhere to the OSHA Bloodborne Pathogens Standard to avoid exposure.

The hospital or reference laboratory test for detecting the HIV antibody in serum is the enzyme-linked immunosorbent assay (ELISA) test, with a confirmatory test called the Western immunoblot method.

CLIA-waived HIV tests are also available that detect the presence of the HIV antibody in blood and oral specimens. One test, the ORA Quick (OraSure Technologies, Bethlehem, Penn.), uses a specimen obtained by thoroughly swabbing the outer gums (both upper and lower). The swabbing device is then inserted into a vial containing a developer solution that provides results that can be read in 20 minutes. A positive test result shows reddish-purple lines in a small window in the testing device. Internal and external controls are provided in the kit and must be run and logged as in other procedures.

Fecal Occult Blood Testing Using iFOB Kits

The QuickVue iFOB test (Fig. 7-7) is a rapid immunochemical diagnostic tool intended to detect the presence of blood in stool specimens. The significance of blood in fecal matter was discussed in Chapter 6.

This new immunochemical method of testing for fecal occult blood uses the following supplies, as seen in Fig. 7-7: (a) The **specimen collection tube and probe** in which the patient pierces a fecal specimen with the blue inner probe located inside the tube. (b) After mixing the specimen with the buffer solution in the tube, the collection tube is then mailed to the office or laboratory in the **mailer pouch.** (c) The liquid specimen is then added to the **test kit** and is interpreted the same way as the QuickVue *H. pylori* Test. A video demonstration of the entire procedure is available at the following website: http://www.quidel.com/assets/swf/iFOBTrainingvideoHQ.htm.

CLIA-Waived Immunology Tests

PROCEDURE 7-1 SureStep Pregnancy Test Procedure

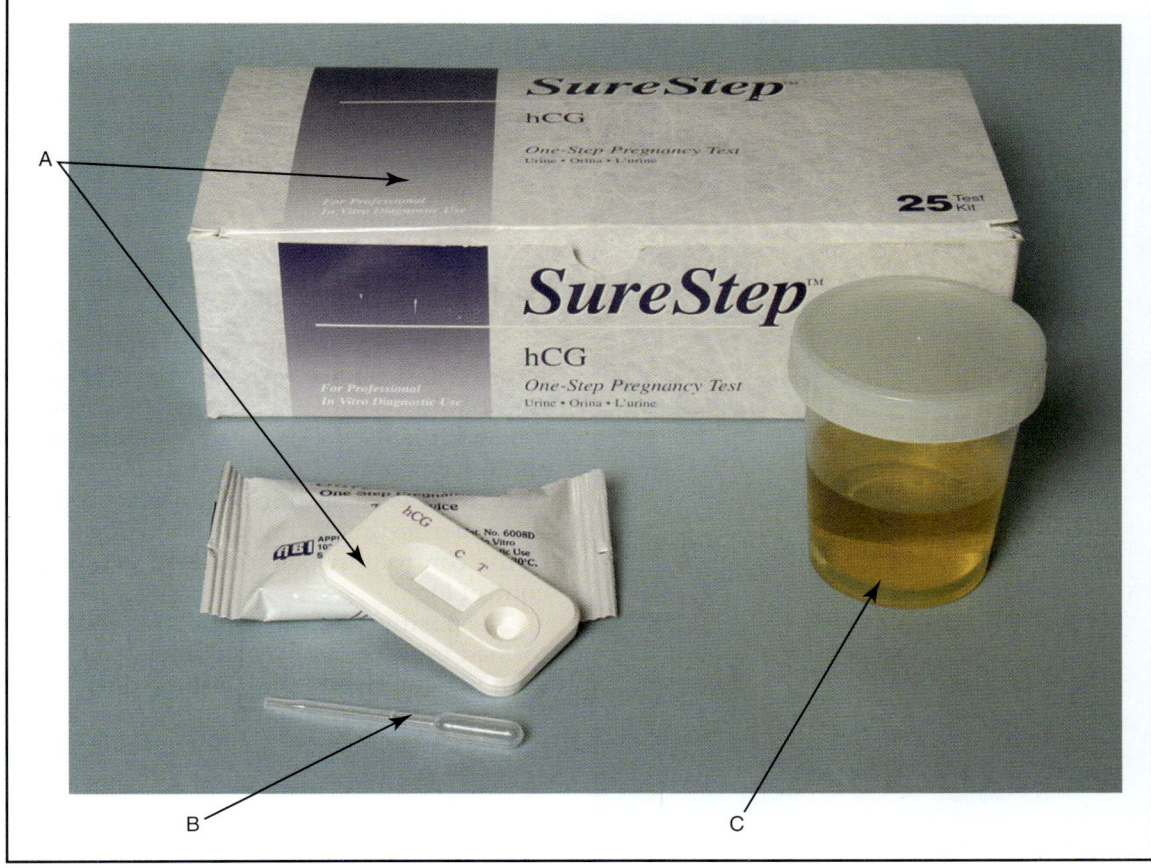

A. SureStep pregnancy test. *a*, Test device; *b*, pipette; *c*, urine specimen.

Equipment and Supplies (Fig. A)— Preanalytical

- Test device from foil package stored in SureStep box
- Pipette from foil-wrapped package
- Urine specimen
- Gloves (not pictured)

Procedure—Analytical

1. Sanitize the hands, and apply gloves.
2. Remove the test device from its protective pouch, and label it with the patient's identification. Bring it to room temperature before opening to prevent condensation.
3. Draw the urine sample to the line marked on the pipette, approximately 0.2 mL. Use separate pipettes and test devices for each specimen and control.
4. Dispense the entire contents of the pipette into the sample well.
5. Wait for the pink bands to appear.
   - High concentrations of HCG can be observed as soon as 40 seconds.
   - Low concentrations may need 5 minutes of reaction time.
   - Do not interpret results after 10 minutes.
6. At 5 minutes, read and record the results (Fig. B).
   - Positive test result: Two distinct pink bands appear, one in the patient test region (T) and one in the control region (C).
   - Negative test result: Only one pink band appears in the control region (C). No pink band is apparent in the patient test region (T).
   - Invalid: Pink bands are absent from the control region. Repeat the test with a new device. If the problem persists, call for technical assistance.

(Continued)

PROCEDURE 7-1 SureStep Pregnancy Test Procedure—cont'd

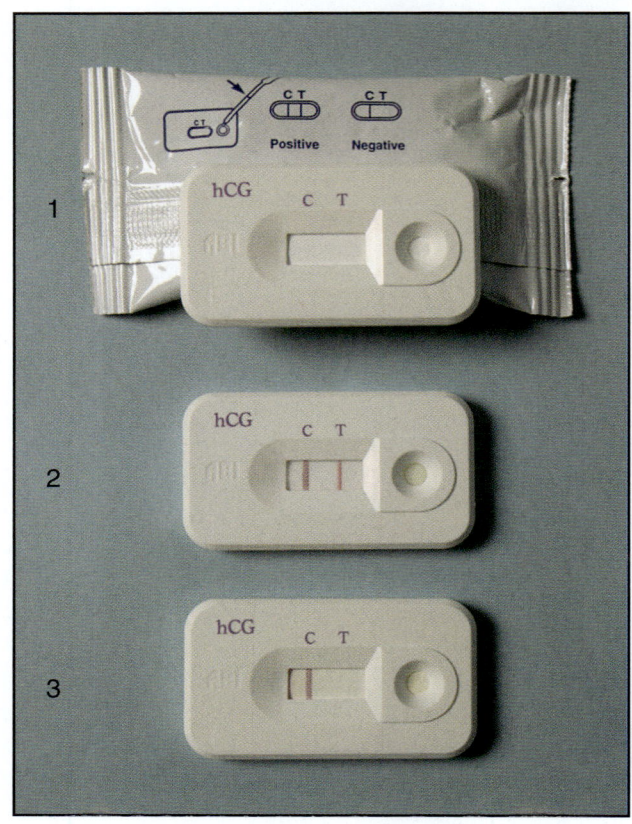

B. SureStep pregnancy test results. *1,* Test device before adding specimen (C: control; T: specimen travels through test area; well: holds specimen); *2,* positive reactions in test area and control area (two pink bands); *3,* negative reaction in test area and positive reaction in control area.

Follow-up—Postanalytical

- Properly dispose of biohazard waste material, and disinfect the work area.
- Remove personal protective equipment, and sanitize the hands.
- Chart results.

Quality Control Procedure

In addition to the internal control region built into the test device, external positive and negative liquid controls should be performed when a new kit is used. Also, each operator of the test should perform a positive and negative control once with each testing method to confirm that his or her testing technique is correct. The results of the control tests should be logged in the HCG control log.

The positive liquid control procedure is performed in the same way as the patient procedure, with a new pipette and testing device. Observe and record the results in 5 minutes. Repeat the procedure with a drop of well-mixed negative control.

CLIA-Waived Immunology Tests

PROCEDURE 7-2 QuickVue+ Mononucleosis Test Procedure

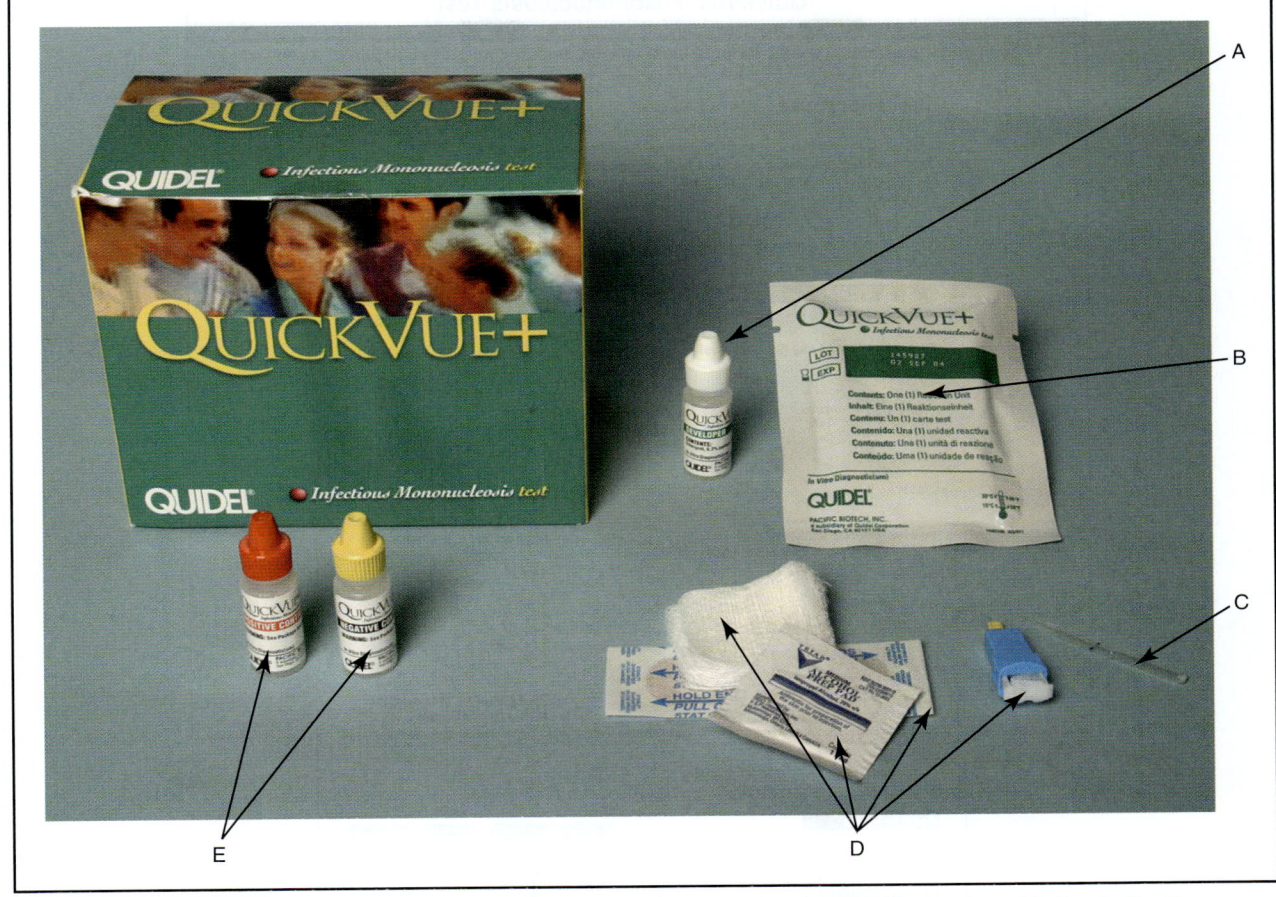

A. QuickVue+ infectious mononucleosis test kit. *a,* Developer; *b,* reaction unit; *c,* capillary tube with line indicating volume of blood; *d,* capillary puncture supplies; *e,* positive and negative liquid controls.

Equipment and Supplies (Fig. A)—Preanalytical

QuickVue+ mononucleosis test kit containing the following:
- Developer
- Individually wrapped reaction units
- Capillary tubes (for capillary specimens) and pipettes (for venous specimens)
- Capillary puncture supplies or venipuncture supplies
- Positive and negative liquid controls

The kit also includes the following:
- Instruction insert and pictorial flowchart (Fig. B)

Procedure—Analytical

1. Sanitize the hands, and apply gloves.
2. Remove the test device from its protective pouch, and label it with the patient's identification.
3. Draw a capillary sample to the line marked on the capillary tube (Fig. C).
   - If using whole blood from a venous specimen, use the pipette provided in the kit.
   - Use separate pipettes and devices for each specimen and the controls.
4. Dispense all the blood from the capillary tube into the "Add" well, or transfer a large drop from the venous whole blood specimen with the pipette.
5. Add 5 drops of developer to the "Add" well. Hold the bottle vertically above the well, and allow drops to fall freely.
6. Read the results at 5 minutes (Fig. D). The "Test Complete" line must be visible by 10 minutes.
7. Interpretation of results:
   - Positive result: A vertical line in any shade of blue forms a plus sign in the "Read Result" window along with a blue "Test Complete" line. Even a faint blue vertical line should be reported as a positive.

(Continued)

PROCEDURE 7-2 QuickVue+ Mononucleosis Test Procedure—cont'd

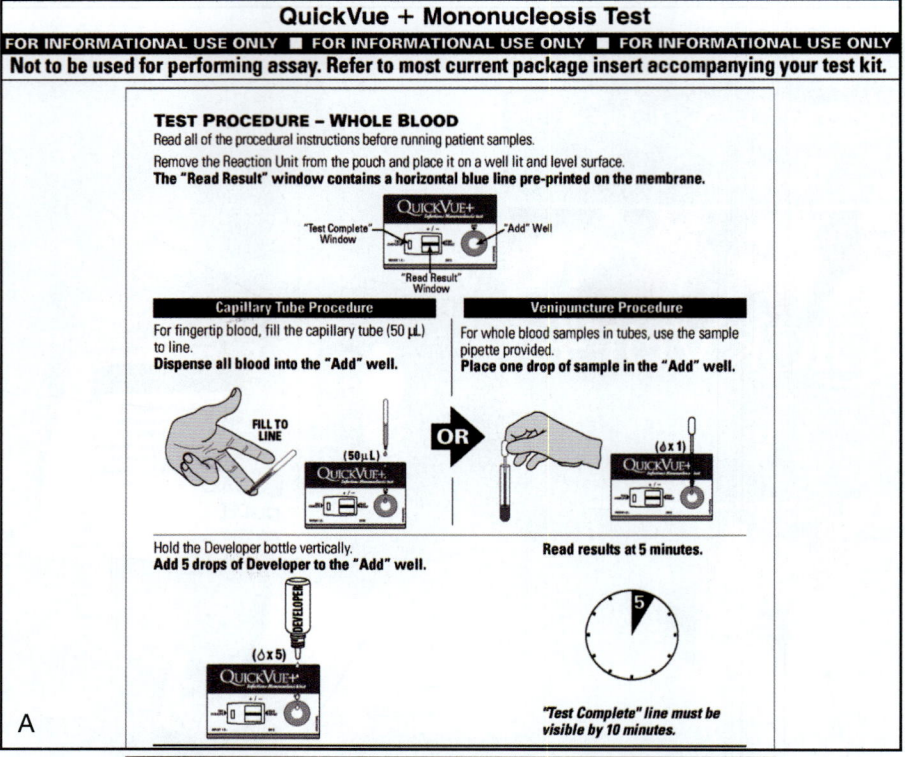

QuickVue + Mononucleosis Test

FOR INFORMATIONAL USE ONLY ■ FOR INFORMATIONAL USE ONLY ■ FOR INFORMATIONAL USE ONLY
Not to be used for performing assay. Refer to most current package insert accompanying your test kit.

TEST PROCEDURE – WHOLE BLOOD
Read all of the procedural instructions before running patient samples.
Remove the Reaction Unit from the pouch and place it on a well lit and level surface.
The "Read Result" window contains a horizontal blue line pre-printed on the membrane.

Capillary Tube Procedure
For fingertip blood, fill the capillary tube (50 μL) to line.
Dispense all blood into the "Add" well.

Venipuncture Procedure
For whole blood samples in tubes, use the sample pipette provided.
Place one drop of sample in the "Add" well.

Hold the Developer bottle vertically.
Add 5 drops of Developer to the "Add" well.

Read results at 5 minutes.

"Test Complete" line must be visible by 10 minutes.

A

INTERPRETATION OF RESULTS
FOR PATIENT SAMPLES, POSITIVE AND NEGATIVE CONTROLS

Positive Result
Any shade of a blue vertical line forming a (+) sign in the "Read Result" window along with the blue "Test Complete" line, is a positive result. **Even a faint blue vertical line should be reported as a positive.**

Negative Result
No blue vertical line in the "Read Result" window along with the blue "Test Complete" line, is a negative result.

Invalid Result
Test results are invalid:
■ If after 10 minutes no signal is observed in the "Test Complete" window. (View #1.)
■ If after 10 minutes a blue color fills the "Read Result" window. (View #2.)

An invalid result indicates either the test was not performed correctly or the reagents are not working properly.

Should an invalid result occur, re-test the sample using a new Reaction Unit.

If the problem continues, contact Technical Support toll-free in the U.S. at (800) 874-1517. Outside the USA, contact your local representative.

LIMITATIONS
1. As is the case of any other diagnostic procedure, the results obtained by this kit yield data that must be used in addition to other information available to the physician.
2. QuickVue+ Infectious Mononucleosis test is a qualitative test for the detection of IM heterophile antibodies.
3. A negative result may be obtained from patients at the onset of the disease due to antibody concentration below the sensitivity of this test kit. If symptoms persist or increase in intensity, the test should be repeated.
4. Some segments of the population who contract Infectious Mononucleosis do not produce measurable levels of heterophile antibodies. Approximately 50% of children under 4 years of age who have IM may test as IM heterophile antibody negative.[4]

B

B. Instructions for QuickVue+ mononucleosis test from package insert. (From Bonewit-West K: *Clinical procedures for medical assistants*, ed 7, St Louis, 2008, Saunders.)

PROCEDURE 7-2 QuickVue+ Mononucleosis Test Procedure—cont'd

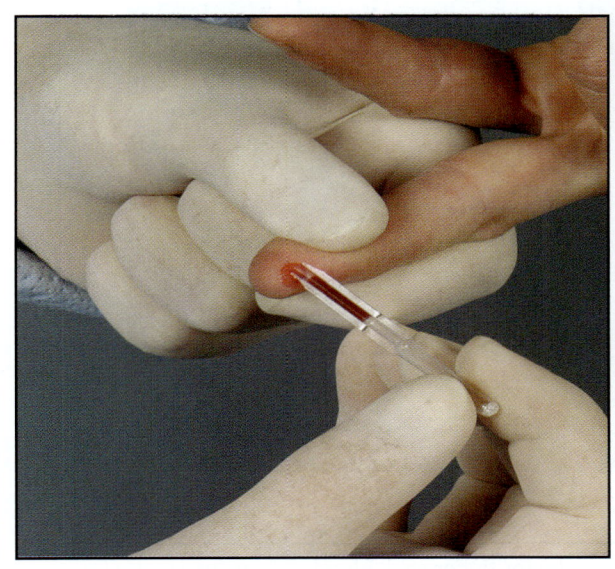

C. Collecting capillary blood to the black line on the disposable capillary tube.

- Negative result: No blue vertical line appears, leaving a minus sign in the "Read Result" window along with a blue "Test Complete" line.
- Invalid result: After 10 minutes, no line is observed in the "Test Complete" window, or a blue color fills the "Read Result" window. If either of these occurs, the test must be repeated with a new reaction unit. If the problem continues, request technical support.

Follow-up—Postanalytical

- Properly dispose of biohazard waste material, and disinfect the work area.
- Remove personal protective equipment, and sanitize the hands.

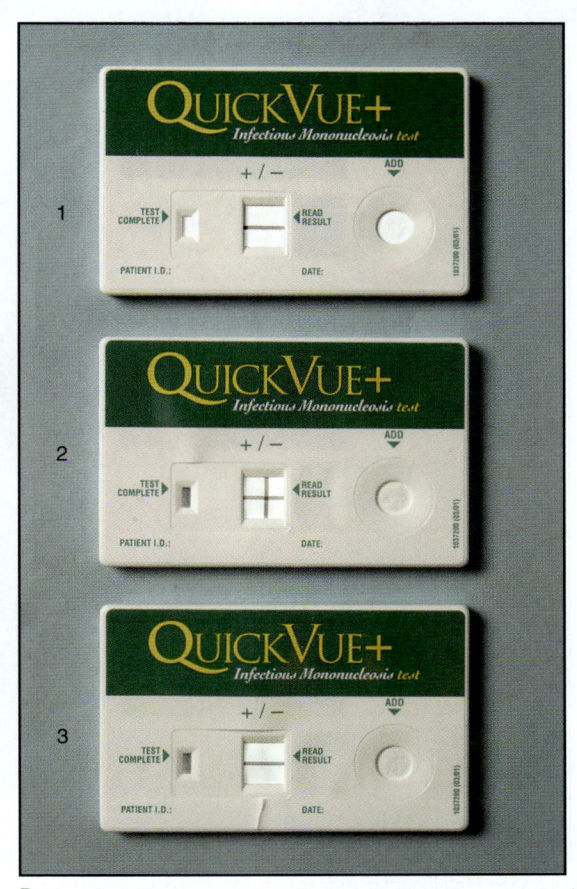

D. Results of mononucleosis test. *1*, Reaction unit before testing; *2*, positive result and "test complete" result; *3*, negative result and "test complete" result.

Quality Control Procedures

The internal control occurs in the "Test Complete" window built into each reaction unit. External positive and negative liquid controls are provided with each new kit. Each operator of the test should perform a positive and negative control once to confirm that his or her testing technique is correct and log the control results in the control log. External controls should also be tested and logged when a new kit is used.

PROCEDURE 7-3 QuickVue *Helicobacter pylori* gII Test (CLIA-Waived) Procedure

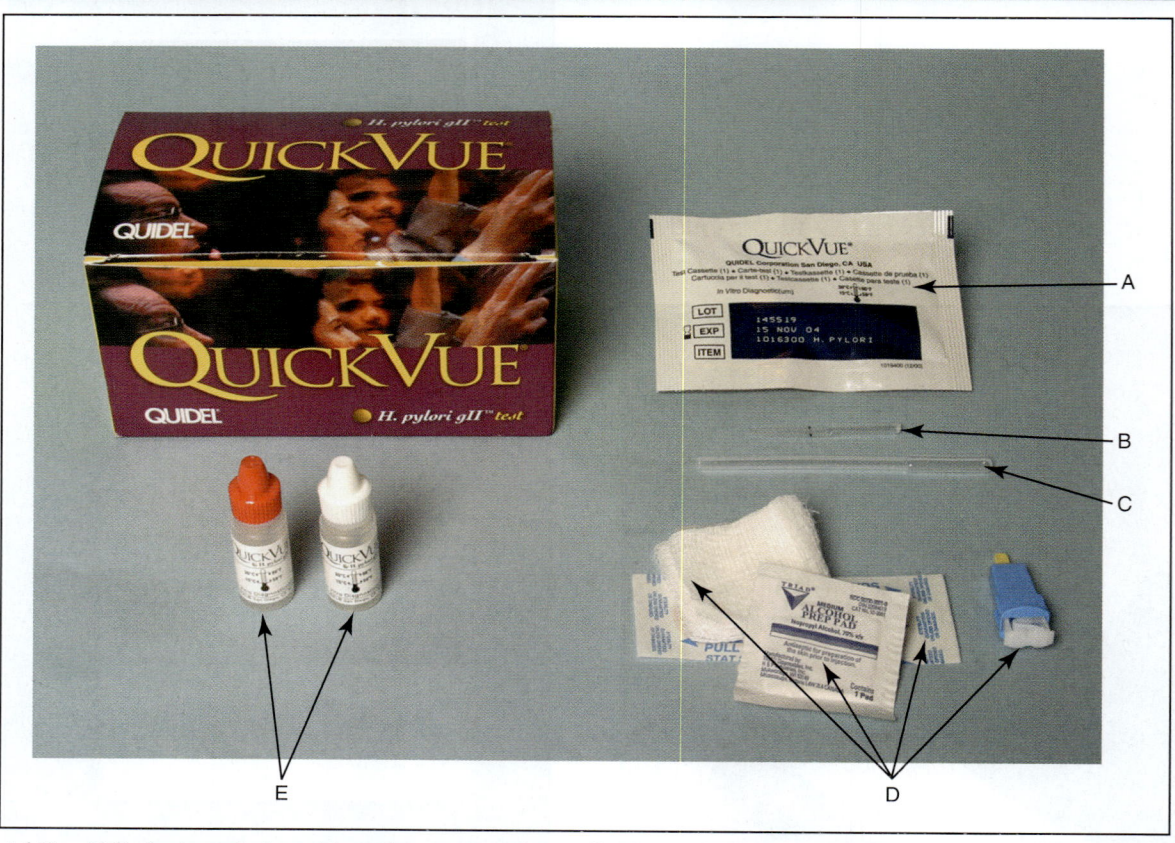

A. QuickVue *Helicobacter pylori* test kit. *a*, Test cassette; *b*, capillary tube for finger stick blood; *c*, transfer pipette for venous blood; *d*, capillary puncture supplies; *e*, liquid controls (external).

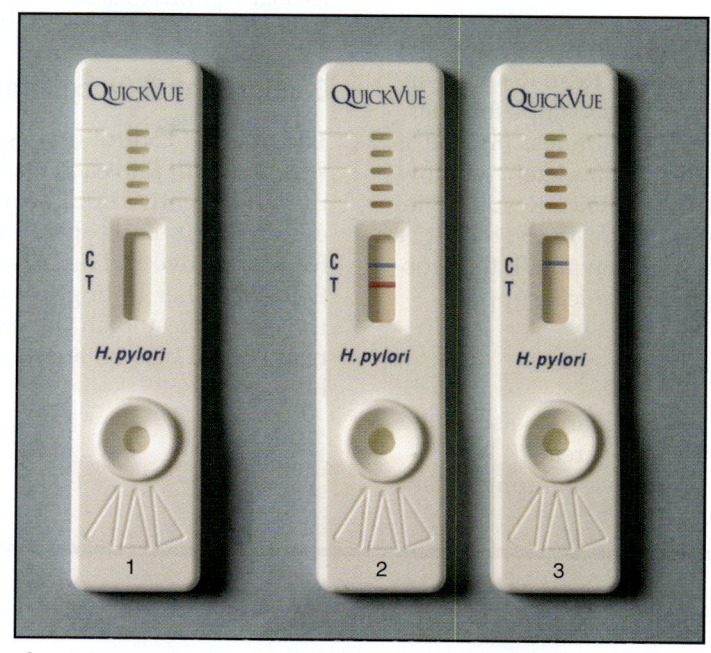

B. *Helicobacter pylori* test results. *1*, Test cassette before adding specimen; *2*, positive result: pink band in test area and blue internal control band; *3*, negative result: no band in test area and blue internal control band.

Advanced Concepts 225

PROCEDURE 7-3 QuickVue *Helicobacter pylori* gII Test (CLIA-Waived) Procedure—cont'd

Equipment and Supplies (Fig. A)—Preanalytical

- Foil-wrapped test cassette
- Capillary tube for finger stick blood
- Transfer pipette for venous blood
- Capillary puncture supplies
- Positive and negative external liquid controls
- Gloves and OSHA disposal equipment (not pictured)

Procedure—Analytical

1. Sanitize the hands, and apply gloves.
2. Add 1 drop of venous whole blood (using disposable dropper in the kit), 1 capillary tube (from kit) of whole blood from a finger stick (see Procedure 7-2), or 2 hanging drops of whole blood from a finger stick to the round sample well on the test cassette.
3. Do not move the test cassette until the assay is complete. Read and record the results of the test after 10 minutes or less (Fig. B).
   - Positive result: A pink line appears next to the letter T and a blue line next to the letter C.
- Negative result: Only a blue line forms next to the letter C. The blue line is the internal control indicating that the capillary flow occurred and the functional integrity of the strip was maintained. If the blue line does not show, the test results are invalid and should not be reported.
3. Discard all the test materials in the appropriate biohazard containers.
4. Remove and discard gloves in the biohazard container, sanitize the hands, and chart the results.

Follow-up—Postanalytical

- Properly dispose of biohazard waste material, and disinfect the work area.
- Remove personal protective equipment, and sanitize the hands.

Quality Control Procedure

The external positive and negative controls should be performed when a new kit is used and with each new operator of the test method. The procedure is done by adding 2 drops of the positive control to a test well and reading and recording the results after 5 minutes. The same procedure is done with the negative control.

ADVANCED CONCEPTS

Agglutination Reactions (Non–CLIA-Waived Tests)

Agglutination is the visible clumping together of blood cells or other particulate matter, such as latex beads. Agglutination is caused by antibodies adhering to their antigens. This type of antibody is referred to as an *agglutinin*. An antibody/antigen reaction produces a visible, latticelike network of cells or beads that have agglutinated and fallen out of solution. The agglutination reaction can be seen on a slide or in a test tube and becomes visible to the naked eye as the slide or tube is tilted or centrifuged. Agglutination reactions require interpretation that is beyond the scope of CLIA-waived testing. They are therefore usually performed in hospital and reference laboratories.

The most common antibody/antigen reactions are seen in immunohematology laboratories (also referred to as *blood banks*). Immunohematology uses agglutination testing to determine blood types for transfusions, paternity determinations, mother/baby blood compatibility, and forensic investigations.

ABO Blood Typing

The reasons for determining blood type are to provide safe blood transfusions, to prevent hemolytic disease in the newborn, to identify parentage, and for forensic (criminal) reasons. More than 300 types of inherited blood antigens are found on RBCs. The ABO and Rh blood types are most important because of their intense antigenic responses when transfused or transmitted into incompatible recipients.

Karl Landsteiner discovered the ABO blood groups in the early 1900s. He determined that two inherited antigens are present on the surface of RBCs: A and B. The presence or absence of each antigen produces the four blood types: A, B, AB, and O. Landsteiner also determined that individuals produce a natural antibody against any antigen absent on their RBC surface. Therefore a type A person has A antigens on his or her RBCs and produces anti-B antibodies in the plasma. A type B person has B antigens on

TABLE 7-2 Summary of ABO Blood Types

Blood Type	Antigens on Cells	Antibodies in Plasma	Transfusion Compatibility
A	A antigens	Anti-B antibodies	Can receive A or O
B	B antigens	Anti-A antibodies	Can receive B or O
AB	A and B antigens	No antibodies	Can receive A, B, AB and O Universal recipient
O	No antigens	Anti-A and anti-B	Can receive only O Universal donor

his or her RBCs and anti-A antibodies in the plasma. A type AB person has both A and B antigens on his or her RBCs and no antibodies in the plasma. A type O person has neither A nor B antigens on his or her RBCs and has both anti-A and anti-B antibodies in the plasma. Table 7-2 provides a summary of these characteristics.

In the immunohematology department, agglutination testing is performed to determine blood types and the compatibility between a donor's blood and a recipient's. If a blood antigen comes in contact with its corresponding antibody, the result is agglutination (clumping) of the RBCs, which eventually leads to hemolysis (breakdown) of the RBCs. These dangerous reactions occur when the wrong type of blood is administered to a patient during a blood transfusion. For example, if a type A person is given type B blood, the recipient's blood, containing anti-B antibodies, would agglutinate the donor's RBCs containing the B antigen. The clumped RBCs would be unable to pass through the kidneys, which might lead to kidney failure. The universal donor is type O because *no antigens* are present on the donor's RBCs, and the universal recipient is AB because *no antibodies* are present in the recipient's plasma.

An **ABO Blood Typing Test** procedure check sheet is provided in the workbook and is demonstrated in Procedure 7-4, located at the end of this section.

Rh System

The Rh or D antigen is also found on the surface of RBCs. A person with the Rh antigen is referred to as *Rh positive*. In the United States 85% of the population is Rh positive. An individual who does not have the Rh antigen is referred to as *Rh negative*. An Rh-negative person has no naturally occurring anti-D antibodies. However, anti-D antibody production may be induced *after* an Rh-negative person is mistakenly transfused with Rh-positive blood or after an Rh-negative mother has carried an Rh-positive baby. In both cases the Rh-positive cells have a strong antigenic effect in the Rh-negative recipient. The Rh negative recipient starts producing anti-Rh antibodies against Rh positive cells.

An **Rh Blood Typing Test** procedure check sheet is provided in the workbook and is demonstrated in Procedure 7-5, located at the end of this section.

Hemolytic Disease of the Newborn and RhoGAM

Hemolytic disease of the newborn (HDN), or **erythroblastosis fetalis,** is a hemolytic anemia in newborns resulting from maternal–fetal blood group incompatibility. Fig. 7-8 illustrates the way an Rh-negative mother becomes sensitized to her first baby's Rh-positive blood cells after delivery. Subsequent pregnancies with Rh-positive babies activate the anti-Rh antibody response. The anti-Rh antibodies cause the destruction of the baby's RBCs. The clinical manifestations in the Rh-positive newborn include severe anemia, jaundice, and enlargement of the liver and spleen. These can lead to cardiac failure, respiratory distress, and death.

HDN can be prevented by the injection of anti-Rh gamma globulin (RhoGAM) during and after the pregnancy of an Rh-negative mother. RhoGAM prevents the mother from becoming sensitized to the Rh antigen.

Enzyme-Linked Immunosorbent Assay: Quantitative Analysis

The term **immunosorbent** pertains to the attachment of an antigen or antibody to a solid surface such as latex beads, wells in plastic dishes, or plastic cartridges (devices capable of absorbing the antigen or antibody). In the ELISA method, an antigen is fixed to a well in a plastic dish. A serum specimen is added to the well to test for a particular antibody. The well is then rinsed to remove anything that did not bind. Next, an enzyme/antibody complex is added that will further bind to the human antibody if present, and the well is rinsed again to remove any enzyme/antibody that was not bound. The final step uses an enzyme color developer that reacts with the enzyme, if present, and produces a color change. If the serum contained the antibody specific to the antigen, a color change occurs. The more antibody is present, the

Advanced Concepts

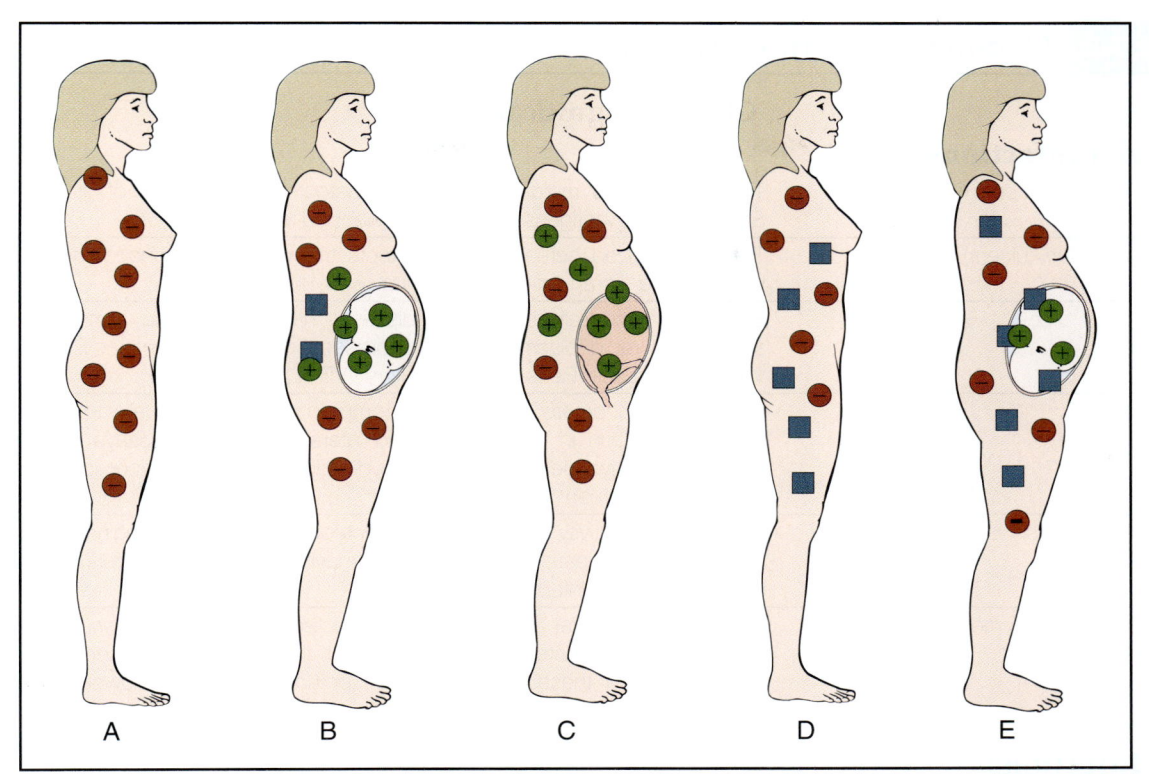

Fig. 7-8. Hemolytic disease of the newborn in the second pregnancy of an Rh-negative mother carrying two Rh-positive babies. **A,** Rh-negative woman before first pregnancy, with Rh-negative red blood cells (RBCs) and no anti-Rh antibodies. **B,** First baby with Rh-positive RBCs begins to sensitize mother in utero, causing the production of anti-Rh antibodies *(blue squares)*. **C,** After birth, more Rh-positive cells enter the mother's bloodstream. **D,** Rh-negative mother reacts, producing more anti-Rh antibodies *(blue squares)*. **E,** Second baby's Rh-positive RBCs are hemolyzed by the mother's antibodies *(blue squares)*. (From Stepp CA, Woods M: *Laboratory procedures for medical office personnel*, Philadelphia, 1998, Saunders.)

darker the color produced. This quantitative method of indirectly measuring antibodies is non–CLIA waived and is performed in reference and hospital laboratories. NOTE: This is the method of in vitro testing used in allergy testing.

Antibody Titers

Reference and hospital laboratories perform both agglutination and ELISA tests with moderately complex equipment to determine the quantity of antibodies in question. Another quantitative method to determine the amount of a specific antibody in the blood is the **titer** (a quantitative test that measures the amount of antibody that reacts with a specific antigen). Quantitative antibody information can provide the physician with additional information regarding the extent of acquired immunity. For example, a physician might order a series of Rh titers to measure the number of anti-Rh antibodies in an Rh-negative pregnant woman's serum. The Rh antibody titers could then be used to monitor the degree of sensitivity the mother might develop against her Rh-positive baby's cells during the pregnancy. If the titer rises, she has an immunity built up against the baby's Rh-positive cells and appropriate measures to protect the baby must be taken.

Summary of Immunological Tests

The ability to detect specific antibodies and antigens associated with disease has made immunology a rapidly growing biomedical science. Table 7-3 describes CLIA-waived and non–CLIA-waived immunology tests commonly ordered for diagnosing bacterial, viral, and other immune-related disorders.

TABLE 7-3 Common Immunology Tests

Tests	Clinical Significance
Bacterial Infections	
Group A *Streptococcus* (strep throat, fever)	The CLIA-waived rapid screening test detects the presence of group A *Streptococcus* antigens in a throat-swabbed specimen.
Helicobacter pylori (ulcers)	The CLIA-waived screening test detects the antibodies specific for *H. pylori* in the blood of an infected individual with ulcers.
Syphilis	Syphilis is a sexually transmitted disease. Three immunology tests for syphilis are rapid plasmin reagin, fluorescent treponemal antibody, and the Venereal Disease Research Laboratory (VDRL) test.
Chlamydia	*Chlamydia trachomatis* is the most common cause of sexually transmitted venereal infection in the world. Rapid lateral flow immunoassays are available for the qualitative detection of chlamydia directly from endocervical swab and cytology brush specimens.
Gardnerella vaginalis (vaginal infection)	This enzyme activity test is used to detect *G. vaginalis* in vaginal fluid specimens from patients suspected of having bacterial vaginosis, the most common vaginal infection.
Borrelia burgdorferi (Lyme disease)	Lyme disease is transmitted by ticks infected with *B. burgdorferi*. The immunology tests used are either the ELISA or the indirect fluorescent antibody test. If either of these tests is positive or uncertain, it is followed by the Western immunoblot.
Viral Infections	
Respiratory syncytial virus (RSV)	RSV is a highly contagious virus that causes acute respiratory illness. It is the most important cause of bronchiolitis and pneumonia in infants.
Epstein–Barr virus (EBV) (mononucleosis)	The CLIA-waived mononucleosis test detects the heterophile antibody associated with EBV infections.
Influenza A and B	The CLIA-waived rapid screening test detects the presence of influenza A and B in nasal-swabbed or nasal wash specimens.
HIV/AIDS	The CLIA-waived test detects antibodies in blood or oral cells that are specific for HIV-1.
Rubella (German measles)	The test is given to evaluate whether a woman is immune to rubella (as a result of childhood exposure or immunization) or presently infected with the disease. If a woman is not immune and becomes infected during pregnancy, the rubella virus could cause birth defects in the fetus.
Hepatitis C (bloodborne pathogen)	The "silent killer," hepatitis C is a growing public health concern. An at-home test provides a confidential hepatitis C result.
Varicella zoster (chickenpox and shingles)	Immunofluorescence is a diagnostic technique used to identify antibodies to a specific virus. In the case of herpes zoster, ultraviolet rays are applied to a preparation composed of cells taken from the herpes blisters. The specific characteristics of the ultraviolet light as seen through a microscope identify the presence of the antibodies. This test is less expensive and more accurate than a culture, and the results are faster.
Other Antigenic Substances	
HCG hormone (pregnancy test)	HCG is produced by the placenta during pregnancy.
CA 125 (ovarian cancer)	This test detects the ovarian cancer antigen.
Prostate-specific antigen (PSA) (prostate cancer)	The PSA and percent-free PSA blood tests aid in the detection and treatment of prostate cancer.
Bladder tumor–associated antigen (BTA)	The BTA stat test was the first tumor marker test to be placed in the CLIA-waived category by the Centers for Disease Control and Prevention. The test detects BTA in the urine of persons being monitored for recurrent bladder cancer.

Advanced Concepts

TABLE 7-3	Common Immunology Tests—cont'd
Tests	**Clinical Significance**
Rheumatoid factor (arthritis)	Rheumatoid arthritis is a chronic inflammatory disease that affects the connective tissue of the body and leads to crippling deformities. Most patients with this disease develop an antibody called *rheumatoid factor* that can be detected immunologically.
Fecal occult blood (screening for colon cancer)	The iFOB test is highly sensitive to blood on the feces. If positive, the patient will be evaluated as to what is causing the bleeding in the colon.

ELISA, Enzyme-linked immunosorbent assay; *HIV*, human immunodeficiency virus; *AIDS*, acquired immune-deficiency syndrome.

PROCEDURE 7-4 Agglutination Slide Testing Procedure for ABO Blood Typing

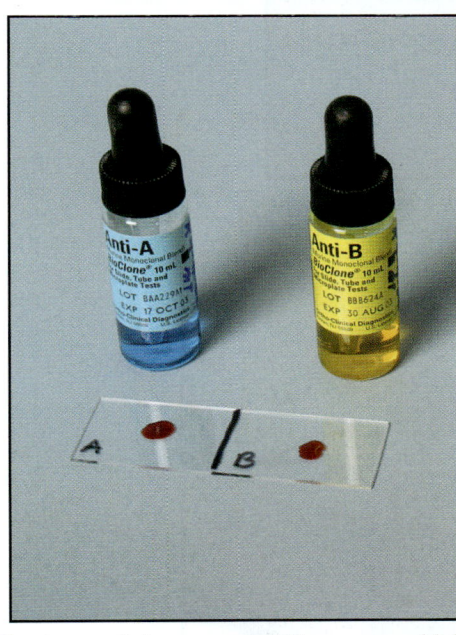

A. ABO setup: anti-A serum, anti-B serum, and labeled slide with drops of blood.

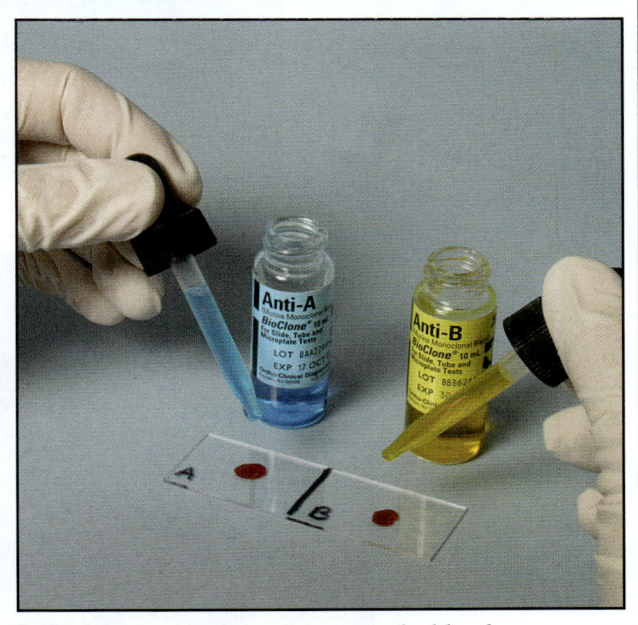

B. Add a drop of each antiserum to the blood.

Equipment and Supplies—Preanalytical

- Anti-A serum (blue bottle)
- Anti-B serum (yellow bottle)
- Slide marked A on the left and B on the right
- Wooden applicator sticks
- Capillary puncture supplies (lancet, alcohol, gauze, bandage)
- Personal protective equipment (gloves, gown, face shield or free standing shield)
- Biohazard sharps containers

Procedure—Analytical

1. Sanitize the hands, and apply gloves.
2. Place 2 drops of whole blood from a capillary puncture or an anticoagulated venous blood specimen on the slide: 1 drop on the left "A" side and the other drop on the "B" side (Fig. A).
3. Place a drop of anti-A serum on the blood on the left side and a drop of anti-B serum on the blood on the right (Fig. B). Do not allow the droppers to touch the blood because the blood cells will contaminate the antisera.

(Continued)

PROCEDURE 7-4 Agglutination Slide Testing Procedure for ABO Blood Typing—cont'd

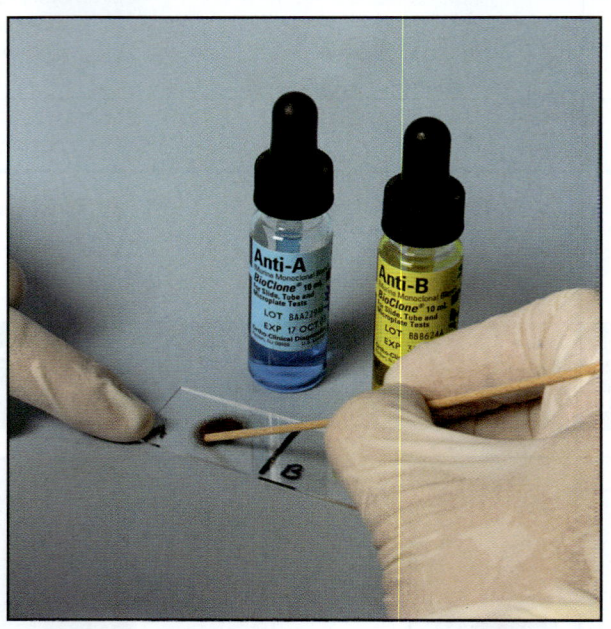

C. Mix the blood and anti-A with a wooden applicator stick.

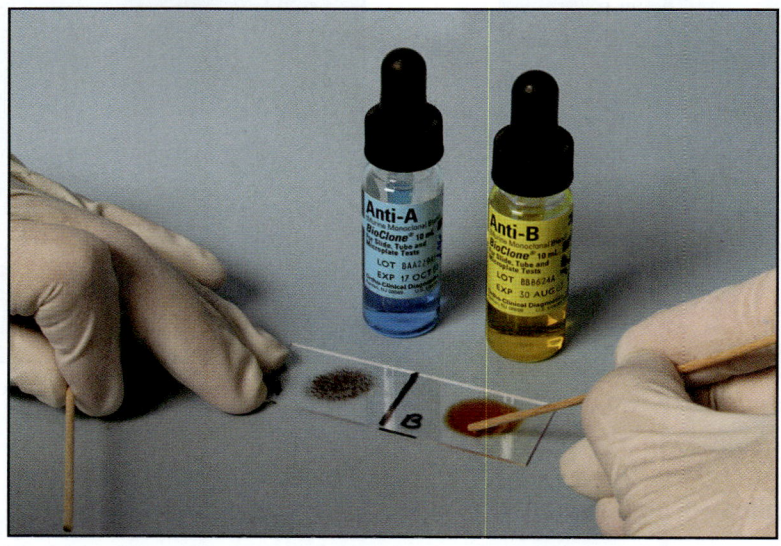

D. Mix the blood and anti-B with another wooden stick. The cells mixed with anti-A have agglutinated, whereas the cells mixed with anti-B have not.

4. Stir each side with its own wooden applicator stick until thoroughly mixed (Fig. C). Tilt the slide to see whether the cells agglutinate.
5. Results can be read immediately at room temperature. In Fig. D agglutination can be seen on the left anti-A side and no agglutination on the right anti-B side. Fig. E lists all the possible ABO blood type reactions. What blood type is the blood in Fig. E?

Follow-up—Postanalytical

- Properly dispose of biohazard waste material, and disinfect the work area.
- Remove personal protective equipment, and sanitize the hands.

Advanced Concepts

PROCEDURE 7-4 Agglutination Slide Testing Procedure for ABO Blood Typing—cont'd

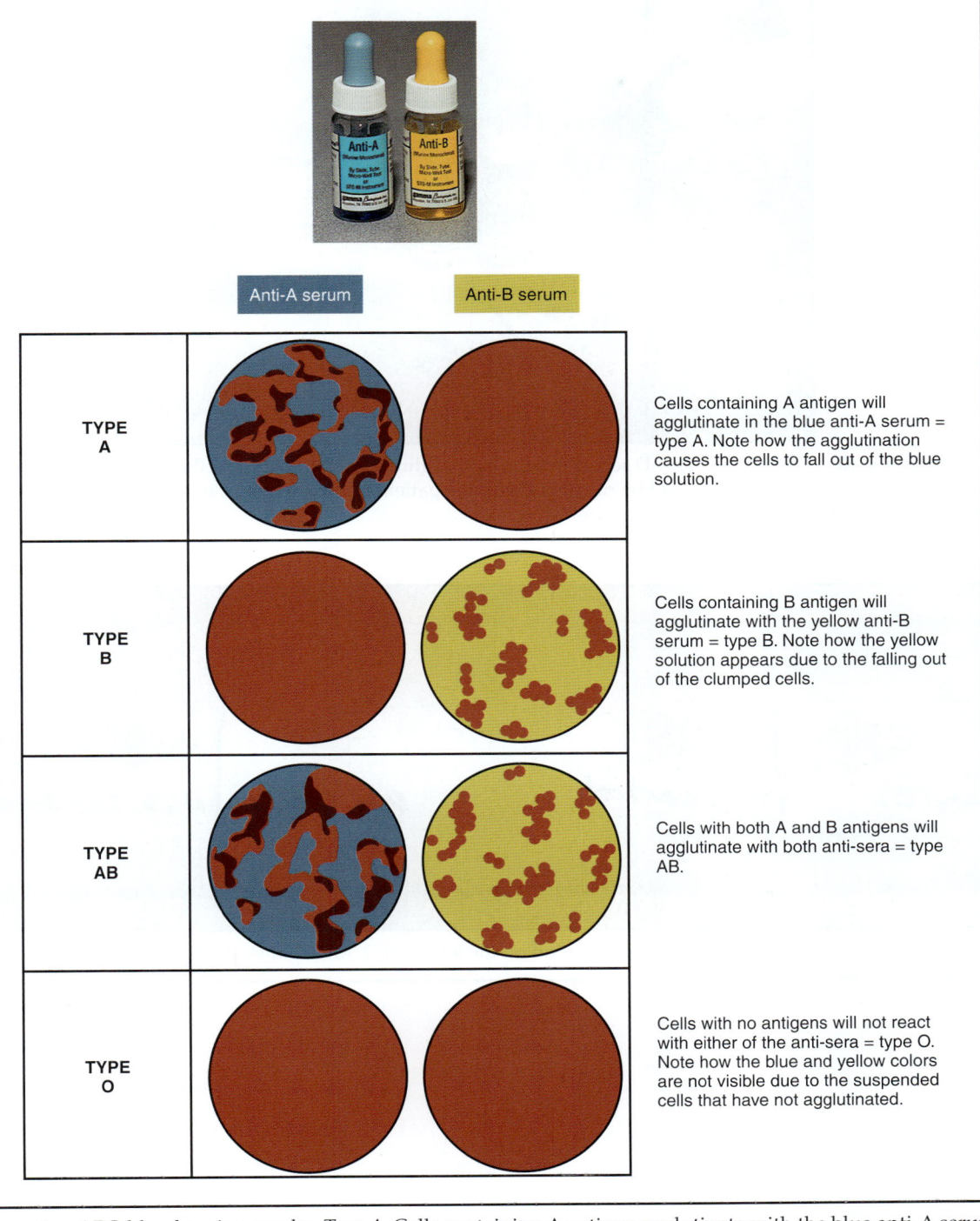

	Anti-A serum	Anti-B serum	
TYPE A	agglutinated	no reaction	Cells containing A antigen will agglutinate in the blue anti-A serum = type A. Note how the agglutination causes the cells to fall out of the blue solution.
TYPE B	no reaction	agglutinated	Cells containing B antigen will agglutinate with the yellow anti-B serum = type B. Note how the yellow solution appears due to the falling out of the clumped cells.
TYPE AB	agglutinated	agglutinated	Cells with both A and B antigens will agglutinate with both anti-sera = type AB.
TYPE O	no reaction	no reaction	Cells with no antigens will not react with either of the anti-sera = type O. Note how the blue and yellow colors are not visible due to the suspended cells that have not agglutinated.

E, Interpreting ABO blood typing results. *Type A,* Cells containing A antigen agglutinate with the blue anti-A serum. Agglutination causes the cells to fall out of the blue solution. *Type B,* Cells containing B antigen agglutinate with the yellow anti-B serum. The yellow solution appears because of the falling out of the clumped cells. *Type AB,* Cells with both A and B antigens agglutinate with both antisera. *Type O,* Cells with no antigens do not react with either antiserum. The blue and yellow are not visible because of the suspended cells that have not agglutinated. (From Stepp CA, Woods M: *Laboratory procedures for medical office personnel,* Philadelphia, 1998, Saunders.)

PROCEDURE 7-5 Rh Blood Typing Procedure by the Slide Method

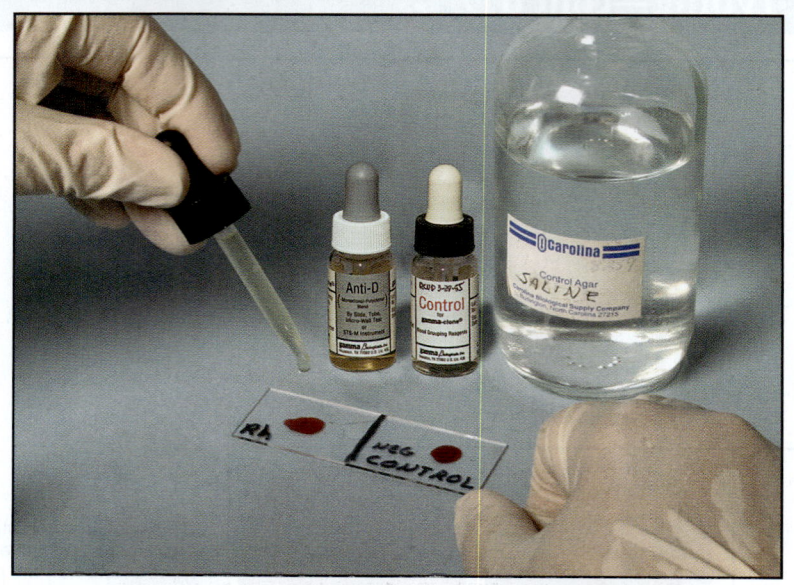

A. Rh blood typing. Rh slide test uses anti-D serum *(left)*, which agglutinates Rh-positive cells when warmed for 2 minutes. An Rh-negative control *(right)* should be run along with the patient's specimen to rule out false-positive reactions. NOTE: Saline may also be used as a negative control.

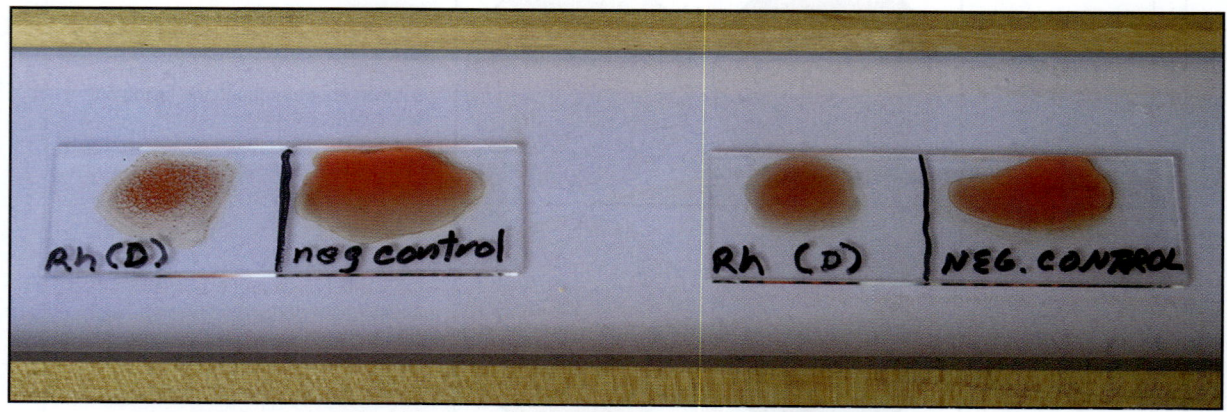

B. Rh blood typing results. *1*, Rh positive (agglutination on the left side); *2*, Rh negative (no agglutination on either side).

Advanced Concepts

PROCEDURE 7-5 Rh Blood Typing Procedure by the Slide Method—cont'd

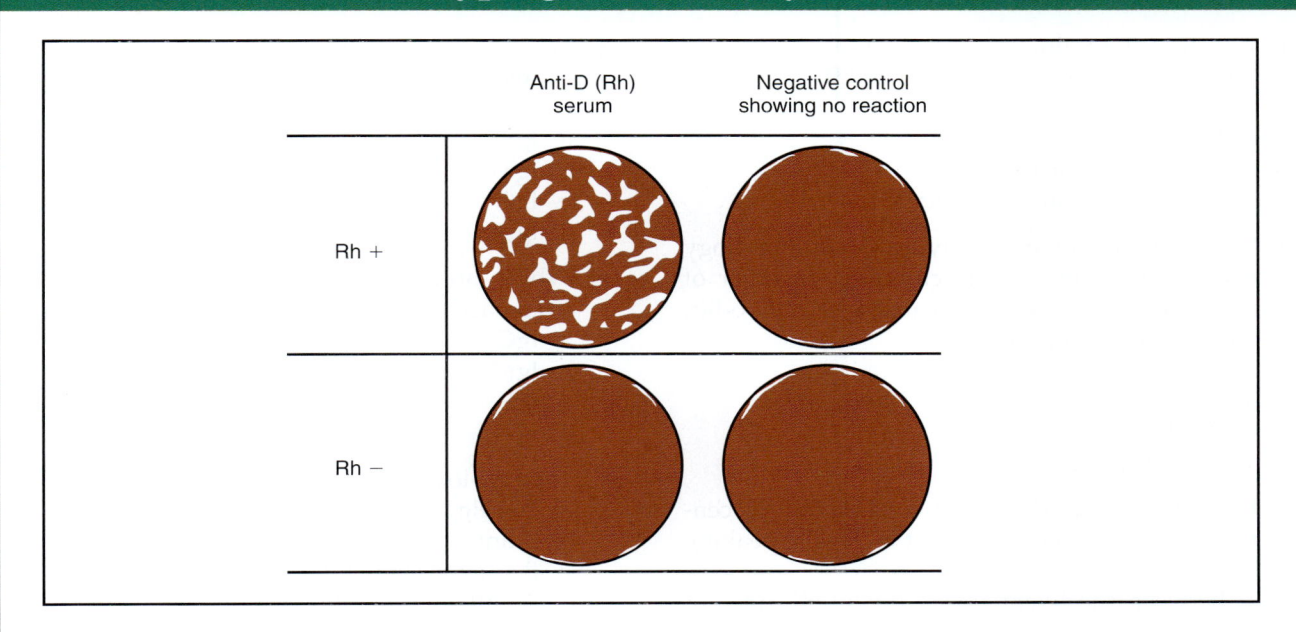

	Anti-D (Rh) serum	Negative control showing no reaction
Rh +	(agglutination)	(no reaction)
Rh −	(no reaction)	(no reaction)

Equipment and Supplies—Preanalytical

- Anti-D serum
- Negative control serum
- Slide marked with "Rh" or "D" on the left and "Control" on the right
- Slide warmer
- Wooden applicator sticks
- Capillary puncture supplies (lancet, alcohol, gauze, bandage)
- Personal protective equipment (gloves, gown, face or workstation shield)
- Biohazard sharps containers

Procedure—Analytical

1. Sanitize the hands, and apply gloves.
2. Place a drop of blood on each side of the labeled slide.
3. Add the anti-D serum and negative controls on each drop of blood, and mix thoroughly with the wooden applicators (Fig. A).
4. Heat and tilt the slide for 2 minutes. A strong Rh positive will agglutinate immediately, whereas a weak Rh positive may take the entire 2 minutes on a heated surface to demonstrate the antibody/antigen agglutination reaction. Therefore watch carefully while tilting the heated slide back and forth to see if and when the cells begin to clump. If the cells do not clump and demonstrate the same reaction as the negative control after 2 minutes, the blood is identified as Rh negative. If agglutination (clumping) occurs, the blood is identified as Rh positive.

Fig. B shows the two possible Rh reactions: agglutination on the left, indicating an Rh positive result, and no agglutination on the right, indicating an Rh negative result.

Follow-up—Postanalytical

- Properly dispose of biohazard waste material, and disinfect the work area.
- Remove personal protective equipment, and sanitize the hands.

Review Questions

1. Which of the following is the causative agent of infectious mononucleosis?
   a. Variola major
   b. Epstein–Barr virus
   c. Cytomegalovirus
   d. Human immunodeficiency virus

2. Which of the following types of immunology tests involves the visible clumping together of blood cells or latex beads caused by antibodies adhering to their antigens?
   a. Titer
   b. EIA
   c. Agglutination
   d. All the above

3. HCG is produced by the developing placenta during pregnancy with the levels peaking _____.
   a. between the twentieth and eightieth days of pregnancy
   b. between the thirtieth and seventieth days of pregnancy
   c. between the tenth and sixtieth days of pregnancy
   d. between the fiftieth and eightieth days of pregnancy

4. Which of the following cells differentiate into plasma cells and memory cells, with the subsequent production of antibodies produced by the plasma cells?
   a. B cells
   b. T cells
   c. Natural killer cells
   d. All the above

5. Which of the following nonspecific immunity mechanisms involves the process of certain cells engulfing and destroying microorganisms and cellular debris?
   a. Normal flora
   b. Phagocytosis
   c. Intact skin and mucous membranes
   d. Inflammation

6. Which two of the five types of antibodies are elevated in acute allergic reactions and subsequent encounters?
   a. IgE
   b. IgM
   c. IgG
   d. IgA

7. Which antibody protects mucous membranes from bacterial and virus infections?
   a. IgG
   b. IgM
   c. IgE
   d. IgA

8. Type A blood consists of _____.
   a. B antigens and anti-B antibodies
   b. A antigens and anti-B antibodies
   c. B antigens and anti-A antibodies
   d. A antigens and anti-A antibodies

9. Which of the following pregnancy scenarios could be a problem for the baby?
   a. mother Rh positive and fetus Rh positive
   b. mother Rh negative and fetus Rh negative
   c. mother Rh positive and fetus Rh negative
   d. mother Rh negative and fetus Rh positive

10. Name the antigens present in a B-positive individual.

Advanced Concepts

Answers to Review Questions

1. b
2. c
3. d
4. a
5. b
6. a and c
7. d
8. b
9. d
10. B and Rh antigens

Websites

The National Primary Immunodeficiency Resource Center (NPI) is the central resource and clearinghouse on primary immunodeficiency, serving researchers, scientists, physicians, government, industry, patients, and their families. Click "related links" on the home page for access to additional sites related to the immune system and immunology:
www.info4pi.org/index.cfm?CFID=8903943&;CFTOKEN=22787603

Link to laboratory that performs IgA, IgG, and IgE testing for food and inhalant allergies:
www.usbiotek.com

Quidel-sponsored video on how to perform and read Quidel's CLIA-waived influenza test:
www.flutest.com/flu-facts/animation2b.htm

Links to all Quidel point-of-care test kits, including chlamydia, streptococcus A, *H. pylori* gII, influenza A and B, OneStep HCG urine, and infectious mononucleosis:
http://www.quidel.com/products/

Links to the Applied Biotech line of point-of-care products for testing for infectious diseases (mononucleosis, streptococcus, and *H. pylori*), pregnancy, and drug abuse:
http://www.invernessmedicalpd.com/point_of_care.aspx

Links to all Thermo BioStar kits for waived and moderately complex testing. The waived tests available are for HCG, streptococcus A, and mononucleosis:
www.pointofcare.net/vendors/thermobiostar.htm

Primary Care rapid diagnostic test products available from Becton Coulter:
www.beckman.com/products/discipline/Clinical_Diagnostics/eli.html

Information on iFOB testing:
http://www.quidel.com/assets/swf/iFOBTrainingvideoHQ.htm

Videos on T-cells:
http://video.google.com/videosearch?q=t-cells&oe=utf-8&rls=org.mozilla:en-US:official&client=firefox-a&um=1&ie=UTF-8&ei=QAmuSuqdMY22sgOKk-WKBQ&sa=X&oi=video_result_group&ct=title&;resnum=14#

CHAPTER 8

Microbiology

Objectives
After completing this chapter you should be able to:

Fundamental Concepts
1. Classify microorganisms into the categories of virus, bacteria, fungi, and parasites, and describe the general characteristics of each category.
2. Perform a throat swab specimen collection according to the stated task, conditions, and standards listed in the Learning Outcome Evaluation in the student workbook.
3. Describe the proper collection and transportation procedures for microbiological specimens.
4. Explain the importance of Gram staining in microbiology.
5. Prepare and perform a Gram stain on a bacterial smear according to the stated task, conditions, and standards listed in the Learning Outcome Evaluation in the student workbook.
6. Recognize gram-positive and gram-negative bacteria, and describe their morphological characteristics.
7. Describe the procedures for acid-fast stains, wet mounts, and KOH preparation.
8. Explain the cellulose tape procedure for the identification of pinworms.

CLIA-Waived Microbiology Tests
1. Describe the diseases caused by group A Streptococci.
2. Perform a rapid group A Streptococcus test and a rapid influenza A and B test according to the stated task, conditions, and standards listed in the Learning Outcome Evaluation in the student workbook.

Advanced Concepts
1. List and describe the types of culture media and their uses.
2. Identify the large equipment, inoculating equipment, and incinerating equipment used in microbiology laboratories.
3. Discuss culture plate streaking methods for colony isolation and colony counting.
4. Explain the function of sensitivity testing.
5. List pathogenic bacteria, fungi, and parasites frequently seen in the physician's office laboratory.
6. List some of the emerging infectious diseases.
7. Discuss some of the organisms that could be used in bioterrorism.

Key Terms

aerobic requiring oxygen for growth
aerosols fine particles suspended in air
agar gelatinous substance obtained from seaweed that is liquid when heated and becomes solid when cooled; used in culture media
anaerobic able to grow and function in the absence of oxygen
binary fission asexual reproduction in which the cell splits in half
capnophilic requiring some carbon dioxide to grow
colony visible mass of bacteria formed on a culture medium by one bacterium growing and replicating
culture the reproduction of microorganisms in a laboratory culture medium
eukaryotic pertaining to organisms that possess a true nucleus with a nuclear membrane and organelles
expectoration coughing up of sputum and mucus from the trachea and lungs

facultative anaerobe organism that grows with or without oxygen
fastidious requiring special nutrients or conditions for growth
gram-negative having the pink/red color of the counterstain used in Gram's method of staining microorganisms
gram-positive retaining the purple color of the stain used in Gram's method of staining microorganisms
Gram stain method of staining microorganisms that serves as a primary means of identifying and classifying bacteria
hyphae tubelike filaments
infection disease that occurs when pathogenic microorganisms invade the body and overcome its natural defense mechanisms
inoculation process of transferring microorganisms into or on a culture medium for growth
malaise feeling of weakness, distress, or discomfort

> ### Key Terms—cont'd
>
> **media (singular: medium)** liquid, semisolid, or solid substances containing nutrients needed to grow microorganisms
> **microaerophilic** requiring reduced oxygen for growth
> **microbiology** study of microorganisms, including bacteria, fungi, protozoa, and viruses
> **microorganism** any tiny, usually microscopic entity capable of carrying on living processes
> **morbidity** the rate at which an illness occurs
>
> **mortality** the rate of deaths
> **myalgia** diffuse muscle pain
> **mycelium** mass of hyphae that some fungi produce
> **Petri dish** dish containing medium in which to grow microorganisms
> **peptidoglycan** component made of polysaccharides and peptides that gives rigidity to the bacterial cell wall
> **prokaryotic** pertaining to unicellular organisms that do not have a true nucleus with a nuclear membrane

FUNDAMENTAL CONCEPTS

Overview of Microbiology

Microbiology is the study of microorganisms, including bacteria, fungi, protozoa, and viruses. According to *Mosby's Medical Dictionary*, a **microorganism** is "any tiny, usually microscopic entity capable of carrying on living processes." Microorganisms were first discovered in 1676, when a Dutch linen merchant and self-made microbiologist named Anthony van Leeuwenhoek created a magnifying glass through which they could be observed.

Microorganisms are found everywhere—in the air, soil, and water. Some microorganisms are involved in the decomposition of waste and the natural recycling process of life and death. Microorganisms that are normally found in and on the human body are referred to as *normal flora* or *normal biota*. Normal flora assist in preventing the growth and spread of disease-causing microorganisms. An example of protective normal flora is the bacteria *Lactobacillus*, which creates an acidic environment in the female vagina. Certain antibiotics destroy *Lactobacillus*, thereby allowing opportunistic infections such as candidiasis (caused by the yeast *Candida albicans*) to take hold.

Research has determined that fewer than 1% of all microorganisms are pathogens. When pathogenic microorganisms invade the body and overcome its natural defense mechanisms, as discussed in Chapter 7, an **infection** occurs. Some infections are contagious, which means they can spread from person to person.

The role that pathogenic microorganisms play in causing disease should be understood, as well as the means to prevent the spread of these organisms. Table 8-1 shows a timeline of efforts to control infectious diseases throughout history.

When a patient contracts an infection, the first step is to identify the pathogenic organism that is causing the problem, then find the appropriate treatment to bring the infection under control. Following is an overview of how microorganisms are classified.

Classification of Microorganisms

Although the more complex microorganism identification procedures are not performed in all laboratories, it is important to have a general knowledge of the classification, nomenclature, structure, and growth requirements of pathogenic microorganisms. Microorganisms are categorized as viruses, bacteria, fungi, or parasites.

Viruses

Viruses are the smallest microorganisms, consisting of either ribonucleic acid (RNA) or deoxyribonucleic acid (DNA) molecules. They are so small they can be seen only under a very high magnification using an electron microscope. They need to live in a host cell and use the host cell's metabolic machinery to multiply. Therefore, unlike bacteria and other microorganisms, viruses must be grown inside tissue cells rather than on typical **culture media** (liquid, semisolid, or solid substances containing nutrients needed to grow microorganisms).

Bacteria

Bacteria are classified as **prokaryotic,** which means they are unicellular organisms that do not have a true nucleus with a nuclear membrane. Bacteria do have a cell membrane and a cell wall. They reproduce by **binary fission,** asexual reproduction in which the cell splits in half. Bacteria can reproduce very rapidly on the culture media containing nutrients for their growth. They are able to form **colonies** (visible masses of bacteria formed on a culture medium by one bacterium growing and replicating itself). **Culture** is the reproduction of microorganisms in a laboratory culture medium.

Fungi

Fungi (singular: fungus) are **eukaryotic,** which means they possess a true nucleus with a nuclear membrane. They lack chlorophyll, can be grown on media, and are generally classified as molds or yeasts. Yeasts are single cells that reproduce by budding, in which a new cell forms on the surface of the yeast, grows, pinches off, and becomes a separate cell. They form

TABLE 8-1 History of Infection Control

1300s	Quarantine practices began. Passengers on ships were not allowed to disembark for 40 days after anchoring to protect coastal cities from epidemics of plague. The Latin word *quaresma*, from which "quarantine" is derived, means 40.
1600s	Bubonic plague killed half the population of Europe. Latin as a spoken language disappeared as a result. During this period, infectious diseases were believed to be caused by poisonous vapors, sin, God, and foreigners.
1800s	The germ theory and Koch's postulates proved that microorganisms caused many diseases. Industrialization and immigration in the United States caused overcrowding in many cities. Inadequate waste disposal systems and unsafe drinking water led to outbreaks of diseases such as cholera, dysentery, tuberculosis, typhoid fever, yellow fever, and malaria. In 1878, after a yellow fever epidemic, the U.S. Congress passed the Federal Quarantine Legislation, which called for federal involvement in quarantine activities. In the late 1800s patients with infectious disease were isolated by disease in wards or floors. Although nursing books from this period discuss aseptic techniques, approximately 40% of maternal deaths were caused by pregnancy complications that occurred because aseptic procedures were not practiced.
1900s	In 1910 a cubicle system of isolation was introduced, consisting of multiple-bed wards, nurses changing gowns between patients, antiseptic hand-washing techniques, and the disinfection of objects that patients had touched. In 1928 Alexander Fleming discovered penicillin. This antibiotic was first used in the 1940s by the U.S. military to treat sick and wounded solders. A 33-year-old woman was the first civilian to be treated with penicillin when her temperature rose to 107° F after she was hospitalized for more than a month with a streptococcal infection. She recovered from the infection, later met Sir Alexander Fleming, and died at the age of 90.
1950s	*Staphylococcus* infections acquired in the hospital were still causing the loss of limbs and death. Hospitals for infectious diseases began closing, except for tuberculosis sanatoriums.
1960s	Tuberculosis sanatoriums began to close.
1970s	In 1970 seven isolation categories for grouping patients with infectious diseases were developed by the Centers for Disease Control (CDC). In 1975 hospitals across the nation developed infection-control manuals.
1980s	New nosocomial infections arose, such as those caused by multidrug-resistant organisms and new pathogens. In 1985 the human immunodeficiency virus (HIV) epidemic began, and Universal Precautions were introduced.
1990s	Multidrug resistance, the rise of tuberculosis, shorter hospital stays, the overuse of antibiotics, and new diseases such as those caused by Hantavirus and the Ebola virus were some of the medical issues of this decade. In 1991 the Occupational Safety and Health Administration (OSHA) Bloodborne Pathogens Standard was instituted. In 1997 the CDC revised isolation guidelines and introduced Standard Precautions (a combination of Universal Precautions and Body Substance Isolation) and Transmission-Based Precautions.
2000s	The CDC has stated that airplanes have replaced ships as the dominant vehicles for the international transmission of diseases. Emerging infectious diseases: avian flu, swine flu (influenza A—H1N1), hepatitis C, methicillin-resistant *Staphylococcus aureus*, C.Diff

colonies with a smooth, creamy appearance on culture media. In contrast, molds are made up of **mycelium,** which consists of tubelike structures called **hyphae,** and have a fuzzy or woolly appearance.

Parasites

Parasites are organisms that live in or on a host and derive nourishment from the host. They can be one-celled protozoa (e.g., amoeba) or many-celled organisms such as helminths (roundworms, tapeworms, and flukes).

Nomenclature of Microorganisms

More than 250 years ago Carl von Linné, a Swedish botanist, created a nomenclature system for all living things. In this system each plant and animal has a name with two parts: genus (group) and species (kind). The standard rule is to capitalize the genus name and write the species name in lowercase. The genus and species names are always underlined or italicized, as in *Staphylococcus aureus*.

Structural Characteristics of Bacteria

Bacteria are classified and identified according to their shapes and growing patterns. Fig. 8-1 illustrates three growing patterns of the circular cocci (diplococci, streptococci, and staphylococci), as well as rod-shaped bacilli and spiral-shaped spirilla.

Coccus

The coccus (plural: cocci) is a round bacteria that grows in a variety of formations, depending on the division pattern of the cocci and whether the cocci remain attached afterwards. Cocci can be found as singles, pairs (diplococci), tetrads (patterns of four), chains (e.g., *Streptococcus*), clusters (e.g., *Staphylococcus*, seen as grapelike clusters).

The most common species of *Staphylococci* are *epidermidis* and *aureus*. *Staphylococcus epidermidis* is found normally on the surface of the skin and the mucous membrane of the mouth. *S. aureus*, on the other hand, is commonly associated with pathogenic conditions such as boils, carbuncles, pimples, impetigo, abscesses, wound infections, and even food poisoning.

Streptococci are cocci arranged in chains. Although some *Streptococci* are part of normal flora, some cause pathogenic conditions such as strep throat, scarlet fever, and rheumatic fever, which are discussed later in this chapter. In addition, *Streptococcus* can cause carbuncles, impetigo, pneumonia, puerperal sepsis (infection after childbirth), and erysipelas (infectious skin disease).

Bacillus

The bacillus (plural: bacilli) is rod shaped and can also be described as coccobacillus when it appears as a combination of cocci and bacilli (rod-shaped but rounded on the ends) or diplobacillus (when it is arranged in pairs).

Bacilli cause diseases such as urinary tract infections, botulism, tetanus, gas gangrene, gastroenteritis, typhoid fever, pertussis (whooping cough), bacillary dysentery, diphtheria, tuberculosis, leprosy, and the plague.

Spirillum

Spirillum (plural: spirilla) is a spiral-shaped microorganism that can be a gently curved rod or look more like a corkscrew or a spring. Some spiral bacteria are *Treponema pallidum*, which causes syphilis, and *Vibrio cholerae*, which causes cholera.

Other Bacterial Structures

Some bacteria have the following additional structures:

- *Flagella* are projections that resemble whips and allow the organism to be motile. Flagella can be seen with the aid of certain stains.
- Some bacteria have *capsules* that surround the cell wall. Organisms with capsules are virulent because antibiotics have difficulty penetrating the capsule.
- Some bacteria produce *spores* when conditions become unfavorable for growth. Spores are resistant to heat, cold, chemicals, and certain conditions. They convert back to a reproductive stage when conditions improve. Some spores survive for many years. Examples of bacteria that can produce spores are *Clostridium tetani* (causes tetanus, or lockjaw), *Clostridium botulinum* (causes botulism), and *Bacillus anthracis* (causes anthrax).

Collecting, Transporting, and Processing Microbiology Specimens

Collection of microbiological specimens requires the use of infection control techniques and precautions to prevent infecting yourself or others. The following precautions should be observed at all times:

- Wear the appropriate personal protection devices.
- Disinfect specimen containers after collection.
- Put the specimens in transport bags after collection.
- Wash the hands after specimen collection.

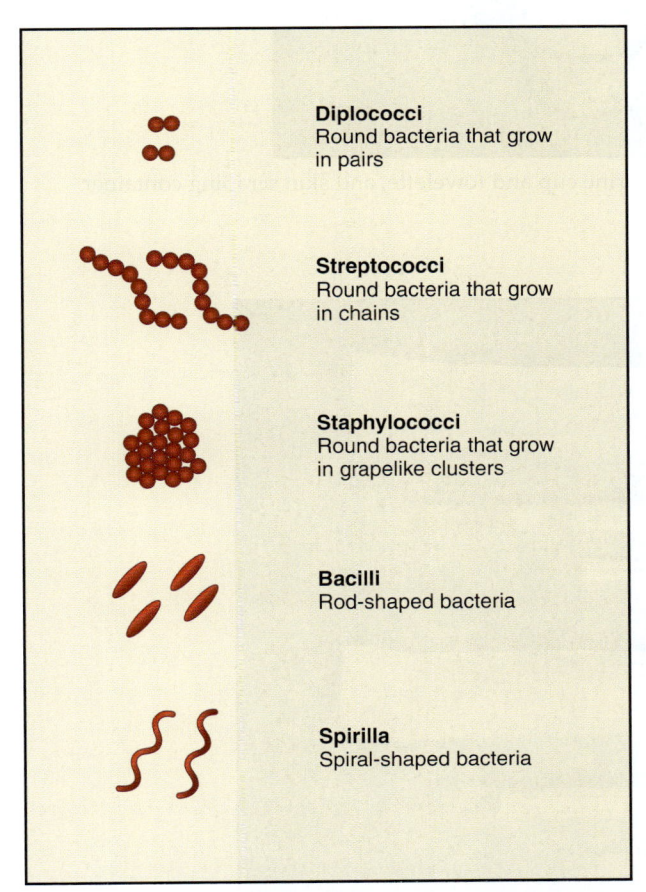

Fig. 8-1. Classification of bacteria by shape. (From Bonewit-West K: *Clinical procedures for medical assistants*, ed 7, Philadelphia, 2008, Saunders.)

As with all specimen collections, the results are only as good as the specimen collected. The ideal time to collect a microbiologic specimen is *before* antibiotics have been administered because the antibiotics will kill the microbes that are needed to be grown and identified.

Specific containers are used to transport a variety of specimens, such as blood cultures, body fluids, skin scrapings, exudates from deep wounds or abscesses, sputum from the lungs, and feces and urine specimens (Fig. 8-2). The specific directions for collecting these specimens will be discussed later in the chapter.

Collecting a microbiological specimen from the following sites generally involves applying a swab to the infected area: eyes, rectum, urogenital areas, throat, and wounds. The microbiology specimens must be processed as soon as possible. Transport systems provide the conditions microorganisms need to survive during the transport to the laboratory. These transport systems contain maintenance media that prevent the microorganisms from dying or multiplying. Two examples of transport systems are shown in Fig. 8-3. The system at the top of the picture includes a blue-handled Dacron swab on

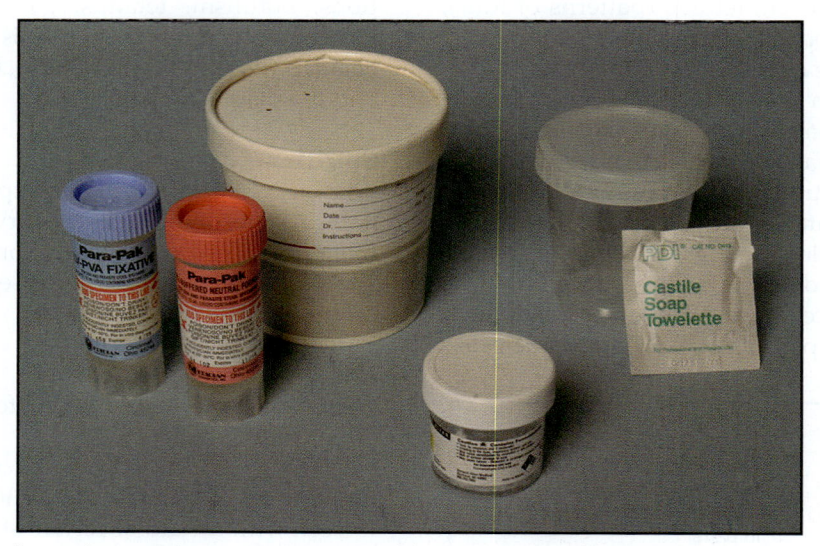

Fig. 8-2. Ova and parasite container, sputum cup, sterile urine cup and towelette, and skin scraping container.

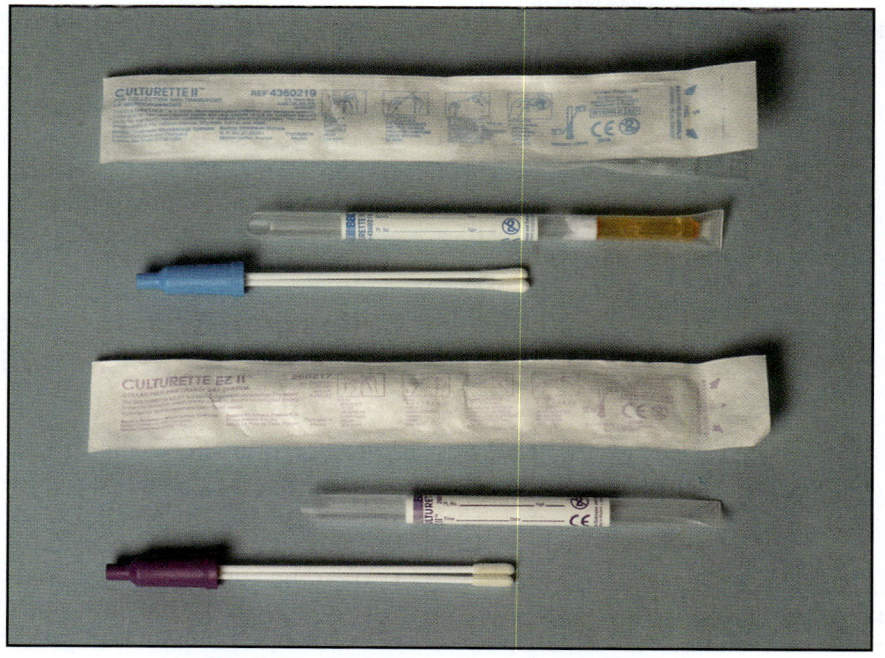

Fig. 8-3. Two specimen transport systems.

a plastic stick. When the specimen is obtained, the swab is put into the holder and the bottom of the tube is squeezed, releasing the transport media onto the swab to maintain the organisms. The swab with the purple handle, at the bottom of the picture, contains dried nutrient media. The transport system to be used will depend on the type of specimen collected or the specific organisms for which the culture was ordered.

Collecting a Throat Specimen

The swabbed throat specimen collection is one of the most common microbiology procedures performed in the physician's office laboratory (POL). The specimen is tested for possible streptococcal infections.

The **Collecting a Throat Specimen** procedure check sheet is provided in the workbook and is demonstrated in Procedure 8-1, located at the end of this section.

Collecting a Blood Culture Specimen

Blood cultures are collected in containers such as BACTEC bottles (Becton Dickinson, Franklin Lakes, NJ) (Fig. 8-4). Approximately 10 mL of blood is required for each bottle when collecting blood from an adult. (NOTE: The aerobic bottle grows oxygen-dependent bacteria and must be drawn first when using the butterfly method of draw, and the anaerobic bottle grows bacteria that grow best in the absence of oxygen. It is drawn second. Also displayed are the Vacutainer tubes with their light yellow caps.) Pediatric patients generally need 1 to 3 mL for one aerobic bottle or the culture tube. When a patient has a fever of unknown origin, the physician often orders a blood culture to determine whether microorganisms are present in the blood. A specific aseptic preparation of the puncture site and the equipment is required when drawing blood cultures. The anaerobic bottle is filled first unless the butterfly method is used, in which case the aerobic bottle is filled first because of the air in the tubing.

Collecting a Urine Culture Specimen

When a urinary tract infection is present, the physician will typically order a urine culture and sensitivity to determine the type of pathogen causing the infection and the antibiotic that will most effectively treat the infection. The patient is instructed to collect a clean-catch midstream urine into a sterile specimen container, as described in Chapter 3. If the urine specimen must be transported to the microbiology lab, the urine can be transferred into a sterile Vacutainer tube with the appropriate preservatives, as seen in Fig. 8-5, *A* and *B*.

Collecting a *Chlamydia* Specimen

Another type of transport media is that used for *Chlamydia* organisms (Fig. 8-6). Chlamydia is a sexually transmitted disease caused by *Chlamydia trachomatis*, a tiny **gram-negative** (having the pink/red color of the counterstain used in Gram's method of staining microorganisms) intracellular bacterium that requires a host cell for growth. Women with this disease may have no symptoms or may have dysuria; itching; irritation of the genital area; and an odorless, yellowish vaginal discharge. Left untreated, chlamydia can cause pelvic inflammatory disease and infertility. The symptoms in men are mild dysuria and a thin, watery discharge from the penis. If not treated in men, the disease can cause epididymitis, which could result in infertility. Using a sterile swab, the physician collects a specimen from the female endocervical canal or the male urethra. The swab is placed in a tube containing a transport medium to preserve the specimen and is sent to a reference laboratory for testing. Testing for *Chlamydia* is most frequently done using a DNA-probe test (test based on DNA detection).

Collecting a *Gonorrhea* Specimen

The JEMBEC transport system (Becton Dickinson) (Fig. 8-7) consists of a JEMBEC plate, a small white pill, and a plastic bag. It is used for transporting and growing *Neisseria gonorrhoeae*, the gram-negative diplococcus that causes gonorrhea. When activated, the pill creates a 10% carbon dioxide atmosphere that this organism needs for growth. Gonorrhea is a sexually transmitted disease of the genitourinary tract. Women either show no symptoms or have dysuria and a yellow discharge. If untreated, the infection can result in pelvic inflammatory disease, which could lead to infertility. Men infected with gonorrhea have dysuria and may have a whitish discharge from the penis that may become thick and creamy. In untreated men epididymitis may occur, which can lead to infertility. Like *Chlamydia*, *N. gonorrhoeae* can be diagnosed with a DNA probe, which tests for the presence of the gonorrhea gene. The collection procedure is the same as for *Chlamydia*.

Collecting a Fecal Specimen for Ova and Parasites

Another transport method is ova and parasite collection kits, which consist of two containers, one with formalin and one with polyvinyl alcohol (Fig. 8-8). The containers must be filled to the appropriate line with a fecal specimen. The kit is used for the preservation of parasites.

242 CHAPTER 8   Microbiology

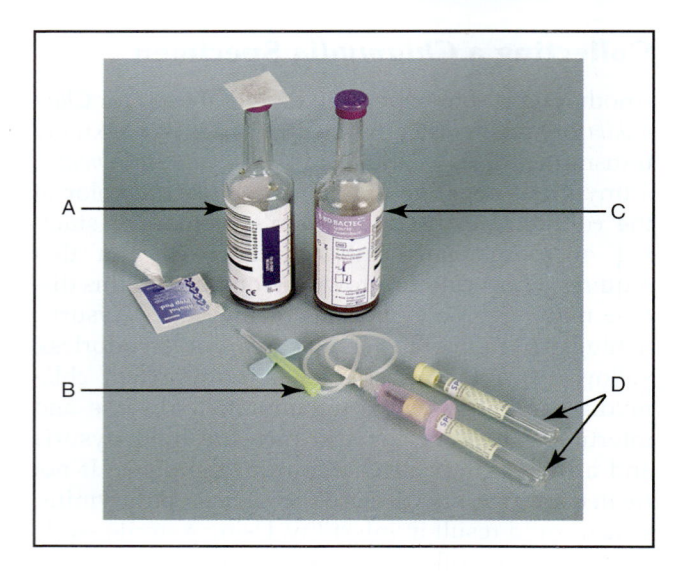

Fig. 8-4. Blood culture equipment. The aerobic bottle **(A)** grows oxygen-dependent bacteria and is drawn first when using the butterfly method of draw **(B)**, and the anaerobic bottle **(C)** grows bacteria that grow best in the absence of oxygen. It is drawn second. There are also blood culture Vacutainer tubes **(D)** that have a light yellow stopper for pediatric patients. (Courtesy Zack Bent.)

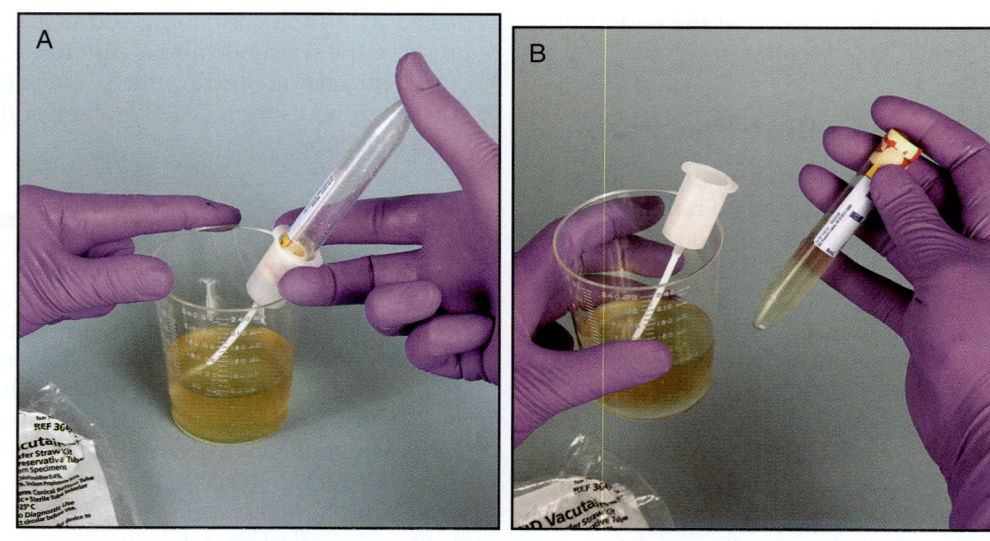

Fig. 8-5. Preparing a clean-catch midstream urine for transport. **A,** The white sterile "straw" and Vacutainer holder with a needle inside are inserted into the urine. The Vacutainer tube is pushed into the needle, causing the urine to fill the tube. **B,** The filled Vacutainer tube in then labeled and sent to the lab. (Courtesy Zack Bent.)

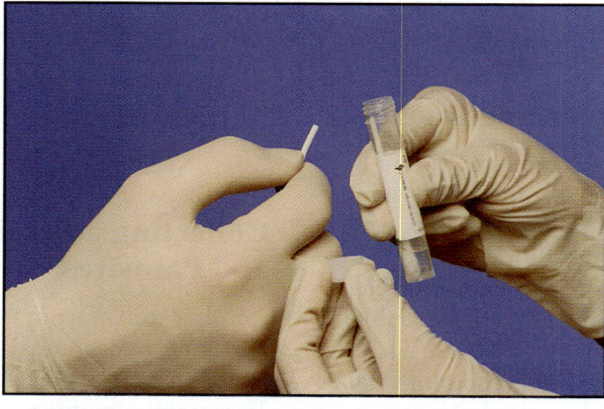

Fig. 8-6. Chlamydia transport medium. The shaft of the swab is broken off at the score line. (From Bonewit-West K: *Clinical procedures for medical assistants*, ed 7, St Louis, 2008, Saunders.)

Fundamental Concepts

Transporting Specimens by Mail

When specimens are transported by mail, they must be packed in the correct container (Fig. 8-9). The specimen is placed in a container, which is then placed inside a mailing container. A biohazard emblem must be affixed to every container, including the outside one.

Microbiology Smears, Stains, and Wet Mounts

After the microbiology specimen is collected, the next step is to identify the infectious microorganism microscopically. A portion of the specimen is generally smeared onto a slide or placed into a solution on a slide. The smeared specimen is then fixed to the slide and stained to demonstrate its staining characteristics.

Gram Stain

More than 100 years have passed since the **Gram stain** was developed by Dr. Hans Christian Gram. Gram stain is defined by *Mosby's Medical Dictionary* as a "method of staining microorganisms...that serves as a primary means of identifying and classifying bacteria." The Gram stain reaction is still used today to distinguish between **gram-positive** (retain-

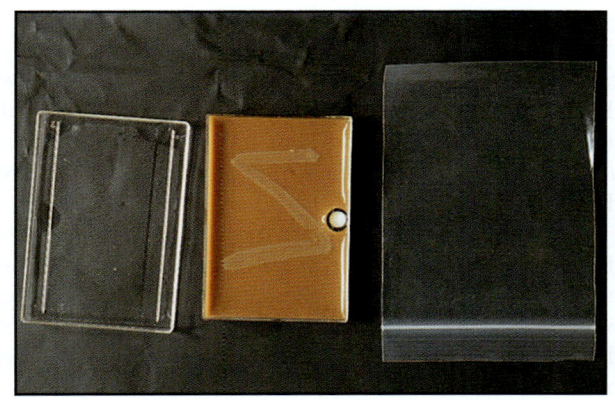

Fig. 8-7. JEMBEC transport system. (From Mahon CR, Manuselis G: *Textbook of diagnostic microbiology,* ed 3, St Louis, 2006, Saunders.)

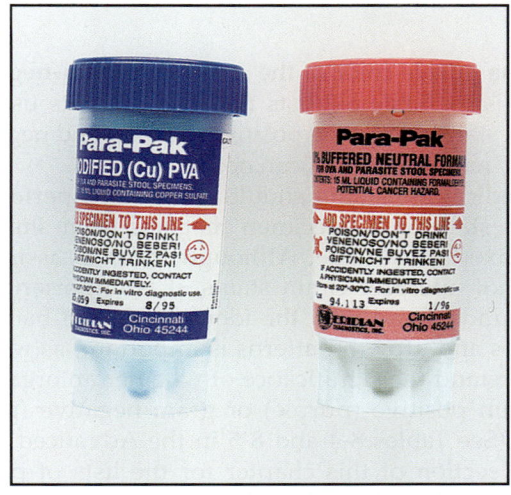

Fig. 8-8. Ova and parasite collection kit. (From Young AP, Kennedy DB: *Kinn's the medical assistant: an applied learning approach,* ed 10, St Louis, 2007, Saunders. Courtesy Meridan Bioscience, Inc.)

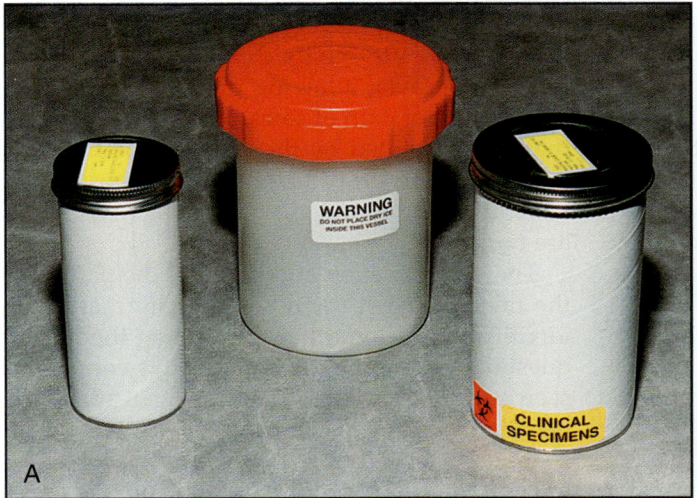

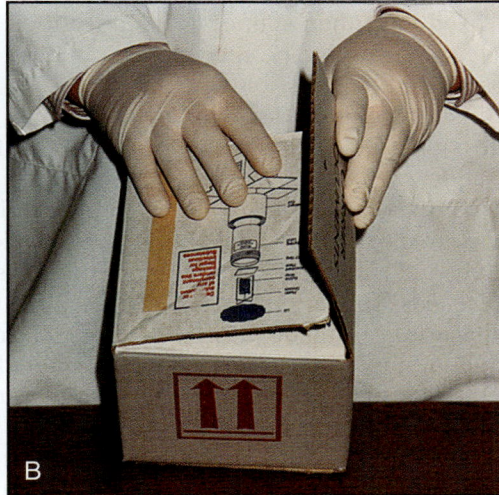

Fig. 8-9. Specimen mailing containers. (From Young AP, Kennedy DB: *Kinn's the medical assistant: an applied learning approach,* ed 10, St Louis, 2007, Saunders.)

TABLE 8-2 Gram Stain Reactions

Stain Step	Staining Reagent	Color of Gram-Positive Organism	Example Gram-Positive Cocci (GPC)	Color of Gram-Negative	Example Gram-Negative Bacilli (GNB)
1. Primary stain	Crystal violet	Purple	● ● ●	Purple	
2. Mordant	Gram's iodine	Purple	● ● ●	Purple	
3. Decolorizer	Acetone or ethyl alcohol	Purple	● ● ●	Colorless	
4. Counterstain	Safranin	Purple	● ● ●	Pink/red	

ing the purple color of the stain) and **gram-negative** organisms. Table 8-2 lists the four reagents used in Gram staining and the positive (purple) and negative (pink/red) results that can occur.

Medical assistants should be able to perform a Gram stain on a specimen that has been smeared and fixed on a slide. Although medical assistants will not interpret Gram stains, it is important that they understand why the identification of bacterial shapes and growth patterns is important, as well as understand the significance of whether an organism is gram positive (purple) or gram negative (pink/red). (See Tables 8-4 and 8-5 in the Advanced Concepts section of this chapter for the lists of pathogenic bacilli and cocci, with their Gram reactions in Column 3 of the tables.)

Smear Preparation

The bacterial specimen must be smeared onto a glass slide, fixed, and then stained to identify it as gram positive or negative. The specimen is obtained from the following three possible sources:
1. A direct smear is made by rolling a specimen swab onto a glass slide. All areas of the swab must touch the slide.
2. A colony of bacteria growing on a culture plate is transferred to a glass slide. This is done by taking a colony and rubbing it into a drop of normal saline on the glass slide.
3. A smear may be made from a liquid media culture. Either a sterile swab or a sterilized inoculating needle is dipped in the culture broth, then rolled or placed on the glass slide.

The smear is allowed to dry and is then heat fixed either by running it through a natural gas Bunsen burner or by placing the slide on an electric incinerator for a few seconds (do not overheat because this could cause distortion of the bacterial cells). Heat fixing kills the microorganisms and causes the swabbed material to stick to the slide before staining. The methanol fixative used in blood smears may also be used to affix the smear to the slide.

The most critical step in the Gram stain procedure is the decolorizing step. If the decolorizing is not done for a sufficient length of time, everything will be purple, and, conversely, if decolorizing is done for too long a duration, everything will be pink/red.

Gram-positive organisms stain purple because a large **peptidoglycan** layer is present in their cell walls that holds the crystal violet stain. Peptidoglycan is a component made of polysaccharides and peptides that gives rigidity to the bacteria's cell walls. Gram-negative organisms, on the other hand, have a small layer of peptidoglycan. In addition, they have an outer layer of lipoprotein and lipopolysaccharides (lipids) that are soluble in the decolorizing solution. When the decolorizer is applied, it punches holes in the lipid portion of the gram-negative outer layer, allowing the crystal violet to seep out. A counterstain of safranin stains all the material that is not stained by the crystal violet. At the end of the staining procedure, the gram-positive organisms are purple and the gram-negative organisms are pink/red.

The gram reaction and shape of the pathogen give the microbiologist the necessary information to help identify the bacteria that are causing the infection in question. For example, gram-positive cocci (GPC) are seen as purple, circular bacteria (Fig. 8-10), and gram-negative bacilli (GNB) are seen as pink/red, rod-shaped bacteria (Fig. 8-11). *N. gonorrhoeae* (Fig. 8-12) are gram-negative cocci (GNC) that appear as pairs of pink/red diplococci shaped like kidney beans and facing each other.

Fundamental Concepts

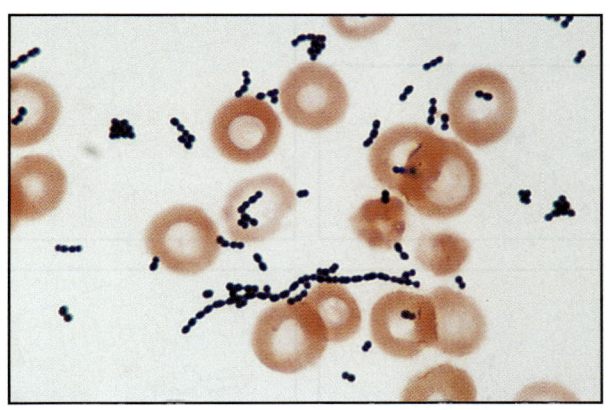

Fig. 8-10. Gram-positive cocci (GPC) in chains (streptococci). (From Young AP, Kennedy DB: *Kinn's the medical assistant: an applied learning approach*, ed 10, St Louis, 2007, Saunders.)

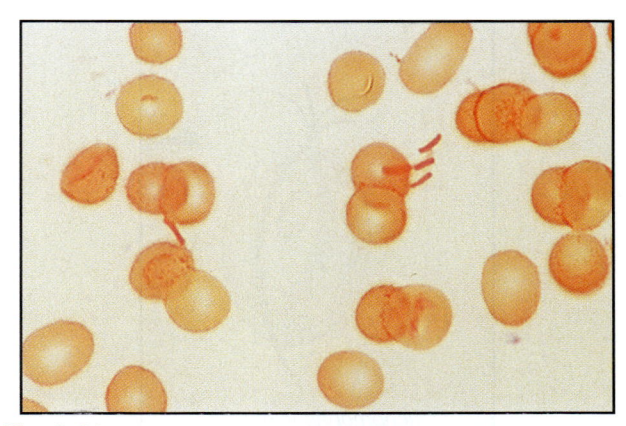

Fig. 8-11. Gram-negative bacilli (GNB). (From Young AP, Kennedy DB: *Kinn's the medical assistant: an applied learning approach*, ed 10, St Louis, 2007, Saunders.)

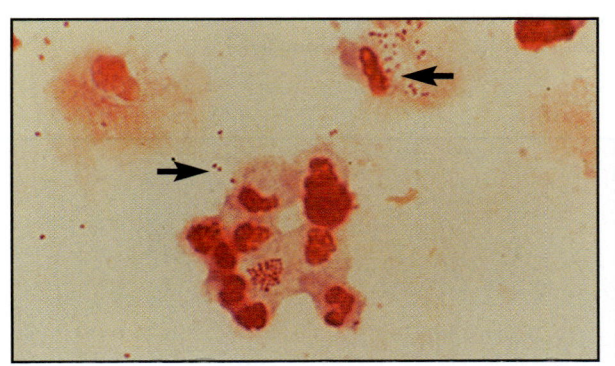

Fig. 8-12. Gram-negative cocci (GNC) in pairs (diplococci). (From Mahon CR, Manuselis G: *Textbook of diagnostic microbiology*, ed 3, St Louis, 2006, Saunders.)

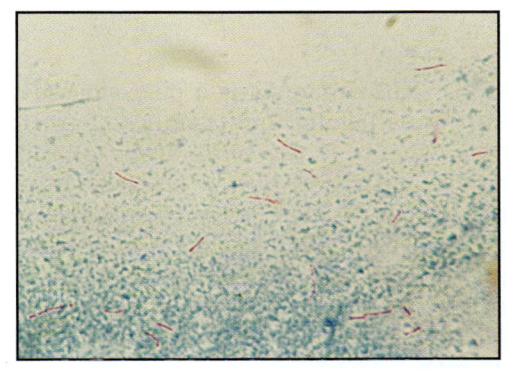

Fig. 8-13. Mycobacterium tuberculosis in acid-fast stain. (From Young AP, Kennedy DB: *Kinn's the medical assistant: an applied learning approach*, ed 10, St Louis, 2007, Saunders.)

The Gram stain procedure check sheet is provided in the workbook and is demonstrated in Procedure 8-2, located at the end of this section.

Acid-Fast Stains

The acid-fast stain is used to microscopically search for microorganisms in the *Mycobacterium* genus referred to as acid-fast bacilli (AFB), which resist decolorization with acid alcohol. *Mycobacterium tuberculosis* causes tuberculosis (TB), a lung infection in which tubercles (nodules) are formed. Symptoms include night sweats, pulmonary hemorrhage, and **expectoration** of purulent sputum. Another species, *Mycobacterium avium* complex, disseminates throughout the body in patients with acquired immunedeficiency syndrome (AIDS). Both mycobacterial diseases have been on the increase with the spread of AIDS.

Although AFB staining is not done in a POL, medical assistants should understand how the stain is done and recognize the appearance of the stained AFB organism. Two methods of AFB staining break down the wax in the AFB cell wall: the Ziehl–Neelsen stain, which uses heat, and Kinyoun, a cold stain that mixes a detergent with the dye. Both methods use carbolfuchsin solutions for the primary stain, decolorize with acid alcohol, and counterstain with methylene blue. When the stain is complete, the acid-fast organisms appear as red beaded rods (Fig. 8-13). The slide is observed under the oil immersion objective.

Fluorescent staining is another method. Auramine or auramine–rhodamine fluorochrome stain is used. It is viewed under a fluorescence microscope equipped with the appropriate filter system for this type of stained smear. The stain may be screened at a lower magnification, which allows more fields to be examined in a shorter period of time. TB organisms appear as bright yellow-orange bacilli against a dark background.

Wet Mounts

Wet mounts are done to view organisms in their living state. One type of wet mount determines the motility of a parasite, *Trichomonas vaginalis*

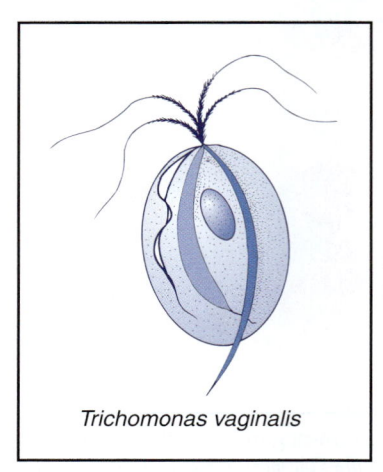

Fig. 8-14. Trichomonas vaginalis. (From Stepp CA, Woods M: *Laboratory procedures for medical office personnel*, Philadelphia, 1998, Saunders.)

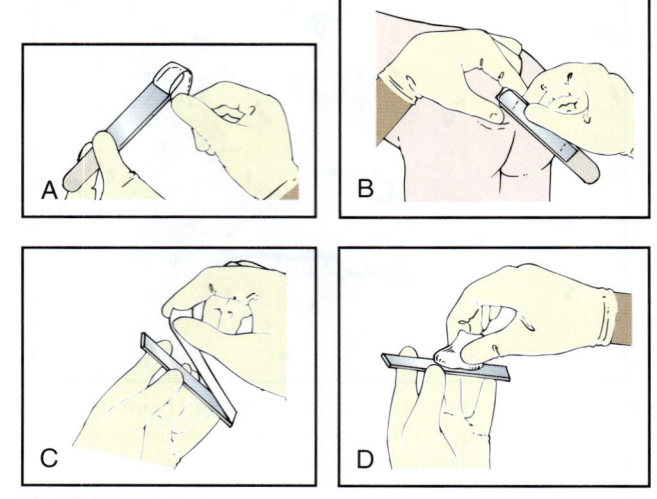

Fig. 8-15. Cellulose tape test for pinworms. (From Young AP, Kennedy DB: *Kinn's the medical assistant: an applied learning approach*, ed 10, St Louis, 2007, Saunders.)

(Fig. 8-14). This organism is a pear-shaped protozoa with four flagella that give it a characteristic jerky movement. *T. vaginalis* is one of the most common sexually transmitted diseases. In women the infection is located primarily in the vagina, where it causes itching and a frothy, creamy discharge. Men are usually asymptomatic and serve as carriers. The organism is found in urine or vaginal specimens in women and urine or prostatic sections in men.

Wet mounts are also done to detect the presence of "clue cells," vaginal epithelial cells covered with *Gardnerella vaginalis*, a gram-negative coccobacillus. This organism is found in almost 100% of women who have bacterial vaginosis. Infected women produce a watery exudate that lacks white blood cells and usually has a fishy odor, and the clue cells are covered by the *Gardnerella* organism.

The **Wet Mount** procedure check sheet is provided in the workbook and is demonstrated in Procedure 8-3, located at the end of this section.

KOH Preparation

Another type of microbiology slide identification is the KOH (potassium hydroxide) preparation. KOH is an alkaline solution that breaks down protein material, facilitating the identification of any fungus that may be present in skin scrapings or mucus. A KOH preparation shows fungal hyphae from skin dermatophyte infections, as well as yeast such as *C. albicans*. Although the KOH preparation may be done by a medical assistant, it is interpreted by a trained laboratorian or physician.

The **KOH Preparation** procedure check sheet is provided in the workbook and is demonstrated in Procedure 8-4, located at the end of this section.

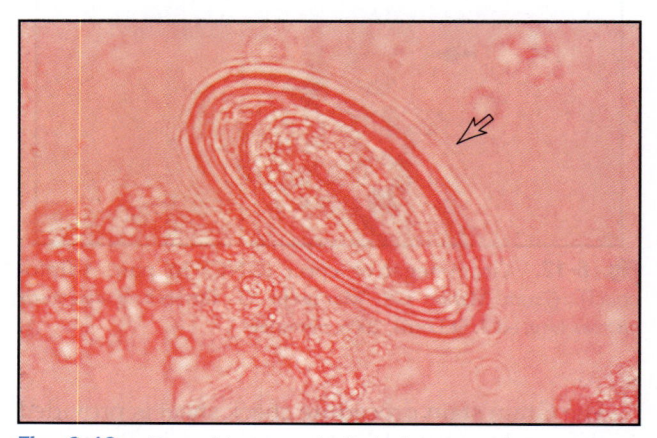

Fig. 8-16. *Enterobius vermicularis* (pinworm) egg. (From Young AP, Kennedy DB: *Kinn's the medical assistant: an applied learning approach*, ed 10, St Louis, 2007, Saunders.)

Pinworm Specimen Collection and Microscopic Results

Enterobius vermicularis is a tiny roundworm known commonly as *pinworm*. The female pinworm normally lays her eggs during the nighttime hours in the anal area of the human host. This causes itching, and the host scratches this area, infecting the hands and fingernails. The identification test is performed by using either swabs coated with petroleum jelly or cellulose tape.

The *cellulose tape test* consists of placing cellulose tape (sticky side) over the patient's anal area and then placing the tape sticky-side-down on a glass slide (Fig. 8-15). A physician or trained laboratorian examines the tape microscopically for *E. vermicularis* eggs (Fig. 8-16).

PROCEDURE 8-1 Procedure for Collecting a Throat Specimen

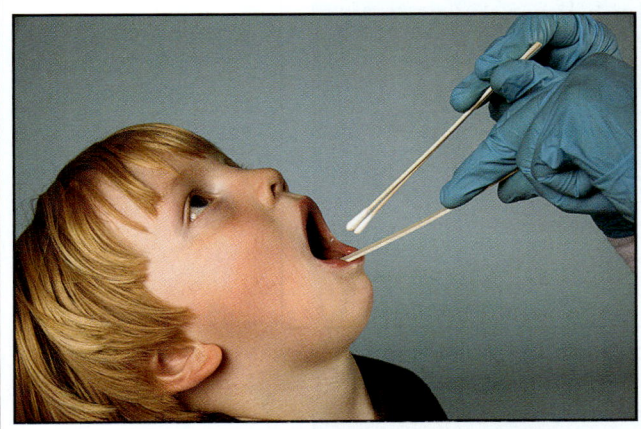

A. Have the patient sit with head back. Use a sterile tongue depressor to hold down the tongue and have the patient say, "ahh" while inserting the two sterile swaps to the back of the throat. (Courtesy Zack Bent.)

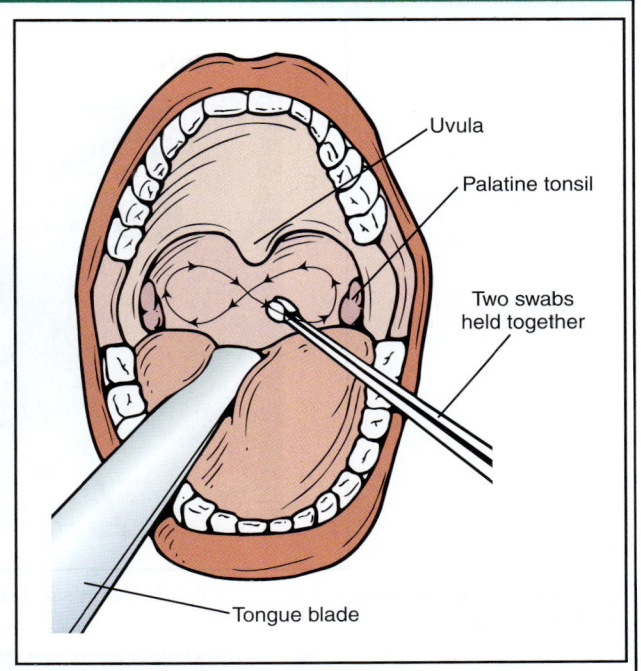

B. Figure-8 technique for obtaining a throat specimen. (From Stepp CA, Woods M: *Laboratory procedures for medical office personnel*, Philadelphia, 1998, Saunders.)

Equipment and Supplies

- Gloves
- Sterile Dacron swabs (not cotton because it inhibits *Streptococcus* growth)
- Swab container
- Tongue depressor

Procedure

1. Sanitize the hands, and apply gloves.
2. Aseptically (following techniques that prevent contamination) remove the sterile swab from the package, holding it by the tip.
3. Have the patient sit with head back. Use a sterile tongue depressor to hold down the tongue, and have the patient say, "ahh" (Fig. A).
4. Rotate the swab on the back of the throat (Fig. B) in a circular motion or figure-eight pattern, and place it in the appropriate container. Do not touch the teeth or the back of the tongue because these areas have normal flora. Two swabs may be used at the same time, as seen in Fig. A.
5. Depending on the microbiology requisition, one swab may be used for a rapid strep test and the other will be placed in a sterile culture transportation tube as seen in Fig. 8-3.
6. Remove gloves (unless the rapid test is done immediately after specimen collection), sanitize the hands, and chart the collection procedure.

Fig. A courtesy Zack Bent.

PROCEDURE 8-2 Gram Stain Procedure

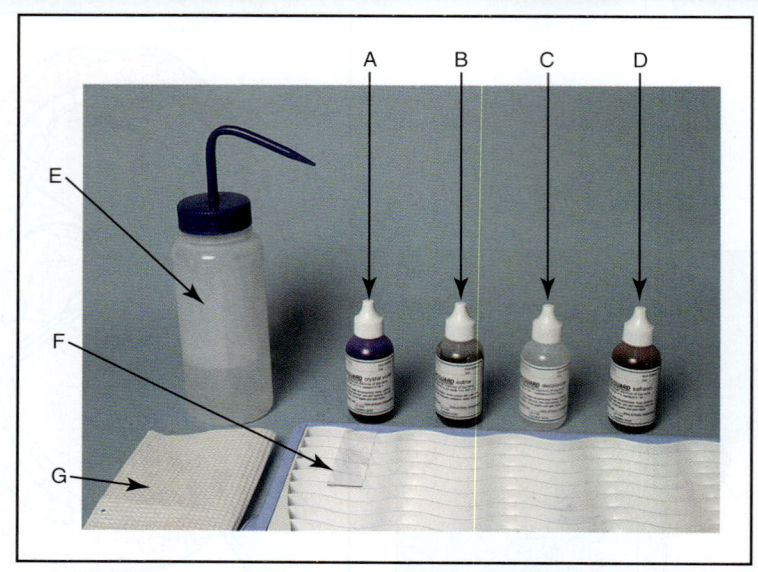

A. Gram stain equipment. *a,* Crystal violet; *b,* Gram's iodine; *c,* decolorizer; *d,* safranin; *e,* rinse water; *f,* staining rack; *g,* bibulous paper.

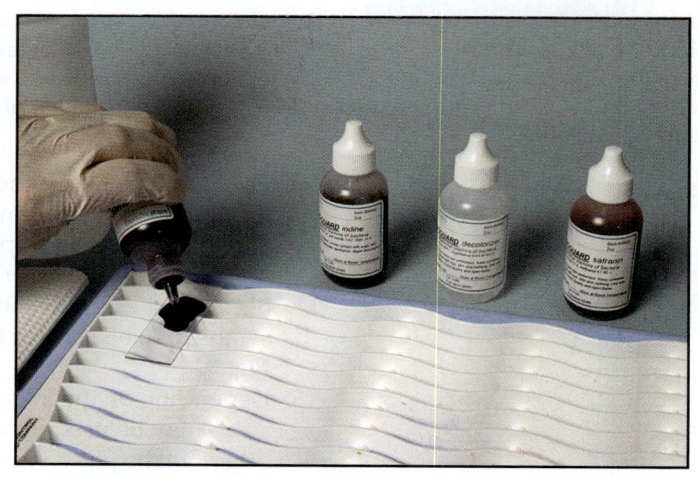

B. Apply crystal violet onto the smeared fixed slide, and time for 1 minute.

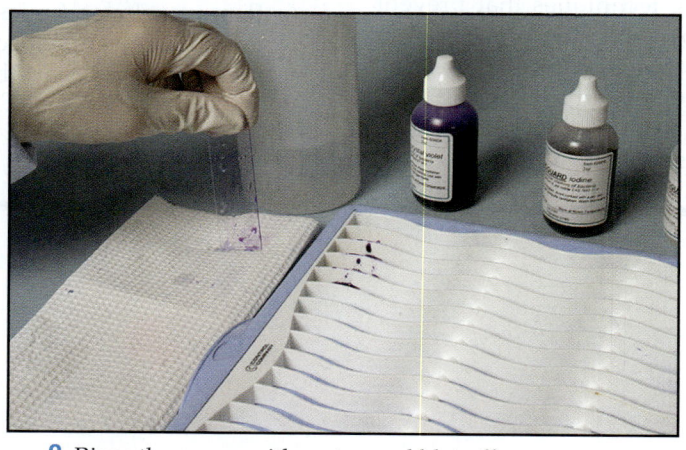

C. Rinse the smear with water, and blot off excess water.

PROCEDURE 8-2 Gram Stain Procedure—cont'd

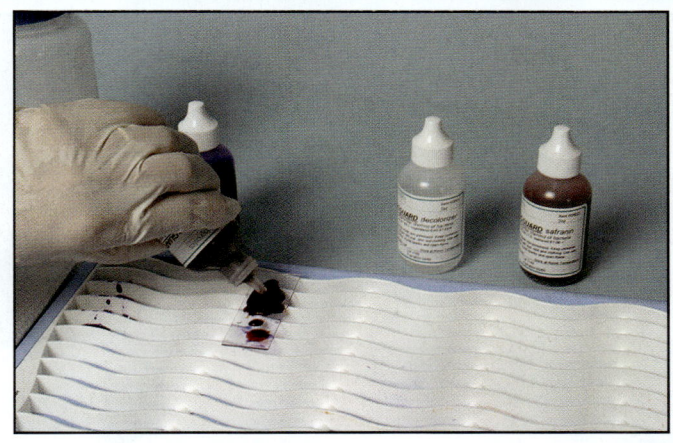

D. Apply Gram's iodine and time for 1 minute, then rinse and blot.

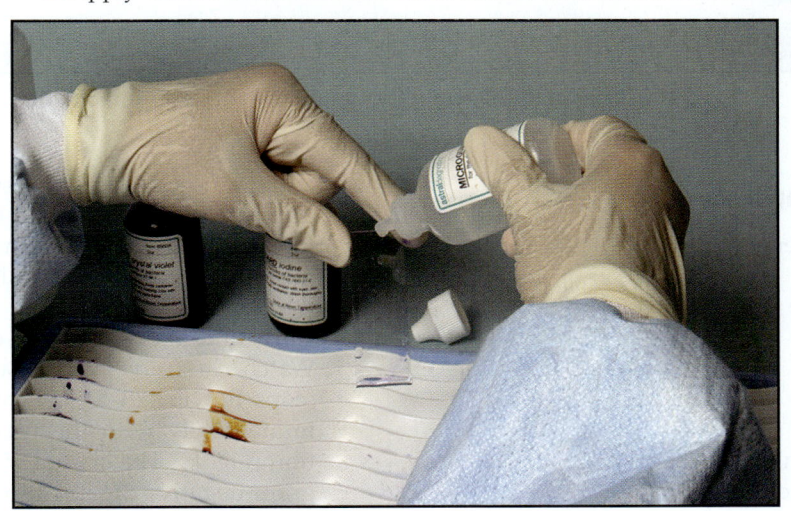

E. Apply decolorizer until all purple dye is removed (approximately 3-5 seconds).

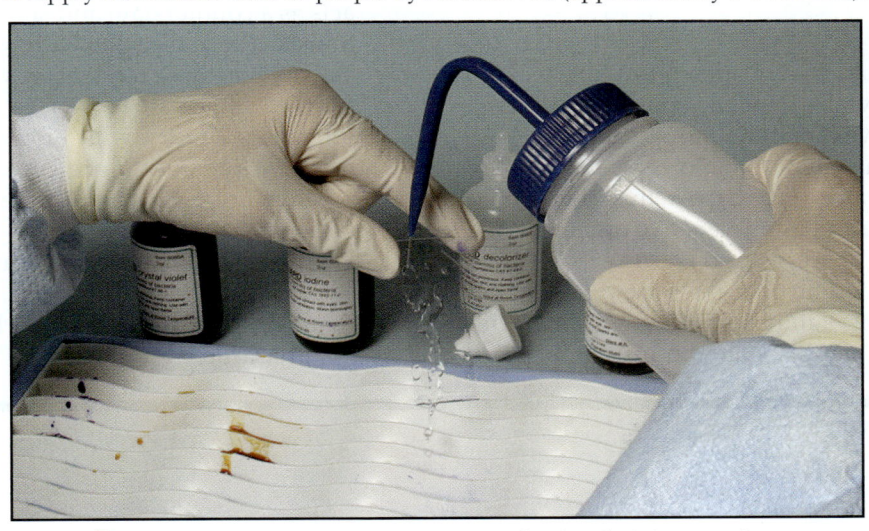

F. Immediately rinse with water to stop the decolorizing reaction.

(Continued)

PROCEDURE 8-2 Gram Stain Procedure—cont'd

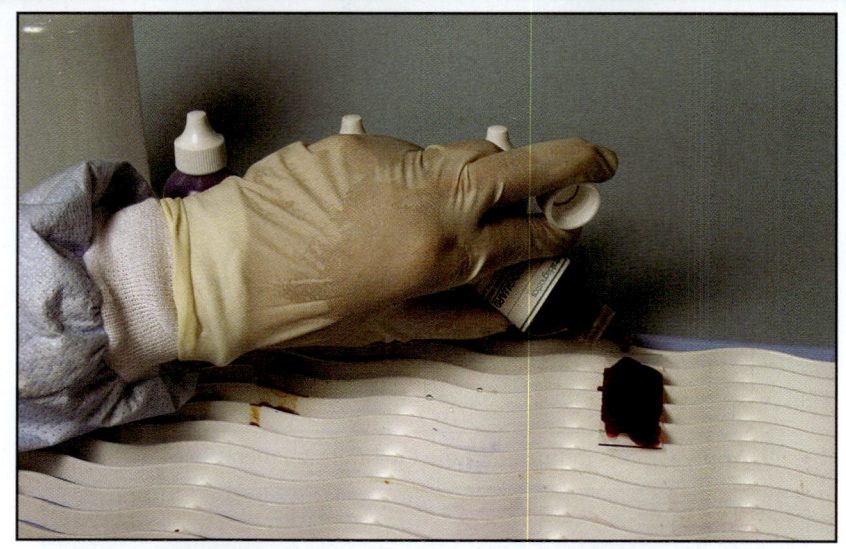

G. Apply the safranin counterstain for 1 minute, then rinse, and blot dry.

Equipment and Supplies (Fig. A)

Gram stain reagents
a) Crystal violet
b) Gram's iodine
c) Decolorizer
d) Safranin
e) Rinse water
f) Staining rack
g) Bibulous (highly absorbent) paper
- Gloves (not pictured)

Procedure

1. Sanitize the hands, and apply gloves.
2. Pour crystal violet over the smeared and fixed slide, and leave it on for 1 minute (Fig. B). Rinse the slide with water. Using forceps, tip the slide to remove water (Fig. C). At this stage, both gram-positive and gram-negative organisms are purple.
3. Pour Gram's iodine over the slide (Fig. D), and leave it on for 1 minute. Rinse the slide with water. Again, at this stage both gram-positive and gram-negative organisms are purple. Iodine acts as a mordant to hold the crystal violet dye in gram-positive organisms.
4. Holding the slide vertically, pour decolorizer, which consists of alcohol or acetone, over the slide, and allow it to run off the slide (Fig. E). Watch carefully to note when the purple dye stops flowing (3 to 5 seconds). Rinse the slide immediately with the water to stop the reaction (Fig. F). The crystal violet is removed from gram-negative organisms during this step.
5. Apply the red dye, safranin (Fig. G). This dye acts as a counterstain and should be left on for 1 minute. Rinse the slide with water. The safranin stains everything red that was no longer stained purple.
6. Blot the slide dry with bibulous paper. Gram-negative organisms are pink/red, and gram-positive organisms are purple at this end stage of Gram staining.
7. Position the slide under the microscope for the physician to view.
8. Remove gloves, sanitize the hands, and chart the procedure.

PROCEDURE 8-3 Wet Mount Procedure

Equipment and Supplies

- Glass slide or slide with a well carved into it
- Cover slip
- Gloves
- Drop of saline
- Specimen

Procedure

1. Sanitize the hands, and apply gloves.
2. Place a small amount of the specimen on the slide or in the slide well.
3. Place a drop of saline (normal) on the specimen and a cover slip over the specimen.
4. Position the slide under the microscope for the physician to view.
5. Remove gloves, sanitize the hands, and chart the procedure.

PROCEDURE 8-4 KOH Preparation Procedure

Equipment and Supplies

- Glass slide
- Cover slip
- KOH
- Scalpel
- Swabs
- Specimen
- Gloves

Procedure

1. Sanitize the hands, and apply gloves.
2. Clean the specimen area with 70% alcohol.
3. The sample of hair, skin, or nail is scraped with a scalpel by the physician. A vaginal swab specimen may also be done by the physician for yeast determination.
4. Place a drop of 10% KOH on the glass slide.
5. Position the specimen in the KOH on the slide.
6. Place a cover slip on the specimen, and let it sit for 30 minutes. The 10% KOH will dissolve all protein material, leaving any fungus to be seen microscopically.
7. Position the slide under the microscope for the physician to view.
8. Remove gloves, sanitize the hands, and chart the procedure.

CLIA-WAIVED MICROBIOLOGY TESTS

Streptococcus Group A Testing

Streptococcus species are gram-positive cocci in chains. Some *Streptococci* are capable of producing hemolytic toxins, which hemolyze red blood cells (RBCs) when grown on blood agar. Part of the identification of *Streptococcus* depends on which of the following types of hemolytic reactions (breaking down red blood cells) occur on blood agar:

- Alpha hemolysis, incomplete hemolysis of RBCs, is seen as a green color around the colonies.
- Beta hemolysis, complete hemolysis of RBCs, is seen as a clear area around the colonies. *Streptococcus pyogenes*, the bacteria that causes strep throat, demonstrates beta hemolysis (Fig. 8-17).
- Gamma hemolysis occurs when no toxin is present and therefore no hemolysis is seen around the colonies.

Streptococcus species can also be divided into groups A through O according to the antigenic properties (the ability to induce the formation of specific antibodies) in their cell walls. This system of classification is named after Dr. Rebecca Lancefield, who identified the various groups. *S. pyogenes* is beta hemolytic and serologically types in group A. This organism, which is often called group A *strep*, causes strep throat, a contagious disease passed from one person to another through droplets of saliva or nasal secretions. The symptoms of strep throat are a very sore throat, a bright red pharynx, white patches on the tonsils, swollen glands in the neck, a tired feeling, and muscular aches.

Some complications of strep throat are scarlet fever, rheumatic fever, and glomerulonephritis. Scarlet fever

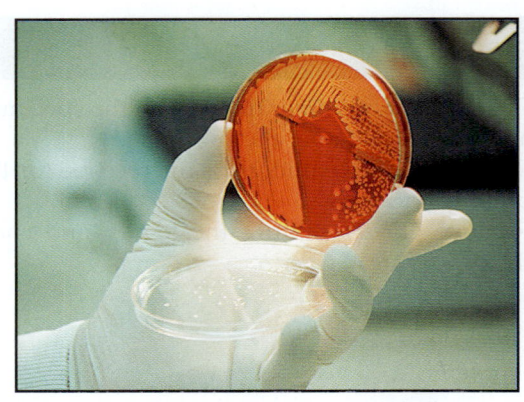

Fig. 8-17. Beta hemolysis. (From Young AP, Kennedy DB: *Kinn's the medical assistant: an applied learning approach*, ed 9, St Louis, 2007, Saunders.)

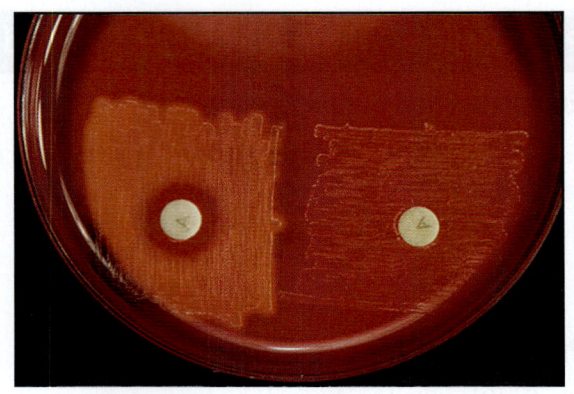

Fig. 8-18. Bacitracin group A test. (From Mahon CR, Manuselis G: *Textbook of diagnostic microbiology*, ed 3, St Louis, 2006, Saunders.)

is a contagious disease characterized by symptoms such as sore throat, fever, enlarged lymph nodes in the neck, flushing of the face, strawberry tongue, and a bright red rash. Rheumatic fever is a systemic inflammatory disease that may affect the brain, heart, joints, skin, or subcutaneous tissues. This disease, which usually occurs in children, may be caused by a delayed reaction to an inadequately treated *S. pyogenes* infection. Glomerulonephritis is an inflammation of the glomerulus of the kidney characterized by decreased urine production, edema, and protein and blood in the urine.

Rapid Strep Testing (CLIA-Waived)

There are many CLIA-waived group A strep kits that test for the extracted antigen. An example is the Acceava Kit (Thermo Electron Corporation).

The **Acceava Strep A Test** procedure check sheet is provided in the workbook and is demonstrated in Procedure 8-5, located at the end of this section.

Bacitracin Method

If the rapid strep test is negative, a culture (with a bacitracin disk) may be done at a reference lab. The specimen might not have contained enough organisms to be detected by the rapid strep test. Preparing the culture consists of swabbing a blood agar culture plate with the throat specimen. The agar is streaked for isolation. A disk impregnated with a specified amount of the antibiotic bacitracin (A disk) is then placed on the swabbed area. The plate is incubated overnight at 37° C. After 24 hours the plate is observed for *S. pyogenes*, which will cause beta hemolysis (clearing of the RBCs) on the blood agar plate. It will also show no growth or beta hemolysis around the bacitracin disk, because strep A is sensitive to the antibiotic. In Fig. 8-18, the positive results of beta hemolysis and inhibited growth around the bacitracin disk are seen on the left, and the negative result of no hemolysis and no inhibited growth around the disk is on the right. If the positive culture is smeared and stained, the bacteria should appear as gram-positive cocci in chains.

Influenza

Influenza is commonly known as the flu. It is caused by a virus that affects the respiratory tract. Symptoms, which last 1 to 2 weeks, are fever (100° to 103° F, higher in children), cough, sore throat, runny or stuffy nose, headache, muscle aches, and fatigue. Gastrointestinal symptoms are rare.

Some individuals with the flu develop complications such as pneumonia. The elderly and people with chronic problems are at greater risk for complications. Three types of influenza exist: A, B, and C. Types A and B cause the winter epidemics that occur almost every year. Type C influenza is milder.

Influenza viruses have the capacity to mutate. One type of mutation is called *antigenic drift,* which refers to a gradual change in the virus strain. Antigenic drift occurs in viruses from one season to another. Another type of mutation, *antigenic shift,* involves an abrupt change in the antigenic properties of the virus. When an antigenic shift occurs, it causes a pandemic, in which large numbers of people contract the disease. The following are examples of past influenza pandemics:

- In 1918 the "swine flu," also known as *Spanish flu* because Spain was one of the countries most seriously affected, killed 500,000 in the United States and 20 million worldwide in only 120 days. This was probably the most devastating epidemic ever to affect the human race.
- In 1957 the "Asian flu" caused 70,000 deaths in the United States.
- In 2005 the "Avian flu" became widespread in humans which included 50 countries in Asia, Europe, and Africa.
- In 2009 the "swine flu," which was referred to as *H1N1,* was considered pandemic.

CLIA-Waived Microbiology Tests

Influenza Testing (CLIA-Waved)

The OSOM influenza A & B test (Genzyme Corporation) is a qualitative lateral flow immunoassay. The kit detects the presence of influenza types A and B.

A nasal swab specimen is collected by inserting a soft foam swab approximately 1 inch into the nose (or until resistance is felt). The swab can then be placed in a dry, closed container for up to 8 hours.

The **OSOM Influenza A & B Test** procedure check sheet is provided in the workbook and is demonstrated in Procedure 8-6, located at the end of this section.

PROCEDURE 8-5 Acceava Strep A Test Procedure

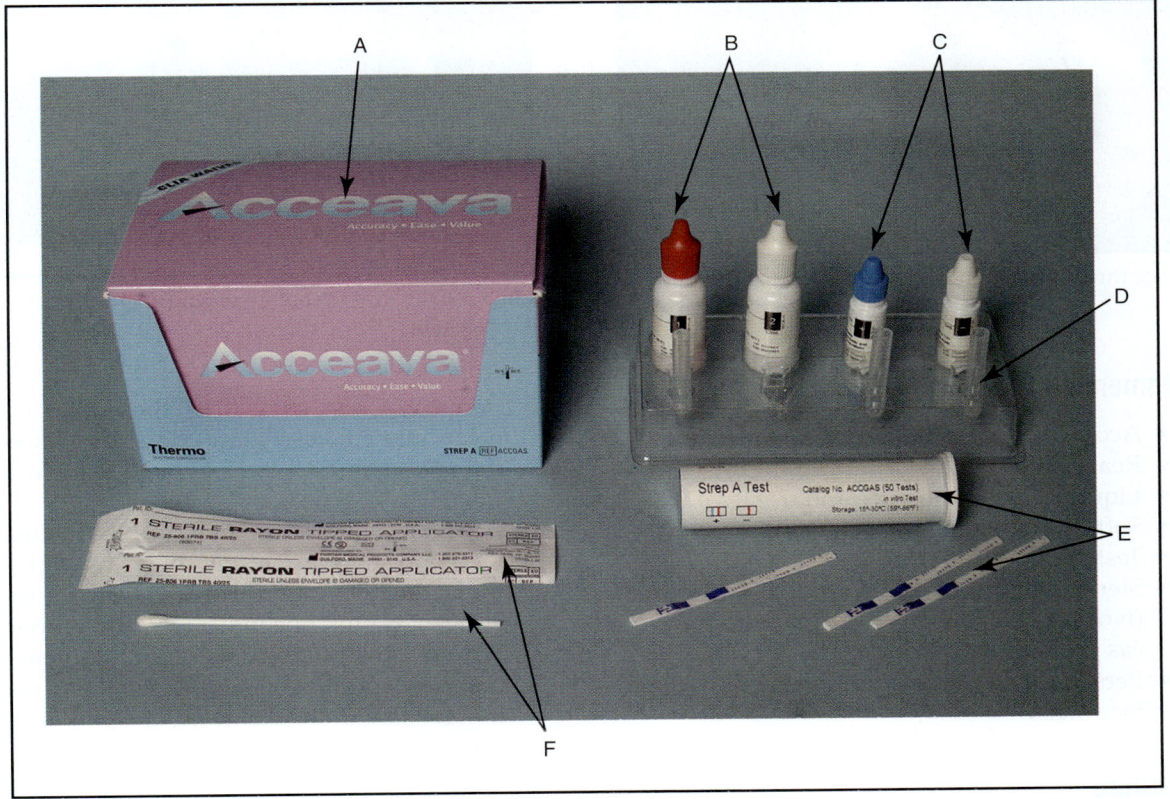

A. Acceava group A strep kit. *a*, Acceava box; *b*, reagents 1 and 2; *c*, positive and negative liquid controls; *d*, testing tubes; *e*, test sticks and container; *f*, sterile swab.

(Continued)

PROCEDURE 8-5 Acceava Strep A Test Procedure—cont'd

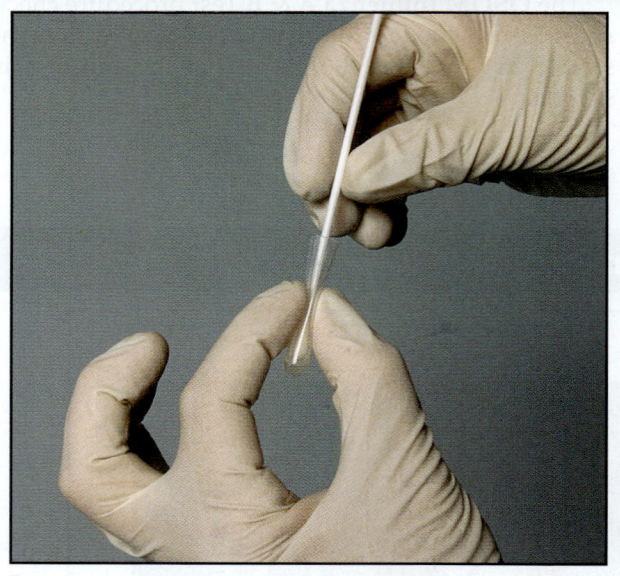

B. Place throat specimen in tube with extraction fluid.

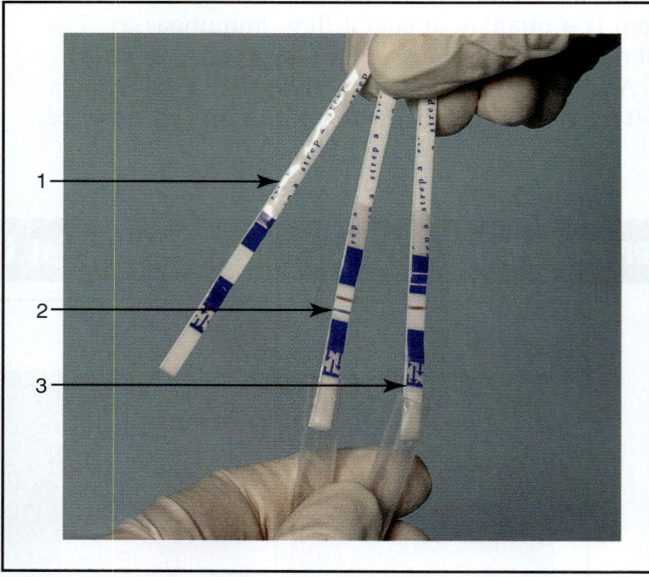

C. Reading results. *1*, Strip before testing; *2*, positive result; *3*, negative result.

Equipment and Supplies (Fig. A)

- Acceava group A *Streptococcus* test kit box
- Reagents 1 and 2
- Liquid controls, positive and negative
- Soft plastic testing tubes
- Test sticks and their container
- Sterile rayon swab taken from wrapper (NOTE: Cotton swabs may inhibit *Streptococcus* growth)
- Personal protective equipment—gloves and face mask

Procedure

1. Sanitize the hands, and apply gloves.
2. Just before testing, add 3 drops of reagent 1 and 3 drops of reagent 2 into a test tube. (The solution should turn light yellow. If it does not, do not proceed with the test.) Immediately put the rayon swab (from the test kit) containing the patient's specimen in the extract solution.
3. Vigorously mix the solution by rotating the swab forcefully against the side of the tube at least 10 times. The best results are obtained when the specimen is vigorously extracted in the solution.
4. Allow the tube containing the swab to stand for 1 minute, then squeeze the swab against the sides of the tube while withdrawing the swab (Fig. B). Discard the swab in a biohazard container.
5. Remove a test stick from the container, and recap immediately. Place the absorbent end of the test stick into the extracted sample in the tube.
6. After 5 minutes read and record the results (Fig. C). A positive test result shows as a blue line indicating the presence of *Streptococcus pyogenes* antigen. A pink line indicates that the specimen flowed up the entire strip and activated the internal control. A negative test result will show no blue line in the test area. The pink line indicates that the internal control worked.
7. Discard all the test materials in the appropriate biohazard containers.
8. Remove and discard gloves in a biohazard container, sanitize the hands, and chart the procedure.

Quality Control Procedures

Internal controls are built into each test strip. The appearance of the pink line indicates that the extracted solution passed through the test area and reacted with the pink antigenic control. If the pink line does not appear, the test is considered invalid.

External positive and negative liquid controls should be performed when a new kit is used. In addition, each operator of the test kit should perform a positive and negative control once with each test kit method to confirm that the testing technique is correct. The controls should be logged.

CLIA-Waived Microbiology Tests

PROCEDURE 8-5 Acceava Strep A Test Procedure—cont'd

The liquid control procedure is performed in the same way as the patient procedure, except for the step in which the patient swab is added to the extract solution. Instead of the patient swab, add 1 drop of well-mixed positive control to the plastic tube along with a sterile swab. Follow the directions in the patient procedure, starting with step 3. Observe and record the results in 5 minutes. Repeat the procedure with a drop of well-mixed negative control.

PROCEDURE 8-6 OSOM Influenza A and B Test Procedure

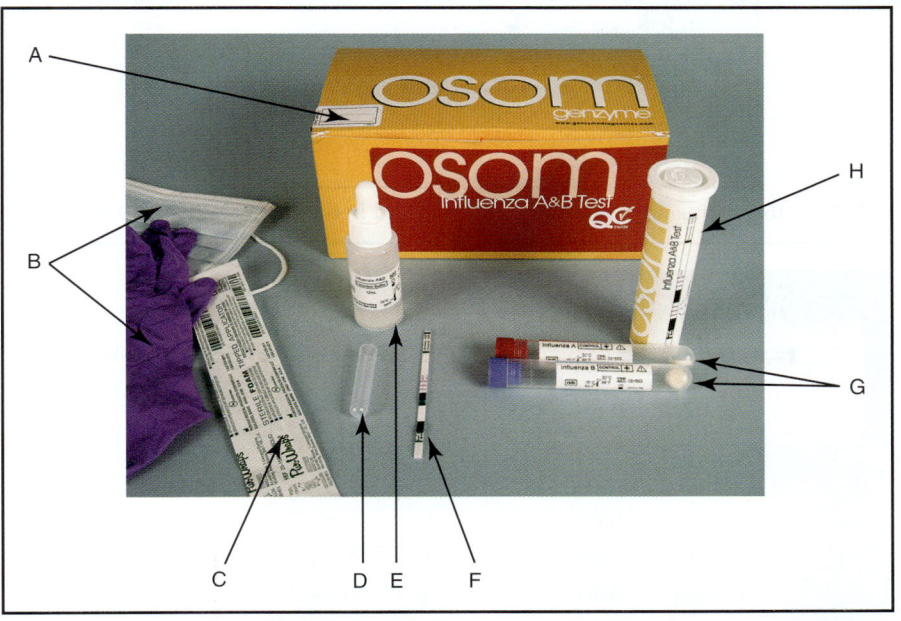

A. OSOM Influenza A & B Test Kit supplies. *a*, OSOM kit; *b*, gloves and face mask; *c*, foam swab; *d*, plastic test tube; *e*, extract solution; *f*, test strip; *g*, control swabs; *h*, container with key to results.

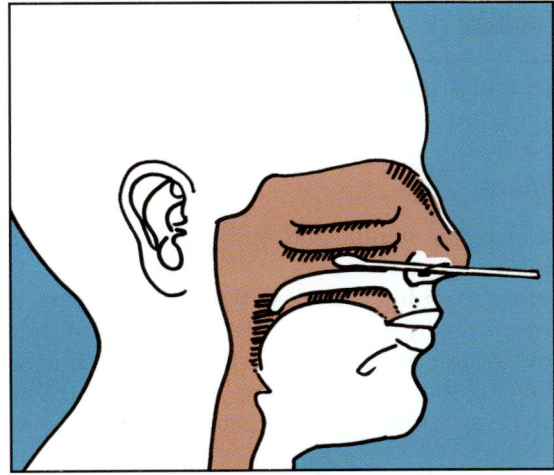

B. Collect the nasal specimen by inserting the foam swab 1 inch into the nostril displaying the most discharge, and gently rotate while rocking it back and forth.

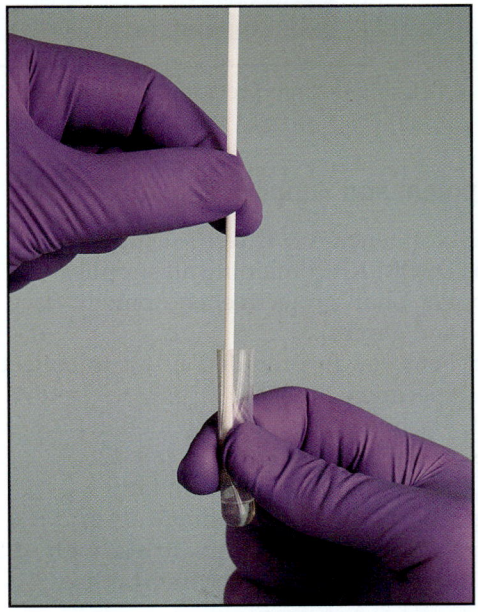

C. After mixing the nasal swab in the buffer extract solution, extract all the solution from the swab by squeezing the swab while removing it from the tube.

(Continued)

PROCEDURE 8-6 OSOM Influenza A and B Test Procedure—cont'd

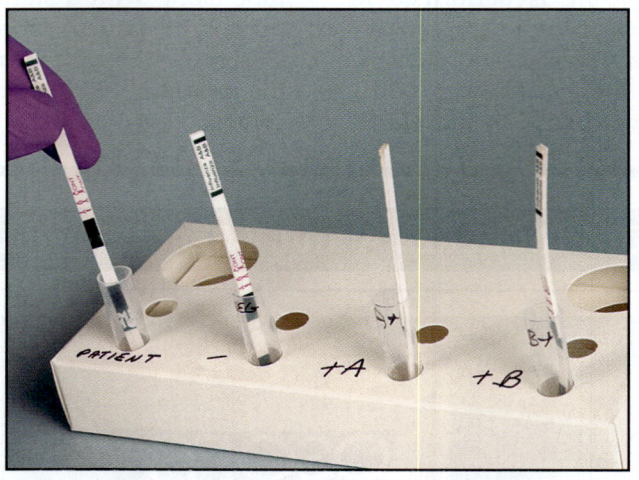

D. Place the testing strip into the extracted fluid in the tube, and wait 10 minutes.

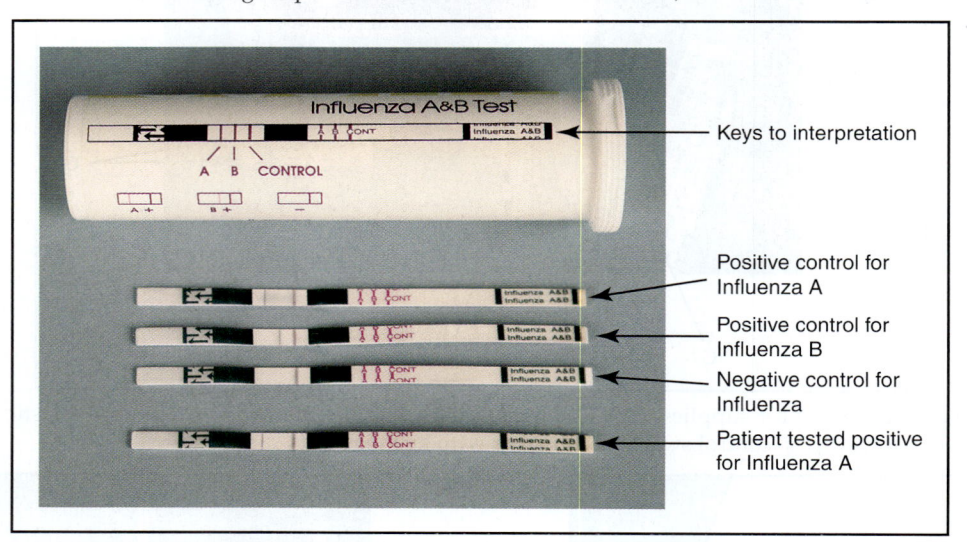

- Keys to interpretation
- Positive control for Influenza A
- Positive control for Influenza B
- Negative control for Influenza
- Patient tested positive for Influenza A

E. Using the interpretation key on the container and the control results, determine the patient's reaction.

Equipment and Supplies (Fig. A)

OSOM Influenza A & B Test Kit supplies.
- a, OSOM Kit containing all supplies
- b, Personal protective equipment (face mask and gloves)
- c, Foam swab provided in kit to collect nasal specimen
- d, Plastic testing tube provided in kit
- e, Extract solution provided in kit
- f, Testing strip provided in kit
- g, Control swabs for influenza A and B
- h, Container of testing strips with diagram showing how to interpret results.

Procedure

1. Sanitize the hands, and apply gloves and face mask.
2. Before running the first patient test from a new test kit, run a negative control test and both of the positive A and the positive B controls to see whether they react correctly. If they check out, then proceed with the patient testing.
3. Insert the foam swab provided in the test kit into the patient's nostril displaying the most secretion. Using a gentle rotation, push the swab until resistance is met at the level of the

(Continued)

Advanced Concepts 257

PROCEDURE 8-6 OSOM Influenza A and B Test Procedure—cont'd

turbinates (at least 1 inch into the nostril; see Fig. B). Rotate the swab a few times against the nasal wall, and gently rock it back and forth.

4. Place the nasal swab into the plastic tube containing the designated amount of extraction buffer solution, and vigorously twist the swab against the sides and bottom of the tube at least 10 times. This disrupts the virus particles and releases the internal viral nucleoproteins into the solution.
5. Extract all the solution from the swab by squeezing the plastic tube against the swab while removing it from the tube, as seen in Fig. C. Dispose of swab properly.
6. Dip the influenza test strip into the tube with the extraction buffer solution with the arrows on the strip pointing down, as seen in Fig. D. It takes 10 minutes for the sample to be absorbed by the strip. During this time the liquid sample migrates across the test areas and control area of the strip, and the colored reactions develop. The nucleoproteins from the virus will react with the reagents on the test strip.
7. Read the test results for Influenza A and B (Fig. E). A positive test result is shown by a pink or purple line in the "A" or "B" test area and a pink line in the internal control area. A negative test result shows no color change in the test area and a pink line in the internal control area.
8. Discard all the test materials in the appropriate biohazard containers.
9. Remove and discard gloves and mask in the biohazard container, sanitize the hands, and chart the results.

Quality Control Procedure

Internal quality controls are built into each strip. The appearance of a pink line in the control area of the strip is the positive control demonstrating that sufficient flow has occurred and the functional integrity of the test strip has been maintained. If the pink line does not appear, the test is considered invalid. A clearing of the background color is the negative internal control and verifies that the test was correctly performed. If background color appears, it will interfere with test interpretation and render the test results invalid.

External quality controls include one influenza A positive control swab and one influenza B positive control swab. The control swabs supplied in the kit are tested following the swab procedure described previously. See Fig. E for the three external control results.

- The presence of a light pink to purple line in the "A" test line position and at the "Control" line position when the influenza A positive control swab is tested indicates that the influenza antigen binding property of the test stick is functional.
- The presence of a light pink to purple line in the "B" test line position and at the "Control" line position when the influenza B positive control swab is tested indicates that the influenza antigen binding property of the test stick is functional.
- The influenza A control swab acts as a negative control for the influenza B antigen, and conversely, the influenza B control swab acts as a negative control for the influenza B antigen.

External positive and negative liquid controls should be performed when a new kit is used. In addition, each operator of the test kit should perform a positive and negative control once with each test kit method to confirm that the testing technique is correct. The control results should be logged.

Figs. A through E courtesy Zack Bent.

ADVANCED CONCEPTS

When a microbiology specimen is sent to a reference laboratory, various steps are followed in the growth, identification, and sensitivity testing of the microorganisms.

Growth Requirements of Bacteria

Identification of bacteria is made on the basis of their growth requirements, particularly their need for oxygen, carbon dioxide, and specific nutrients.

Oxygen Requirements

Of the three gases that are needed for growth—oxygen, carbon dioxide, and nitrogen—oxygen has the greatest impact on an organism's ability to adapt. Organisms can be broken down into the following two types:

- **Aerobic** organisms require oxygen for growth. *Salmonella* (some species cause enteric dysentery) is an example of an aerobe.
- **Anaerobic** organisms can grow and function in the absence of oxygen. *Clostridium tetani* is an

anaerobe found in soil. If this organism gets into a wound deep in the tissue, it will grow and produce a deadly neurotoxin that causes tetanus or lockjaw. Therefore all patients with a puncture wound should receive a tetanus injection.

Anaerobic conditions can be created by placing a gas-generating envelope into a container, adding 10 mL of water, and closing the container with a lid with an airtight seal (Fig. 8-19). The water generates hydrogen and carbon dioxide, which react with the oxygen in the container's air and create an anaerobic atmosphere. More specific organism types include the following:

- A **facultative anaerobe** is an aerobic organism that is also capable of growing in the absence of oxygen. *Staphylococci* are facultative anaerobes.
- **Microaerophilic** organisms require reduced oxygen for growth. *Campylobacter* (an organism that causes enteric dysentery) requires 5% to 6% oxygen.
- **Capnophilic** organisms require some carbon dioxide to grow. An example is *N. gonorrhoeae*, which requires 10% carbon dioxide. A 10% carbon dioxide environment can be created by putting the organism in a closed jar with a burning candle or in a 10% carbon dioxide incubator.

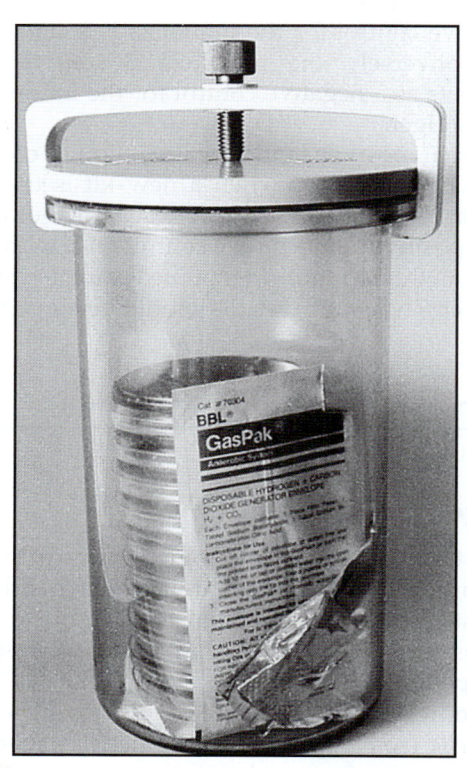

Fig. 8-19. Anaerobic jar. (From Young AP, Kennedy DB: *Kinn's the medical assistant: an applied learning approach*, ed 10, St Louis, 2007, Saunders.)

Nutrient Requirements

The nutrients that most pathogenic bacteria require outside the body are meat extracts, peptone (a nitrogen compound), mineral salts such as sulfates, chlorides, and calcium and sodium phosphates. Some organisms are **fastidious,** which means they require specific nutrients and conditions for growth. An example of a fastidious pathogen is *N. gonorrhoeae*, which requires blood serum, some amino acids, vitamins, and 10% carbon dioxide.

Media Used for Growing Bacteria

Bacteria are grown and isolated on culture media for identification purposes. Media contain essential nutritious substances that allow microorganisms to grow and multiply. Media can be solid, semisolid, or liquid. Solid media contain **agar,** a gelatinous substance obtained from seaweed that is liquid when heated and becomes solid when cooled in a **Petri dish.** When a bacterium is placed on a solid medium, it will grow and replicate until it forms a visible mass of bacteria, or a **colony.** Liquid media such as thioglycolate broth are used to grow most bacteria, including anaerobes.

Growth media can be classified as follows (Fig. 8-20):

- *Selective media* inhibit some bacteria while allowing other types to grow. MacConkey agar is an example of selective media because gram-positive organisms are inhibited from growing on this type of media.
- *Nutrient media* are made of extracts of meat and soybeans. They contain nutrients that keep bacteria alive but do not support fastidious organisms that require special nutrients.
- *Differential media* visually show the metabolic differences among types of bacteria. An example is MacConkey agar, which differentiates

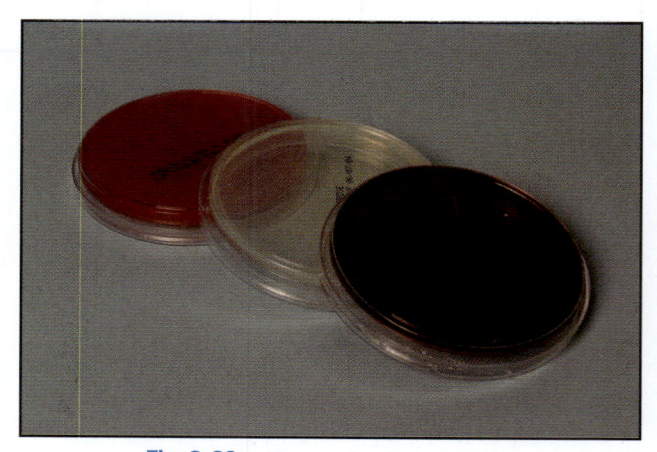

Fig. 8-20. Types of culture media.

Advanced Concepts

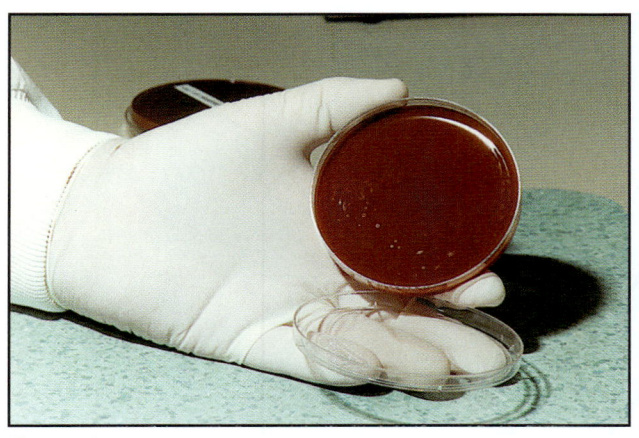

Fig. 8-21. Chocolate agar. (From Stepp CA, Woods M: *Laboratory procedures for medical office personnel*, Philadelphia, 1998, Saunders.)

between bacteria that can ferment the sugar lactose and those that cannot. The lactose fermenters are red and nonfermenters are colorless on this medium.
- *Enriched media* contain enrichment such as blood or yeast extract. Blood agar and chocolate agar are examples of enriched media. Blood agar, also referred to as a *nonselective medium*, is enriched with 5% sheep blood and grows most organisms. Chocolate agar contains blood serum, some amino acids, and vitamins and grows fastidious organisms such as *Neisseria* species (Fig. 8-21).

Microbiology Equipment

Several types of equipment used in a microbiology laboratory are very large and are not usually found in a POL. Other types are used for **inoculation** (the process of transferring microorganisms into or on a culture medium for growth) and incineration of microorganisms.

Large Equipment in a Microbiology Laboratory

Larger equipment commonly used in a microbiology laboratory includes the following:
- Incubator (37° C)—used for growing cultures at body temperature
- Safety hood—built-in area with a fan to pull the airflow away from the operator
- Autoclave—destroys microorganisms by applying steam under pressure
- Refrigerator—for storage of culture plates and supplies
- Microscopes—used to identify microorganisms

Equipment Used to Inoculate Culture Plates

The most common equipment used to transfer microorganisms from specimens to various culture media are inoculation loops and needles. The inoculating loop has a bubble wand at the end that varies in size. One type of inoculating loop is a reusable wire type that is sterilized before and after each use. Another type is a sterile disposable loop (Fig. 8-22). Loops can be calibrated to collect a precise amount of specimen. An example is the urine culture loop, made of platinum, that is calibrated to collect either 0.01 mL or 0.001 mL of urine for culturing. The inoculating needle is straight at the end and is used to pick up colonies of bacteria.

Equipment Used for Incineration

The incineration equipment used to sterilize loops and needles are Bunsen burners and electric incinerators (Fig. 8-23). Bunsen burners produce a flame by igniting natural gas that is connected to the burner. This method is dangerous because of the fire hazard and because the organisms could splatter as they are heated. The electric incinerator is much safer because it prevents splattering.

Culturing Methods

Inoculation of Media

If a patient's clinical signs and symptoms indicate that a bacterial infection is present, the physician orders a "culture and sensitivity" to determine what bacteria are present (culture) and what antibiotics will kill them (sensitivity).

After microbiology specimens are collected, they are placed on the correct media according to the source of the specimen. If the specimen is sent to the laboratory on a swab or a sterile swab is dipped into the specimen (e.g., sputum), the swab is rolled in the upper quadrant of a solid-medium Petri dish so that all sides of the swab touch the medium. If the specimen is liquid, an inoculating loop is used. The loop must be sterilized first by placing it in a Bunsen burner or incinerator until it is red and then allowing it to cool. The sterilized loop is placed in the liquid specimen and applied to the upper quadrant of the solid culture medium.

The following two techniques are used for spreading a specimen:
- The isolation technique, or *quadrant technique*, consists of using the sterilized loop to spread the specimen over four areas of the plate to establish isolated colonies of bacteria that can be used for identification (Fig. 8-24). Better isolation is

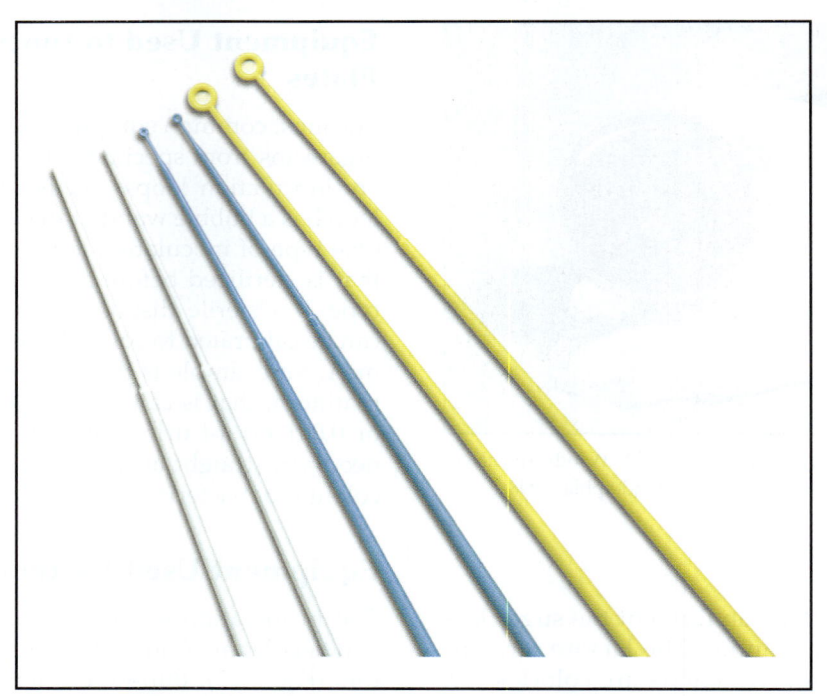

Fig. 8-22. Disposable inoculating loops. (From Young AP, Kennedy DB: *Kinn's the medical assistant: an applied learning approach*, ed 10, St Louis, 2007, Saunders. Courtesy Simport Plastics, Beloeil, Quebec.)

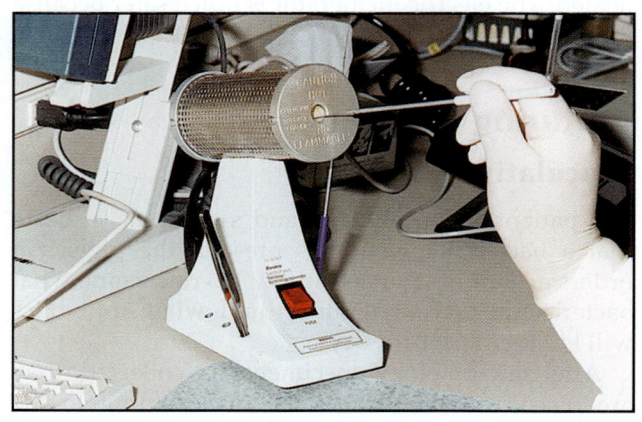

Fig. 8-23. Reusable loops and incinerator. (From Stepp CA, Woods M: *Laboratory procedures for medical office personnel*, Philadelphia, 1998, Saunders.)

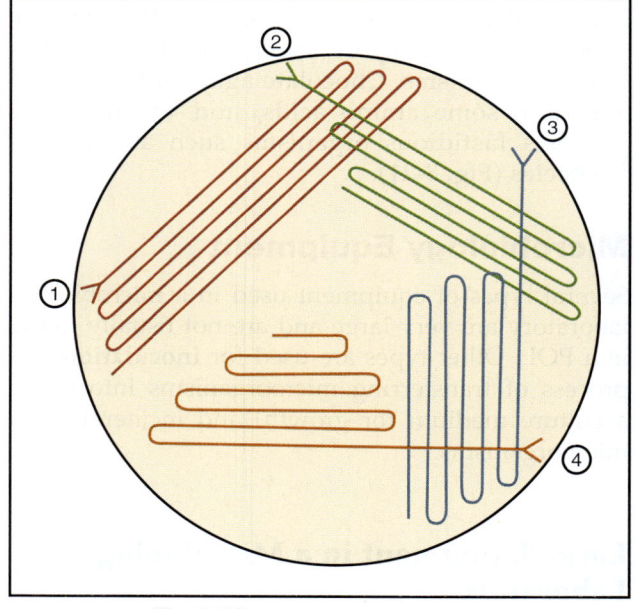

Fig. 8-24. Quadrant streaking.

achieved if the streak lines are kept close together and the loop is sterilized between quadrants.
- The *colony count*, or *lawn technique*, involves streaking the entire plate (Fig. 8-25). The lawn method is used for antibiotic testing and consists of using a swab that has been dipped in a broth containing only one kind of organism (pure culture) and swabbing the entire plate. In the colony count method, the whole plate is streaked with a calibrated loop so that the colonies that grow on the plate can be counted.

After the specimens are streaked onto the appropriate media plates, the plates are placed in an incubator with the correct amount of atmospheric gases to grow the organisms. The temperature of the incubator is usually 37° C, which is body temperature.

Urine Culture

A urine culture commonly involves performing a colony count to evaluate urinary tract infections. The urine must be collected by the midstream

Advanced Concepts

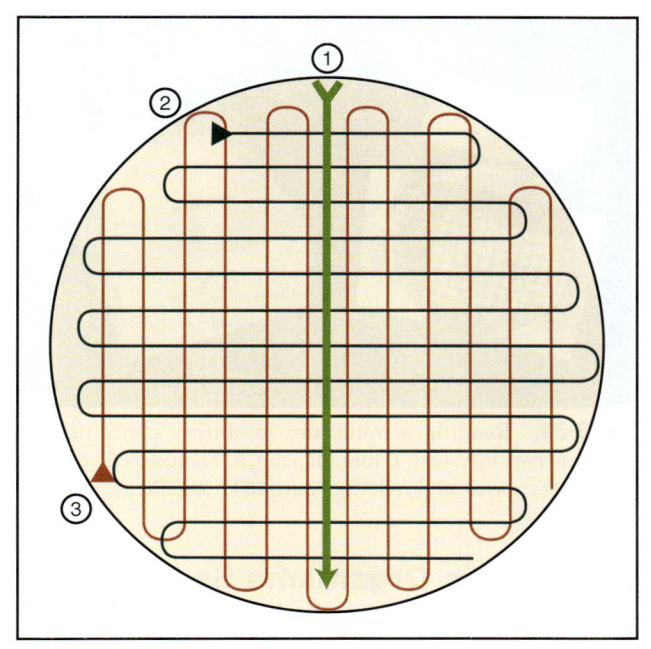

Fig. 8-25. Lawn spread or colony count streaking.

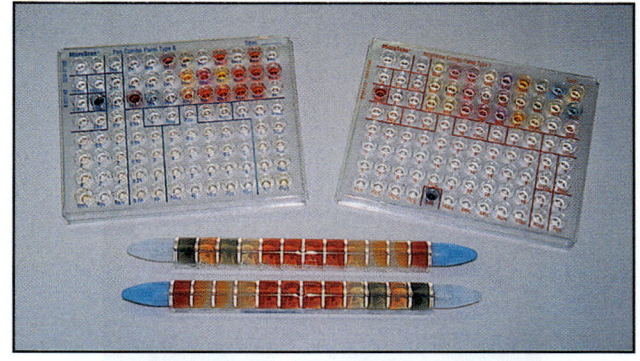

Fig. 8-26. MicroScan and Enterotube identification kits. (From Stepp CA, Woods M: *Laboratory procedures for medical office personnel*, Philadelphia, 1998, Saunders.)

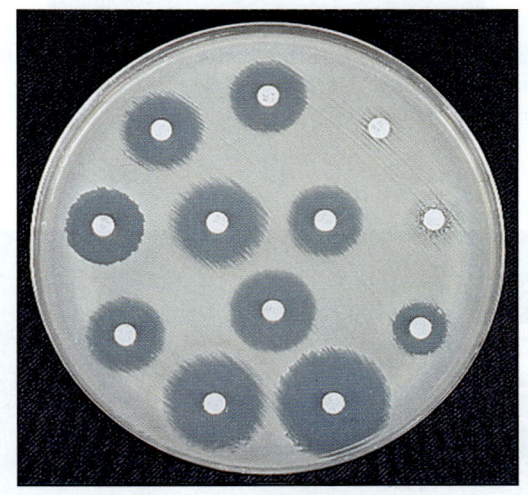

Fig. 8-27. Kirby–Bauer sensitivity test. (From Mahon CR, Manuselis G: *Textbook of diagnostic microbiology*, ed 3, St Louis, 2006, Saunders.)

clean-catch method. Following the colony count technique described previously, a calibrated loop (usually one containing 0.001 mL of specimen) is used to cover the entire culture medium plate with the urine. After the urine is incubated overnight, the colonies that form on the medium are counted. The number of colonies is multiplied by 1000 (if a 0.001-mL calibrated loop is used). Fewer than 10 colonies (10,000 per milliliter) is normal. Between 10 and 100 colonies (10,000 to 100,000 colonies per milliliter) is considered suspicious. More than 100 colonies (100,000 colonies per milliliter) indicates an infection.

Biochemical Testing

Bacteria are identified biochemically by using a pure culture that consists of only one kind of bacteria.
- Testing with enzymes takes only a few minutes. A catalase test, for example, differentiates between *Streptococcus* (negative for the enzyme catalase) and *Staphylococcus* (positive for catalase).
- Testing methods such as MicroScan (Baxter Healthcare Corp., Deerfield, Ill.) and Enterotube (Roche Inc., Nutley, N.J.) take a longer time to establish sufficient growth for testing (Fig. 8-26).
- Automated instruments such as Vitek (BioMérieux, Durham, N.C.), MicroScan, and Autobac (Pfizer Diagnostics) are used to identify bacteria. Other automated instruments, such as BACTEC (Becton Dickinson), can test for bacteria in blood cultures.

Sensitivity Testing

Physicians often order sensitivity tests to determine the type of antibiotics that would be most effective at treating patients' bacterial infections. One of the methods used for sensitivity testing is the Kirby–Bauer method. A liquid nutrient broth is inoculated with a pure culture of the bacteria grown to a specific turbidity, or cloudiness. The bacteria is then spread over the whole plate (lawn method) of the appropriate media. The Kirby–Bauer apparatus fits over the media plate and drops disks containing a specific amount of antibiotic on the bacteria. After the plates are incubated overnight, each disk on the plate is checked for zones of inhibition. The zones are measured in millimeters, compared with the manufacturer's values, and recorded as *S* (sensitive), *I* (intermediate), or *R* (resistant) (Figs. 8-27 and 8-28).

For the physician the best antibiotic is the one that is most sensitive, showing no growth of bacteria

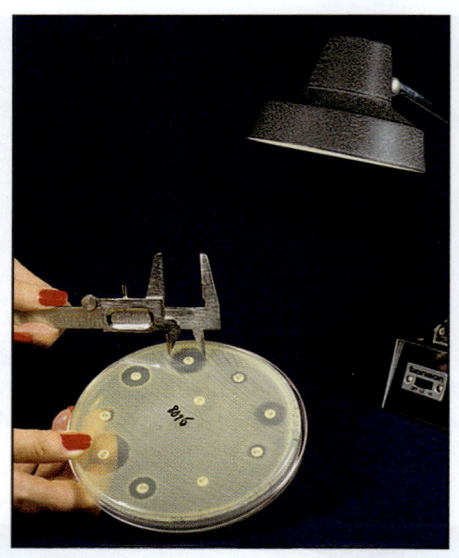

Fig. 8-28. Reading a Kirby–Bauer sensitivity test. (From Mahon CR, Manuselis G: *Textbook of diagnostic microbiology*, ed 3, St Louis, 2006, Saunders.)

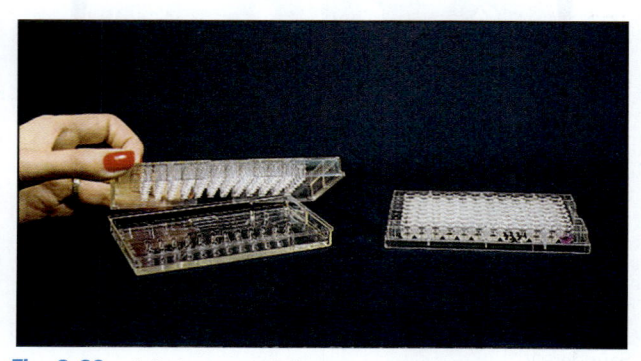

Fig. 8-29. Minimum inhibitory concentration (MIC) sensitivity test. (From Mahon CR, Manuselis G: *Textbook of diagnostic microbiology*, ed 3, St Louis, 2006, Saunders.)

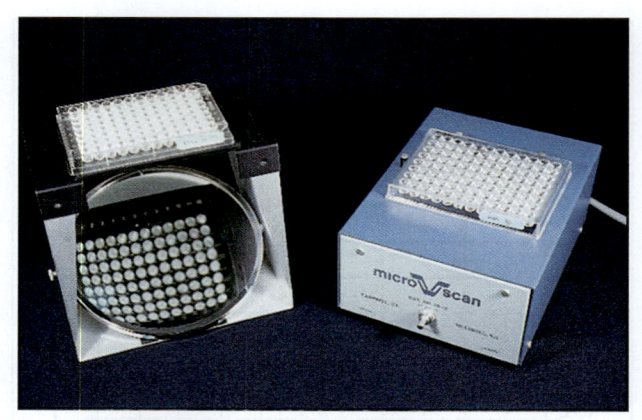

Fig. 8-30. Reading a minimum inhibitory concentration (MIC) sensitivity test. (From Mahon CR, Manuselis G: *Textbook of diagnostic microbiology*, ed 3, St Louis, 2006, Saunders.)

around the disk. It should also be the least toxic to the patient and the patient's normal flora, and it should be the most cost-effective.

Another sensitivity method consists of measuring the minimum inhibitory concentration (MIC) (Figs. 8-29 and 8-30). A liquid nutrient broth is inoculated with a pure culture of the bacteria grown to a specified turbidity. The wells in the plates contain serially diluted antibiotic solution (concentration levels are decreased in a series of proportional amounts). The same amount of bacteria is added to each well. For each antibiotic the first well of dilution that does not show any growth is the MIC. This method tells the physician exactly how much antibiotic is required to inhibit the growth of the bacteria. The interpretation can be done either by the manual method or by automated technology.

Pathogenic Organisms Seen Frequently in Physician Office Laboratories

Medical assistants should understand some of the common causes of diseases frequently seen in patients in physicians' offices. Tables 8-3 to 8-8 list common diseases caused by bacteria, fungi, and parasites. (See Tables on pp. 263-268 and Atlas on p. 269.)

Pathogenic Bacteria

The following are bacterial infections most commonly seen in the POL:
- Strep throat—*S. pyogenes,* gram-positive cocci in chains
- Urinary tract infections—*Escherichia coli, Proteus* spp., *Klebsiella* spp., *Pseudomonas aeruginosa;* all gram-negative bacilli.
- Pneumonia—*Streptococcus pneumoniae,* gram-positive diplococci (look like cat eyes) (Fig. 8-31)
- Wound infections—*S. aureus,* gram-positive cocci in clusters (Fig. 8-32). NOTE: Because of the danger of methicillin-resistant *Staphylococcus aureus* (MRSA), strict aseptic technique is necessary to prevent nosocomial infections.
- Gonorrhea—*N. gonorrhoeae,* gram-negative diplococci (kidney-bean shape, facing each other) (Fig. 8-33)
- Chlamydia—*C. trachomatis,* group of bacteria that can reproduce only in a cell

Pathogenic Fungi

The following are fungal infections commonly seen in POLs:
- Yeast infections—*C. albicans,* oval-shaped organisms that take up crystal violet and can be seen budding

TABLE 8-3 Common Diseases Caused by Bacilli

Disease	Organism	Description	Transmission	Symptoms	Tests/ Specimens	Prevention and Immunization
Tuberculosis	*Mycobacterium tuberculosis*	Acid-fast branching bacilli, anaerobic	Inhalation	Pulmonary: cough, hemoptysis, sweats, weight loss May affect other systems	Sputum for culture, radiographs, skin tests	BCG vaccine (not routinely given in the United States)
Urinary tract infections	*Escherichia coli*, *Proteus* spp., *Klebsiella* spp., *Pseudomonas aeruginosa*	Gram-negative bacilli, many flagellated	Ascends urethra; catheterization	Cystitis: frequency, burning, blood in urine Pyelonephritis: flank pain, fever	Clean-catch urine for culture and analysis	Good personal hygiene (always wipe from front to back)
C. diff infection	*Clostridium difficile*	Spore-forming, gram-positive, anaerobic bacilli	Nosocomial direct contact with contaminated equipment and hands. Patients on antibiotic therapy are susceptible.	Diarrhea, fever, nausea, belly pain, colitis	Stool culture and toxin confirmation followed by endoscopy	Antibiotics taken only as prescribed; proper washing of hands and equipment after bowel movements
Legionnaires' disease	*Legionella pneumophila*	Gram-negative bacillus (stains poorly with usual methods)	Grows freely in water (air-conditioning systems)	Pneumonia-like symptoms	Sputum, blood	Isolation
Tetanus (lockjaw)	*Clostridium tetani*	Gram-positive spore-forming bacilli; anaerobic	Open wounds, fractures, punctures	Toxin affects motor nerves; muscle spasms, convulsions, rigidity	Blood	DPT vaccine in childhood; T or Td every 10 years
Gas gangrene	*Clostridium perfringens*	Gram-positive spore-forming bacilli; anaerobic	Wounds	Gas and watery exudate in infected wound	Swab, aspirate of wound for culture	Proper wound care
Botulism	*Clostridium botulinum*	Gram-positive spore-forming bacilli; anaerobic	Improperly cooked canned foods	Neurotoxin affects speech, swallowing, vision; paralysis of respiratory muscles; death	Contaminated food, blood	Botulinus antitoxin; canned goods boiled for 20 minutes before tasting or eating
Diphtheria respiratory secretions	*Corynebacterium diphtheriae*	Gram-positive bacilli; club shaped		Sore throat, fever, headache, gray membrane in throat	Swabs; Gram stain, culture; Schick test for immunity	DPT in childhood

(Continued)

TABLE 8-3 Common Diseases Caused by Bacilli—cont'd

Disease	Organism	Description	Transmission	Symptoms	Tests/ Specimens	Prevention and Immunization
Whooping cough	*Bordetella pertussis*	Gram-negative bacilli	Respiratory sections	Upper respiratory tract symptoms; high-pitched crowing "whoop"	Swabs for culture	DPT in childhood
Plague	*Yersinia pestis*	Gram-negative bacilli	Flea bite from infected rodents	Fever and chills, delirium; enlarged, painful lymph nodes	Sputum for culture, blood	Vaccine, rodent control

BCG, Bacille Calmette-Guérin vaccine; *DPT*, diphtheria–pertussis–tetanus vaccine; *T*, tetanus (toxoid); *Td*, tetanus and diphtheria (toxoids). Modified from Young AP, Kennedy DB: *Kinn's the medical assistant: an applied learning approach*, ed 10, St Louis, 2007, Saunders.

- Dermatophyte infections (athlete's foot, jock itch, ringworm)—*Trichophyton* spp., *Microsporum* spp., and others (see hyphae in KOH preparation)

Parasites and Protozoa

The following are pathogenic parasites frequently seen in the POL:
- Pinworm—*E. vermicularis*
- Giardiasis—*Giardia lamblia,* protozoan flagellate that causes gastrointestinal symptoms (Fig. 8-34)
- Trichomonas—*T. vaginalis*
- Lice—*Pediculus humanus* (body louse) (Fig. 8-35), *Phthirus pubis* (crab louse, or crab) (Fig. 8-36)

Emerging Infectious Diseases

The relation between microorganisms and diseases is not fixed. New infectious diseases may emerge suddenly, whereas others seem to disappear and then reemerge. According to most experts, the rate at which infectious diseases emerge and reemerge has risen in recent years. Some of the most important reasons for this trend are the growth of human populations, the rise in international travel, and environmental changes. Table 8-9 on p. 270 lists some emerging diseases and the microorganisms that cause them (causative agents).

Bioterrorism

As a result of the bioterrorism threats that occurred in the aftermath of 9/11, all laboratories (including POLs) should perform a risk assessment. Laboratories must identify procedures and methods that have the potential to produce **aerosols** (fine particles suspended in the air). The use of biosafety cabinets or hoods when performing tasks is one way to avoid exposure to aerosols. The Centers for Disease Control and Prevention recommend referring any suspicious organisms or substances to the proper authorities and practicing the proper biosafety techniques at all times.

Most of the bacteria, viruses, and toxins used as bioterrorism agents can be spread by an aerosol route, which is very stable. They also produce high **morbidity** (rate of illness) and **mortality** (rate of deaths) rates. Other bioterrorism agents are transmitted person to person, and some are difficult to treat.

Agents Used in Bacterial Bioterrorism

Anthrax (See Atlas on p. 271)

Anthrax, caused by *Bacillus anthracis,* is a very old disease—the fifth plague of the Bible (Fig. 8-37). It is a disease of livestock, which become infected after feeding on plants contaminated with the organism. Human beings contract the disease mostly through contact with infected animals or animal products. On Gram stain the organism is a gram-positive bacillus. *Endospores,* as seen in the spore stain, can live for 40 years (Fig. 8-38). The spores must be ground into a very fine powder before they can penetrate deep into the lungs and cause infection.

Three forms of anthrax can be contracted in human beings: cutaneous, inhalation (or pulmonary), and gastrointestinal.
- *Cutaneous anthrax*—Blisters form and develop into blackened craters, called *eschars* (Fig. 8-39). These may heal spontaneously or be treated with penicillin. If the anthrax organism enters the blood and produces substantial quantities of toxin, however, antibiotics are no longer effective.

Advanced Concepts

TABLE 8-4 Common Diseases Caused by Cocci

Disease	Organism	Description	Transmission	Symptoms	Specimens	Tests	Prevention
Pneumonia	*Streptococcus pneumoniae*	Gram-positive encapsulated cocci in pairs	Direct contact, droplets	Productive cough, fever, chest pain	Sputum, bronchoscopy secretions	Culture, Gram stain	Vaccine
Strep throat	*Streptococcus pyogenes* (group A strep)	Gram-positive cocci in chains	Direct contact, droplets, fomites	Severe sore throat, fever, malaise	Direct swab	Rapid strep test, throat culture	None
Wound infection, abscesses, boils	*Staphylococcus aureus* and Methicillin-resistant *Staphylococcus aureus* (MRSA)	Gram-positive cocci in clusters	Direct contact, fomites, carriers; poor hand washing	Area red, warm, swollen; pus; pain; ulceration or sinus formation	Deep swab, aspirate of drainage	Culture and sensitivity (aerobic and anaerobic)	None
Staphylococcal food poisoning	*Staphylococcus aureus*	Gram-positive cocci in clusters	Poor hygiene and improper refrigeration of foods	Vomiting, abdominal cramps, diarrhea	Suspected food, stool	Culture of food (organism will not be found in stool)	Properly refrigerated food to prevent toxin production
Toxic shock	*Staphylococcus aureus*	Gram-positive cocci in clusters	Use of absorbent pack materials (e.g., tampons, nasal packs)	Fever, headache, nausea, vomiting, delirium, low blood pressure	Swab, blood	Culture and serology	Frequent changing of tampons, packing material
Gonorrhea	*Neisseria gonorrhoeae*	Gram-negative cocci in pairs; intracellular in white blood cells	Sexually transmitted	Women: pelvic pain, discharge; may be asymptomatic Men: urethral drip, pain on urination	Swab of cervix, urethra; rectal and pharyngeal swabs in homosexuals	Gram stain, culture	Avoidance of unprotected sex
Meningococcal meningitis	*Neisseria meningitidis*	Gram-negative diplococci	Respiratory tract secretions	High fever, headache, projectile vomiting, delirium, neck and back rigidity, convulsions, petechial rash	Nasopharyngeal swabs, cerebrospinal fluid, blood	Gram stain, culture, cell counts and chemistries	Vaccine, prophylactic antibiotics

Modified from Young AP, Kennedy DB: *Kinn's the medical assistant: an applied learning approach*, ed 10, St Louis, 2007, Saunders.

TABLE 8-5 Common Diseases Caused by Spirilla

Disease	Organism	Description	Transmission	Symptoms	Tests/Specimens	Prevention and Immunization
Syphilis	*Treponema pallidum*	Spirochete	Sexually, congenitally	Primary: painless sore (chancre) Secondary: generalized rash involving palms and soles of feet Congenital: birth defects	Blood for serological tests: VDRL, RPR, FTA-ABS	Avoidance of unprotected sex
Lyme disease	*Borrelia burgdorferi*	Spirochete	Tick bite	Fever, joint pain, red bull's-eye rash	Swab for culture	Avoidance of tick-infested areas
Pyloric ulcers	*Helicobacter pylori*	Gram-negative, spiral-shaped	Unknown, possibly food and water	Burning pain in stomach, especially between meals	Stomach biopsy for staining and culture; stool for EIA testing	Unknown
Food poisoning (most common cause in United States)	*Campylobacter jejuni*	Paired gram-negative curved rods forming a seagull shape	Contaminated food, water, and milk	Bloody or watery diarrhea	Stool for dark field microscopy	Sanitary food preparation and control of water and milk supplies

VDRL, Venereal Disease Research Laboratory; *RPR*, rapid plasma reagin (test); *FTA-ABS*, fluorescent treponemal antibody absorption (test); *EIA*, enzyme immunoassays.
From Young AP, Kennedy DB: *Kinn's the medical assistant: an applied learning approach*, ed 10, St Louis, 2007, Saunders.

TABLE 8-6 Diseases Caused by Rickettsia, Chlamydia, and Mycoplasma

Disease	Organism	Transmission	Symptoms	Tests/Specimens
Rocky Mountain spotted fever	*Rickettsia rickettsii*	Tick bite	Headache, chills, fever, characteristic rash on extremities and trunk	Blood for serological tests, skin biopsy for direct fluorescent microscopy
Typhus	*Rickettsia prowazekii*	Tick bite	Fever, rash, confusion	Blood for serology
Atypical (walking) pneumonia	*Mycoplasma pneumoniae*	Respiratory secretions	Fever, cough, chest pain	Blood, sputum
Nongonococcal urethritis and vaginitis	*Chlamydia trachomatis*	Sexual	May be asymptomatic	Swabs for culture and serological testing
Inclusion conjunctivitis, pneumonia		Congenital	Severe conjunctivitis in newborns; afebrile pneumonia in newborns	

From Young AP, Kennedy DB: *Kinn's the medical assistant: an applied learning approach*, ed 10, St Louis, 2007, Saunders.

Advanced Concepts

TABLE 8-7 Common Diseases Caused by Fungi

Disease	Organism	Predisposing Conditions and Transmission	Symptoms	Tests/Specimens
Thrush (oral yeast), vulvovaginal candidiasis, or Monilia (vaginal yeast)	Candida spp. (yeast)	Oral: during birth; other: after antibiotic therapy, oral birth control, severe diabetes	White, cheesy growth	Swab for KOH prep, culture
Athlete's foot, jock itch, ringworm (tinea)	Trichophyton spp., Microsporum spp., and others (skin fungi)	Opportunistic; direct contact; clothing; prolonged exposure to moist environment	Hair loss, thickening of skin, nails; itching; red, scaly patches	Skin scraping for KOH prep; skin, hair for culture
Histoplasmosis	Histoplasma capsulatum	Inhalation of dust contaminated with bird or bat droppings	Mild, flulike to system	Serological, culture of biopsy material
Cryptococcosis	Cryptococcus neoformans	Contact with poultry droppings	Cough, fever, malaise; can become systemic	Sputum culture
Sporotrichosis	Sporothrix schenckii	Farmers, florists, people exposed to soil	Skin lesions that spread along lymphatics, can become systemic	Cerebrospinal fluid culture, India ink direct examination, scrapings, serological KOH, potassium hydroxide
Pneumocystis pneumonia	Pneumocystis carinii	Widely prevalent in animals; occurs in debilitated persons, immunosuppressed; common in patients with acquired immune-deficiency syndrome (AIDS)	Pneumonia-like	Biopsy

From Young AP, Kennedy DB: *Kinn's the medical assistant: an applied learning approach*, ed 10, St Louis, 2007, Saunders.

- *Inhalation or pulmonary anthrax:* Naturally occurring pulmonary anthrax is rare. It can be an occupational hazard for those who work with contaminated wool and inhale the spores (hence the nickname "woolsorter's disease"). Before September 2001 the last case of inhalation anthrax in the United States occurred in 1978. In September and October 2001, anthrax was spread through letters in the mail. The cutaneous form developed in a number of people, and at least 10 contracted the inhalation form. Six of those 10 survived, probably because they were treated early with combinations of antibiotics—ciprofloxacin or doxycycline along with one or more other antibiotics effective against anthrax.
- *Gastrointestinal anthrax:* Intestinal eschars, similar to those produced by cutaneous anthrax, are characteristic of this disease. It can progress to generalized toxemia. The mortality rate is 50% to 100% despite treatment.

Plague

In the Middle Ages between a quarter and a third of the population of Europe was killed by the plague. In 1891 approximately 6 million people died as a result of the plague in India. Currently, only a dozen cases are reported in the United States each year. The plague is known as the "black death" because in its later stages, in untreated patients, the blood vessels are destroyed and subcutaneous bleeding leads to black spots on the skin.

Yersinia pestis, the causative agent of the plague, is a gram-negative bacillus that may resemble a safety pin (bipolar staining). The disease primarily affects rodents, but it is transferred to human beings by flea bites. Two forms of the plague are the following:

- Bubonic plague results from flea bites. The incubation period is 2 to 6 days. The symptoms are sudden headache, fever, **malaise** (feeling of weakness, distress, or discomfort), **myalgia** (diffuse muscular pain), and tender lymph nodes (buboes).

TABLE 8-8 Common Protozoan and Parasitic Diseases

Disease	Organism	Transmission	Symptoms	Tests/Specimens
Malaria	*Plasmodium* spp. (protozoa)	Bite of the *Anopheles* mosquito	Chills, fever (cyclic)	Blood: examination of stained blood for parasites
Toxoplasmosis	*Toxoplasma gondii* (protozoa)	Fecal contamination (cat litter), congenital	Febrile illness, rash; congenital: jaundice, enlarged liver and spleen, brain abnormalities	Skin test
Amoebic dysentery	*Entamoeba histolytica* (protozoa)	Fecal contamination of food and water	Bloody diarrhea, cramping, fever	Stool for O&P
Giardiasis	*Giardia lamblia* (protozoa)	Common in intestinal tract, opportunistic; contaminated surface water	Asymptomatic to severe diarrhea and abdominal discomfort	Stool for O&P, intestinal biopsy, string test
Trichinosis	*Trichinella spiralis* (roundworm)	Ingestion of undercooked pork or bear meat	Nausea, fever, diarrhea, muscle pain and swelling, edema of face	Biopsy, blood tests
Tapeworm	*Taenia* spp. *Diphyllobothrium latum*	Undercooked meats (beef and pork) Undercooked fish; common among Norwegians, Japanese	Abdominal discomfort, diarrhea, weight loss; as above, may become anemia	Stool for O&P Stool for O&P
Pinworm	*Enterobius vermicularis* (roundworm)	Fecal–oral	Severe rectal itching, restlessness, insomnia	Adhesive tape applied to perianal region for ova
Scabies	Itch mite: *Sarcoptes scabiei*	Direct contact, clothing, bedding	Nocturnal itching, skin burrows	Skin scrapings for parasites
Lice	*Pediculus humanus*, *Pthirus pubis* (crabs)	Direct contact, clothing, bedding, furniture (can transmit other diseases by bite)	Intense itching, skin lesions	Finding adult lice or eggs (nits) on body or hair

O&P, Ova and parasites.
From Young AP, Kennedy DB: *Kinn's the medical assistant: an applied learning approach*, ed 10, St Louis, 2007, Saunders.

- Pneumonic plague is spread person to person by respiratory droplets or develops from bubonic plague into a systemic infection that affects the lungs. If the disease is not treated, the mortality rate is 100%.

Tularemia

Tularemia is caused by *Francisella tularensis*, a gram-negative bacillus. Human beings are usually infected after being bitten by infected rabbits or ticks. The disease is characterized by fever and flulike symptoms. The patient may develop ulcerated skin lesions with localized lymph node enlargement as the result of direct contact.

Pneumonic tularemia may result from exposure to aerosols. The incubation period is 3 to 5 days, with the abrupt onset of chills, fever, headache, myalgia, and nonproductive cough. The mortality rate is 30% if the disease is untreated and less than 10% if treated.

Viruses Used in Bioterrorism

Smallpox

Some historians believe that smallpox has killed more people than any other disease (300 million deaths in the twentieth century). As of 1980 smallpox was declared eradicated, thanks to vaccination programs around the world. This victory over smallpox could be in jeopardy if it were to be used as a weapon of bioterrorism.

The severity of the disease depends on the virus that is causing it. *Variola major*, the most virulent strain, causes severe blistering and high fever and kills approximately half of those affected. *Variola minor* is a milder form, with a mortality rate of less than 1%. Some of the complications of smallpox are encephalitis, keratitis, and infections of pregnancy.

A vaccine made from live *Vaccinia* virus (not *Variola*) is available and is given intradermally with a bifurcated needle. After vaccination a pustular lesion develops, with induration surrounding a scab.

Advanced Concepts

Common Pathogenic Organisms

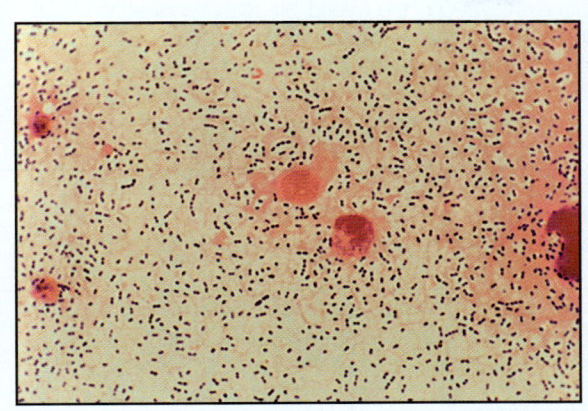

Fig. 8-31. *Streptococcus pneumoniae* Gram stain. (From Mahon CR, Manuselis G: *Textbook of diagnostic microbiology*, ed 3, St Louis, 2006, Saunders.)

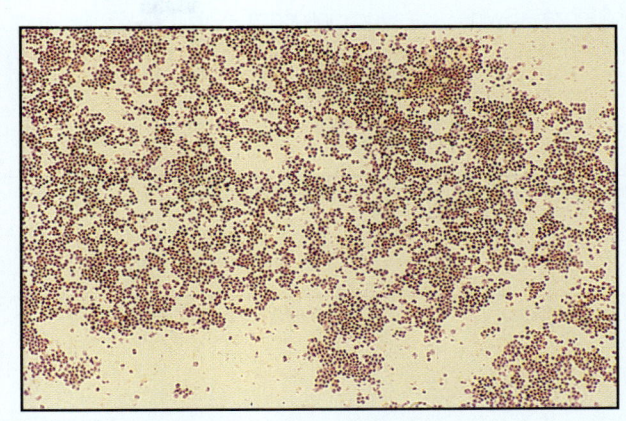

Fig. 8-32. *Staphylococcus aureus* Gram stain. (From Mahon CR, Manuselis G: *Textbook of diagnostic microbiology*, ed 3, St Louis, 2006, Saunders.)

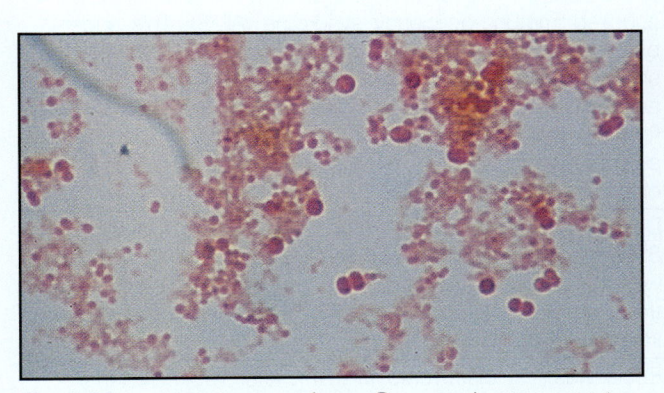

Fig. 8-33. *Neisseria gonorrhoeae* Gram stain. (From Mahon CR, Manuselis G: *Textbook of diagnostic microbiology*, ed 3, St Louis, 2006, Saunders.)

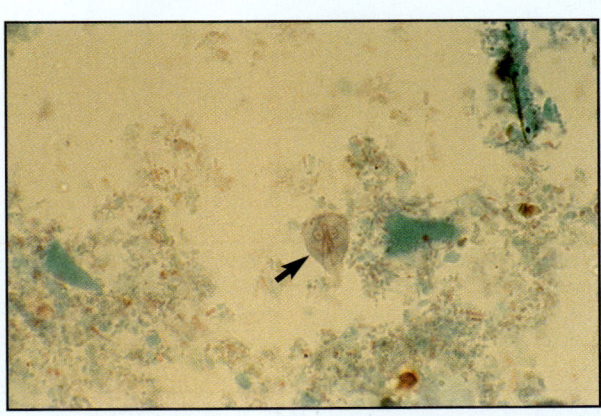

Fig. 8-34. *Giardia lamblia* smear. (From Mahon CR, Manuselis G: *Textbook of diagnostic microbiology*, ed 3, St Louis, 2006, Saunders.)

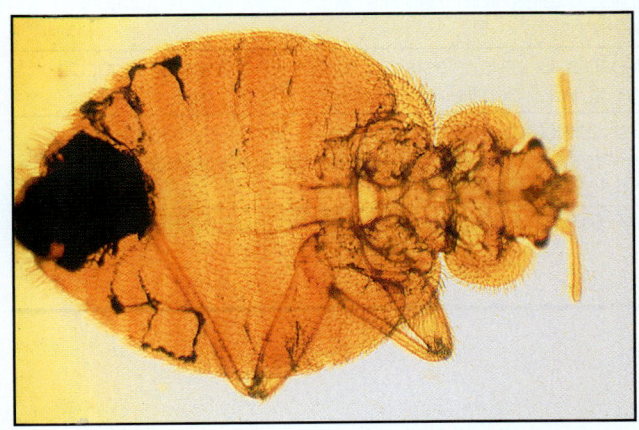

Fig. 8-35. Body louse. (From Stepp CA, Woods M: *Laboratory procedures for medical office personnel*, Philadelphia, 1998, Saunders.)

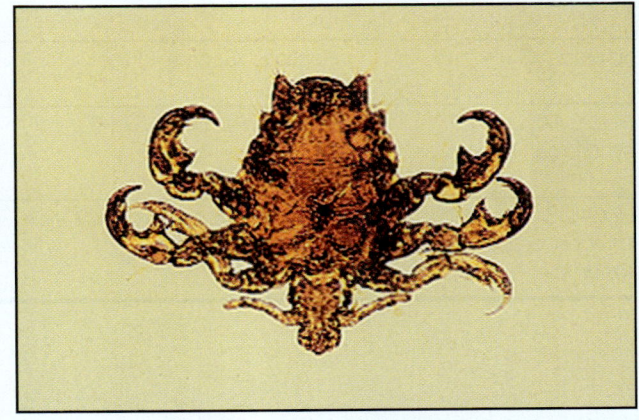

Fig. 8-36. Pubic louse, also called crab louse. (From Mahon CR, Manuselis G: *Textbook of diagnostic microbiology*, ed 3, St Louis, 2006, Saunders.)

TABLE 8-9 Some Emerging Infectious Diseases

Disease	Causative Agent	Description
Influenza—Swine	Influenza A (H1N1)	On June 11, 2009, the World Health Organization (WHO) signaled that a pandemic of 2009 H1N1 flu was under way. The virus had mutated genes from former flu viruses that normally circulated in pigs in Europe and Asia and in bird (avian) genes and human genes. Scientists called this a "quadruple reassortant" virus.
Influenza—Avian	Influenza A (H5N1)	In 1997 a novel strain of flu virus was discovered in poultry in South Asia and China. In 2005 it became widespread in humans, including those in 50 countries in Asia, Europe, and Africa.
C-diff colitis	Clostridium difficile	Major cause of colitis and antibiotic-induced diarrhea. It produces two toxins, which cause inflammation of the intestinal wall (colitis) along with diarrhea, abdominal pain, and fever. It is one of the most common hospital (nosocomial) infections around the world. As of 2009, it was becoming resistant to most antibiotics. Treatment is by discontinuing antibiotics and starting specific anticlostridial antibiotics, such as metronidazole.
MRSA	Methicillin-resistant Staphylococcus aureus	In 2005 the Centers for Disease Control and Prevention reported more deaths attributed to MRSA than to acquired immune-deficiency syndrome (AIDS). This superbug caused nosocomial wound infections such as toxic shock syndrome, scalded skin syndrome, scarlet fever, erysipelas and impetigo, and pneumonia. The antibiotic-resistant staph also emerged in the community, causing skin infections, such as pimples and boils, to occur in otherwise healthy people.
Severe acute respiratory syndrome (SARS)	Coronavirus	During November 2002 through July 2003, a total of 8098 people worldwide became sick with SARS, which was accompanied by either pneumonia or respiratory distress syndrome (probable cases), according to the World Health Organization.
Ebola	Ebola virus	Ebola was first discovered in 1977 after two simultaneous outbreaks in Africa (Sudan and Congo). It causes fever, extensive bleeding, and destruction of internal organs.
Hantavirus pulmonary syndrome	Sin nombre virus	Hantavirus was first isolated in 1993 in the southwestern United States from patients with highly fatal respiratory infections.
Hepatitis C	Hepatitis C virus	Hepatitis C virus infects up to 3% of the world's population. It was identified in 1989.
Hemolytic uremic syndrome	Escherichia coli O157:H7	First detected in 1982, hemolytic uremic syndrome is a life-threatening condition characterized by severe anemia and kidney failure.
HIV/AIDS (acquired immune deficiency syndrome)	Human immunodeficiency virus	HIV, first discovered in 1981, is the cause of AIDS.

Advanced Concepts

Viral Hemorrhagic Fever

Viral hemorrhagic fever is thought by some to be the most lethal disease known to man. The Ebola virus is one of the causes of hemorrhagic fever and is classified in one of the four families that include hemorrhagic viruses (Ebola is in the Filoviridae family). Ebola was first discovered in 1977 after two simultaneous outbreaks of the fever in Africa (Sudan and Congo). In 1995 an outbreak of viral hemorrhagic fever in Kikwit, Democratic Republic of the Congo, took 190 lives. The fever is spread by direct contact with infected blood or body parts. In the Kikwit outbreak, Ebola was spread when bodies were prepared for burial and organs were manually removed. The disease is characterized by high fever, extensive bleeding, and destruction of internal organs.

Biological Toxin Used in Bioterrorism

Botulism

Clostridium botulinum produces a neurotoxin, botulinum, which is the most poisonous natural substance known. It causes dry mouth, dilated pupils, and a progressive muscle weakness that leads to respiratory failure and death. There are seven types of botulism toxin, but types A, B, and E are most commonly associated with human disease. Toxin A is the most potent. A lethal dose of botulinum toxin is measured in nanograms, an amount that cannot be seen.

Anthrax

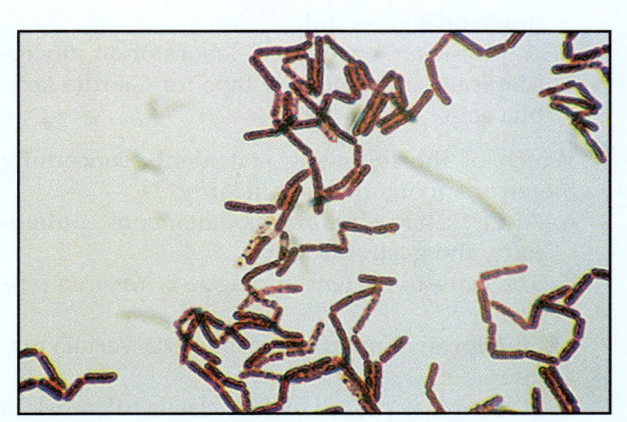

Fig. 8-37. *Bacillus anthracis* Gram stain. (From Mahon CR, Manuselis G: *Textbook of diagnostic microbiology*, ed 3, St Louis, 2006, Saunders.)

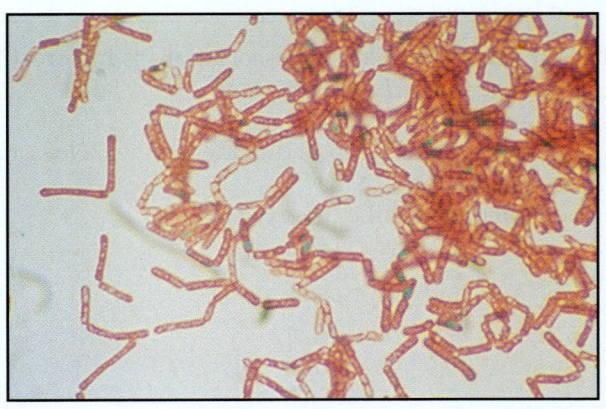

Fig. 8-38. *Bacillus anthracis* endospores seen in spore stain. (From Mahon CR, Manuselis G: *Textbook of diagnostic microbiology*, ed 3, St Louis, 2006, Saunders.)

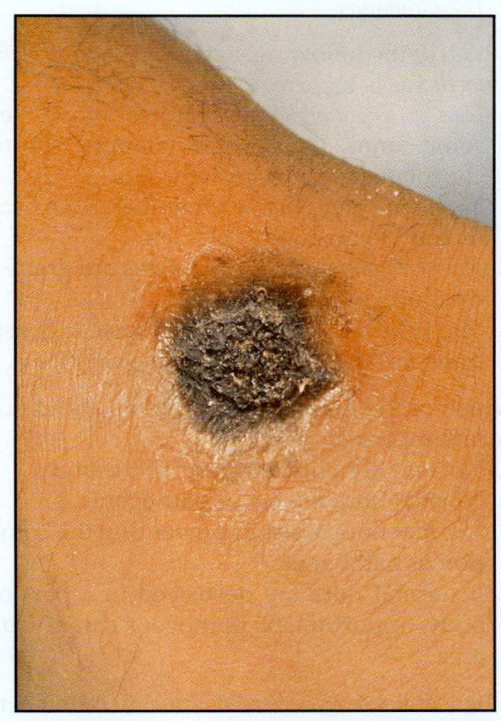

Fig. 8-39. Cutaneous anthrax eschar. (Courtesy the Centers for Disease Control and Prevention.)

Review Questions

1. Which of the following statements is incorrect?
   a. The most important step in the Gram stain procedure is the decolorizer step.
   b. If too much decolorizer has been applied, at the end of the Gram stain procedure all the organisms will be pink/red.
   c. At the end of the decolorizer step, the gram-positive organisms are purple and the gram-negative organisms are colorless.
   d. If too little decolorizer has been applied, at the end of the Gram stain procedure all the organisms will be pink/red.

2. Which of the following organisms is gram positive? (Hint: Check "Pathogenic Bacteria" and Tables 8-3 and 8-4.)
   a. *Escherichia coli*
   b. *Proteus*
   c. *Staphylococcus*
   d. *Pseudomonas*

3. Which of the following statements about *Neisseria gonorrhoeae* is incorrect?
   a. *Neisseria gonorrhoeae* requires blood serum, some amino acids, and vitamins (found in chocolate agar) for growth.
   b. *Neisseria gonorrhoeae* requires 10% carbon dioxide for growth.
   c. *Neisseria gonorrhoeae* organisms are gram-positive cocci in pairs.
   d. The JEMBEC transportation system is used to transport and grow *Neisseria gonorrhoeae*.

4. Which of the following statements about normal flora is incorrect?
   a. Normal flora inhabit parts of the body.
   b. Normal flora are never pathogenic.
   c. Normal flora assist in preventing the colonization of pathogens.
   d. If normal flora are destroyed in a part of the body, opportunistic pathogens can invade the area.

5. When collecting a throat specimen for a rapid strep test, which of the following steps is incorrect?
   a. Use a cotton swab.
   b. Have the patient sit with head back.
   c. Use a sterile tongue depressor to hold down the tongue, and have patient say "ahh."
   d. Rotate the swab on the back of throat in a circular motion or figure-of-eight pattern.

6. In the aftermath of the 9/11 bioterrorism threats, all laboratories (including POLs) should do which of the following?
   a. Identify procedures and methods that have the potential to produce aerosols.
   b. Refer any suspicious organisms or substances to the proper authorities.
   c. Use proper biosafety techniques at all times.
   d. All of the above.

7. Which of the following statements about pinworm testing is incorrect?
   a. The female pinworm normally lays her eggs during the night in the anal area of the human host.
   b. The cellulose tape test consists of pressing cellulose tape (sticky side) over the patient's anal area.
   c. The tape is placed with the tape sticky side down on a glass slide.
   d. A physician or trained laboratorian microscopically examines the tape for Giardia lamblia eggs.

8. Which of the following statements concerning bioterrorism organisms is incorrect?
   a. Anthrax has three forms: cutaneous, pulmonary, and gastrointestinal.
   b. The causative agent of plague is Yersinia pestis.
   c. Smallpox is caused by the bacteria Variola major.
   d. Tularemia is caused by Francisella tularensis, a gram-negative bacillus.

9. Name the three sources from which smears on slides are made.
   a. _____
   b. _____
   c. _____

10. Which of the following associations is incorrect?
    a. anaerobe/*Clostridium tetani*
    b. aerobe/oxygen
    c. capnophilic (carbon dioxide–loving)/*Neisseria gonorrhoeae*
    d. microaerophilic/no oxygen

Answers to Review Questions

1. d
2. c
3. c
4. b
5. a
6. d
7. d
8. c
9. specimen—direct smear using swabbed specimen; colony growing on a solid medium; liquid medium with growth
10. d

Websites

The Public Health Image Library is a great site for microbiology pictures. Click "continue" to enter the PHIL directory and search for microbiology pictures:
http://phil.cdc.gov/Phil/home.asp

American Society for Microbiology:
www.asm.org/

Information on group A streptococcal infections from the National Institute of Allergy and Infectious Diseases:
www.niaid.nih.gov/factsheets/strep.htm

Information on MRSA:
http://www.cdc.gov/mrsa/mrsa_initiative/skin_infection/index.html

Great slideshow on MRSA:
http://www.medicinenet.com/mrsa_picture_slideshow/article.htm

Information on Swine Flu (H1N1):
http://www.cdc.gov/h1n1flu/qa.htm

World Health Organization:
www.who.int/en/

National Institute of Allergy and Infectious Diseases listing of emerging diseases:
http://www3.niaid.nih.gov/topics/emerging/list.htm

Information on bioterrorism from Centers for Disease Control and Prevention:
http://www.bt.cdc.gov/bioterrorism/

CHAPTER 9

Toxicology

Objectives
After completing this chapter you should be able to:

Fundamental Concepts
1. List the most common illicit drugs used in the United States.
2. Describe the widely used and abused legal drug ethanol (alcohol).
3. Identify the types of specimens commonly used for drug testing.
4. Explain why urine specimens are so good for drug screening tests.
5. Describe and/or perform proper collection of urine and blood specimens used for drug testing and monitoring.

CLIA-Waived Immunology Tests
1. Describe and/or perform urine drug screening and monitoring testing for addictive drugs of abuse.
2. Explain a positive drug test result in a urine specimen.

Advanced Concepts
1. Define and elaborate on therapeutic drug monitoring.
2. List examples of therapeutic drugs that may require monitoring.
3. Describe the five steps in pharmacokinetics.
4. Discuss the meaning of "drug half-life."
5. List the most common poisonous metals, and cite a source for each.

Key Terms

absorption passage of a substance through the surface of the body into body fluids and tissues
buprenorphine an FDA-approved drug for treating opioid drug addiction
cannabinoid marijuana
distribution the blood then carries the drug through the body
idiosyncrasy an abnormal susceptibility to a drug or other agent that is peculiar to the individual
liberation the release of a prescribed drug from its dosage
metabolite a substance produced by the metabolism of a drug in the body
opiates methadone and morphine
pharmacokinetics the movement of drugs through the body from the time of introduction to elimination
qualitative drug screening a measurement that determines if a substance is present or absent
quantitative drug screening a precise measurement of the amount of a substance present in the specimen
toxicity the level at which a drug becomes poisonous in the body

FUNDAMENTAL CONCEPTS

Overview of Toxicology

The toxicology department in the medical laboratory tests the levels of both therapeutic drugs and drugs of abuse to determine their presence and/or their harmful or "toxic" effect on the body. These departments may also test for other poisons, such as lead. In the toxicology laboratory, tests are generally performed using blood or urine specimens and sometimes saliva, sweat, or stomach contents. A toxicology test may be for one specific drug or more than 20 drugs.

Drugs may be accidentally or deliberately injected, inhaled, swallowed, or **absorbed** through the skin or mucous membranes. **Toxicity** is the level at which a drug becomes poisonous in the body.

The medical assistant may be responsible for collecting the urine or blood specimen, which is then sent to the toxicology lab, also for testing the specimen for screening or monitoring purposes. The following are common reasons for performing drug screening tests:

- To determine the cause of bizarre behavior, unconsciousness, or life-threatening symptoms in an emergency situation in which drug overdose may be a possibility.
- To test for drug use in the workplace or in schools, particularly among bus and truck drivers, child-care workers, and public safety workers. These professions generally require a urine or blood drug test as part of the application process and may also require employees to undergo periodic drug testing.
- To test athletes for drugs that enhance their athletic ability.

The fundamental concepts section of this chapter includes an overview of the common drugs of abuse that can become toxic and/or addictive when taken incorrectly. It then describes proper collection of urine and blood specimens used for drug testing. When testing for drugs of abuse, the medical assistant must ensure that collection of the specimen adheres to the legal "chain of custody" guidelines certifying that the collection of the specimen was witnessed and there was no opportunity for the specimen to be tampered with in any way.

The CLIA-waived section presents in-office drug screening tests and the procedure for monitoring patients on **buprenorphine** (a Food and Drug Administration [FDA]–approved drug for treating drug addiction).

The advanced concepts section presents the principles of therapeutic drug monitoring and collecting a blood specimen for lead poisoning.

Drugs of Abuse

There are thousands of drugs available worldwide. Over-the-counter (OTC) drugs fill the shelves of pharmacies and are useful for many minor medical conditions. Unfortunately, these drugs may have toxic effects on the body if taken incorrectly. Three causes of drug toxicity with OTCs are overdosage, interactions with other drugs, or **idiosyncrasy** (an abnormal susceptibility to a drug or other agent that is peculiar to the individual). The medical assistant should be mindful of these possibilities and faithfully record any OTC drugs that are being taken.

Any drug can be abused, but "drugs of abuse" are considered to be those that are illegally obtained for recreational purposes or to satisfy an addiction. Some therapeutic drugs may be misused or become addictive over time. Table 9-1 lists the 13 most common illicit or addictive drugs of abuse. Note the number of these drugs that also have medical uses when taken appropriately.

Each of the drugs in Table 9-1 produces a specific **metabolite,** the substance produced by **metabolism** (breaking down) of the drug in the body. The metabolite is then excreted in the urine. These metabolites can be tested **qualitatively** in the same way that the urine dipstick tested for various analytes (e.g., glucose, protein). Urine is generally the specimen of choice for screening drugs of abuse because it is easily obtained and it is relatively simple to perform multiple drug tests at the same time. Table 9-2 lists the time intervals for detecting various drugs in urine. Also, see Procedure 9-1, located at the end of this section.

If a **quantitative** result is necessary to determine the amount of the drug that is in the patient, a blood specimen would also be used because its dilution stays constant. The dilution of the drug in the urine volume varies depending on water intake and output. The blood specimen is commonly ordered by law enforcement officials who need to know the actual amount of a specific illicit drug after it has tested positive in the urine.

The most common legal drug of abuse in America is ethanol, also known as grain alcohol. It is found in beer, wine, and distilled liquors. Table 9-3 lists the approximate ethanol content in alcoholic beverages. Ethanol depresses the central nervous system and may lead to coma, progressing to death at the following "panic" levels:

> $> 2000\ \mu g/mL$ in the blood, or $> 1600\ \mu g/mL$ in the urine

Alcohol is one of the few drugs that has a direct correlation between blood levels and impaired driving ability. Drug alcohol testing for prosecution of an accused drunk driver is strictly regulated by law (see Procedure 9-2).

TABLE 9-1 Common Drugs of Abuse Detected on Multiple Drug Urine Screening Tests[*]

Drug and (Test Code)	Street Name	Source/Route	Medical Use/Brand Names	Side Effects, Risks/Overdose
1. Cocaine (COC)	Rock, crack, coke, blow, nose nachos, hooter, yeyo	Coca bush leaves refined/Nasal administration, smoked	Topical anesthetic, natural stimulant, anesthetic, vasoconstrictor, painkiller, appetite suppressant, altitude sickness/Less addictive derivatives for anesthesia: Benzocaine, Lidocaine, Cepacol, Dermaplast, Lanocane	Perforation of nasal septum, renal failure, hyperthermia, cardiac arrest, seizures, dermatitis, tetany, septicemia, respiratory arrest, dehydration, sleep disorders, depression, impulsiveness, hostility, impaired memory/**Overdose:** fever, unresponsiveness, difficulty breathing, unconsciousness, stroke, death
2. Amphetamine (AMP)	Black beauties, Christmas trees, dexies, speed, double trouble, gaggler, beanies	Made in illegal laboratories/Smoked, injected, snorted	Appetite suppressant, central nervous system stimulant/Adderall, Citramine, Dexalone, Tamphetamin, Zamitam	Dependence, increased blood pressure, increased respiration, dilated pupils, sweating, tremors/**Overdose:** seizures, cardiac arrest
3. Methamphetamine (mAMP) Ecstasy XTC (MDMA)	Cat, crank, glass, speed, ice, love, Disco biscuits, Molly	Made in illegal laboratories/Oral, powder inhalant, crystals smoked,	Nasal decongestant/Desoxyn, No medical use	Dependence, psychosis, decreased appetite, restlessness, anxiety, heart failure, extreme fatigue, hunger, mental depression, dysrhythmias, lethargy, skin pallor, fits of rage/**Overdose:** seizures, cardiac arrest
4. Marijuana (THC) Hashish	Pot, weed, joint, reefer, roach, dope Hashish, hash oil, ganja	Cannabis sativa, hemp plant flowers and leaves/Smoked, eaten, injected	Pain relief (colitis), treatment of glaucoma, appetite stimulant, reduction of nausea from chemotherapy, euphoria, detachment, relaxation/Marinol, Dronabinol	Talkativeness, slowed time perception, inappropriate hilarity, paranoia, confusion, anxiety, short-term memory loss, impaired lung structure, chromosomal mutation, micronucleic white blood cells, cancer, lack of motivation
5. Methadone (MTD)	Fizzies, chocolate chip cookies, juice, wafer	Laboratory manufactured/Oral, injection, powder	Treatment for narcotic addiction, pain/Methadose, Dolophine	Also addictive/can result in respiratory and cardiac arrest and death if stopped suddenly
6. Opiates (OPI 2000) (also see MOP 300)	Smack, horse, chiva, junk, black tar, gunpowder, courage pills, bomb	Poppy refined/nasal, oral, intravenous injection, dermal patch	Potent painkiller, heroin, morphine, codeine, fentanyl/Demerol, Darvon, Vicodin, Dilaudid	Addiction in hospitals, constipation, dermatitis, malnutrition, hypoglycemia, dental caries, amenorrhea, acquired immunodeficiency syndrome (from sharing needles)

(Continued)

Fundamental Concepts

TABLE 9-1 Common Drugs of Abuse Detected on Multiple Drug Urine Screening Tests*—cont'd

Drug and (Test Code)	Street Name	Source/Route	Medical Use/Brand Names	Side Effects, Risks/Overdose
7. Oxycodone (OXY)	Oxy, OC, blues, killers, kickers hillbilly percs	Semisynthetic similar to codeine/Oral, injection	Moderate to heavy pain relief/OxyContin, Percodan, Percocet	Addiction in patients on long-term pain therapy
8. Barbiturates (BAR)	Barbs, pinks, blockbusters, Christmas trees, goofballs, red devils, reds and blues, yellowjackets	Laboratory manufactured/Oral, intravenous injection	Depressant, sedative, hypnotic, anticonvulsant/Seconal, Amytal, Nembutal	Dullness, apathy, dependence/**Overdose:** respiratory arrest, coma, death
9. Benzodiazepines (BZO)	Roofies, downers, tranks, benzos	Laboratory manufactured/Oral, injection	Treatment for anxiety, seizures, sleeplessness, muscle relaxant/Valium, Xanax, Restoril, Versed	Carefree, detached, sleepy, disoriented, unconsciousness, amnesia, diminished reflexes/**Overdose:** coma, can be lethal when combined with alcohol
10. Buprenorphine (BUP)	Bupe, Subs	Laboratory manufactured	Analgesic, treatment for opioid addiction/Buprenex, Suboxone, Subutix	Euphoria, respiratory depression, sedation/Causes severe respiratory depression when combined with benzodiazepines
11. Tricyclic antidepressants (TCA)	Yellow	Laboratory manufactured/Oral, injection	Treatment for depression, attention-deficit/hyperactivity disorder, migraines/Adapin, Norpramin, Anafranil, Pamelor, Tofranil, Elavil	Blurred vision, constipation and dry mouth, anxiety, restlessness, difficulty urinating, weight gain, drowsiness, muscle twitches, weakness, sweating, nausea, dizziness, cognitive and memory difficulties, increased heart rate, irregular heart rhythms, panic attacks, hostile/angry feelings, impulsive actions, severe restlessness, very rapid speech
12. Lysergic acid diethylamide (LSD) Salfia	Acid, the Beast, California sunshine Shrooms	Illicit laboratories, peyote (mescaline), psilocybin mexicana (mushroom), fungus on grains/Ingested orally	No medical use	Hallucinations, anxiety, depression, confusion, paranoia, panic attacks, impaired memory, inability to reason, flashbacks, increased blood pressure, high temperature, dilated pupils, increased heart rate, psychosis, flashbacks

(Continued)

TABLE 9-1 Common Drugs of Abuse Detected on Multiple Drug Urine Screening Tests*—cont'd

Drug and (Test Code)	Street Name	Source/Route	Medical Use/Brand Names	Side Effects, Risks/Overdose
13. Phencyclidine (PCP)	Angel dust, peace pill, rocket fuel, wack, ozone, fry	Illegal laboratories/Oral, intravenous, sniffed, smoked	No medical use	Hallucinations, acute anxiety, dulled thinking, poor memory, depression, severe brain damage, hepatitis, respiratory arrest, panic reaction, confusion, blurred vision, high blood pressure/**Overdose:** violence, psychoses, self-injurious behavior, suicide

*Numbers 1 through 9 are the screened drugs for patients on Number 10, buprenorphine therapy (see Procedure 9-3).

TABLE 9-2 Typical Time Intervals for Detecting Drugs in Urine

Drug	Time Found in Urine
Alcohol	6 hours to 1 day
Amphetamines	4 hours
Barbiturates	24 hours to 4 days
Benzodiazepines	Short-term therapeutic use: 3 days; long-term chronic use: 4 to 6 weeks
Cannabinoids	1 hour to 3 days
Cocaine	2 to 3 days
Codeine	4 hours
LSD	1 to 4 days
Marijuana (THC)	Casual use: up to 7 days; chronic use: up to 30 days or longer
MDMA (Ecstasy)	1 to 4 days
Methadone	1 to 7 days
Methamphetamine	1 to 4 days
Opiates	1 to 4 days
PCP	Casual use: up to 7 days; chronic use: up to 30 days
Tricyclic antidepressants	1 to 9 days

Modified from Stepp CA, Woods M: *Laboratory procedures for medical office personnel*, Philadelphia, 1998, Saunders.

TABLE 9-3 Approximate Ethanol Content in Alcoholic Beverages

Beverage	Ethanol Content (%)
Beer	3-6
Ciders	4-5
Wines	8-15
Sherry, Madeira, Port	18-20
Whiskey, gin	40-45
Vodka	40-50
Brandy	45-50
Rum	50-70

From Calbreath DF: *Clinical chemistry*, 1992, Philadelphia, Saunders.

PROCEDURE 9-1 Assisting with Urine Collection for Drug Screening

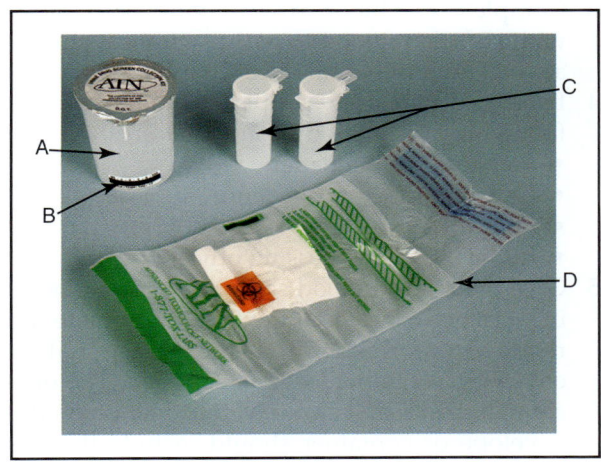

A. *a*, urine drug screening collection kit specimen cup; *b*, temperature indicator on collection cup; *c*, urine specimen containers to be sent to the lab; *d*, plastic sealable pouch for the two urine specimen containers and the chain of custody documents.

Equipment and Supplies for Collecting and Processing Urine Specimen (Fig. A)

a) urine drug screening collection kit specimen cup
b) temperature indicator on collection cup
c) urine specimen containers to be sent to the laboratory
d) plastic sealable pouch for the two urine specimen containers and the chain of custody documents

Procedure

1. Sanitize the hands, and apply gloves.
2. Explain to the patient the purpose of the test and the procedure to be followed for a midstream clean-catch specimen collection (see Chapter 3).
3. Obtain a signed consent form from the patient
4. A trained professional must witness the actual voiding of at least 50 mL of urine into the specimen cup provided in the urine collection drug kit.
5. Originate the chain of custody document at the time of the sample collection. The person who witnessed the voiding must sign the document, as must every other person who handles the sample.
6. After the collection, verify the temperature of the urine as seen on the indicator at the bottom of the cup, and document it. NOTE: If the temperature of the urine specimen is out of range (too cold), a second specimen must be collected. If the donor refuses to provide the second specimen under direct observation, the collection would be considered "refusal to test."
7. Transfer the specimen to the two containers that must be labeled with the following information:
   - Full name of the patient
   - Date and time of collection
   - Your initials
   - Initials of the witnessing officer
8. Place the two sample containers into the sealed plastic pouch, mark it with a notary-style seal or with tamper-proof tape to protect the integrity of the sample, and send the specimen to the toxicology laboratory.
9. If you are trained and qualified to do the testing, proceed with the testing according to laboratory and state regulations.
10. After both the initial and confirmatory testing is complete, mark the urine sample, reseal it, and securely store it for a minimum of 30 days or for the length of time specified by laboratory protocols.
11. Clean or discard all equipment and supplies according to safety guidelines.
12. Remove gloves, and wash hands.

Fig. A courtesy Zack Bent.

PROCEDURE 9-2 Assisting with Blood Collection for Alcohol Testing

Equipment and Supplies

- Gray-topped Vacutainer tubes
- Venipuncture needle and holder (or syringe and transfer device)
- Nonvolatile disinfectant (e.g., benzalkonium [Zephiran] or aqueous thimerosal [merthiolate])
- Gauze
- Tourniquet
- Gloves
- Legally authorized transportation envelope, container, or plastic pouch

Patient Preparation

1. An officer of the law will be present to act as a witness to the procedure.
2. The patient will probably still be under the influence of alcohol, so explain what you will be doing in as brief and concise a manner as possible. NOTE: Do not allow yourself to become irritated by the speech or mannerisms of the patient. Treat the patient with the respect and dignity with which you treat all your patients.

Blood Collection Procedure

NOTE: The Department of Justice for each state has established uniform standards for the collection, handling, and preservation of blood samples used for alcohol testing. If you are authorized to obtain specimens for forensic analysis, check your laboratory's procedure manual so that you perform the collection *exactly* as required by the uniform standards established for your state.

1. Sanitize hands, and apply gloves.
2. Prepare the draw site using Zephiran, aqueous Merthiolate, or another aqueous disinfectant. *Do not use alcohol or other volatile organic disinfectants to clean the skin site.*
3. Complete the blood draw, filling both tubes with sufficient blood to permit duplicate blood alcohol determinations (see Chapter 5).
4. Label the two gray-stoppered tubes with the following information:
    - Full name of the patient
    - Date and time of collection
    - Your initials
    - Initials of the witnessing officer
5. Give the labeled blood samples to the witnessing officer, who will immediately complete the required information on the transportation envelope, container, or plastic pouch. The officer will then seal it securely. Information on the envelope or container should include the following:
    - The full name of the patient
    - Whether the patient is alive or dead
    - The submitting agency
    - The geographical location where the blood was drawn (e.g., hospital, clinic, jail)
    - The name of the person drawing the blood sample
    - The date and time the blood sample was drawn
    - The signature of the witnessing officer
6. Once the envelope or container is sealed, it must not be opened, except for analysis. Each person who is subsequently in possession of the sealed sample must sign his or her name in the space provided on the envelope or container (chain of custody). The integrity of the sample *must* be safeguarded.
7. Remove gloves, and wash hands.

CLIA-WAIVED DRUG SCREENING TESTS

Some offices may perform drug screening tests for companies as part of pre-employment physicals or as a requirement for insurance or government mandates (e.g., the federally mandated testing of transportation workers).

Although plasma samples provide the best diagnostic and quantitative results, CLIA-waived urine test kits are available to provide an initial screening for the presence of a variety of drugs, including amphetamines, marijuana **(cannabinoid),** cocaine, and **opiates** (e.g., methadone and morphine). The urine drug testing kits generally contain a rapid drug screening device and a wide-mouth collection container. Be sure to read the step-by-step instructions on the package inserts. Generally, the instructions require that the operator dip the testing device into the urine and observe the qualitative reactions in a specified time. The results are reported as positive, negative, or inconclusive, which requires confirmation testing. Be sure to follow the shipping instructions if the screening device indicates the presence of drugs in the sample or if the results are inconclusive.

CLIA-waived saliva alcohol tests are also available for facilities that screen clients or patients for alcohol. These qualitative tests generally consist of a test strip that turns shades of green or blue if alcohol is present in the subject's saliva.

A growing number of drug screening products are also FDA approved for home use. (For a list of the drugs that may be detected in urine, saliva, hair and breath, see the website at the end of the chapter.) Schools, employers, and the Department of Transportation (DOT) may also use these products to randomly monitor their students and employees. NOTE: If performing drug testing for the DOT in the office, the physician must be a certified Medical Review Officer (MRO). As an MRO, the licensed physician is responsible for receiving laboratory results and interpreting and evaluating an individual's positive test result.

Most rapid urine drug tests are immunoassay tests based on the principle of competitive binding. Drugs that may be present in the urine specimen compete against their respective drug conjugate for binding sites with their specific antibody. During testing the urine specimen migrates upward on the test strip by capillary action. If the drug in question has a sufficiently high concentration, it will saturate all the binding sites of the antibody so that it will not react in the drug–protein conjugate test area of the strip. Therefore, if the drug is present in the urine, the test area will show no reaction. (NOTE: The immunoassay results discussed in Chapter 7 had an opposite positive reaction.) Conversely, if the drug is not present, it will not saturate the antibody sites and the antibody will then react in the test area, causing a colored line to appear. The control area (C) of the strip indicates that the proper volume of urine migrated through the test area and the color caused by the antibody conjugation worked. (NOTE: The colored line in the internal control area does not represent a positive reaction, as in other immunoassays, because a positive reaction in this method inhibits the formation of a colored band.) See Fig. D in Procedure 9-3, which demonstrates these results.

Physicians who treat opioid addiction using buprenorphine must monitor their patients using CLIA-waived urine drug screening test kits. These physicians are authorized by the FDA and the Substance Abuse and Mental Health Services Association (SAMHSA) to treat and monitor up to 30 patients. (For more information on buprenorphine treatment, see the websites at the end of this chapter.) The urine test cassettes detect the presence of nine addictive drugs in addition to buprenorphine and assist the physician in monitoring the patient's drug use and treatment progress. Table 9-1 lists each drug with its three- or four-digit testing code along with the drug's street name, source, method of administration, medical use, side effects and overdose information. Table 9-2 shows the time intervals for detecting various drugs in urine.

PROCEDURE 9-3 Urine Drug Panel Testing Procedure

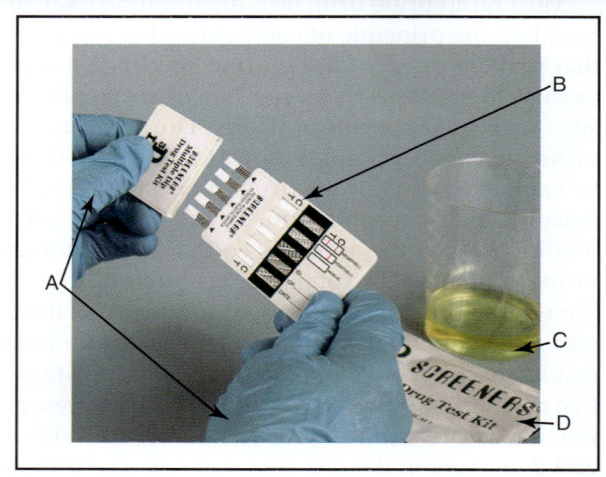

A. *a*, Gloves; *b*, test card with multiple test strips (five tests are on each side of the card); *c*, fresh urine specimen, or specimen that has been stored at 2° to 8° Centigrade (refrigerated) for up to 48 hours then brought to room temperature; *d*, metal pouch that stored the card at 2° to 30° Centigrade.

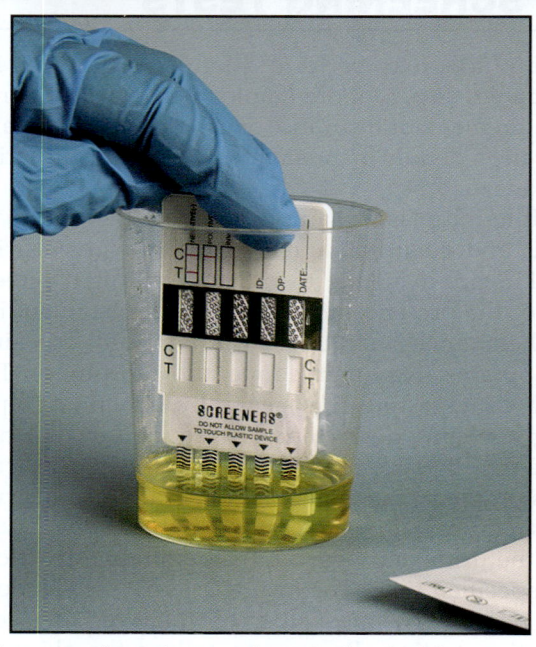

B. Immerse the strips to at least the level of the wavy lines on the strips but not above the arrows on the test card for 10 to 15 seconds.

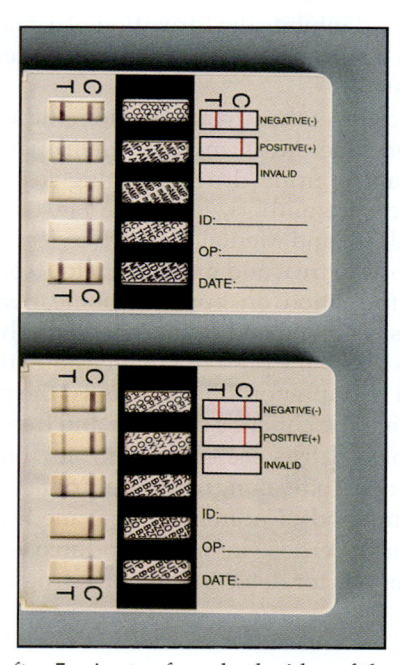

C. Results after 5 minutes from both sides of the card showing six negative results (testing area shows two colored bands) and four positive results (the testing areas have only one colored band in the control area).

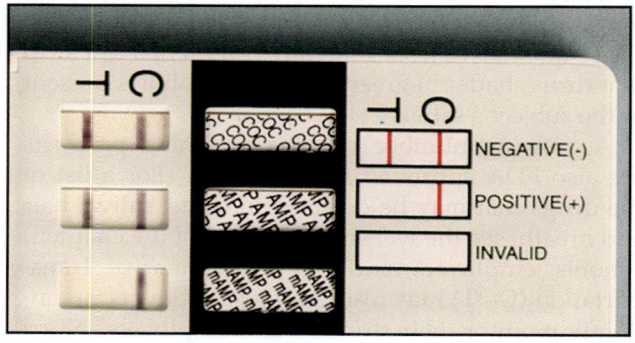

D. Close-up on first three drug results: COC = Cocaine is negative; AMP = Amphetamine is negative; mAMP = Methamphetamine is positive.

Equipment and Supplies (Fig. A)

a. Gloves
b. Test card with multiple test strips (five tests are on each side of the card)
c. Fresh urine specimen or specimen that has been stored at 2° to 8° Centigrade for up to 48 hours and then brought to room temperature
d. Metal pouch that stored the card at 2° to 30° Centigrade (check expiration date)

Procedure

1. Sanitize the hands, and apply gloves.
2. Remove the test device from its protective pouch, and label it with the patient's identification.

NOTE: If the specimen has been stored in the refrigerator, bring it to room temperature before opening to prevent condensation.

Advanced Concepts

PROCEDURE 9-3 Urine Drug Panel Testing Procedure—cont'd

3. Remove the cap from the end of the test card. (Fig. A)
4. With the arrows pointing toward the urine specimen, immerse the strips of the test card vertically into the urine specimen for at least 10 to 15 seconds. **Immerse the strips to at least the level of the wavy lines on the strips but not above the arrows on the test card. (Fig. B).**
5. Place the test card on a nonabsorbent surface, and wait for the colored lines to appear.
6. At 5 minutes, read and record the results (Fig. C).
   - Positive test result: One distinct pink band appears in the control region (C), no line in the test region (T)
   - Negative test result: Two pink bands appear, one pink band in the control region (C) and one pink band in the patient test region (T).
   - Invalid: Pink bands are absent from the control region. Repeat the test with a new device. If the problem persists, call for technical assistance.
7. See Fig. D for close-up results on the following three drugs:
   - COC = Cocaine is negative
   - AMP = Amphetamine is negative
   - mAMP = Methamphetamine is positive

Quality Control Procedure

In addition to the internal control region built into the test device, external positive and negative liquid controls should be performed when a new kit is used. Also, each operator of the test should perform a positive and negative control once with each testing method to confirm that his or her testing technique is correct. The results of the control tests should be logged in the drug screening control log.

The positive liquid control procedure is performed in the same way as the patient procedure, with a new testing card. Observe and record the results within 5 minutes. Repeat the procedure with a drop of well-mixed negative control.

ADVANCED CONCEPTS

Therapeutic Drug Monitoring

Therapeutic drug monitoring (TDM) is the process of measuring either the effects of a drug on a patient or the actual levels of a drug being administered to a patient. For example, we have already seen how to monitor the *effect* of insulin therapy by performing blood glucose levels, and we monitored the *effect* of coumadin therapy by testing the patient's protime and INR ratio. In this chapter we will learn the importance of monitoring therapeutic drug levels in the patient's blood and/or urine.

Most prescribed drugs have a therapeutic range that must be maintained for successful therapy. If a patient's drug level falls outside of the range, it may become ineffective if too low or toxic if too high. Table 9-4 lists therapeutic ranges and toxic levels for various drugs. Therapeutic ranges and the subsequent monitoring of the drug levels in the body give the physician guidelines for prescribing the medication and fine-tuning the exact effective amount of medication to keep the patient within the range.

It is very important to collect the blood sample for TDM at a certain time—either before or after administering the drug. Otherwise, the test results will be useless and unreliable, or even worse, they may prompt the physician to initiate inappropriate treatment.

Common Therapeutic Drugs That Are Tested for Toxicity

Amikacin	Paracetamol
Caffeine	Phenobarbitone
Carbamazepine	Phenytoin
Cyclosporine	Primidone
Digoxin	Salicylic acid
Ethosuximide	Theophylline
Gentamicin	Tobramycin
Lithium	Valproic acid
Methotrexate	

Pharmacokinetics

For a better understanding of how drugs are utilized by the body, here is a brief look at the five stages of **pharmacokinetics** (the movement of drugs through the body from the time of introduction to elimination).

Liberation

Liberation is the release of a drug from its dosage form. For a drug to be liberated, it must first go into a body by way of a solution. For example, eye drops

TABLE 9-4 Drug Categories Showing Therapeutic Ranges and Toxic Levels

Drug	Therapeutic Range	Toxic Level
Antibiotics		
Ampicillin	20-25 µg/mL	35 µg/mL
Gentamicin	4-8 µg/mL	12 µg/mL
Kanamycin	20-25 µg/mL	35 µg/mL
Tobramycin	2-8 µg/mL	12 µg/mL
Anticonvulsants		
Carbamazepine (Tegretol)	2-10 µg/mL	12 µg/mL
Ethosuximide (Zarontin)	40-80 µg/mL	100 µg/mL
Phenobarbital (Luminal)	10 µg/mL	>55 µg/mL
Phenytoin (Dilantin)	10-20 µg/mL	>20 µg/mL
Primidone	1 µg/mL	>10 µg/mL
Antidepressants and Antipsychotics		
Amitriptyline (Elavil)	100-250 ng/mL	>300 ng/mL
Diazepam (Valium)	5-70 ng/mL	>70 ng/mL
Imipramine (Tofranil)	100-250 ng/mL	>300 ng/mL
Lithium (Lithonate)	0.8-1.4 mEq/L	1.5 mEq/L
Antirheumatics		
Salicylate (aspirin)	2-30 mg/dL	>40 mg/dL
Acetaminophen (Tylenol)	0-25 mg/mL	>150 µg/mL
Barbiturates		
Amobarbital (Amytal)	7 µg/mL	30 µg/mL
Pentobarbital (Nembutal)	10 µg/mL	55 µg/mL
Secobarbital (Seconal)	3 µg/mL	10 µg/mL
Cardiotonics		
Digoxin	0.5-2 µg/mL	>2.5 µg/mL
Disopyramide	2-4.5 µg/mL	>9 µg/mL
Lidocaine	2-6 µg/mL	>9 µg/mL
Procainamide (Pronestyl)	4-8 µg/mL	>12 µg/mL
Quinidine	2.3-5 µg/mL	>5 µg/mL

Modified from Stepp CA, Woods M: *Laboratory procedures for medical office personnel*, Philadelphia, 1998, Saunders.

go into solution in the tears of the eye. Swallowed medication goes into solution in the gastric fluid. Liquid injections are inserted into the skin, muscle, or vein.

Absorption and Distribution

Absorption is the movement of the drug from some body surface (i.e., the skin or mucous membrane) through the tissues and into the blood (also called *uptake*). The blood then carries the drug through the body **(distribution)** until it finds its target (e.g., antibiotics find the pathogen, anticonvulsants and antidepressants find the brain, cardiotonics the heart and vessels).

Metabolism and Elimination

Next, the drug needs to be broken down **(metabolism)**, which generally occurs in the liver. Once it is broken down, the drug metabolite is **eliminated** by way of the bile from the liver or urine from the kidneys. Drug metabolites may also be excreted through the skin by way of sweat, the lungs by way of expired air, or the salivary or mammary glands.

Drug Half-Life and Specimen Collection

The amount of time necessary to eliminate 50% of a drug is referred to as its *half-life*. The half-life cycle varies for each individual depending on sex, age, body weight, and health status. For example, children and the elderly are more prone to experiencing toxic levels of therapeutic drugs on account of their size and altered metabolic rates. All these factors have an effect on whether a drug is prescribed, when to test for the drug, and what type of specimen is tested (e.g., urine, blood).

Drugs of abuse are generally tested using urine specimens for the qualitative result and blood for the quantitative result. Therapeutic drug monitoring generally uses blood specimens taken in a gold gel tube (serum separator tube) or a light green heparin tube with gel (plasma separator tube). NOTE: Do *not* use a lithium heparin tube when monitoring blood lithium levels. Be sure to refer to the laboratory manual when collecting toxicology specimens that are sent to the toxicology department of reference labs and hospitals. See the website listed at the end of the chapter for additional information on TDM testing and specimen collection.

Other Toxicology Tests

Other conditions in which a medical assistant may be asked to collect specimens for toxicology or perform drug screening tests are as follows:
- Chronic lead poisoning from the lead-based paint found in old homes. Fig. 9-1 shows the royal blue–topped tube needed for a lead test specimen. NOTE: The royal blue–topped tube has a red strip on the label indicating that it has no additive (similar to the red-topped tubes) and should therefore be drawn in the same order as red-topped tubes. Also, refer to the laboratory manual for any other directions regarding collection and processing of the specimen.
- Acute iron poisoning in children who have taken adult iron tablets is a stat test.
- Chronic exposure to mercury and arsenic poisoning tests
- Forensic drug tests for court purposes
- Urine screening testing on pregnant mothers for drugs of abuse
- Urine and blood drug testing for on-the-job injuries to rule out impaired employee

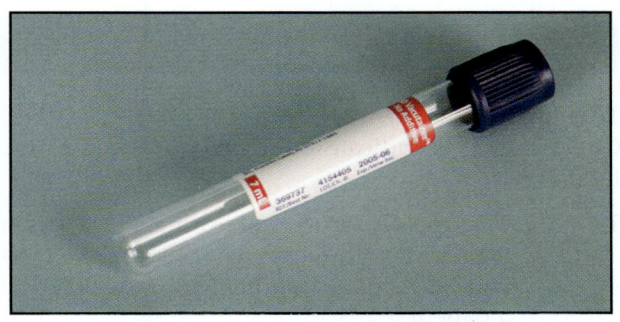

Fig. 9-1. Royal blue Vacutainer tube for lead toxicology test. Note the red band on the label, which indicates it has no additives and is therefore drawn in the order of a red Vacutainer tube. (Courtesy Zack Bent.)

SUMMARY

We are constantly exposed to harmful and poisonous substances. Even prescription medications may be harmful if not used as directed. The physician needs to know whether a drug is at its therapeutic level or whether the drug level is becoming toxic. Toxicology is the study and monitoring of these drugs as well the identification of drugs of abuse. The medical assistant must be aware of the proper timing and specifics of collecting toxicology specimens, as well as the legal processing of specimens that may contain illicit drugs (i.e., chain of custody protocol).

Review Questions

True or False
Circle T or F to indicate the correct answers to the following:

T F 1. Therapeutic drug monitoring (TDM) is a way for the physician to measure the effects and levels of a drug being administered to a patient.

T F 2. Pharmacokinetics is the study of drugs.

Fill in the Blanks
Complete the following statements:

3. _____ is the term meaning the release of the drug from its dosage.

4. The movement of a drug from solution to the blood is called _____.

5. The distribution of a drug throughout the body by way of the blood is called _____.

6. The term for the breakdown of a drug within the body is _____.

7. The two main organs that eliminate drugs are the _____ and the _____.

8. The time it takes to eliminate 50% of any drug is called its _____.

9. Poisonous metals may include _____, _____, _____, and _____.

10. The most widely used and abused legal drug in society is _____.

11. Methamphetamine is also known as _____, or _____.

12. Two examples of opiate-derived drugs are _____ and _____.

Multiple Choice
Circle the letter that represents the single best answer:

13. Drugs may be excreted through all of the following *except*:
    a. Skin
    b. Sweat
    c. Stool
    d. Tears
    e. Lungs

14. Forensic laboratories often prefer _____ for quantitative drug testing.
    a. Urine
    b. Serum
    c. Plasma
    d. Whole blood
    e. Breath

Answers to Review Questions

1. T
2. F (It is the mechanism of the drug's action in the body from introduction to elimination.)
3. liberation
4. absorption
5. distribution
6. metabolism
7. kidney and liver
8. half-life
9. lead, arsenic, mercury, and iron
10. alcohol
11. crank, speed
12. morphine, codeine, and heroin
13. c
14. c

Websites

U.S. Department of Justice—Drug Enforcement Administration—Office of Diversion Control. An excellent website for finding information on drugs of abuse, it provides an alphabetical index of all drugs and chemicals of concern.
http://www.deadiversion.usdoj.gov/drugs_concern/index.html

Drug testing site for safer schools:
http://www.keystosaferschools.com/drug_testing_specifics.htm#druglist-mor

Drugs that may be detected in urine, saliva, hair, and breath:
http://www.drugalcoholtestkits.com/fs_search.asp?testtypes=urine&portalid=GOO

U.S. Department of Health and Human Services and SAMHSA's National Clearing House for Alcohol and Drug Information:
http://ncadi.samhsa.gov/

Information on drug addiction treatment using buprenorphine:
http://buprenorphine.samhsa.gov/bwns_locator/dr_facilitylocatordoc.htm

Website for Screeners Dip Drug Test Kit:
http://www.lifelinemedical.net/ddd_dip_drug_test.html

Website with links to therapeutic drug monitoring (TDM) testing and specimen collection information:
http://www.questdiagnostics.com/common/sitesearch/jsp/cm_ss_srch.jsp

APPENDIX A

Reference Values

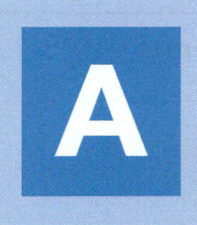

Urine Reference Values*: For Chapter 3

Analyte	Conventional Units	SI Units
Acetone and acetoacetate, qualitative	Negative	Negative
Albumin		
Qualitative	Negative	Negative
Quantitative	10-100 mg/24 h	0.15-1.5 µmol/d
Amylase/creatinine clearance ratio	0.01-0.04	0.01-0.04
Bilirubin, qualitative	Negative	Negative
Creatinine	15-25 mg/kg/24 h	0.13-0.22 mmol/kg/d
Glucose (as reducing substance)	<250 mg/24 h	<250 mg/d
Hemoglobin and myoglobin, qualitative	Negative	Negative
pH	4.6-8.0	4.6-8.0
Protein, total		
Qualitative	Negative	Negative
Quantitative	10-150 mg/24 h	10-150 mg/d
Protein/creatinine ratio	<0.2	<0.2
Specific gravity		
Random specimen	1.003-1.030	1.003-1.030
24-hour collection	1.015-1.025	1.015-1.025
Urobilinogen	0.5-4.0 mg/24 h	0.6-6.9 µmol/d

*Values may vary depending on the method used.
From *Mosby's dictionary of medical, nursing, and health professions*, ed 8, St Louis, 2008, Mosby.

Hematology Reference Values: For Chapter 5

Test	Conventional Units	SI Units
Cell Counts		
Erythrocytes		
Males	4.6-6.2 million/mm³	4.6-6.2 × 10¹²/L
Females	4.2-5.4 million/mm³	4.2-5.4 × 10¹²/L
Children (varies with age)	4.5-5.1 million/mm³	4.5-5.1 × 10¹²/L
Leukocytes, total	4500-11,000/mm³	
Leukocytes, differential counts		
Myelocytes	0%	0/L
Band neutrophils	3%-5%	150-400 × 10⁶/L
Segmented neutrophils	54%-62%	3000-5800 × 10⁶/L
Lymphocytes	25%-33%	1500-3000 × 10⁶/L
Monocytes	3%-7%	300-500 × 10⁶/L
Eosinophils	1%-3%	50-250 × 10⁶/L
Basophils	0%-1%	15-50 × 10⁶/L
Platelets	150,000-400,000/mm³	150-400 × 10⁹/L
Reticulocytes	25,000-75,000/mm³	25-75 × 10⁹/L
Coagulation tests		
Bleeding time (template)	2.75-8.0 min	2.75-8.0 min
Coagulation time (glass tube)	5-15 min	5-15 min
D-Dimer	<0.5 µg/mL	<0.5 mg/L
Factor VIII and other coagulation factors	50%-150% of normal	0.5-1.5 of normal
Fibrin split products (Thrombo–Wellco test)	<10 µg/mL	<10 mg/L
Fibrinogen	200-400 mg/dL	2.0-4.0 g/L
Partial thromboplastin time, activated (aPTT)	20-35 s	20-35 s
Prothrombin time (PT)	12.0-14.0 s	12.0-14.0 s
Corpuscular values of erythrocytes		
Mean corpuscular hemoglobin (MCH)	26-34 pg/cell	26-34 pg/cell
Mean corpuscular volume (MCV)	80-96 µm³	80-96 fL
Mean corpuscular hemoglobin concentration (MCHC)	32-36 g/dL	320-360 g/L
Hematocrit		
Males	40-54 mL/dL	0.40-0.54
Females	37-47 mL/dL	0.37-0.47
Newborns	49-54 mL/dL	0.49-0.54
Children (varies with age)	35-49 mL/dL	0.35-0.49
Hemoglobin		
Males	13.0-18.0 g/dL	8.1-11.2 mmol/L
Females	12.0-16.0 g/dL	7.4-9.9 mmol/L
Newborns	16.5-19.5 g/dL	10.2-12.1 mmol/L
Children (varies with age)	11.2-16.5 g/dL	7.0-10.2 mmol/L
Hemoglobin A1c	3%-5% of total	0.03-0.05 of total
Sedimentation rate (ESR)		
Westergren: Males	0-15 mm/h	0-15 mm/h
Females	0-20 mm/h	0-20 mm/h

From Rakel RE: *Conn's current therapy 2009*, Philadelphia, 2010, Saunders.

Blood Chemistry Reference Values: For Chapter 6

Analyte	Conventional Units	SI Units
Acid phosphatase, serum (thymolphthalein monophosphate substrate)	0.1-0.6 U/L	0.1-0.6 U/L
Alanine aminotransferase (ALT) serum (SGPT)	1-45 U/L	1-45 U/L
Albumin, serum	3.3-5.2 g/dL	33-52 g/L
Alkaline phosphatase (ALP), serum		
Adult	35-150 U/L	35-150 U/L
Adolescent	100-500 U/L	100-500 U/L
Child	100-350 U/L	100-350 U/L
Anion gap, serum, calculated	8-16 mEq/L	8-16 mmol/L
Aspartate aminotransferase (AST) serum (SGOT)	1-36 U/L	1-36 U/L
Bilirubin, serum		
Conjugated	0.1-0.4 mg/dL	1.7-6.8 µmol/L
Total	0.3-101 mg/dL	5.1-19.0 µmol/L
Calcium, serum	8.4-10.6 mg/dL	2.10-2.65 mmol/L
Chloride, serum or plasma	96-106 mEq/L	96-106 mmol/L
Cholesterol, serum or ethylenediaminetetraacetic acid (EDTA) plasma		
Desirable range	<200 mg/dL	<5.20 mmol/L
Low-density lipoprotein (LDL) cholesterol	60-180 mg/dL	1.55-4.65 mmol/L
High-density lipoprotein (HDL) cholesterol	30-80 mg/dL	0.80-2.05 mmol/L
Creatine kinase (CK), serum		
Males	55-170 U/L	55-170 U/L
Females	30-135 U/L	30-135 U/L
Creatinine, serum	0.6-1.2 mg/dL	50-110 µmol/L
Gamma-glutamyltransferase (GGT), serum	5-40 U/L	5-40 U/L
Glucose, fasting, plasma or serum	70-115 mg/dL	3.9-6.4 nmol/L
Iron, serum	74-175 µg/dL	13-31 µmol/L
Lactate dehydrogenase (LD), serum	110-220 U/L	110-220 U/L
Phosphate, inorganic, serum		
Adult	3.0-4.5 mg/dL	1.0-1.5 mmol/L
Child	4.0-7.0 mg/dL	1.3-2.3 mmol/L
Potassium		
Serum	3.5-5.0 mEq/L	3.5-5.0 mmol/L
Plasma	3.5-4.5 mEq/L	3.5-4.5 mmol/L
Protein, serum, electrophoresis		
Total	6.0-8.0 g/dL	60-80 g/L
Albumin	3.5-5.5 g/dL	35-55 g/L
Globulins		
Alpha$_1$	0.2-0.4 g/dL	2.0-4.0 g/L
Alpha$_2$	0.5-0.9 g/dL	5.0-9.0 g/L
Beta	0.6-1.1 g/dL	6.0-11.0 g/L
Gamma	0.7-1.7 g/dL	7.0-17.0 g/L
Sodium, serum or plasma	135-145 mEq/L	135-145 mmol/L
Thyroxine (T$_4$), serum	4.5-12.0 µg/dL	58-154 nmol/L
Triglycerides, serum, 12-h fast	40-150 mg/dL	0.4-1.5 g/L
Triiodothyronine (T$_3$), serum	70-190 ng/dL	1.1-2.9 nmol/L
Triiodothyronine uptake, resin (T$_3$RU)	25%-38%	0.25-0.38
Urea, serum or plasma	24-49 mg/dL	4.0-8.2 nmol/L
Urea nitrogen, serum or plasma	11-23 mg/dL	8.0-16.4 nmol/L

From *Mosby's dictionary of medical, nursing, and health professions*, ed 8, St Louis, 2008, Mosby.

Tests of Immunological Function Reference Values: For Chapter 7

Test	Conventional Units	SI Units
Complement, serum		
C3	85-175 mg/dL	0.85-1.75 g/L
C4	15-45 mg/dL	150-450 mg/L
Total hemolytic (CH$_{50}$)	150-250 U/mL	150-250 U/mL
Immunoglobulins, serum, adult		
IgG	640-1350 mg/dL	6.4-13.5 g/L
IgA	70-310 mg/dL	0.70-3.1 g/L
IgM	90-350 mg/dL	0.90-3.5 g/L
IgD	0.0-6.0 mg/dL	0.0-60 mg/L
IgE	0.0-430 ng/dL	0.0-430 µg/L

From *Mosby's dictionary of medical, nursing, and health professions*, ed 8, St Louis, 2008, Mosby.

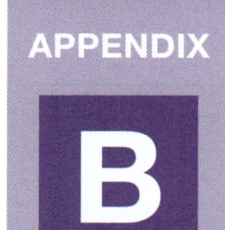

APPENDIX B: Herb/Laboratory Test Interactions

Herb/Laboratory Test Interactions

Herb	Test Affected	Results
Aloe	Serum potassium	↓ Test values
Angelica	Plasma partial thromboplastin time (PTT)	↑ In clients taking warfarin concurrently
	Prothrombin time (PT) and plasma International Normalized Ratio	↑ In clients taking warfarin concurrently
Astragalus	Semen specimen analysis	↑ Sperm motility in vitro
Cascara	Serum and 24-hour urine estrogens	↑ or ↓ Test values
Chaparral	Alanine aminotransferase (ALT)	
	Aspartate aminotransferase (AST)	
	Total bilirubin	
	Urine bilirubin	
Chaste tree	Serum prolactin	↓ Test values
Chromium	Blood glucose	↓ Test values
	High-density lipoprotein (HDL) levels	↑ Test values
	Triglycerides	↓ Test values
Coffee	AST	↓ Test values in alcoholics
	Secretion provocation test	↑ Test values
	Serum 2-hour postprandial glucose	False ↑ if caffeine is ingested during test
	Specimen infertility screen	Possible ↓ in number of motile sperm with heavy coffee consumption
Comfrey	ALT	↑ Test values
	AST	↑ Test values
	Total bilirubin	↑ Test values
Cranberry	Urine pH	↓ pH
Echinacea	ALT	↑ Test values
	AST	↑ Test values
	Lymphocyte counts	↑ Lymphocyte counts
	Serum immunoglobin E (IgE)	↑ Test values
	Blood erythrocyte sedimentation rate (ESR)	↑ ESR
	Specimen semen analysis	High doses of herb interfere with sperm enzyme activity
Ephedra	AST	↑ Test values
	ALT	↑ Test values
	Total bilirubin	↑ Test values
	Urine bilirubin	↑ Test values
Fenugreek	Total cholesterol	↓ Total cholesterol
	Blood glucose	↓ Test values
	Low-density lipoprotein (LDL) cholesterol	↓ LDL cholesterol
Feverfew	Blood platelet aggregation	↓ Test values
	PT	↑ Values in clients taking warfarin concurrently
	PTT	↑ Values in clients taking warfarin concurrently
Figwort	Blood glucose	↓ Test values

(continued)

Herb/Laboratory Test Interactions—Cont'd

Herb	Test Affected	Results
Garlic	LDL cholesterol	↓ Test values with aged extract taken continuously
	Platelet aggregation	↓ Test values with aged extract taken continuously
	Triglycerides	↓ Test values with aged extract taken continuously
	Blood lipid profile	↓ Test values
	PT	↓ Test values
	Serum IgE	↓ Test values
Ginger	PTT	↑ Values in clients taking warfarin concurrently
	PT	↑ Test values
Ginkgo	PT	↑ Test values
	Blood salicylate	↑ Test values
	Platelet activity	↓ Platelet activity
	PTT	↑ Bleeding
	Acetylsalicylic acid tolerance test	↑ Bleeding
Ginseng	Blood glucose	↓ Test values
	PTT	↓ Test values
	Serum and 24-hour urine estrogens	Additive effects to estrogen
	Serum digoxin	Falsely ↑ test values
Goldenseal	Bilirubin	↑ Test values
	Blood osmolality	↑ Test values
	Serum or urine plasma sodium	↑ Test values
Guar gum	Blood cholesterol	↓ Test values
	Blood glucose levels	↓ Test values
Gymnema	Blood glucose	↓ Test values
	LDL cholesterol	↓ Test values
	Total cholesterol	↓ Test values
Hawthorn	Serum digoxin	Falsely ↑ test values
Lecithin	Blood lipid profile	↓ Total cholesterol test values
Licorice	Blood anion gap	↓ Test values
	Qualitative urine myoglobin	Possible positive test result
	Serum or urine plasma sodium	↑ Test values (hypernatremia)
	Serum myoglobin	Possible positive test result
	Serum potassium	↓ Test values
	Serum prolactin (human prolactin)	↓ Test values
Mayapple	Red blood cells (RBCs)	↓ Test values
Mistletoe	ALT	↑ Test values
	AST	↑ Test values
	Total bilirubin	↑ Test values
	Urine bilirubin	↑ Test values
	Lymphocyte counts	↑ Lymphocyte counts
	RBCs	↓ Test values
Mugwort	Serum bilirubin: total, direct (conjugated), and indirect (unconjugated)	Possible ↑ direct bilirubin
Pennyroyal	ALT	↑ Test values
	AST	↑ Test values
	Total bilirubin	↑ Test values
	Urine bilirubin	↑ Test values
	RBCs	↓ Test values
Plantain	Blood glucose	↓ Test values
	Cholesterol: total, LDL, HDL ratio tests	↓ Test values
	Serum digoxin	Falsely ↑ test values
Poppy	Urine heroin	False-positive test result
	Urine morphine	False-positive test result
Pycnogenol	Blood platelet aggregation	↓ Test values

Herb/Laboratory Test Interactions—Cont'd

Herb	Test Affected	Results
Rauwolfia	Gastric analysis results	↑ Test values
	Basal nocturnal acid output	↑ Test values
	Serum or urine plasma sodium	↑ Test values (hypernatremia)
	RBCs	↓ Test values
	Urine vanillylmandelic acid	↓ Test values
	Serum gastrin	↓ Test values
Saw palmetto	Bleeding time	↑ Bleeding time
	Specimen semen analysis	Metabolic changes in sperm
Schisandra	ALT	↓ Test values
	AST	↓ Test values
Senna	Serum and 24-hour urine estriol	↓ Test values
Siberian ginseng	Serum androstenedione	↑ Test values
	Blood glucose levels	↓ Test values
Skullcap	ALT	↑ Test values
	AST	↑ Test values
	Total and urine bilirubin	↑ Test values
Soy	HDL cholesterol	↑ Test values
	LDL cholesterol	↓ Test values
	Triglycerides	↓ Test values
	Total cholesterol	↓ Test values
Squill	RBCs	↓ Test values
St. John's wort	Growth hormone (somatotropin)	↑ Test values
	Serum prolactin	↓ Test values
	Theophylline (aminophylline)	↓ Test values
	Serum iron	↓ Test values
	Serum digoxin	↓ Digoxin peak and trough concentrations
Valerian	ALT	↑ Test values
	AST	↑ Test values
	Total bilirubin	↑ Test values
	Urine bilirubin	↑ Test values

From Skidmore-Roth L: *Mosby's handbook of herbs and natural supplements*, ed 4, St Louis, 2009, Mosby.

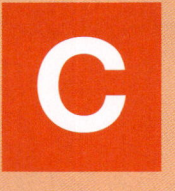

APPENDIX C: Common Laboratory Tests

Values may vary according to laboratory and are for reference only. Results of one test alone usually are not conclusive and should be considered with results of other diagnostic procedures, the signs and symptoms, and the physical examination to arrive at a diagnosis.

URINE STUDIES: CHAPTER 3

Urinalysis

A screening test that uses a urine specimen can give a picture of the patient's overall state of health and the state of the urinary tract. Measurements include pH and specific gravity of the urine and the presence of ketones, protein, sugars, bilirubin, and urobilinogen. Color and odor are noted, as is the presence of abnormal blood cells, casts, bacteria, other cells, and crystals.

A routine urinalysis should reveal normal results.

Characteristics

Color and clarity: pale to darker yellow and clear
Odor: aromatic
Chemical nature: pH is generally slightly acidic, approximately 6.5
Specific gravity: 1.003-1.030, reflecting amount of waste, minerals, and solids in urine

Constituent Compounds

Protein: none or small amount
Glucose: none
Ketone bodies: none
Bile and bilirubin: none
Casts: none, or small amount of hyaline casts
Nitrogenous wastes: ammonia, creatinine, urea, and uric acid
Crystals: none to trace
Fat droplets: none

Culture and Sensitivity of Urine

Culture: A sample of urine specimen is placed in or on culture medium to see whether microbial growth occurs. If growth occurs, the pathogenic microbe is identified.

Sensitivity: A portion of the specimen is placed on a sensitivity disk that has been impregnated with specific antibiotics to determine the antibiotic to which the pathogen is resistant or to which it will be responsive. Normal results show no growth.

Growth indicates pathogens residing in the urinary tract. Sensitivity will identify antimicrobials to which pathogens are sensitive.

HEMATOLOGY: CHAPTER 5

Complete Blood Count

The complete blood count (CBC) is the evaluation of cellular components of the blood. It includes red blood cell count, red blood cell indexes, white blood cell count, white blood cell differential, hemoglobin, hematocrit, and platelet count. It is sometimes referred to as *hemogram*. Often, the differential must be ordered specifically as CBC with differential.

Red Blood Cell Count

Red blood cell (RBC) count is the count of erythrocytes in a specimen of whole blood.

Normal RBC counts are as follows:
Adult male: 4.6 to 6.1 million/μL
Adult female: 4.0 to 5.5 million/μL
Infants and children: 3.8 to 5.5 million/μL
Newborns: 4.8 to 7.1 million/μL

An elevated RBC count may indicate erythmia, polycythemia, erythrocytosis, dehydration, burns, anoxia, diarrhea, cardiovascular disease, poisoning, and pulmonary disease. A reduced RBC count may indicate anemia, bone marrow suppression, hemorrhage, liver diseases, thyroid disorders, cardiovascular disease, vitamin deficiency, and ingestion of certain drugs. When the RBC count is abnormal, cell morphology should be examined. As with most blood tests, results should be evaluated with other tests, along with signs and symptoms, to determine a diagnosis.

Hemoglobin

Hemoglobin (Hgb) is the measurement of the oxygen-carrying pigment of the red blood cells.

Normal values for Hgb are as follows:
Adult male: 14.0 to 18.0 g/dL
Adult female: 12.0 to 16.0 g/dL
Infants and children: 11.5 to 15.5 g/dL
Newborns: 14.5 to 22.5 g/dL

An elevated Hgb value may indicate congestive heart failure, chronic obstructive pulmonary disease, dehydration, burns, diarrhea, erythrocytosis, high altitudes, and thrombotic thrombocytopenia. A reduced Hgb may indicate iron-deficiency anemia, hemorrhage, hemolytic reaction to drugs or chemicals, liver diseases, systemic lupus erythematosus, and pregnancy.

Hematocrit

Hematocrit (HCT) is the measurement of the percentage of red blood cells in a volume of whole blood.

Normal hematocrit values are as follows:
Adult male: 37% to 52%
Adult female: 36% to 48%
Infants and children: 28% to 45%
Newborns: 48% to 69%

An elevated HCT value may indicate dehydration, burns, diarrhea, eclampsia, pancreatitis, shock, and polycythemia. A reduced HCT value may indicate anemia, bone marrow hyperplasia, congestive heart failure, fluid overload, burns, thyroid disorders, pancreatitis, pregnancy, pneumonia, and ingestion of certain drugs.

White Blood Cell Count

White blood cell (WBC) count is the count of white blood cells in a whole blood specimen.

Normal values are as follows:
Adult male: 4500 to 11,000/μL
Adult female: 4500 to 11,000/μL
Infants and children: 6000 to 17,500/μL
Newborns: 9000 to 30,000/μL

An elevated WBC count may indicate acquired hemolytic anemia, anorexia, abscess, appendicitis, bacterial infections, bronchitis, burns, biliary disorders, respiratory disorders, disorders of the gastrointestinal tract, renal disorders, blood disorders, lactic acidosis, poisoning, pregnancy, sepsis, shock, tonsillitis, trauma, uremia, and ingestion of certain drugs. Similar to an abnormal RBC count, a differential should be evaluated, and, as with most blood tests, results should be evaluated with other tests, along with signs and symptoms, to determine a diagnosis. A decreased WBC count may indicate acquired immune-deficiency syndrome (AIDS), anemia, chemical toxicity, Hodgkin's disease, influenza, Legionnaires' disease, radiation therapy, shock, septicemia, vitamin B_{12} deficiency, cirrhosis, hepatitis, hypothermia, leukopenia, tuberculosis, and ingestion of certain drugs.

Differential White Blood Cells (Differential Leukocyte Count)

A differential leukocyte count is an assessment by percentage of leukocyte distribution in a specimen of 100 WBCs.

Normal granulocytes levels are as follows:
Segmented neutrophils (SEGs), adult: 50% to 62%
Band neutrophils (bands), adult: 3% to 6%
Eosinophils (EOS), adult: 0% to 3%
Basophils (BASOS), adult: 0% to 0.75%
Monocytes (MONOS), adult: 3% to 7%
Lymphocytes (LYMPHS), adult: 25% to 40%

Increased neutrophils may indicate allergies, asthma, acute infections, appendicitis, burns, diabetic acidosis, cardiovascular disorders, disorders of the gastrointestinal tract, leukemia, respiratory disorders, poisoning, pyelonephritis, septicemia, tonsillitis, and ingestion of certain drugs. A decrease in neutrophils may indicate endocrine disorders, anaphylactic shock, carcinoma, chemotherapy, anemia, pneumonia, septicemia, radiation therapy, and ingestion of certain drugs.

Increased bands primarily indicate pharyngitis. Increased segmented neutrophils primarily indicate pernicious anemia.

Increased eosinophils may indicate allergies, asthma, cancer, dermatitis, diverticulitis, eczema, Hodgkin's disease, leukemia, parasitic infection, pernicious anemia, radiation therapy, sickle-cell anemia, tuberculosis, and ingestion of certain drugs. Reduced eosinophils may indicate aplastic anemia, congestive heart failure, eclampsia, infections, stress, and ingestion of certain drugs.

Increased basophils may indicate allergic reactions, Hodgkin's disease, hypothyroidism, radiation therapy, sinusitis, urticaria, and ingestion of certain drugs. Decreased basophils may indicate acute infections, anaphylactic shock, endocrine disorders, pregnancy, radiation therapy, stress, and ingestion of certain drugs.

Increased lymphocytes may indicate endocarditis, infectious mononucleosis, leukocytosis, lymphocytic leukemia, syphilis, toxoplasmosis, and ingestion of certain drugs. Decreased lymphocytes may indicate aplastic anemia, Hodgkin's disease, immunoglobulin deficiencies, leukemia, renal failure, systemic lupus erythematosus, uremia, and ingestion of certain drugs.

Increased monocytes may be indicative of Epstein–Barr virus, Hodgkin's disease, leukemia, rheumatoid arthritis, syphilis, systemic lupus erythematosus, tuberculosis, and ingestion of certain drugs. Decreased monocytes primarily indicate aplastic anemia and hairy cell leukemia.

Platelet Count (Thrombocyte Count)

The platelet count is the count of platelets in a whole blood specimen. Normal adult values are 150,000 to 400,000/mm^3.

Increased platelet count may indicate anemia, carcinoma, fractures, liver disorders, heart disease, hemorrhage, acute infection, inflammation, leukemia, pancreatitis, pregnancy, rheumatoid arthritis, surgery, and ingestion of certain drugs. A decreased platelet count may indicate anemia, bone marrow disorders, autoimmune disorders, severe burns, carcinoma, liver disorders, diffuse intravascular coagulation, hemolytic disease of the newborn, infections, radiation therapy, leukemia, and ingestion of certain drugs.

CLOTTING AND COAGULATION STUDIES: CHAPTER 5

Partial Thromboplastin Time

Partial thromboplastin time (PTT) is an evaluation of the functioning of the coagulation sequence. PTT is a screening process used to detect coagulation disorders and monitor the effectiveness of heparin therapy.

Normal values or standardized times must be checked with the laboratory because various processes may be used.

Increased standardized times may indicate cardiac surgery, diffuse intravascular coagulation, abruptio placentae, factor defects, hemodialysis, obstructive jaundice, vitamin K deficiency, presence of circulating anticoagulants, and ingestion of certain drugs. Decreased standardized times indicate acute early hemorrhage and extensive cancer.

Prothrombin Time

Prothrombin time (PT) is a measurement of the time taken for clot formation after the addition of reagent tissue thromboplastin and calcium to citrated plasma. In the clotting process, PT converts to thrombin. Adequate vitamin K is necessary for adequate PT production. This test helps in the evaluation of the clotting mechanism and in monitoring oral anticoagulant therapy. Normal values are 11.0 to 13.0 seconds but may vary by laboratory.

An increase in PT time may indicate vitamin K deficiency, liver disorders, anticoagulant therapy, prothrombin deficiency, salicylate intoxication, diffuse intravascular coagulation, systemic lupus erythematosus, clotting disorders, biliary obstruction, congestive heart failure, pancreatitis, snakebite, vomiting, toxic shock syndrome, and ingestion of certain drugs. A reduced PT time may indicate limited to deep vein thrombosis, myocardial infarction, peripheral vascular disease, spinal cord injury, pulmonary embolism, and ingestion of certain drugs.

Bleeding Times

Bleeding time is a screening test for coagulation disorders, a measurement of the time required for the platelet clot to form. Normal time at most laboratories is 3 to 10 minutes.

Increased bleeding times indicate several disorders, including thrombocytopenia, diffuse intravascular coagulation, aplastic anemia, platelet dysfunction, vascular disease, leukemia, liver disorders, aspirin ingestion, and ingestion of certain drugs. Decreased bleeding time is clinically insignificant.

Erythrocyte Sedimentation Rate

Erythrocyte sedimentation rate (ESR) is the rate at which red blood cells (erythrocytes) fall out of well-mixed whole blood to the bottom of the test tube. An alteration in blood proteins occurs during inflammatory and necrotic processes, causing an aggregation of red cells, thereby making them heavier and causing them to fall rapidly when placed in a special vertical test tube. A higher ESR is the result of faster settling of the cells. Although not diagnostic of any particular disease process, an elevated ESR gives an indication of an ongoing disease process.

Normal values by the Westergren method are as follows:
  Adult male: 0 to 15 mm/hr
  Adult female: 0 to 20 mm/hr
  Children: 0 to 10 mm/hr

Normal values by the Wintrobe method are as follows:
  Adult male: 0.41 to 0.51 mm/hr
  Adult female: 0.36 to 0.45 mm/hr

Increased ESRs may indicate collagen diseases, infectious processes, inflammatory disorders, cancer, heavy metal poisoning, toxemia, pelvic inflammatory disease, anemia, pain, pregnancy, pulmonary embolism, renal disorders, arthritis, subacute bacterial endocarditis, and ingestion of certain drugs. Decreased levels may be found in congestive heart failure and ingestion of certain drugs.

BLOOD CHEMISTRIES: CHAPTER 6

Chemistries

Normal chemistry profiles may contain blood serum levels for albumin, alkaline phosphatase, aspartate aminotransferase, bilirubin, calcium, creatinine, lactate dehydrogenase, phosphorus, total protein, urea nitrogen, and uric acid.

Albumin

Albumin measures one of two major protein factions of blood. Normal values are 3.5 to 5.0 g/dL.

Increased levels of serum albumin may indicate dehydration, diarrhea, meningitis, carcinoma, myeloma, nephrosis, nephrotic syndrome, peptic ulcers, pneumonia, rheumatic fever, systemic lupus erythematosus, uremia, vomiting, and ingestion of certain drugs. Below-normal levels of serum albumin may indicate ascites, alcoholism, burns, congestive heart failure, Crohn's disease, diabetes mellitus, edema, hypertension, kidney disorders, gastrointestinal disorders, trauma, stress, and ingestion of certain drugs.

Alkaline Phosphatase

Alkaline phosphatase measures the enzyme found in bone, liver, intestine, and placenta. Normal values are 35 to 150 U/L.

Elevated alkaline phosphatase levels may indicate alcoholism, liver disorders, diabetes mellitus, fractures, gastrointestinal disorders, endocrine disorders, hepatitis, Hodgkin's disease, leukemia, neoplasms, myocardial infarction, bone disorders, disorders of the pancreas, kidney disorders, and ingestion of certain drugs. Below-normal levels of alkaline phosphatase may indicate pernicious anemia, cretinism, hypothyroidism, malnutrition, nephritis, and ingestion of certain drugs.

Aspartate Aminotransferase

Aspartate aminotransferase (AST) measures the enzyme found primarily in the heart, liver, and muscle. Normal values are 1 to 36 U/L.

Elevated AST levels may indicate myocardial infarction, alcoholism, liver disorders, insult and injury to tissue (including trauma), cerebral and pulmonary infarctions, and ingestion of certain drugs. Reduced AST levels may indicate diabetic ketoacidosis, liver disease, uremia, and ingestion of certain drugs.

Bilirubin

A by-product of hemoglobin breakdown, bilirubin is produced in the liver, spleen, and bone marrow.
Normal values are as follows:
Total, adult: less than 1.5 mg/dL
Direct, adult: 0.0 to 0.3 mg/dL
Indirect, adult: 0.1 to 1.0 mg/dL
Total bilirubin is divided into direct bilirubin, primarily secreted by the intestinal tract, and indirect bilirubin, primarily circulating in the bloodstream. Obstructive or hepatic jaundice results in an increased amount of direct bilirubin entering the bloodstream rather than entering the gastrointestinal tract and being filtered and eliminated by the kidneys. Conditions that cause an increase in direct bilirubin include biliary obstruction, pancreatic cancer (head of pancreas), cirrhosis, hepatitis, and ingestion of certain drugs. Hemolytic jaundice causes the indirect bilirubin to accumulate in the blood because of the increased breakdown of Hgb. Conditions that cause an increase in direct bilirubin levels include pernicious and sickle-cell anemia, autoimmune hemolysis, cirrhosis, hepatitis, intracavity and soft tissue hemorrhage, myocardial infarction, septicemia, hemolytic transfusion reaction, and ingestion of certain drugs.

Calcium

Calcium measures blood serum calcium levels. Normal values are 8.2 to 10.2 mg/dL.

Calcium acts in bone formation, impulse conduction, myocardial and skeletal muscle contractions, and the blood clotting process. Elevated serum calcium levels may indicate endocrine disorders, hepatic disease, respiratory acidosis, leukemia, neoplasms, blood disorders, respiratory disorders, and ingestion of certain drugs. Reduced serum calcium levels may indicate alkalosis, bacteremia, burns, chronic renal disease and other renal disorders, endocrine disorders, osteomalacia, rickets, vitamin D deficiency, and ingestion of certain drugs.

Creatinine

Creatine measurement is an indicator of renal function.
Normal values are as follows:
Adult male: 0.6 to 1.2 mg/dL
Adult female: 0.5 to 1.1 mg/dL
Serum creatinine is continually excreted by the renal system, and elevated levels indicate a slowing of glomerular filtration. Other conditions that may contribute to elevation of serum creatinine include congestive heart failure, diabetes mellitus, kidney disorders, hypovolemia, metal poisoning, endocrine disorders, subacute bacterial endocarditis, systemic lupus erythematosus, and ingestion of certain drugs. Decreased serum creatinine levels indicate diabetic ketoacidosis and muscular dystrophy.

Lactate Dehydrogenase

Lactate dehydrogenase measures the body tissue intracellular enzyme released after tissue damage. Normal values are 110 to 220 U/L.

Elevated lactate dehydrogenase levels may indicate alcoholism, anoxia, burns, cardiomyopathy, cerebrovascular accident, cirrhosis, congestive heart failure and myocardial infarction, neoplasms, anemias and leukemia, renal disorders, muscle and bone pain, respiratory disorders, shock, trauma, and ingestion of certain drugs. Decreased levels of lactate dehydrogenase develop after radiation and after the ingestion of oxalates.

Total Protein

Total protein is a reflection of the total amounts of albumin and globulins in blood serum. Normal values are 6.0 to 8.0 g/dL.

Increased total protein may indicate Addison's disease, Crohn's disease, dehydration, diarrhea, renal disease, vomiting, protozoal diseases, and ingestion of certain drugs. Decreased total protein may indicate burns, cholecystitis, cirrhosis, congestive heart failure, diarrhea, hyperthyroidism, edema, leukemia, peptic ulcer, nephrosis, malnutrition, ulcerative colitis, and ingestion of certain drugs.

Urea Nitrogen/Blood Urea Nitrogen

Blood urea nitrogen is the assessment of the urea content in the blood that indicates the functioning of the renal glomeruli. Normal values are 10 to 23 mg/dL.

An elevated urea nitrogen level can be attributable to prerenal (inadequate renal circulation or abnormally high levels of blood protein), renal (impaired renal filtration and excretion), or postrenal (lower urinary tract obstruction) causes.

Uric Acid

Uric acid is an end product of the metabolism of purines.

Normal values are as follows:
Adult male: 3.4 to 7.0 mg/dL
Adult female: 2.4 to 6.0 mg/dL

Elevated uric acid levels may indicate gout; hyperuricemia; hemolytic, pernicious, and sickle-cell anemia; arteriosclerosis; arthritis; congestive heart failure; dehydration; diabetes mellitus; fasting; exercise; hypothyroidism; intestinal obstruction; acute infections; lead poisoning; leukemia; neoplasms; nephritis; polycystic kidney; renal failure; starvation; stress; uremia; urinary obstruction; and ingestion of certain drugs. Reduced uric acid levels may indicate acromegaly, carcinomas, Hodgkin's disease, pernicious anemia, and ingestion of certain drugs.

Thyroid Function Tests

Thyroid function tests are an evaluation of all three thyroid levels and are important in diagnosing thyroid disorders.

Thyroid Thyroxine (T_4)

The hormone thyroxine is produced in the thyroid gland from iodide and thyroglobulin in response to stimulation by thyroid-stimulating hormone (TSH) produced by the pituitary gland. T_4 stimulates T_3 to be produced. It also stimulates the basal metabolism. In the process of negative feedback, circulating levels of T_4 influence the levels of TSH. Normal values are 5.0 to 12.0 µg/dL.

Increased levels of T_4 usually indicate the presence of hyperfunctioning thyroid disorders, including Graves' disease, hyperthyroidism, thyrotoxicosis, and ingestion of certain drugs. Decreased levels of T_4 indicate hypothyroid disorders, including acromegaly, cretinism, and goiter, as well as hypothyroidism, liver disease, endocrine disorders, gastrointestinal tract disorders, pituitary tumor, and ingestion of certain drugs.

Triiodothyronine (T_3)

T_3 stimulates the basal metabolic rate for metabolism of carbohydrates and lipids, protein synthesis, vitamin metabolism, and bone calcium release. Normal values are 80 to 230 ng/dL.

An increase in T_3 levels may indicate Graves' disease, hyperthyroidism, thyrotoxicosis, and ingestion of certain drugs. Decreased levels of T_3 may indicate iodine and thyroid deficiency disorders, including goiter and myxedema, renal failure, starvation, thyroidectomy, and ingestion of certain drugs.

Thyroid-Stimulating Hormone

TSH, produced in the anterior lobe of the pituitary gland, stimulates the production and release of T_3 and T_4 by the thyroid gland. Normal values are less than 10 µU/mL.

An increase in TSH levels may indicate Addison's disease, goiter, hyperpituitarism, hypothyroidism, thyroiditis, and ingestion of certain drugs. A decrease in TSH may indicate Hashimoto thyroiditis, hyperthyroidism, and hypothyroidism.

Lipid Profile

A lipid profile consists of the comparison of results of four serum lipids, total cholesterol, triglycerides, high-density lipoproteins (HDLs), and low-density lipoproteins (LDLs). One consideration is the ratio of HDL to LDL; the recommended ratio is 3.4:5.0.

Common Laboratory Tests

Total Cholesterol

Total cholesterol is a widely distributed sterol that facilitates the absorption and transport of fatty acids. Found in foods of animal origin, cholesterol is continuously synthesized in the body.

Normal values are as follows:
Less than 29 years: less than 200 mg/dL
30 to 39 years: less than 225 mg/dL
40 to 49 years: less than 245 mg/dL
More than 50 years: less than 265 mg/dL

Elevated serum cholesterol levels may indicate atherosclerosis, coronary artery disease, congestive heart failure, biliary disorders, kidney disorders, lipid disorders, and ingestion of certain drugs. Decreased levels of serum cholesterol may indicate anemia, carcinoma, cirrhosis, liver disease, hepatitis, endocrine disorders, gastrointestinal tract disorders, and ingestion of certain drugs.

Triglycerides

Triglycerides, the principal lipids in blood, are simple fat compounds of three molecules of fatty acid: oleic, palmitic, or stearic.

Normal values for an adult male are as follows:
20 to 29 years: 10 to 157 mg/dL
30 to 39 years: 10 to 182 mg/dL
40 to 49 years: 10 to 193 mg/dL
50 to 59 years: 10 to 197 mg/dL
More than 59 years: 10 to 199 mg/dL
Normal values for an adult female are as follows:
20 to 29 years: 10 to 100 mg/dL
30 to 39 years: 10 to 110 mg/dL
40 to 49 years: 10 to 122 mg/dL
50-59 years: 10 to 134 mg/dL
More than 59 years: 10 to 147 mg/dL

Elevated triglyceride levels may indicate arteriosclerosis, myocardial infarction, aortic aneurysm, hypercholesterolemia, hyperlipoproteinemia, alcoholism, diabetes mellitus, gout, renal disease, starvation, and malnutrition. Decreased triglyceride levels may indicate cirrhosis, malabsorption, hyperalimentation, and ingestion of certain drugs.

High-Density Lipoprotein Cholesterol

HDL transports cholesterol and other lipids to the liver for excretion. HDL is believed to reduce the risk of coronary artery disease.

Normal values are as follows:
Adult male: 30 to 70 mg/dL
Adult female: 30 to 85 mg/dL

Increased levels of HDL may indicate alcoholism, hepatic disorders, cirrhosis, and ingestion of certain drugs. Reduced levels of HDL may indicate arteriosclerosis, hypercholesterolemia, hyperlipoproteinemia, coronary artery disease, diabetes mellitus, liver disease, kidney disease, bacterial infections, and ingestion of certain drugs.

Low-Density Lipoprotein Cholesterol

LDL has a high cholesterol content and delivers lipids to body tissues. Normal values are 80 to 190 mg/dL.

Elevated LDL levels may indicate diabetes mellitus, anorexia nervosa, renal failure, hepatic disease, and ingestion of certain drugs. Decreased levels of LDL may indicate hyperlipoproteinemia, arteriosclerosis, pulmonary disease, stress, and the ingestion of certain drugs.

Electrolytes

Electrolyte measurement is a blood serum test for chloride, potassium, sodium, and carbon dioxide.

Chloride

Chloride is an anion found predominantly in extracellular spaces. Normal values are 97 to 106 mEq/L.

Increased chloride blood serum levels may indicate metabolic disorders, dehydration, diabetes insipidus, hyperventilation, hyperparathyroidism, acidosis, respiratory alkalosis, congestive heart failure, Cushing's disease, nephritis, renal failure, and ingestion of certain drugs. Reduced blood serum levels of chloride may indicate metabolic alkalosis, diabetes, severe vomiting, burns, overhydration, salt-losing diseases, some diuretic therapies, central nervous system disorders, diaphoresis, fasting, fever, heat exhaustion, acute infections, gastric obstructions, uremia, and ingestion of certain drugs.

Potassium

Potassium is the main cation of intracellular fluid. Potassium is important in nerve conduction, muscle function, osmotic pressure, acid–base balance, and myocardial activity. Normal values are 3.5 to 5.3 mEq/L.

Increased potassium blood serum levels may be the result of renal failure, dehydration, burns, trauma, chemotherapy, metabolic acidosis, Addison's disease, uncontrolled diabetes, dialysis, hemolysis, intestinal obstruction, sepsis, shock, pneumonia, uremia, and ingestion of certain drugs. Reduced potassium blood serum levels may be the result of alkalosis, anorexia, vomiting, diarrhea, malabsorption, starvation, diuresis, excessive sweating, draining wounds, severe burns, endocrine disorders, pancreatitis, gastrointestinal stress, and ingestion of certain drugs.

Sodium

Sodium is the major cation of extracellular fluid and the main base in the blood. Its functions include chemical maintenance of osmotic pressure, acid–base balance, and nerve transmission. Normal values are 135 to 145 mEq/L.

Increased blood serum levels of sodium may be the result of severe burns; congestive heart failure; excessive fluid loss caused by vomiting, diarrhea, or sweating; Addison's disease; nephrotic syndrome; pyloric obstruction; diabetes insipidus; hypertension; hypovolemia; toxemia; malabsorption syndrome; diuresis; edema; hypothyroidism; and ingestion of certain drugs. Decreased blood serum levels of sodium may be the result of bowel obstruction, dehydration, coma, Cushing's disease, diabetes mellitus, glomerulonephritis, hyperthermia, myxedema, certain renal conditions, and ingestion of certain drugs.

Carbon Dioxide

Carbon dioxide in normal blood plasma comes from bicarbonate. Normal values are 20 to 30 mEq/L.

Increased carbon dioxide blood serum levels may be the result of emphysema, aldosteronism, mercurial diuretics, severe vomiting, airway obstruction, bradycardia, cardiac disorders, renal disorders, and ingestion of certain drugs. Decreased carbon dioxide blood serum levels may be the result of severe diarrhea, diabetic acidosis, salicylate toxicity, starvation, acute renal failure, alcoholic ketosis, dehydration, high fever, head trauma, malabsorption syndrome, uremia, and ingestion of certain drugs.

GLUCOSE MONITORING: CHAPTER 6

Glucose Tolerance Test

The glucose tolerance test (GTT) evaluates patients who have symptoms of diabetes mellitus or diabetic complications. It also screens for gestational diabetes. The test measures blood glucose levels at the following intervals: fasting, 30 minutes, 1 hour, 2 hours, and 3 hours after ingestion of a dose of glucose. Urine samples are also taken at these intervals.

Normal values are as follows:
Fasting: 70 to 110 mg/dL
30 minutes: 110 to 170 mg/dL
1 hour: 120 to 170 mg/dL
2 hour: 70 to 120 mg/dL
3 hour: 70 to 120 mg/dL
All urine samples should test negative for glucose.

Increased glucose values or decreased glucose tolerance may indicate diabetes mellitus, excessive glucose ingestion, certain endocrine disorders, hepatic damage, postgastrectomy, central nervous system lesions, pancreatitis, pheochromocytoma, and ingestion of certain drugs. Decreased glucose values or increased glucose tolerance may indicate Addison's disease, hypoglycemia, malabsorption, pancreatic disease, liver disease, hypoparathyroidism, hypopituitarism, and ingestion of certain drugs.

Fasting Blood Glucose Levels

Fasting blood glucose is the amount of glucose found in the blood after 8 hours of fasting. Normal serum values are 70 to 110 mg/dL.

Increased levels of blood glucose may indicate diabetes mellitus, excessive glucose ingestion, certain endocrine disorders, hepatic damage, postgastrectomy, central nervous system lesions, pancreatitis, pheochromocytoma, and ingestion of certain drugs. Decreased glucose values may indicate Addison's disease, hypoglycemia, malabsorption, pancreatic disease, liver disease, hypoparathyroidism, hypopituitarism, and ingestion of certain drugs.

Two-Hour Postprandial

Two-hour postprandial measures blood glucose levels 2 hours after ingestion of a normal meal, usually the noon meal. Normal values are 65 to 139 mg/dL.

Increased postprandial levels of blood glucose may indicate diabetes mellitus, excessive glucose ingestion, certain endocrine disorders, hepatic damage, postgastrectomy, central nervous system lesions, pancreatitis, pheochromocytoma, and ingestion of certain drugs. Decreased postprandial glucose values may indicate Addison's disease, hypoglycemia, malabsorption, pancreatic disease, liver disease, hypoparathyroidism, hypopituitarism, and ingestion of certain drugs.

Glycosylated Hemoglobin/ Glycohemoglobin/Hemoglobin A1c

Glycohemoglobin is a measurement of the blood glucose bound to hemoglobin; it gives an overall view of the past 120 days of glucose saturation. Normal values are 5.5% to 8.5%.

Increased glycohemoglobin levels may indicate poorly controlled diabetes mellitus, iron deficiency anemia, splenectomy, alcohol or lead toxicity, and hyperglycemia. Decreased levels of glycohemoglobin may indicate hemolytic anemia, chronic blood loss, chronic renal failure, and pregnancy.

TOXICOLOGY STUDIES: CHAPTER 9

Toxicology studies are conducted on blood, primarily plasma, and urine. Blood levels of various medications are checked for toxic levels to determine whether the medications are at therapeutic level or are at or approaching a toxic level. Blood alcohol levels are the preferred method of screening for blood alcohol content to provide the desired quantitative information. Urine drug screens are used to detect the presence of various drug substances, primarily drugs of common abuse or illegal origin, as well as screening for blood alcohol. Drugs detected by urine screening include depressants, hallucinogens, sedatives, and stimulants.

BLOOD (DRUG) MONITORING TESTS: CHAPTER 9

Drug Levels

Common blood serum testing for therapeutic drugs includes digoxin, digitoxin, theophylline, lidocaine, lithium, and various drugs for therapeutic or toxic levels.

Digoxin

Digoxin is a cardiac glycoside used to treat congestive heart failure and cardiac arrhythmias. Blood level studies produce information about the therapeutic or toxic levels. The normal therapeutic level is 0.8 to 2 ng/mL.

Levels greater than 2 ng/mL indicate drug toxicity. Medical intervention is necessary to return levels to the therapeutic range. Levels less than 0.8 ng/mL indicate that more digoxin is necessary to achieve the expected therapy.

Digitoxin

Digitoxin is a cardiac glycoside used to treat congestive heart failure and cardiac arrhythmias. Blood level studies provide information about the therapeutic or toxic levels. The normal therapeutic level is 20 to 35 ng/mL.

Levels greater than 35 ng/mL indicate a toxicity of the drug. Medical intervention is necessary to return levels to the therapeutic range. Levels less than 20 ng/mL indicate that more digitoxin is necessary to achieve the expected therapy.

Theophylline

Theophylline, a bronchodilator, is used to treat asthma and obstructive respiratory disorders. Blood level studies give information about the therapeutic or toxic levels. The normal therapeutic level is 8 to 20 µg/mL.

Levels greater than 20 µg/mL indicate drug toxicity. Medical intervention is necessary to return levels to the therapeutic range. Levels less than 8 µg/mL indicate that more theophylline is necessary to achieve the expected therapy.

Lidocaine

Lidocaine is used to treat ventricular arrhythmias. Blood level studies give information about the therapeutic or toxic levels. The normal therapeutic level is 1.5 to 6 µg/mL.

Levels greater than 6 µg/mL indicate drug toxicity. Medical intervention is necessary to return levels to the therapeutic range. Levels less than 1.5 µg/mL indicate that more lidocaine is necessary to achieve the expected therapy.

Lithium

Lithium is used to treat bipolar disorders. The normal therapeutic level is 0.6 to 1.2 mEq/L.

Levels greater than 1.2 mEq/L indicate drug toxicity. Medical intervention is necessary to return levels to the therapeutic range. Levels less than 0.6 mEq/L indicate that more lithium is necessary to achieve the expected therapy.

Alcohol Levels

Normal alcohol levels are 0%. Each state has established the content of alcohol in the blood considered "legally drunk or intoxicated." Refer to state guidelines for these levels.

From Frazier MS, Drzymkowski JW: *Essentials of human diseases and conditions*, ed 4, St Louis, 2008, Saunders.

APPENDIX D: Frequent Medical Diagnoses and Laboratory Tests

When caring for the patient, the physician or nurse practitioner can use a number of laboratory tests and diagnostic procedures to make a diagnosis of what has caused the illness and determine the seriousness or extent of the disease. In the following table, common medical conditions are listed with the tests specific to that diagnosis. Generally, when particular tests can confirm or support the diagnosis, the list is somewhat shorter. For conditions in which no specific tests are available, a longer list of tests provides partial information.

Essential parts of the diagnostic process begin with the patient's history and the physical examination. The physician or nurse practitioner uses this important initial information as a guide to determine what is wrong. The diagnostic procedures and laboratory tests selected confirm or support the diagnosis by providing measurable, objective data. The physician or nurse practitioner uses all the data, in totality, to arrive at a definitive diagnosis.

Common Medical Diagnoses	Common Tests Used
Acquired immunodeficiency syndrome	Human immunodeficiency virus (HIV) antibody screen/enzyme-linked immunosorbent assay Western blot HIV antigen p24 antigen HIV-DNA amplification CD4 T-lymphocyte count Viral load
Addison's disease	Adrenocorticotropic hormone, plasma Corticotropin stimulation test Cortisol, serum or plasma Electrolytes, serum Growth hormone, serum Osmolality, urine Sodium, urine Thyroid-stimulating hormone, serum Thyroxine, serum
Aldosteronism	Adrenal vein catheterization for renin Aldosterone, serum or plasma Aldosterone, urine Computed tomography (CT) scan of the abdomen Electrolytes, serum Potassium, urine Renin, plasma Sodium, urine
Alzheimer's disease	Lumbar puncture Cerebrospinal fluid analysis Beta amyloid$_{(1-42)}$ Positron emission tomography (PET) scan
Anemia	Complete blood count (CBC) Hemoglobin Hematocrit Red blood cell morphology, peripheral blood Red blood cell indexes Reticulocyte count Biopsy, bone marrow

Frequent Medical Diagnoses and Laboratory Tests

Common Medical Diagnoses	Common Tests Used
Anemia, iron deficiency	CBC Red blood cell morphology, peripheral blood Ferritin, serum Iron, serum Transferrin, serum Total iron binding capacity Biopsy, bone marrow Occult blood, feces
Anemia, sickle-cell	Sickle-cell test Hemoglobin electrophoresis CBC Red blood cell morphology, peripheral blood In pregnancy: amniocentesis with amniotic fluid analysis for chromosome and genetic analysis
Aneurysm, aortic	Radiograph, abdomen CT scan, abdomen Aortography Magnetic resonance imaging (MRI), abdomen Transesophageal ultrasound
Angina	Cardiac markers Cardiac catheterization Echocardiogram Electrocardiogram Holter monitoring Lipids, serum Stress testing, cardiac Thallium stress testing
Appendicitis	CBC White blood cell count White blood cell differential, peripheral blood CT scan, abdomen Ultrasound, abdomen
Arthritis, rheumatoid	CBC Erythrocyte sedimentation rate C-reactive protein Rheumatoid factor Arthrocentesis with synovial fluid analysis Radiograph, joint
Ascariasis	Ova and parasites, feces CBC Eosinophil count
Asthma	Allergen identification Arterial blood gases Eosinophil count Culture, sputum Pulmonary function studies Radiograph, chest
Bronchitis	Arterial blood gases Culture, bacterial, sputum Culture, viral, sputum Radiograph, chest
Cancer, bone	Radiograph, bone Bone scan, nuclear Computed tomography, bone MRI, bone, extremity Biopsy, bone

Common Medical Diagnoses	Common Tests Used
Cancer, bone marrow (see *Leukemia*)	
Cancer, breast	Mammography Biopsy, breast Estrogen and progesterone receptor assay Carcinogenic embryonic antigen, serum Cancer antigen 15-3 Bone scan
Cancer, cervix	Papanicolaou smear Cervicovaginal cytology Human papilloma virus DNA probe Colposcopy Ultrasound, pelvic
Cancer, colorectal	Occult blood, feces Colonoscopy Sigmoidoscopy Barium enema Carcinogenic antigen 19-9 Carcinogenic antigen 125
Cancer, esophagus, stomach	Occult blood, feces Esophagogastroduodenoscopy with biopsy for cytology Upper gastrointestinal series Carcinoembryonic antigen Carcinogenic antigen 19-9 CT scan, chest, abdomen
Cancer, liver	Liver biopsy with cytology studies Ultrasound, abdominal CT scan, abdominal MRI, abdominal Alkaline phosphatase Carcinoembryonic antigen
Cancer, lung	Bronchial brushings for cytology Bronchial washings for cytology Cytology, sputum CT scan, chest Fine-needle biopsy, lung Open lung biopsy Transbronchial fine-needle aspiration Radiograph, chest
Cancer, pancreas	Percutaneous needle aspiration biopsy, pancreas, with cytology CA 19-9, serum CT scan, abdomen Carcinoembryonic antigen Ultrasound, pancreas Endoscopic retrograde cholangiopancreatography with pancreatic cytology Bilirubin, serum, urine Alkaline phosphatase
Cancer, prostate	Alkaline phosphates, serum Biopsy, prostate Prostate-specific antigen, serum
Cancer, renal	Fine-needle aspiration biopsy, kidney MRI, abdomen Ultrasound, abdomen
Cancer, testicular	Ultrasound, testes Alpha fetoprotein, serum Beta human chorionic gonadotropin Radiograph, chest CT, abdomen, pelvis

Frequent Medical Diagnoses and Laboratory Tests

Common Medical Diagnoses	Common Tests Used
Cancer, thyroid	Calcitonin, serum or plasma Fine-needle biopsy, thyroid
Cholecystitis/cholelithiasis	Ultrasound, gallbladder Liver/gallbladder radionuclide scan CT scan, abdomen MRI, cholangiography Oral cholecystography Endoscopic retrograde cholangiography Percutaneous transhepatic cholangiography
Chronic obstructive lung (pulmonary) disease	Arterial blood gas Electrocardiogram CBC Culture, sputum Pulmonary function studies Radiograph, chest
Cirrhosis, liver	Alanine aminotransferase Aspartate aminotransferase Protein, total, serum Albumin, serum Prothrombin time Sodium, serum Bilirubin, total, direct, indirect, serum Liver biopsy Liver/spleen scan Paracentesis with peritoneal fluid analysis Ultrasound, liver CT, abdomen
Colitis, ulcerative	Occult blood, feces CBC Total serum protein Albumin, serum Sigmoidoscopy with biopsy and cytology studies Barium enema Colonoscopy
Coronary artery disease	Cardiac catheterization Cardiac markers Electrocardiogram Stress testing, cardiac
Coronary artery disease, risk for	Cholesterol total, serum or plasma C-reactive protein Homocysteine, plasma Lipids, serum
Crohn's disease	Barium enema Upper gastrointestinal series with small bowel series CBC Protein, total, serum Occult blood, feces
Cushing's syndrome	Cortisol, free, urine Cortisol, serum or plasma Metyrapone test MRI, head Potassium, urine
Cystic fibrosis	Chloride sweat test Cystic fibrosis DNA amplification Fat, fecal Pulmonary function tests Radiograph, chest In pregnancy: amniocentesis with amniotic fluid analysis and chromosomal analysis

Common Medical Diagnoses	Common Tests Used
Deep vein thrombosis (see *Thrombophlebitis*)	
Dehydration	Electrolyte panel, serum Sodium, serum, urine Urea nitrogen, serum Creatinine, serum Urinalysis Specific gravity, urine Osmolality, serum, urine CBC Hemoglobin Hematocrit
Diabetes insipidus	Albumin, serum Antidiuretic hormone, plasma Electrolytes, serum Fluid deprivation test MRI, pituitary and hypothalamus Osmolality, serum Osmolality, urine Specific gravity, urine
Diabetes mellitus	Anion gap Electrolytes, serum Glucose, fasting, whole blood Glycosylated hemoglobin assay Ketone bodies, blood Ketones, urine Osmolality, plasma
Disseminated intravascular coagulation	Disseminated intravascular screen, serum D-dimer and fibrin split products Fibrinogen Partial thromboplastin time Prothrombin time CBC Platelet count Red blood cell morphology, peripheral blood

Fetal maturity	Fetal fibronectin, cervicovaginal secretions
	 Amniocentesis with amniotic fluid analysis:
	  Lecithin/sphingomyelin ratio
	  Phosphatidylglycerol
	  Pulmonary surfactant

Gastritis	*Helicobacter pylori* antibody, serum *Helicobacter pylori* antigen, serum Esophagogastroduodenoscopy with biopsy for cytology
Gastroesophageal reflux disease	Barium swallow Esophagoscopy with esophageal biopsy and cytological examination Esophageal manometry pH monitoring Bernstein acid perfusion test
Gonorrhea	Genital culture, *Neisseria gonorrhoeae* *Neisseria gonorrhoeae* RNA detection, secretions Throat culture, *Neisseria gonorrhoeae* Rectal culture, *Neisseria gonorrhoeae*
Gout	Uric acid, serum, urine Urinalysis Arthrocentesis with synovial fluid analysis

Common Medical Diagnoses	Common Tests Used
Heart failure (also called *congestive heart failure*)	Albumin, serum CBC Creatinine, serum or plasma Echocardiogram Electrolytes, serum Electrolytes, urine Thyroid-stimulating hormone Radiograph, chest
Hepatitis	Alanine aminotransferase Aspartate aminotransferase Bilirubin, total, direct, indirect, serum Hepatitis A antibody Hepatitis B, core antibody Hepatitis B DNA detection Hepatitis B surface antibody Hepatitis C virus serology Liver biopsy with cytology examination
Histoplasmosis infection	CBC Peripheral blood smear Fungal culture, blood, sputum, bronchial lavage, cerebrospinal fluid, urine Cytology examination, oral ulcers or sores Bronchoscopy with transbronchial biopsy, fine-needle aspiration, and cytology studies
HIV infection (see *Acquired immunodeficiency syndrome*)	
Hodgkin's disease	CBC Lymph node biopsy Liver biopsy Bone marrow biopsy CT scan, thorax, abdomen, pelvis
Hyperosmolar coma	Anion gap Arterial blood gases Electrolytes, serum Glucose, fasting, plasma Ketones, serum Ketones, urine Osmolality, serum Osmolality, urine
Hyperparathyroidism	Calcium, serum Calcium ionized, serum Calcium urine Parathyroid hormone, serum Phosphorus, serum Vitamin D, serum or plasma
Hypertension	Creatinine, serum or plasma Protein, urine Renal biopsy Renin, plasma Urea nitrogen, serum or plasma Sodium, serum or plasma Urinalysis

Common Medical Diagnoses	Common Tests Used
Hyperthyroidism	CT scan, thyroid
	MRI, thyroid
	Radionuclide scan (^{131}I, ^{123}I)
	Thyroid antibodies
	Thyroid-stimulating hormone
	Thyroxine, free, serum
	Thyroxine, total, serum
	Triiodothyronine, serum
Hypoparathyroidism	Calcium, ionized, serum
	Calcium, serum
	Calcium, urine
	Parathyroid hormone, serum
	Phosphorus, plasma
Hypopituitarism	Adrenocorticotropic hormone
	Cortisol, serum or plasma
	CT scan, head
	Follicle-stimulating hormone
	Luteinizing hormone
	Metyrapone stimulation test
	MRI, head
	Thyroid-stimulating hormone
Hypothyroidism	Cholesterol, serum or plasma
	Thyroid-stimulating hormone
	Thyroid antibodies
	Thyroxine, free, serum
	Thyroxine, total, serum
	Triiodothyronine, serum
	Ultrasound of the thyroid
Kidney stones	Calcium, serum
	CT scan, kidneys
	Intravenous pyelogram
	Kidney stone analysis
	Phosphorus, serum
	pH, urine
	Retrograde pyelogram
	Ultrasound, renal
	Uric acid, serum
	Uric acid, urine
	Urinalysis
Leukemia	CBC
	White blood count
	White blood cell differential count, peripheral blood
	Platelet count
	Bone marrow aspiration and biopsy
	Chromosome analysis, bone marrow
Lyme disease	Lyme disease antibody
	Lyme disease DNA detection
	Biopsy of lesion with bacterial culture for *Borrelia burgdorferi*
	Arthrocentesis with synovial fluid analysis and culture
Lymphoma	CBC
	White blood cell differential, peripheral blood
	Biopsy, bone marrow
	Biopsy, lymph node(s)
	Lumbar puncture, with cerebral fluid analysis: chemistry analysis, protein electrophoresis, cytology

Frequent Medical Diagnoses and Laboratory Tests

Common Medical Diagnoses	Common Tests Used
Melanoma	Biopsy, lesion or tumor, with microscopic pathology and chromosome analysis Biopsy, lymph node(s)
Meningitis	CT scan, brain Lumbar puncture with cerebral fluid analysis Cerebrospinal fluid culture, fungal, bacterial Culture: blood, nasopharyngeal, sputum, urine, skin lesion
Multiple myeloma	CBC Erythrocyte sedimentation rate Urinalysis Protein electrophoresis, serum: immunoglobulin (Ig) A, D, E, G, M Protein, total, serum Protein electrophoresis, urine Biopsy and aspiration, bone marrow Radiograph, bones MRI, bones
Multiple sclerosis	MRI Lumbar puncture with cerebrospinal fluid analysis Electroencephalogram
Myocardial infarction, acute	Cardiac markers Echocardiogram Electrocardiogram Thallium scan Erythrocyte sedimentation rate
Myocarditis	Culture, bacterial, blood Erythrocyte sedimentation rate Fine needle biopsy, myocardium White blood cell count
Nephrosis	Albumin, serum Antinuclear antibody Cholesterol, serum or plasma Complement components Creatinine clearance Glucose, plasma Glycosylated hemoglobin Osmolality, urine Protein electrophoresis, serum Protein, serum Protein, urine Urinalysis
Osteoporosis	Bone density scan (dual energy x-ray absorptiometry, CT) Calcium, serum, urine Parathyroid hormone, serum Radiograph, bone
Pancreatitis	Amylase, serum, urine Lipase, serum CBC White blood count Hematocrit Calcium, serum Glucose, plasma Urea nitrogen, serum Triglycerides, serum Radiograph, abdomen CT, pancreas

Common Medical Diagnoses	Common Tests Used
Peptic ulcer	*Helicobacter pylori* antigen, serum *Helicobacter pylori* antibody, serum Occult blood, feces Esophagogastroduodenoscopy with biopsy Ulcer biopsy: urease test, culture, cytology, DNA identification Upper gastrointestinal series
Peripheral arterial occlusive disease	Duplex Doppler ultrasound Arterial plethysmography Magnetic resonance angiography, extremity Arteriography
Peritonitis, acute	Laparotomy, diagnostic Peritoneal aspiration and bacterial culture Peritoneal fluid analysis and cytology Radiograph, abdomen
Pheochromocytoma	Catecholamines, plasma Catecholamines, urine Clonidine suppression test CT scan, chest and/or abdomen Cytology Glucagon stimulation test Metanephrine, urine or plasma MRI, chest and abdomen Vanillylmandelic acid, urine Radiograph, chest and abdomen

Pneumonia	CBC
	Culture, bacterial
	  Abscess
	  Biopsy
	  Blood
	  Sputum
	Culture, influenza viral
	Culture, viral
	Gram stain, sputum
	Sputum cytology
	Radiograph, chest

Preeclampsia	CBC Urea nitrogen, serum Urinalysis Creatinine clearance, urine Albumin, serum, urine Protein, urine Electrolytes, serum Prothrombin time Partial thromboplastin time Alanine aminotransferase Aspartate aminotransferase
Prostatitis	Bacterial culture, urine and/or prostatic secretions Biopsy, prostate (transurethral) Culture, urine Prostate-specific antigen Urinalysis

Frequent Medical Diagnoses and Laboratory Tests

Common Medical Diagnoses	Common Tests Used
Renal failure	Albumin, serum Anion gap Biopsy, renal Calcium, serum Creatinine clearance Creatinine, serum or plasma Electrolytes, serum Erythropoietin, serum Osmolality, urine Protein, urine Sodium, urine Specific gravity, urine Ultrasound, kidney Urea nitrogen, serum or plasma Urea nitrogen/creatinine ratio Urinalysis
Rheumatic fever	CBC White blood count C-reactive protein, serum Culture, oropharyngeal (throat) Group A beta hemolytic streptococcus screen, throat secretions Erythrocyte sedimentation rate Streptozyme, serum Electrocardiogram Antistreptolysin O antibody titer, serum
Sarcoidosis	CBC White blood count Calcium, serum Angiotensin converting enzyme, serum Alkaline phosphatase, serum Biopsy: liver, lymph node, or skin Fiberoptic bronchoscopy, with transbronchial fine-needle biopsy or aspiration Radiograph, chest Pulmonary function tests
Seizure	Electroencephalogram Glucose, plasma Sodium, serum Magnesium, serum Calcium, serum Osmolality, serum Toxicology, screen, urine MRI, brain Lumbar puncture with cerebrospinal fluid culture: bacterial, viral
Severe acute respiratory syndrome (SARS)	SARS antibody titers, serum SARS polymerase chain reaction (PCR) RNA detection, blood, feces, sputum Nasopharyngeal swab, SARS PCR viral RNA detection Oropharyngeal swab, SARS PCR viral RNA detection Bronchoscopy with bronchoalveolar lavage, tracheal aspirate: SARS PCR viral RNA detection Thoracentesis with pleural fluid aspirate: SARS PCR viral RNA detection
Syndrome of inappropriate secretion of antidiuretic hormone	Antidiuretic hormone, plasma Electrolytes, serum Osmolality, serum Osmolality, urine Sodium, urine Specific gravity, urine Urea nitrogen, serum or plasma Uric acid, serum

Common Medical Diagnoses	Common Tests Used
Syphilis	Darkfield examination, syphilis Fluorescent treponemal antibody, absorbed, serum Microhemagglutination, *Treponema pallidum*, serum Venereal Research Disease Laboratory test, serum, cerebrospinal fluid Biopsy, skin lesion, lymph node
Systemic lupus erythematosus	CBC White blood cell count, blood White blood cell differential, peripheral blood Urinalysis Anti-DNA Antinuclear antibody Complement, total, serum Complement C_3, serum Complement C_4, serum Antiphospholipid antibody, serum Smith and ribonucleoprotein (RNP) antibodies Creatinine, serum Creatinine clearance, urine Protein, urine Biopsy, kidney
Thalassemia	CBC Fetal hemoglobin, blood Hemoglobin electrophoresis
Thrombophlebitis	Duplex ultrasound, vein Venography Plethysmography, venous Hypercoagulation panel: protein C, protein S, serum
Toxoplasmosis	*Toxoplasma gondii* antibodies (IgM, IgG), serum Biopsy, lymph node with tissue culture PCR amplification DNA, blood, amniotic fluid Bronchoscopy with bronchoalveolar lavage, culture Lumbar puncture with cerebrospinal fluid cytology
Tuberculosis, pulmonary	Acid–base stain, sputum Culture, sputum Bronchoscopy, fiberoptic Transbronchial biopsy/washing Radiograph, chest
Urinary tract infection	Bacterial culture, urine Gram stain, urine Intravenous pyelogram (for recurrent infections) Urinalysis
Valvular heart disease	Cardiac catheterization Echocardiogram, transthoracic, transesophageal Electrocardiogram Radiograph, chest
Wilson's disease	Ceruloplasmin, serum Copper, serum, urine Liver biopsy Alanine aminotransferase Alkaline phosphatase Aspartate aminotransferase Bilirubin, total, serum

From Malarkey LM, McMorrow ME: *Saunders nursing guide to laboratory and diagnostic tests*, St Louis, 2005, Saunders.

Glossary

absorbance photometry indirect measurement of the amount of light that a solution absorbs

absorption passage of a substance through the surface of the body into body fluids and tissues

accuracy (correctness) when controls consistently fall within two standard deviations of the mean

active immunity long-term protection against future infections resulting from the production of antibodies formed naturally during an infection or artificially by vaccination

aerobic requiring oxygen for growth

aerosols fine particles suspended in air

agar gelatinous substance obtained from seaweed that is liquid when heated and becomes solid when cooled; used in culture media

agglutination clumping together of blood cells or latex beads caused by antibodies adhering to their antigens

ambulatory setting outpatient facility versus hospital or bedridden setting

anaerobic able to grow and function in the absence of oxygen

analyte the substance being tested, such as glucose or cholesterol in a blood specimen

anemia condition in which the red blood cell or hemoglobin level is below normal

anion negatively charged ion

anisocytosis abnormal variances in red blood cell size

antecubital space area in front of the elbow

antibodies immunoglobulins produced specifically to destroy foreign invaders

antigens substances that are perceived as foreign to the body and elicit an antibody response

anuria no flow of urine

arteries blood vessels that carry blood away from the heart

atherosclerosis formation of plaque along the inside walls of blood vessels

autoimmune diseases destructive tissue diseases caused by antibody/self-antigen reactions

band immature neutrophil whose nucleus has not segmented (also called *stab*)

bar code a pattern of narrow and wide bars and spaces encoded with its own particular meaning, just as words in a language are made up of letters and symbols

baso- prefix meaning alkaline

basophil white blood cell with large granules that stain dark blue

Beer–Lambert law law stating that intensity of color change is directly proportional to the concentration of an analyte in a solution

Bence Jones protein protein found in the urine of patients with multiple myeloma

bilirubin waste product from the breakdown of hemoglobin

binary fission asexual reproduction in which the cell splits in half

biohazard danger related to the exposure to infectious and bloodborne pathogens

bloodborne pathogens infectious microorganisms transmitted by the blood or bloody body fluid from an infected host into the blood of a susceptible host

Bloodborne Pathogens Standard rigorous standard of policies and procedures developed by the Occupational Safety and Health Administration to protect employees who work in occupations that put them at risk of exposure to blood or other potentially infectious materials

buffy coat narrow middle layer of white blood cells and platelets in a centrifuged whole blood specimen

buprenorphine an FDA-approved drug for treating opioid drug addiction

calibration the process of setting an instrument to respond accurately to the test reagents or devices

cannabinoid resembling marijuana

capillaries microscopic blood vessels that contain a mixture of arterial and venous blood

capillary action process by which blood flows freely into a capillary tube in microcollection procedures

carbohydrates sugars and starches

casts elements excreted in the urine in the shape of the renal tubules and ducts

catalysts chemicals that produce specific changes in other substances without being changed themselves

cation positively charged ion

cell-mediated immunity T-lymphocytic cell response to antigens

certificate of waiver (CoW) CLIA document that allows a facility to perform only waived tests

chemical hazard danger related to exposure to toxic, unstable, explosive, or flammable substances

chromatographic pertaining to a visual color change that appears when an enzyme-linked antibody/antigen reaction takes place

chronic disorders long-lasting, debilitating conditions

CLIA-waived tests tests that provide simple, unvarying results and require a minimal amount of judgment and interpretation

clinical diagnosis diagnosis based on the patient's initial signs and symptoms

clinical laboratory a facility or an area within a medical setting in which materials or specimens from the human body are examined or analyzed

clot activator chemical additive that speeds up the clotting of a blood specimen

coagulation clotting ability of blood

colony visible mass of bacteria formed on a culture medium by one bacterium growing and replicating

complement proteins proteins that stimulate phagocytosis and inflammation and are capable of destroying bacteria

contaminated an area that has been in contact with infectious materials or surfaces where infectious organisms may reside

control sample a manufactured specimen that has a known value of the analyte being tested

C-reactive protein (CRP) protein associated with myocardial infarctions (heart attacks)

critical value a test result far from the reference range indicating a threat to a patient's health (also referred to as "panic value")

cross-contamination transmitting a pathogen from one individual to another

culture the reproduction of microorganisms in a laboratory culture medium

cyanotic a condition in which the skin and mucous membranes are blue; caused by an oxygen deficiency

cytoplasm fluid within cells between the nucleus and the outer cell membrane

definitive diagnosis final, confirmed diagnosis based on clinical signs and symptoms and the results of diagnostic tests

diabetes mellitus disease caused by the lack of insulin or the inability to regulate blood sugar levels

differential count procedure for determining the distribution of the five types of leukocytes based on their staining characteristics, shapes, and sizes

distribution the blood then carries the drug through the body

diuresis increase in the volume of urine output

don to put on

dyslipidemia abnormal amounts of fat and lipoproteins in the blood

dysuria painful urination

edema abnormal collection of fluid in interstitial spaces

electrolyte element or compound that forms positively or negatively charged ions when dissolved and can conduct electricity

embolus traveling clot

endogenous cholesterol cholesterol manufactured in the liver

engineering controls efforts and research toward isolating or removing bloodborne pathogens from the workplace (e.g., biohazard disposal containers, safety devices on needles, and sharps containers)

eosino- prefix meaning acid

eosinophil white blood cell with large granules that stain red

erythroblastosis fetalis hemolytic anemia in newborns resulting from maternal–fetal blood group incompatibility

erythroblasts immature red blood cells (also called *rubriblasts*)

erythrocyte sedimentation rate (ESR) rate at which red blood cells settle out of an anticoagulated blood specimen after 60 minutes

eukaryotic pertaining to organisms that possess a true nucleus with a nuclear membrane and organelles

evacuate to remove air to produce a vacuum

exogenous cholesterol cholesterol derived from the diet

expectoration coughing up of sputum and mucus from the trachea and lungs

exposure control plan documented plan provided by a facility to eliminate or minimize occupational exposure to bloodborne pathogens

external controls liquid positive and negative controls tested before the patient specimen to check the reliability of the instrument and the testing technique

facultative anaerobe organism that grows with or without oxygen

fastidious requiring special nutrients or conditions for growth

fibrinogen (factor I) one of two plasma proteins involved in clotting

formed elements cells and cell fragments that can be viewed under the microscope

g/dL grams per deciliter (g/dL), which represents the weight of a substance (g) per volume (dL)

galvanometer instrument capable of measuring the intensity of light

glomerular (Bowman's) capsule cup-shaped structure surrounding the glomerulus that collects the glomerular filtrate

glomerulus structure in the renal corpuscle made up of tangled blood capillaries in which the hydrostatic pressure in the capillaries pushes substances through the capillary pores

glucagon hormone produced by the pancreas to raise blood glucose by converting glycogen into glucose and noncarbohydrates into glucose

glucose sugar

glycogen stored form of glucose found especially in muscles and the liver

glycosuria sugars (especially glucose) in the urine

glycosylated hemoglobin (hemoglobin A1c) hemoglobin A molecule within red blood cells that becomes permanently bound to glucose

gout form of arthritis caused by accumulation of uric acid crystals in the synovial fluid

gram-negative having the pink/red color of the counterstain used in Gram's method of staining microorganisms

gram-positive retaining the purple color of the stain used in Gram's method of staining microorganisms

Gram stain method of staining microorganisms that serves as a primary means of identifying and classifying bacteria

granulocytes white blood cells that contain granules in their cytoplasm: neutrophils, basophils, and eosinophils

Hazard Communication Standard federal law protecting employees' right to know about the dangers of all the hazardous chemicals they may be exposed to under normal working conditions

helper T cells (TH4 or CD4) antigen-activated lymphocytes that stimulate other T cells and help B cells produce their antibodies

hematocrit test that measures percentage of packed red blood cells compared with total blood volume

hematologist one who evaluates the cellular elements of blood microscopically and analytically by using a variety of test methods

hematology study of the visible cellular components in the bloodstream and bone marrow

hematoma tumor or swelling of blood in the tissues (resulting in bruising during blood collection procedures)

hematopoiesis blood production

hematuria intact red blood cells in the urine

hemoconcentration condition in which blood concentration of large molecules such as proteins, cells, and coagulation factors increases

hemocytoblast stem cell that differentiates (changes) and becomes any of the seven visible blood elements found in circulating blood

hemoglobin oxygen-carrying reddish pigment in red blood cells

hemolysis red cells breaking open and releasing hemoglobin

hemostasis the body's ability to initiate a clotting response to stop bleeding and at the same time prevent the blood from forming an unwanted stationary clot

hepatitis A virus (HAV) highly contagious virus that enters the body through the gastrointestinal tract and attacks the liver

hepatitis B virus (HBV) most prevalent bloodborne virus that attacks the liver; an individual can build a protective resistance against this virus by prior immunization or vaccination

hepatitis C virus (HCV) bloodborne virus that attacks the liver and is very likely to reach the chronic stage later in life

heterophile antibody antibody that appears during an Epstein–Barr viral infection (mononucleosis) and has an unusual affinity to antigens on sheep red cells

histamine compound released by injured cells that causes the dilation of blood vessels

homeostasis steady state of internal chemical and physical balance

human immunodeficiency virus (HIV) retrovirus that attacks the immune system by destroying the white blood cells known as CD4+ T lymphocytes

humoral immunity B lymphocytic cell response to antigens resulting in the production of specific antibodies to destroy a foreign invader; also called *antibody-mediated immunity*

humors fluid or semifluid substances found in the body

hyperchromia increase in color (based on hemoglobin concentration)

hyperglycemia elevated blood sugar

hyperinsulinemia excessively high blood insulin levels

hyperlipidemia excessive fat in blood, which gives plasma a milky appearance

hyphae tubelike filaments

hypochromic pertaining to less than normal color

hypoglycemia low blood sugar

hypoxemia lack of oxygen in the blood

iatrogenic caused by treatment or diagnostic procedures

idiosyncrasy an abnormal susceptibility to a drug or other agent that is peculiar to the individual

immunoglobulins antibodies that destroy or render harmless foreign invaders containing antigens

immunosorbent pertaining to the attachment of an antigen or antibody to a solid surface such as latex beads, wells in plastic dishes, or plastic cartridges

infection disease that occurs when pathogenic microorganisms invade the body and overcome its natural defense mechanisms

inflammation overall reaction of the body to tissue injury or invasion by an infectious agent, characterized by redness, heat, swelling, and pain

inoculation process of transferring microorganisms into or on a culture medium for growth

insulin hormone produced by the pancreas to lower blood glucose level by moving glucose into body cells and converting glucose into glycogen for future use

insulin resistance condition in which insulin is not effective at moving the glucose from the blood into the cells (seen in type 2 diabetes)

interferons proteins secreted by infected cells to prevent the further replication and spread of an infection into neighboring cells

internal control built-in positive control used in qualitative tests to prove the device or test kit is working

interstitial fluid all the fluid except blood that is found in the space between tissues; also referred to as *tissue fluid*

in vitro within a laboratory apparatus

in vivo within a host or living organism

ions electrolytes consisting of positively or negatively charged particles

ketoacidosis acidosis caused by an accumulation of ketones in the body as a result of the excessive breakdown of fats; occurs primarily as a complication of type 1 diabetes mellitus

ketonuria ketones in the urine

killer T cells antigen-activated lymphocytes that directly attack foreign antigens and destroy cells that bear the antigens; also called *cytotoxic cells*

kit all components of a test packaged together

laboratory reports results of laboratory tests that have been ordered

laboratory requisitions laboratory orders indicating what tests are to be performed

leukemia various cancers of the white blood cells

leukocytosis abnormal increase in white blood cells

leukopenia abnormal decrease in white blood cells

Levy–Jennings chart a graph used to plot and visualize the results of control samples over time

liberation the release of a prescribed drug from its dosage

lipiduria lipids in the urine

lipoproteins protein-linked lipids

lumen inner tubular space of a needle, vessel, or tube

lymphocyte small, nongranular white blood cell that develops from lymphoblasts in bone marrow

lyse to break open

macrophages large, engulfing cells that come from monocytes when they enter the tissues

malaise feeling of weakness, distress, or discomfort

mean the average test result of a series of control tests

media (singular: medium) liquid, semisolid, or solid substances containing nutrients needed to grow microorganisms

medical assistants multiskilled professionals dedicated to assisting in patient care management in medical offices, clinics, and ambulatory care centers

medical office risk management overseeing the physical and procedural risks that may bring about an injury or legal action against the practice

megakaryocyte large nuclear cell in the bone marrow that fragments its cytoplasm to become platelets

memory B cells antigen-activated B lymphocytes that remember an identified antigen for future encounters

memory T cells antigen-activated T lymphocytes that remember an antigen for future encounters

metabolite a substance produced by the metabolism of a drug in the body

microbiology study of microorganisms, including bacteria, fungi, protozoa, and viruses

microcollection collecting a small amount of blood

microorganism any tiny, usually microscopic entity capable of carrying on living processes

micturition expelling of urine, also referred to as *voiding* and *urination*

monocytes large, nongranular white blood cells that develop from monoblasts in bone marrow

morbidity the rate at which an illness occurs

mortality the rate of deaths

mucous membrane thin sheets of tissue that line the internal cavities and canals of the body and serve as a barrier against the entry of pathogens into the body

myalgia diffuse muscle pain

mycelium mass of hyphae that some fungi produce

myeloblasts stem cells that develop into the three kinds of granulocytes

myoglobin iron-containing, oxygen-binding protein found in muscles

natural killer cells special type of lymphocyte that attacks and destroys infected cells and cancer cells in a nonspecific way

nephron functional unit of the kidney

neutro- prefix meaning neither acid nor alkaline

neutrophil white blood cells with fine granules that stain lavender/pink

nocturia excessive urination at night

nongranulocytes (agranulocytes) white blood cells that may have a few or no granules in their cytoplasm; lymphocytes and monocytes

normal flora nonpathogenic microorganisms that normally inhabit the skin and mucous membranes

normocytes young red blood cells that shed their nuclei before entering the bloodstream

nosocomial infection disease spread within a health care facility

nucleus central controlling structure in the cell

occult hidden or not visible to the naked eye

occupational exposure occurs when blood or other potentially infectious material comes in contact with open skin, eye, or mucous membrane or parenterally in the workplace

oliguria decreased urine volume

opiates methadone and morphine

opportunistic infections infections that occur because of the body's inability to fight off pathogens normally found in the environment

optics check confirming that the light source and light sensor in optical analyzers are working properly

osteomyelitis inflammation of the bone caused by bacterial infection

palpating gently touching and pressing down on an area to feel texture, size, and consistency

panels/profiles a series of tests associated with a particular organ, disease, or metabolic function

parenteral contact when blood enters the body through the skin or mucous membrane by a needle stick, bite, cut, or abrasion

passive immunity short-term acquired immunity created by antibodies received naturally through the placenta (or the colostrum to an infant) or artificially by injection

pathogen disease-causing microorganism

patient compliance a patient's willingness to follow a treatment plan and take an active role in his or her health care

peptidoglycan component made of polysaccharides and peptides that gives rigidity to the bacterial cell wall

percutaneous through the skin

petechiae tiny purple or red skin spots caused by small amounts of blood under the skin; found in those with coagulation problems; condition can lead to excessive bleeding during phlebotomy procedures

Petri dish dish containing medium in which to grow microorganisms

pH scale that measures the level of acidity or alkalinity of a solution

phagocytes cells capable of engulfing and ingesting microorganisms and cellular debris

phagocytosis process of engulfing and digesting microorganisms and cellular debris

pharmacokinetics the movement of drugs through the body from the time of introduction to elimination

-phil suffix meaning attraction

phlebotomy blood collection; derived from the Greek words *phlebo,* meaning vein, and *tomy,* meaning to cut

physical hazards dangers related to electricity, fire, weather emergencies, bomb threats, and accidental injuries

plasma liquid part of whole blood

plasma cells a subgroup of B lymphocytes that produce the antibodies that travel through the blood specifically targeting and reacting with antigens

poikilocytosis abnormal shapes in red blood cells

polychromia increase in color variation (based on hemoglobin concentration)

polycythemia abnormal condition of increased red blood cells

polydipsia excessive thirst

polymorphonuclear having a multishaped, segmented nucleus; sometimes abbreviated as PMN or seg

polyphagia excessive hunger

polyuria passing abnormally large amounts of urine

porphyrin intermediate substance in the formation of heme (part of hemoglobin)

portal of entry any body opening or break in the skin through which an infectious agent enters the body

portal of exit the means by which an infectious agent leaves the host's body, such as through the mouth, broken skin, rectum, or body fluids

precision (reproducibility) ability to produce the same test result each time a test is performed

proficiency testing proving laboratory competency by testing a sample specimen from an outside accreditation agency and obtaining the correct result

prokaryotic pertaining to unicellular organisms that do not have a true nucleus with a nuclear membrane

protected health information (PHI) any health information in any form (written, electronic, or oral) that contains patient-identifiable information (e.g., name, Social Security number, telephone number) that must be kept confidential

proteinuria proteins in the urine

prothrombin (factor II) one of two plasma proteins involved in clotting

ProTime test test for monitoring coagulation times for patients taking anticoagulants

pyuria white blood cells in the urine

qualitative drug screening a measurement that determines if a substance is present or absent

qualitative test test that simply looks for the presence or absence of a substance

quality assurance (QA) overall process to aid in improving the reliability, efficiency, and quality of laboratory testing in general

quality control (QC) process in which known samples (controls) are routinely tested to establish the reliability, accuracy, and precision of a specific test system

quantitative drug screening a precise measurement of the amount of a substance present in the specimen

quantitative test test that produces a numerical value indicating the amount of a substance present

RBC indexes mathematical ratios of the three red blood cell tests (hemoglobin, hematocrit, and red blood cell count)

reagent substance or ingredient used in a laboratory test to detect, measure, examine, or produce a reaction

reducing substance substance that easily loses electrons

reference range the range of analyte values with which the general population will consistently show similar results 95% of the time

reflectance photometry indirect measurement of the light that reflects off a solution

reliability when both accuracy and precision are accomplished

renal corpuscle part of the nephron that contains the glomerulus and glomerular capsule

renal threshold level blood reabsorption limit of a substance and the point at which the substance is then excreted in the urine

renal tubules parts of the nephron composed of proximal convoluted tubules, the nephron loop (loop of Henle), and distal convoluted tubules

reservoir host an infected person who is carrying an infectious agent (pathogen)

reticulocytes newly released red blood cells in the blood that still contain some nuclear DNA

retroperitoneal located behind the peritoneal cavity

rouleaux formation arrangement of red blood cells resembling stacked chips

sediment the material at the bottom of the centrifuged tube of urine

self-antigens substances within the body that induce the production of antibodies that attack an individual's own body tissues; also called *autoantigens*

serology branch of laboratory medicine that performs antibody/antigen testing with serum

serum liquid part obtained when blood is clotted; lacks the clotting factors

specific gravity in urinalysis the weight of urine compared with the weight of an equal volume of water; measures the amount of dissolved substances in urine

standard deviation (SD) statistical term describing the amount of variation from the mean in a data set

Standard Precautions Centers for Disease Control and Prevention recommendations for infection control within health care facilities

supernatant the liquid portion of urine on top of the spun sediment

suppressor T cells antigen-activated lymphocytes that inhibit T and B cells after a sufficient number of cells have been activated

susceptible host an individual who is unable to defend himself or herself against a pathogen

syncope fainting

thrombocytes platelets; cellular fragments that gather at the site of a damaged blood vessel and release clotting chemicals to form a clot

thrombosis abnormal condition of clotting

thrombus unwanted stationary clot

titer a quantitative test that measures the amount of antibody that reacts with a specific antigen

toxicity the level at which a drug becomes poisonous in the body

trans fats synthetic hydrogenated fats

transient microorganisms organisms from contaminated objects or infectious patients that adhere to the skin and can be transmitted to others

transmission the means by which an infectious agent or pathogen is transported from an infected individual to another person by indirect or direct contact

transmittance photometry measurement of the amount of light passing through a solution

troponin I and T heart-specific indicators of a recent myocardial infarction

Universal Precautions assumption that blood or other potentially infectious material from any patient or test kit could be infectious

ureters slender, muscular tubes 10 to 12 inches long that carry the urine formed in the kidneys to the urinary bladder

urethra tube that carries urine to the outside of the body

urethral meatus urethral opening through which urine is expelled

urinary bladder hollow muscular organ that holds urine until it is expelled

vaccination process of injecting harmless or killed microorganisms into the body to induce immunity against a potential pathogen (also called *immunization*)

veins blood vessels that carry blood toward the heart

venipuncture removal of blood from a vein

vitamin K critical element in the production of prothrombin

wheal raised induration

work practice controls policies that are recorded, monitored, and evaluated with a view to protecting employees from exposure to the pathogens in blood or body fluids

Index

A
A blood type, 225–226, 226t
AB blood type, 225–226, 226t
abnormal crystals, microscopic urinalysis, 74–75, 79f
ABO blood types
 agglutination slide testing for, 229b–230b
 overview of, 225–226
 summary of, 226t
abscesses, from cocci, 265t
absorbance photometry, 171, 182
absorption stage, pharmacokinetics, 274–275, 284
Acceava Strep A Test procedure, 252, 253b–255b
acid urine crystals, microscopic urinalysis, 74, 78f
acid-fast bacilli (AFB), 62
acid-fast stains, 245, 245f
acquired immune deficiency syndrome. *see* AIDS (acquired immune deficiency syndrome)
acquired immunity, 212–215, 214f
active immunity
 acquiring, 213–215, 214f
 defined, 209
 overview of, 213, 214f
acute lymphocytic leukemia (ALL), 163
acute myelocytic leukemia (AML), 163
adaptive immunity, 212–215
additive contamination, order of draw in vacuum tubes, 102–104, 104t
additives
 color-coded hemoguard tubes for, 97–98, 98t
 order of draw for filling vacuum tubes, 102–104, 104t
 testing blood chemistry in reference laboratories using, 173
 in vacuum collection tubes, 95–97
aerobic
 defined, 236
 organisms, 257–258
aerosols
 as bioterrorism agent, 264
 defined, 236
AFB (acid-fast bacilli), 62
agar
 defined, 236
 growing bacteria with, 258
 using blood, 251–252, 259
 using chocolate, 259
agglutinin, 225
agglutination
 defined, 209
 overview of, 225
agglutination reaction tests
 ABO blood typing, 225–226, 226t, 229b–230b
 hemolytic disease of newborn and RhoGAM, 226, 227f

agglutination reaction tests *(continued)*
 overview of, 225–226
 Rh system, 226, 232b–233b
AIDS (acquired immune deficiency syndrome)
 diagnosing with acid-fast stains, 62
 as emerging infectious disease, 270t
 immunology test for, 228t–229t
 resulting from HIV, 218
 symptoms of, 19
air bubbles, in capillary tubes, 92
alanine aminotransferase. *see* ALT (alanine aminotransferase)
albumin
 in blood plasma, 173
 liver metabolizing amino acids into, 200
alcohol
 blood collection tests screening for, 280b
 CLIA-waived tests screening for, 281
 ethanol content in beverages, 278t
 impaired driving laws and, 275
 as most common legal drug of abuse, 275
 time intervals for detecting in urine, 278t
alcohol-based hand rubs
 applying, 17, 18f
 on contaminated objects, 17
 hand hygiene with, 17, 17f
alkaline phosphatase (ALP or AP), hepatic panel testing, 200
alkaline urine crystals, microscopic urinalysis, 74, 78f
ALL (acute lymphocytic leukemia), 163
allergens, 209, 215
ALP or AP (alkaline phosphatase), hepatic panel testing, 200
ALT (alanine aminotransferase)
 Cholestech analyzer testing, 183–184
 hepatic panel testing, 200–201
ambulatory care settings
 defined, 1
 monitoring patients in, 18
 overview of, 6–7
 prerequisites to laboratory procedures in, 3
amino acids, liver metabolism of, 200
AML (acute myelocytic leukemia), 163
ammonia odor of urine, 62
amoebic dysentery, 268t
amorphous phosphate crystals, 74, 78f
amorphous urates, 74, 78f
amphetamines, drug urine screening tests for, 276t–278t
ampicillin crystals, 75
anaerobic, 236
anaerobic organisms, 257–258, 258f
analytes
 analyzing specimens with, 3–4
 blood test report showing comprehensive panel of, 4, 5f
 defined, 1

analytes *(continued)*
 disease associations of individual, 201, 202t–204t
 laboratory measurements of, 9–11
 monitoring QC in qualitative tests, 44
 monitoring QC in semiquantitative tests, 44–45
 testing using optics, 45
 testing with Portable Clinical Analyzer, 6
anemia
 CBC test results indicating, 162
 defined, 128
 forms of, 164t
 RBC indices identifying, 159–162
anions, 171, 199
anisocytosis, 128, 139
antecubital space
 defined, 86
 venipuncture in, 89, 89f
anthrax
 Bacillus anthracis causing, 239, 264
 in bioterrorism, 264–268, 271f
antibiotics
 history of, 238t
 sensitivity testing for, 261–262, 261f–262f
 therapeutic drug monitoring of, 283, 284t
antibodies
 acquiring specific immunity, 213–215, 214f
 agglutinin and, 225
 agglutination reaction tests and. *see* agglutination reaction tests
 classes of, 213
 CLIA-waived enzyme-linked immunoassay tests, 215–216
 defined, 209
 ELISA tests, 226–227
 overview of, 210–215
 as third line of defense, 212–215
 vitro allergy tests, 215
 vivo allergy tests, 215
antibody titers, immunological test
 agglutination reactions, 227
 overview of, 227
antibody-mediated (humoral) immunity, 213, 213f–214f
anticoagulant additives
 order of draw for filling vacuum tubes, 102–104, 104t
 in vacuum collection tubes, 95–97, 97f
anticoagulant medications, monitoring thrombosis patient, 3
anticonvulsants, therapeutic drug monitoring, 283, 284t
antidepressants, therapeutic drug monitoring, 283, 284t
antigenic drift, mutation of influenza viruses, 252
antigenic shift, mutation of influenza viruses, 252

Page numbers with "t" denote tables; with "f" denote figures; and with "b" denote boxes.

321

antigens
  agglutination reactions. *see* agglutination reaction tests
  CLIA-waived enzyme-linked immunoassays, 215–216
  defined, 209
  ELISA test and, 226–227
  overview of, 210
  testing for, 210
  in vitro allergy tests and, 215
  in vivo allergy tests and, 215
antimicrobial soap, 17, 17f
antipsychotics, therapeutic drug monitoring, 283, 284t
antirheumatics, therapeutic drug monitoring, 283, 284t
anuria, 51, 55
aplastic anemia, in CBC test results, 162
appearance of urine, urinalysis, 62, 62f
arm, microscope, 36, 37f
arsenic poisoning, toxicology tests for, 285
arteries
  in closed circuit system, 88f
  defined, 86
  layers within, 89f
  overview of, 87
arterioles
  in closed circuit system, 88f
  collecting blood with skin puncture from, 91
  defined, 87
arthritis (rheumatoid factor) test, 228t–229t
artifacts, microscopic urinalysis, 75, 80f
artificial immunity, 213, 214f
-ase suffix, enzymes, 200
Asian flu, 252, 270t
aspartate aminotransferase (AST). *see* AST (aspartate aminotransferase)
AST (aspartate aminotransferase)
  Cholestech analyzer testing, 183–184
  hepatic panel testing, 200–201
atherosclerosis
  defined, 171
  high levels of triglycerides causing, 181
  type 2 diabetes causing, 177
Athlete's foot, 267t
attentiveness, laboratory professional attributes, 8
attitude, laboratory professional attributes, 8
atypical (walking) pneumonia, 266t
aureus, Staphylococci, 239
autoantigens, 210
autoimmune diseases, 209–210
automated hematology systems, CLIA-nonwaived
  Coulter Counter system, 167
  overview of, 165–167
  QBC STAR Centrifugal Hematology system, 166–167, 166f
Avian flu, 252

B

B blood type, 225–226, 226t
B cells
  activated in humoral immunity, 213f
  as third line of defense, 212–215
B lymphocytes, 134, 134f
bacillus (bacilli), characteristics of, 239
Bacillus anthracis, 239, 264
bacitracin method, Streptococcus Group A testing, 252
BACTEC bottles, for blood cultures, 241

bacteria
  biochemical testing of, 261, 261f
  culturing methods. *see* culturing methods
  diseases caused, 263t–264t
  gram-positive bacteria (GNB), 244, 245f
  growth requirements of, 257–258, 258f
  lines of defense against harmful. *see* immune process
  media for growing, 258–259, 258f–259f
  microbiology equipment for, 259, 260f
  microscopic urinalysis of, 75, 79f
  most commonly seen, 262, 269f
  overview of, 237
  structural characteristics of, 239, 239f
bacterial bioterrorism. *see* bioterrorism
bacterial infections
  immunology test for, 228t–229t
  indications of, 163
  most commonly seen, 262, 269f
  QBC STAR giving WBC information on, 166
  sensitivity testing for antibiotics in, 261–262, 261f–262f
bands (immature neutrophils)
  bone marrow cell development with, 133f
  defined, 128
  granulocytes entering bloodstream as, 131–132, 133f
  in hematopoiesis, 130, 131f
  showing in WBCs, 141t
bar codes, in medical laboratories, 32, 48–49, 49f
barbiturates
  drug urine screening tests detecting, 276t–278t
  therapeutic drug monitoring of, 283, 284t
  time intervals for detecting drugs in urine, 276t–278t
base, microscope, 36, 37f
basilic vein, 89
baso- prefix, 128
basophils
  defined, 128
  identifying in white blood cells, 138
  overview of, 132
BBPS (Bloodborne Pathogens Standard)
  avoiding exposure to HIV, 218
  defined, 1
  diseases caused by bloodborne pathogens, 18–19
  federal laws for safety equipment, 89–90
  Hepatitis A virus and, 20t
  instituted in 1991 for infection control, 238t
  overview of, 18–22
  preventive measures, 19–21
  procedure after exposure to blood, 21–22
  risk management during blood collection, 126
Beer-Lambert Law, 171, 181, 182f
Bence Jones protein, 51, 67
benzodiazepines, detecting, 276t–278t
bicarbonate (HCO$_3$-)
  electrolyte panels testing, 199
  renal panel testing, 199
bilirubin
  crystals, 75
  defined, 51
  liver metabolism of, 200
  measuring in urine, 65–66
  urine standing at room temperature changing, 60
  urine urobilinogen levels, 66

billing information, in laboratory requisitions, 9
binary fission, bacterial reproduction, 236–237
biochemical testing, 261, 261f
biohazard bags, 19, 21
biohazard sharps container
  for butterfly method, 118b–123b
  for syringes, 116b–118b
  for Vacutainer needle, 112b–115b
biohazard spill kit, physical hazard training, 26, 26f
biohazards
  defined, 1
  laboratory housekeeping guidelines, 21, 22f–23f
  in medical laboratories, 14
  OSHA training for bloodborne pathogens. *see* BBPS (Bloodborne Pathogens Standard)
  physical hazard training, 25
bioterrorism
  anthrax in, 264–268, 271f
  biological toxin in, 271
  overview of, 264–271
  plague in, 267–268
  smallpox virus in, 268
  tularemia in, 268
  viral hemorrhagic fever in, 271
black death (plague), 267–268
bladder tumor-associated antigen (BTA) test, 228t–229t
bleach
  chemical hazard training for, 23, 24f
  laboratory housekeeping guidelines, 20, 22f
blood
  chemistry. *see* chemistry
  collecting culture specimen, 241, 242f
  in composition of urine, 55
  enzymes panel, possible disease associations, 202t–204t
  flow through kidney, 54
  liquid portion of. *see* plasma
  measuring in urine, 66
  overview of, 129–135, 130f
  preparing smear for observation, 135–139, 136f–138f, 145b–146b
  production of, 130, 131f
blood agar, 251–252, 259
Blood and Body Fluid Exposure Report, 21–22
blood area nitrogen (BUN)
  i-STAT testing, 198
  renal panel testing, 199
blood banks, antibody/antigen reactions in, 225
blood collection
  for alcohol tests, 275, 280b
  blood vessels and. *see* blood vessels
  capillary puncture for. *see* capillary puncture
  federal laws for safety equipment, 89–90
  fundamental concepts, 87–90
  half-life in drugs of abuse and, 285
  preparing specimens for laboratory pickup, 104–123, 104f
  procedure preparation, 90, 90f
  review question answers, 127
  review questions, 126–127
  risk management, 126
  therapeutic drug monitoring and, 283
  venipuncture for. *see* venipuncture
  websites, 127b

blood collection, complications
    areas to avoid, 125
    defined, 123
    excessive bleeding, 125
    failure to obtain blood, 123–124, 124f–125f
    hematomas, 123
    hemolysis, 124–125
    neurological problems, 125
    in patients with IV therapy and edema, 125
    in patients with obesity and mastectomy, 125
    syncope, 124
blood gases
    i-STAT testing of, 198, 198t
    overview of, 201
    possible disease associations, 202t–204t
blood glucose. *see* glucose
blood plasma. *see* plasma
blood vessels
    commonly used veins, 89, 89f
    comparison of blood substances, 87, 89f
    structure of, 87–89, 88f–89f
    types of, 87
bloodborne pathogens. *see also* BBPS (Bloodborne Pathogens Standard)
    as biohazard in medical laboratories, 14
    defined, 1
    diseases caused by, 18–19, 20t
    procedure after exposure to blood, 21–22
bone marrow
    blood cell production in, 130, 130f
    red cell production in, 130–131, 132f
    stem cell's differentiation in, 131f
botulism
    in bioterrorism, 271
    caused by bacilli, 263t–264t
    Clostridium botulinum causing, 239
BTA (bladder tumor-associated antigen) test, 228t–229t
bubonic plague, 238t, 267
buffy coat, 86, 97
BUN (blood area nitrogen)
    i-STAT testing, 198
    renal panel testing, 199
Bunsen burners, microbiology, 259
BUP (buprenorphine)
    CLIA-waived tests for monitoring patients on, 275, 281
    defined, 274
    drug urine screening tests detecting, 276t–278t
butterfly method, venipuncture
    equipment for, 102f–103f
    order of draw for, 102–104
    overview of, 100–101
    procedure for, 118b–123b

C

C. diff infection, caused by bacilli, 263t–264t
Ca (ionized calcium), i-STAT testing of, 198–199
CA 125 (ovarian cancer) antigen test, 228t–229t
calcium oxate crystals, 74, 78f
calibration
    defined, 32
    QA in optical tests, 182
    testing analytes using optics, 45
cancer
    CA 125 antigen test for ovarian, 228t–229t
    lines of defense against. *see* immune process

candidiasis, caused by antibiotics, 237
cannabinoids (marijuana)
    CLIA-waived tests screening for, 281
    defined, 274
    time intervals for detecting drugs in urine, 276t–278t
capillaries
    defined, 86
    layers within, 89f
    overview of, 87
capillary action, 86, 92
capillary puncture
    additional information, 94
    CLIA-waived tests for, 174
    neonatal screening test using, 94–95, 95f–96f, 109b–111b
    order of draw for, 93, 93t
    overview of, 91–95
    procedure for, 106b–108b
    site preparation for, 94
    site selection for, 93–94, 94f
capillary puncture, equipment for
    capillary tubes. *see* capillary tubes
    devices, 91
    microcollection tubes, 92f, 93
    point-of-care testing collection devices for, 91–92, 92f
    procedure for, 106b–108b
capillary tubes
    capillary puncture and, 92–93, 93f
    equipment, 92f
    laboratory metrics for length of, 11
    microcollection tubes vs., 93
capnophilic organisms, 236, 258
capsules, bacterial structure of, 239
carbohydrates
    in blood plasma, 172
    defined, 171
    high triglycerides from diet rich in, 181
cardiac panel, 201, 201f, 202t–204t
cardiotonics, therapeutic drug monitoring, 283, 284t
cardiovascular problems
    Medicare-approved screening for, 184
    poor lipid metabolism linked to, 179–180
    in type 1 diabetes, 177
casts, microscopic urinalysis
    defined, 51
    granular, 74, 77f
    hyaline, 73–74, 77f
    overview, 73–74
    red blood cell, 74, 77f
    renal epithelial cell, 74, 77f
    in urine standing at room temperature, 60
    waxy, 74, 77f
    white blood cell, 74, 77f
catalysts
    blood plasma, 172
    defined, 171
catheterization, for urine specimens, 56
cations, 171, 199
caudate epithelial cells, 73, 76f
CaviWipes, 20, 22f
CBC (complete blood count)
    abnormal findings, 162–163, 164t, 165f
    defined, 129
    differential counter for, 130f
    laboratory report form, 161f
    overview of, 159–162
    reference range for, 163t
    requisition form for, 160f
ccs (cubic centimeters), laboratory metrics for liquids, 11

CD4 (helper T cells)
    in cell-mediated immunity, 212
    defined, 209
    HIV destroying, 218
CDC (Centers for Disease Control and Prevention)
    bioterrorism, 264
    history of infection control, 238t
    needle sticks, 89–90
    personal protective equipment, 18
    Standard Precautions for infection control, 15–18
C-diff colitis, as emerging infectious disease, 270t
cell-mediated immunity, 209, 212–213, 212f
cells, microscopic urinalysis
    epithelial, 73, 76f
    overview, 73
    red blood, 73, 76f
    white blood, 73, 76f
cellulose tape test, pinworms, 246
Centers for Disease Control and Prevention. *see* CDC (Centers for Disease Control and Prevention)
Centers for Medicare and Medicaid Services (CMS), 33
centrifuges, 104–123, 104f
Certificate of Accreditation, 33–35
Certificate of Compliance, 33–35
Certificate of Waiver laboratories. *see* CoW (Certificate of Waiver) laboratories
chemical hazards
    defined, 1
    inventory sheet for, 5f, 23
    in medical laboratories, 14
    safety training in laboratory, 22–24
chemical spill kit, 26, 27f
chemical urinalysis
    automated click method, 64, 64f
    becoming proficient at, 52, 67f
    overview of, 62–64, 63f
    quality assurance, 62–64
    reagent strip quality control, 63–64, 63f, 68b–71b
chemistry, 162
    blood chemistry specimens, 173–174
    blood glucose tests. *see* glucose screening/monitoring tests; glucose tests, CLIA-waived
    blood plasma, 172–173, 173f
    fundamental concepts, 172–181
    glucose metabolism. *see* glucose metabolism
    laboratory report, 9, 12f
    lipid metabolism and testing, 179–181, 180f
    reference laboratory specimens for blood chemistry tests, 173–174, 174f–175f
    specimens, 173–174
    tests granted waived status, 34t–35t
    websites, 208b
chemistry, CLIA-waived tests
    in ambulatory care setting, 6
    becoming proficient at, 184–198
    fecal occult blood, Guaiac method, 184, 194b–198b
    glucose, 183, 185b–189b
    i-STAT blood analyzer, 198t, 146, 147f, 174, 198–207, 198t, 205b
    lipids and glucose, Cholestech method, 183–184, 190b–194b
    list of, 34t–35t
    metabolic panels. *see* metabolic panels, basic and comprehensive

chemistry, CLIA-waived tests *(Continued)*
　monitoring QC results with Westgard's rules, 182–183
　overview of, 181–198
　Piccolo, 199
　principle of photometers and spectrophotometers, 181–183, 182f
　QA when using optical instruments, 182
　specimens for, 174
　summary of, 184, 201–207
chickenpox (varicella zoster) test, 228t–229t
Chlamydia
　diseases caused by, 266t
　immunology test for, 228t–229t
　as most commonly seen disease, 262
　specimen collection, 241, 242f
chloride (CL-)
　electrolyte panel testing of, 199
　renal panel testing of, 199
chloride (CL), i-STAT testing of, 198–199
chocolate agar, 259
Cholestech LDX analyzer, 174, 183–184, 190b–194b
cholesterol
　crystals, 75, 79f
　lipid metabolism and, 180
　routinely tested in lipid panel, 180–181
　testing with Cholestech LDX, 67–72, 183–184
　total cholesterol/high-density lipoprotein ratio, 181
chromatographic, 209, 215–216
chronic disorders, 1, 3
chronic lymphocytic leukemia (CLL), 163
chronic myelocytic leukemia (CML), 163
CK or CPK (creatine kinase), hepatic panel testing, 201
Cl (chloride), i-STAT testing of, 198–199
Cl-(chloride)
　electrolyte panel testing of, 199
　renal panel testing of, 199
clean-catch midstream urine specimen
　equipment for, 56f
　overview of, 56
　procedure for, 57b–59b
clear appearance of urine, 62, 62f
CLIA government regulations
　Certificate of Waiver, 33, 34t–35t
　high and moderately complex laboratories, 33–35
　levels of complexity and certification, 33–36
　overview of, 33–36
　Provider-Performed Microscopy Procedures Certificate, 35–36, 36t
　review question answers, 50
　review questions, 50
　websites, 50b
CLIA-nonwaived automated systems
　Coulter Counter system, 167f–168f
　QBC STAR Centrifugal Hematology System, 166f
CLIA-waived tests
　accuracy and reliability of, 41
　in ambulatory care settings, 6
　chemistry. *see* chemistry, CLIA-waived tests
　defined, 1, 32
　drug screening, 281–283
　hematology. *see* hematology, CLIA-waived tests
　immunology. *see* immunology, CLIA-waived tests
　microbiology. *see* microbiology, CLIA-waived tests

CLIA-waived tests *(Continued)*
　physician office laboratory performing, 6
　QC for qualitative waived tests, 44, 44f
　QC for quantitative waived tests, 45–48
　QC for semiquantitative waived tests, 44–45
　toxicology, 281–283
　urinalysis. *see* urinalysis, CLIA-waived tests
　websites, 50b
clinical diagnosis
　defined, 171
　definitive, 176
　detecting/confirming with blood chemistry, 173
clinical laboratory, 2
　ambulatory care settings as, 6–7
　defined, 1, 3–4
　documentation in, 9–11
　hospital laboratories as, 6
　laboratory professional attributes, 8–9
　overview of, 3–7
　personnel involved in testing, 8t
　purpose of, 3–4
　reference (or referral) laboratories, 4–6
　review question answers, 31
　review questions, 30
　safety training in. *see* safety training in laboratory
　specimen analysis in, 3–4
　websites, 31b
　why tests are ordered, 3
Clinical Laboratory Improvement Amendments. *see also* CLIA government regulations; CLIA-waived tests
Clinitek urine analyzer, 64, 64f, 70b–71b
Clinitest (Bayer Corporation), 65, 72b
CLL (chronic lymphocytic leukemia), 163
closed circuit system, 87, 88f
Clostridium botulinum, 239, 271
Clostridium tetani, 239
clot activator, 171, 173–174, 174f
clotted blood tubes, 96–97, 97f
cloudy appearance of urine, 62, 62f
cluster, cocci bacterial structure, 239
CML (chronic myelocytic leukemia), 163
CMS (Centers for Medicare and Medicaid Services), 33
coagulation, defined, 1
coagulation testing
　ambulatory care setting, 6
　hematology and, 129
coarse focus adjustment, microscope, 37f, 38
cocaine
　CLIA-waived tests screening for, 281
　drug urine screening tests detecting, 276t–278t
　time intervals for detecting drugs in urine, 278t
coccobacillus, 239
coccus (cocci)
　characteristics of, 239
　diseases caused by, 265t
　gram-negative cocci (GNC), 244, 245f
　gram-positive cocci (GPC), 244, 245f
coding, testing analytes using optics, 45
ColoCARE method, fecal occult blood testing, 184, 194b–198b
colon cancer, screening for. *see* fecal occult blood testing
colonies, bacteria forming, 236–237

colony count (lawn) technique, inoculation of media
　overview of, 260, 261f
　urine culture involving, 260–261, 273b
color of urine, 61–62, 61f
color-coded blood collection hemoguard tubes, 97–98, 98t
ColoScreen III method, fecal occult blood testing, 194b–198b
commitment, of laboratory professionals, 8
complement proteins (switched with), 209, 211–212
complete blood count. *see* CBC (complete blood count)
complexity testing, CLIA
　Certificate of Waiver, 33
　high and moderate, 33–35
　overview of, 50
　provider-performed microscopy, 35–36
computer printout laboratory reports, 9, 12f
condenser, microscope
　adjusting, 37–38, 37f
　overview of, 37–38, 37f
　settings, 38b–40b
confidentiality, HIPAA Privacy Rule, 48
container labels, hazardous chemicals, 23, 24f
containers, urine specimen, 55–56, 55f
contaminated, defined, 1
contaminated needles
　laboratory housekeeping guidelines, 21
　preventing exposure incidents, 19, 21f
contaminated objects, alcohol-based hand rubs for, 17
control sample, 32, 44
correctness (accuracy)
　analyzing control results, 47, 47f
　defined, 32
Coulter Counter system, 167, 167f–168f
CoW (Certificate of Waiver) laboratories
　defined, 32
　good laboratory practices for, 41, 42f
　as least regulated, 41
　regulations for certification, 33–36
　tests granted waived status, 34t–35t
C-reactive protein (CRP)
　defined, 1
　monitoring patient treatment for heart disease, 3
creatine kinase (CK or CPK), hepatic panel testing, 201
creatinine, renal panel testing, 199
crenated RBCs, 73
critical value, as test result, 1, 4
cross-contamination, 1, 17
CRP (C-reactive protein)
　defined, 1
　monitoring patient treatment for heart disease, 3
cryptococcosis, fungi causing, 267t
crystals, microscopic urinalysis
　abnormal, 74–75, 79f
　acid urine, 74, 78f
　alkaline urine, 74, 78f
　overview, 74–75
culture, defined, 236
culture media
　defined, 237
　growing bacteria with, 258–259, 258f–259f
　inoculation of, 259–260, 260f–261f
culturing methods
　inoculation of media, 259–260, 260f–261f
　microbiology, 259–260, 260f–261f
　urine culture, 260–261, 273b

cutaneous anthrax, 264, 271f
cyanotic sites
  for capillary punctures, 93–94
  defined, 86
cystine crystals, 74–75
cytoplasm, 128, 132

D

decolorizing step, Gram stain procedure, 244
definitive diagnosis, 171, 176
deoxyribonucleic acid. *see* DNA (deoxyribonucleic acid)
Department of Health and Human Services (HHS), 2, 33
Department of Transportation (DOT), drug screening tests for home use, 281
dermatophyte infections, 264
dexterity, of laboratory professionals, 9
diagnosis. *see* clinical diagnosis
diagnostic tests
  in hospital laboratories, 6
  reasons for ordering, 3
  in reference laboratories, 4–6
Diff device
  preparing blood smear with, 135–136, 136f
  staining procedure, 145b–146b
differential count procedure, 128, 136–139, 138f
differential media, growing bacteria, 258–259
diplococci, 239
diphtheria, caused by bacilli, 263t–264t
disinfectants, laboratory housekeeping guidelines, 20
distribution stage, pharmacokinetics, 274, 284
diuresis, 51, 55
DM (diabetes mellitus)
  analyzing by measuring reference range, 4
  blood glucose tests for. *see* glucose screening/monitoring tests
  comparing type 1 and type 2, 178t
  defined, 1
  insulin-dependent (type 1), 177, 178t
  Medicare-approved screening for, 184
  monitoring patient treatment for, 3
  non-insulin-dependent (type 2), 177, 177f, 178t
  overview of, 176–178
  prediabetes, 177
  renal panel testing in, 199
  transient diabetes, 178
DNA (deoxyribonucleic acid)
  diagnosing Chlamydia with DNA-probe test, 241
  diagnosing Gonorrhea with DNA-probe test, 241
  in viruses, 237
documentation
  laboratory measurements, 9–11
  of laboratory professionals, 9
  laboratory reports, 9
  laboratory requisitions, 9
  overview of, 9–11
  procedure after exposure to blood, 21–22
  risk management practices, 48
don (putting on PPE), 2, 27b–30b
DOT (Department of Transportation), drug screening tests for home use, 281
drug screening tests, 34t–35t, 275

drugs of abuse, 275–281, 276t–278t
dyslipidemia, 171, 177
dysuria, 51

E

Ebola virus
  in bioterrorism, 271
  as emerging infectious disease, 270t
EBV (Epstein-Barr virus)
  causing mononucleosis, 217
  immunology test for, 228t–229t
Ecstasy (MDMA), detecting in urine, 276t–278t
Ecstasy, screening for, 276t–278t
edema
  defined, 86
  venipuncture precautions in patients with, 125
efficiency, of laboratory professional, 8
electrical equipment, physical hazard training, 24
electrical incinerators, microbiology, 259, 260f
electrolyte panels, 173–174
electrolytes
  defined, 51, 172
  formation of urine and, 54
  i-STAT testing for, 198, 198t
  possible disease associations, 202t–204t
  renal panel testing for, 199
electronic bar codes, requisitions, 9, 11f
electronic medical records, 48
elimination stage, pharmacokinetics, 284–285
ELISA (enzyme-linked immunosorbent assay) test, 218, 226–227
embolus, 128, 139
EMLA (eutectic mixture of local anesthetics), venipuncture, 99–100
endogenous cholesterol, 171, 180
endospores, anthrax, 264, 271f
engineering controls, 2, 19, 21f
enriched media, growing bacteria, 259
Enterobius vermicularis (pinworm) specimen collection, 246–251, 246f
Enterotube identification kit, 261, 261f
enzyme-linked immunoassays, 215–216, 217t
enzyme-linked immunosorbent assay (ELISA) test, 218, 226–227
enzymes, catalysts in metabolic changes, 200
eosino- prefix, 128
eosinophils
  defined, 128
  overview of, 132
  WBC identification, 138
epidermis, Staphylococci, 239
epithelial cells, in microscopic urinalysis, 73, 76f
Epstein-Barr virus (EBV)
  causing mononucleosis, 217
  immunology test for, 228t–229t
equipment, microbiology, 259, 260f
ergonomic practices
  defined, 2
  physical hazard training, 25
erythroblastosis fetalis
  defined, 209
  overview of, 226, 227f
erythroblasts (rubriblasts)
  defined, 128
  red cell production, 130–131
erythrocytes. *see* RBCs (red blood cells)
eschars, cutaneous anthrax, 264, 271f

ESR (erythrocyte sedimentation rate)
  becoming proficient at CLIA-waived tests, 149–159
  CLIA-waived test for, 164t
  defined, 128
  false decreased rates, 148
  false increased rates, 148
  other interferences, 148
  overview of, 148–149, 148f
  SEDIPLAST system procedure, 148–149, 155b–156b
ethanol
  content in alcoholic beverages, 278t
  as most common legal drug of abuse, 275
eukaryotic
  defined, 236
  fungi as, 237–238
eutectic mixture of local anesthetics (EMLA), venipuncture, 99–100
evacuated vacuum tubes, 86, 95
excessive bleeding, from phlebotomy, 125
excessive scatter, 46, 46f
exogenous cholesterol, 171, 180
expectoration, 236, 245
exposure control plan, 1–2
external controls, analyzing
  defined, 32
  with Levy-Jennings charts. *see* Levy-Jennings charts
  overview of, 45–48
  QC monitoring in qualitative tests, 44
eye goggles, 27b–30b
eye wash station, 26, 27f

F

facultative anaerobe, 236, 258
fastidious organisms, 236, 258
fasting blood glucose (FBG) test, 178
fats
  lipids as. *see* lipid metabolism
  liver function in metabolizing, 200
FBG (fasting blood glucose) test, 178
FDA (Food and Drug Administration), and lab test complexity, 33
fecal occult blood testing
  in ambulatory care setting, 7
  ColoCARE method of, 184, 194b–198b
  granted waived status, 34t–35t
  guaiac method of, 184, 194b–198b
  iFOB kits for, 218–225, 218f, 228t–229t
  as qualitative analysis, 181
fecal specimen collection, for ova and parasites, 241, 243f
Federal Quarantine Legislation, 238t
fibrinogen
  in blood plasma, 173
  (factor 1), 128, 139
filtration, urine and, 54
fine focus adjustment, microscope, 37f, 38
fingernail hygiene, safety in laboratory, 18
fingerstick blood samples, glucose monitoring with, 183
first line of defense, immune process, 211
first morning urine specimen, 56
flagella, bacterial structure of, 239
Fleming, Alexander, 238t
fleshy sites, capillary punctures, 93–94
focus, of laboratory professional, 8
folate (folic acid)-deficiency anemia, diagnosing, 162
Food and Drug Administration (FDA), and lab test complexity, 33

food poisoning
  caused by cocci, 265t
  caused by spirilla, 266t
forearm testing, glucose monitoring with, 183
formed elements
  defined, 128
  viewing within blood, 130, 130f
foul odor of urine, 62
foundational structures, microscopes, 36
Francisella tularensis, 268
fungi
  commonly seen in POLs, 262–264
  diseases caused by pathogenic, 267t
  lines of defense against harmful. see immune process
  overview of, 237–238

G

G. vaginalis (vaginal infection) test, 228t–229t
galactosemia, 65
galvanometer, 171, 182
gamma globulins, 173
gamma-glutamyltransferase (GGT), hepatic panel testing, 200
gastrointestinal anthrax, 267
g/dL (grams per deciliter), measuring Hgb, 146
germ theory, 238t
German measles (Rubella) test, 228t–229t
gestational diabetes, testing, 178
GGT (gamma-glutamyltransferase), hepatic panel testing, 200
Giardiasis, 264, 268t
globulins, in blood plasma, 173
glomerular (Bowman's) capsule, 51, 53f, 54
glomerulonephritis, 251–252
glomerulus, 51, 53f, 54
gloves, personal protective, 27b–30b
  defined, 171
glucometers, 183, 185b–186b
glucose
  defined, 2
  i-STAT testing of, 198–207, 198t
  measuring in urine, 64–65
  in venous vs. capillary blood, 87
glucose metabolism. see also glucose screening/monitoring tests
  diabetes mellitus, 176–178
  gestational diabetes, 178
  insulin-dependent diabetes mellitus, 177, 178t
  liver function in, 200
  non-insulin-dependent diabetes mellitus, 177, 177f, 178t
  overview of, 176–179, 176f
  prediabetes, 177
  transient diabetes, 178
glucose screening/monitoring tests
  fasting blood glucose (FBG), 178
  glucose tolerance test (GTT), 176–179
  glycosated hemoglobin, glycated hemoglobin (Hgb A1c), 179
  oral glucose tolerance test (2-hour postprandial blood sugar), 178
  overview of, 178–179
  random glucose test, 178
glucose tests, CLIA-waived
  glycosated hemoglobin (Hgb A1c), 183, 187b–189b
  monitoring devices, 183, 185b–186b
  overview of, 183
  in physician's office laboratory, 174
glucosuria, 64–65
glycosuria, 51, 64–65

glycosylated hemoglobin (Hbg A1c) test
  defined, 171
  overview of, 179
  procedure for, 183, 187b–189b
  specimen collection for, 174
GNB (gram-positive bacteria), 244, 245f
GNC (gram-negative cocci), 244, 245f
Gonorrhea
  caused by cocci, 265t
  most commonly seen in POL, 262
Gonorrhea specimen collection, 241, 243f
gout
  defined, 171
  renal panel testing for, 199
government regulations
  blood collection safety equipment, 89–90
  CLIA. see CLIA government regulations
  neonatal screening f, 94–95
gowns, fluid-impenetrable, 27b–30b
GPC (gram-positive cocci), 244, 245f
Gram stain reaction
  defined, 236
  diseases caused by cocci, 265t
  diseases caused by spirilla, 266t
  overview of, 243–244, 244t
  procedure for, 245, 248b–250b
  smear preparation, 244–245, 245f
gram-negative
  Chlamydia as, 241
  defined, 236
gram-negative cocci (GNC), 244, 245f
gram-positive, defined, 236
gram-positive bacteria (GNB), 244, 245f
granular casts, 74, 77f
granulocytes
  defined, 128
  overview of, 131–134
  QBC STAR information on, 166
  in WBC production, 133f
green-topped vacuum tubes, 174
group A *Streptococcus*, immunology test for, 228t–229t
GTT (glucose tolerance test), 178–179, 179f
guaiac method, fecal occult blood testing, 184, 194b–198b

H

H. (helicobacter) pylori test, 217–218, 224b–225b, 228t–229t
H1N1 flu, 252
hair, physical hazard training, 25
half-life, drug, 285
hand hygiene, 15–18, 17f
Hantavirus pulmonary syndrome, 238t, 270t
HAV (hepatitis A virus)
  bloodborne pathogens causing, 19, 20t
  defined, 2
  procedure after exposure to blood, 22
Hazard Communication Standard, 2, 22–23
hazardous materials information system. see HMIS (hazardous materials information system)
hazards
  safety training in laboratory, 14–26
  types of medical laboratory, 14
hazy appearance of urine, 62, 62f
Hbg A1c test. see glycosylated hemoglobin (Hbg A1c) test
HBV (hepatitis B virus)
  bloodborne pathogens causing, 19, 20t
  defined, 2
  procedure after exposure to blood, 22
  vaccinating health care employees for, 19

HCAIs (health care associated infections)
  chain of infection causing, 15
  defined, 2
  hand hygiene preventing, 16
HCG (human chorionic gonadotropin) test, 216, 228t–229t
HCO₃⁻ (bicarbonate)
  electrolyte panels testing, 199
  renal panel testing, 199
HCT (hematocrit)
  becoming proficient at CLIA-waived tests, 149–159
  for complete blood count, 159
  defined, 128
  general procedure, 151b–152b
  general spun microhematocrit procedures, 147, 148f
  HemataSTAT procedure, 147, 153b–155b
  i-STAT testing of, 198–199, 198t
  overview of, 147
HCV (hepatitis C virus)
  bloodborne pathogens causing, 19, 20t
  defined, 2
  as emerging infectious disease, 270t
  procedure after exposure to blood, 22
  testing, 228t–229t
HDLs (high-density lipoproteins)
  overview of, 180
  routinely tested in lipid panel, 180
  total cholesterol/high-density lipoprotein ratio, 180
HDN (hemolytic disease of newborn)
  antibody titer tests to prevent, 227
  and RhoGAM, 226, 227f
health care associated infections. see HCAIs (health care associated infections)
Health Insurance Portability and Accountability Act. see HIPAA Privacy Rule
heart disease, monitoring patient treatment for, 3
helicobacter (H.) pylori test, 217–218, 224b–225b, 228t–229t
helper T cells (TH4 or CD4)
  in cell-mediated immunity, 212
  defined, 209
  HIV destroying, 218
HemataSTAT procedure, 147, 153b–155b
hematocrit. see HCT (hematocrit)
hematologist, 128
hematologists, 129
hematology
  blood and, 129–135, 130f
  blood production, 130, 131f
  CBC testing. see CBC (complete blood count)
  CLIA-nonwaived automated systems, 165–167, 166f–168f
  defined, 128–129
  hemostasis and, 135f, 139, 144f, 144t
  platelets (thrombocytes), 134–135, 134f–135f
  preparing blood smear, 135–139, 136f–138f, 145b–146b
  RBC identification and description, 139, 139f, 144f
  RBCs, overview of, 130–131, 132f
  review question answers, 170
  review questions, 169
  WBCs, disorders, 163, 165f
  WBCs, granulocytes, 131–134, 131f, 133f
  WBCs, identification and differential, 136–139, 138f
  WBCs, nongranulocytes, 132, 134f
  WBCs, overview, 131–134
  websites, 170b

hematology, CLIA-waived tests
  in ambulatory care setting, 6
  becoming proficient at, 149–159, 149b–159b
  ESR. see ESR (erythrocyte sedimentation rate)
  hematocrit, 147, 148f, 151b–155b
  hemoglobin, 146, 147f, 149b–150b
  list of tests for, 34t–35t
  overview of, 146–159
  prothrombin time, 144f, 149, 157b–159b
hematomas, 86, 123
hematopoiesis, 128, 130, 131f
hematuria, 51
hemoconcentration
  applying tourniquet to avoid, 99, 103f
  defined, 86
HemoCue procedure, 146, 149b–150b
hemocytoblast, 128, 130
hemoglobin. see Hgb (hemoglobin)
hemolysis (hemolyzing)
  defined, 51, 66, 128
  measuring Hgb within RBCs with, 146
  phlebotomy causing, 124–125
hemolytic anemia, CBC testing for, 162
hemolytic disease of newborn. see HDN (hemolytic disease of newborn)
hemolytic uremic syndrome, 270t
HemoSense (INRatio) system for PT testing, 149, 157b–159b
hemostasis, 129
hemostasis, theory of
  coagulation and testing, 139
  overview of, 135f, 139, 144f, 144t
heparin
  Cholestech lipid tests containing, 174
  defined, 139
hepatic panel, 200–201, 202t–204t
hepatitis A virus. see HAV (hepatitis A virus)
hepatitis B virus. see HBV (hepatitis B virus)
hepatitis C virus. see HCV (hepatitis C virus)
hereditary spherocytosis, CBC testing indicating, 162
heterophile antibody, 209, 217
Hgb (hemoglobin)
  becoming proficient at CLIA-waived tests, 149–159
  breaking down into heme and globin, 131, 132f
  in CBC test results, 159
  defined, 128
  HemoCue procedure for, 146, 149b–150b
  Hgb meter and i-STAT methods for, 146, 147f
  i-STAT testing of, 198–199
  overview of, 146
  red cell production and, 130–131, 132f
  testing methods, 146
  venous vs. capillary, 87
(Hgb A1c) glycosylated/glycated hemoglobin test
  CLIA-waived test, 183
  overview of, 179
  procedure for, 187b–189b
Hgb meter, and i-STAT methods, 146, 147f
HHS (Department of Health and Human Services), 2, 33
high power focus, microscope setting, 38b–40b
high-density lipoproteins. see HDLs (high-density lipoproteins)
HIPAA Privacy Rule, 48

histamines
  defined, 209
  released during inflammation, 212
histoplasmosis, fungi causing, 267t
HIV (human immunodeficiency virus)
  bloodborne pathogens causing, 18
  defined, 2
  as emerging infectious disease, 270t
  history of, 238t
  immunology test for, 228t–229t
  procedure after exposure to blood with, 22
  testing for, 218
HMIS (hazardous materials information system)
  labeling hazardous chemicals, 23, 24f
  overview of, 23
homeostasis, 2–4
honesty, of laboratory professional, 9
hormones, in blood plasma, 172
hospital laboratories
  organizational chart for, 7f
  overview of, 6
  regulations for certification, 33–35
housekeeping guidelines, laboratory, 20, 22f–23f
human chorionic gonadotropin (HCG), 216, 228t–229t
human immunodeficiency virus. see HIV (human immunodeficiency virus)
humoral immunity, 213, 213f–214f
humors, 86–87
hyaline casts, 73–74, 77f
hyperchromia, 129
hyperglycemia, 171
hyperinsulinemia
  creating rising triglyceride levels, 181
  defined, 171
  type 2 diabetes beginning with, 177
hyperlipidemia, 171, 181
hyphae, 236–238
hypochromia, RBC identification and description, 139
hypochromic
  defined, 129
  indicating anemia in CBC test results, 162
hypodermic needle, 100
hypoglycemia, 171, 177
hypothyroidism, neonatal screening for, 94–95
hypoxemia, 129, 162

I
iatrogenic
  crystallization of compounds, 74
  defined, 51
icons, labeling chemical hazards, 24, 25f
IDDM (insulin-dependent diabetes mellitus), type1, 177, 178t
idiosyncrasy, drug reaction, 274–275
iFOB (immunoassayed fecal occult blood)
  defined, 209
  fecal occult blood testing with kits for, 218–225, 218f
  screening for colon cancer with, 228t–229t
IGT (impaired glucose tolerance), type 2 diabetes, 177
illuminating structures, microscopes, 36–38
immune process
  acquiring specific immunity, 213–215, 214f
  cell-mediated immunity, 212–213, 212f
  first line of defense, 211

immune process (Continued)
  humoral immunity, 213, 213f
  overview of, 210–215, 211f
  second line of defense, 211–212
  third line of defense, 212–215
immunization
  defined, 210
  development of, 210
immunoassay tests
  fecal occult blood. see iFOB (immunoassayed fecal occult blood)
  rapid urine drug tests as, 281
immunoglobulins
  in blood plasma, 173
  classes of, 213
  defined, 129, 134
immunological memory, 212–215
immunology
  agglutination and. see agglutination reaction tests
  antibody titers, 227
  common tests for, 228t–229t
  defined, 210
  enzyme-linked immunosorbent assay, 226–227
  history of, 210
  immune process. see immune process
  overview of, 210–215
  review question answers, 235
  review questions, (missing section number) page234
  summary of tests for, 227–234
  vitro allergy testing, 215
  vivo allergy testing, 215
  websites, 235b
immunology, CLIA-waived tests
  in ambulatory care setting, 6
  enzyme-linked immunoassays, 215–216, 217t
  fecal occult blood, with iFOB kits, 218–225, 218f
  H. pylori, 217–218, 224b–225b
  HIV, 218
  list of, 34t–35t
  mononucleosis, 217, 221b–223b
  pregnancy, 216–217, 216f, 219b–220b
immunosorbent (switched with), 209
impaired glucose tolerance (IGT), type 2 diabetes, 177
in vitro
  allergy testing, 215
  CLIA-waived enzyme-linked immunoassays, 215, 216f
  defined, 210
in vivo
  allergy testing, 215, 215f
  defined, 210
incineration equipment, microbiology, 259
inclusion conjunctivitis, 266t
infection
  analyzing specimens for, 4
  defined, 236
  historical efforts to control, 237, 238t
  role of pathogenic microorganisms in, 237
  Standard Precautions for infection control, 15–18, 16f
  transmission and chain of, 15, 15f
  WBC counts indicating, 163, 166
infectious diseases, emerging, 264
inflammation, 210–212
influenza
  as emerging infectious disease, 270t
  OSOM A & B Test for, 228t–229t, 253–257, 255b–257b
  overview of, 252–257

inhalation anthrax, 267
inoculating loops, 259
inoculation
   of culture media, 259–260, 260f–261f
   defined, 236
   equipment used for, 259, 260f
INR (internationalized normalized ratio)
   prothrombin time, 149, 157b–159b
   protime test, 139
INRatio (HemoSense) system for PT testing, 149, 157b–159b
insulin
   defined, 171
   resistance, 171, 177
insulin-dependent diabetes mellitus (IDDM), type1, 177, 178t
insurance billing, on requisitions, 9
integrity, of laboratory professional, 9
interferons, 210–212
internal clots. see thrombosis (internal clots)
internal controls, 32, 44
internationalized normalized ratio. see INR (internationalized normalized ratio)
interpersonal communication skills, of laboratory professional, 8
interstitial fluid, 86, 91
IOMED, for venipuncture, 99–100
ionized calcium (Ca), i-STAT testing of, 198–199
ions, blood plasma, 172
iQC (intelligent Quality Control), Piccolo Xpress, 199
iris diaphragm lever, microscope, 37–38, 37f
iron poisoning, toxicology tests for, 285
iron-deficiency anemia, diagnosing, 162
isolation (quadrant) technique, inoculation of media, 259–260, 260f
isopropyl alcohol, for capillary puncture site, 94
i-STAT blood analyzer
   blood chemistry results on, 198t
   defined, 146, 147f
   physician's office laboratory using, 174
   procedure for, 205b
IV therapy, 125

J
jaundice, 66
JEMBEC transport system, 241, 243f
Jenner, Edward, 210
jock itch, fungi causing, 267t

K
K (potassium), i-STAT testing of, 198–199
K+ (potassium), testing, 199
ketoacidosis, 65, 172, 177
ketones
   measuring in urine, 65
   odor of urine indicating, 62
ketonuria, 51
kidney (renal) panel, 199
kidneys
   flow of blood and urine through, 54
   urinary system and, 52–54, 53f
killer T cells (TC), 210, 212
Kirby-Bauer sensitivity testing, 261, 261f–262f
kissing disease (mononucleosis), 217
   overview of, 163, 165f, 217
   test procedure, 217, 221b–223b
kit, defined, 32

KOH (potassium hydroxide) preparation, 246, 251b
Kova System of microscopic urinalysis, 72

L
labeling capillary tubes, 92–93
labeling chemical hazards
   with HMIS system, 23, 24f
   with icons, 24, 25f
   with NFPA system, 24, 25f
   overview of, 23, 24f
labeling urine specimen, 55
laboratory. see also clinical laboratory
   measurements, 9–11
   requisitions. see requisitions
   safety training in, 26, 26f–27f
laboratory reports
   computer printouts of, 9, 12f
   defined, 2
   highlighting critical results on, 4
   measurements in, 9–11, 13t–14t
   overview of, 9
   requisitions requesting, 9, 10f
   stages in laboratory process, 9, 13f
Laboratory Safety Checklist, 26
lactic dehydrogenase (LD), hepatic panel testing, 200
Lactobacillus, 237
laser capillary puncture devices, 91
lateral flow immunochromatographic assay
   common CLIA-waived tests using, 215–216, 217t
   overview of, 215
   pregnancy testing with, 216–217, 216f, 219b–220b
layers, blood vessel, 87
LD (lactic dehydrogenase), hepatic panel testing, 200
LDLs (low-density lipoproteins), 180–181
lead toxicology tests, 285
Leeuwenhoek, Anthony van, 237
Legionnaires" disease, 263t–264t
leucine crystals, 75
leukemia
   defined, 129
   WBC tests indicating, 162
leukocytes
   CBC tests identifying, 162
   measuring in urine, 67
   WBC tests identifying, 138, 138f
leukocytosis, 129, 162
leukopenia, 129, 162
Levy-Jennings charts
   analyzing excessive chatter, 46f
   analyzing results in control, 45f
   analyzing shifts, 47f
   analyzing trends, 46
   defined, 32
   overview of, 46
   Westgard's rules for monitoring QC results, 182–183
liberation stage, pharmacokinetics, 274, 283–284
lice, 264, 268t
light source, microscope, 37–38, 37f
Linné, Carl von, 238
lipid metabolism
   Cholestech test for, 174, 183–184, 190b–194b
   cholesterol, 180, 180f
   lipid panel of tests for, 181
   lipoproteins, 180–181
   overview of, 179–181
   total cholesterol/high-density lipoprotein ratio, 181
   triglycerides, 181

lipiduria, 52
lipoproteins
   defined, 172
   lipid metabolism and, 180–181
   total cholesterol/high-density lipoprotein ratio, 181
liquids, laboratory measurements of, 11
liver
   hepatic panel tests for, 200–201
   monitoring treatment for heart disease, 3
lockjaw (tetanus), 239, 263t–264t
low power focus, microscope setting, 38b–40b
low-density lipoproteins (LDLs), 180–181
LSD (lysergic acid diethylamine), detecting, 276t–278t
lumen, 86, 99
Lyme disease
   caused by spirilla, 266t
   immunology test for, 228t–229t
lymphocytes
   defined, 129
   indications of viral infection, 163, 165f
   overview of, 134, 134f
   WBC test identifying, 138
lyse (break open)
   cells in urine standing at room temperature, 60
   creating red blood cell casts, 74
   defined, 52
   formation of bilirubin, 65

M
macrophages, 129, 134
magnifying structures, microscopes, 36, 38–41
mail, transporting specimens by, 243
mailer pouch, iFOB test, 218–225
malaise, 236, 267
malaria, 268t
marijuana. see cannabinoids (marijuana)
mastectomy patients, venipuncture precautions in, 125
material safety data sheets. see MSDS (material safety data sheets)
MCH (mean cell Hgb), 162
MCV (mean cell volume), 162
MDMA (Ecstasy), detecting in urine, 276t–278t
mean
   analyzing external controls, 45–46
   defined, 32
mean cell Hgb (MCH), 162
mean cell volume (MCV), 162
mechanical controls, microscopes, 36
mechanical holder, microscopes, 36, 37f
media (singular: medium), 237
median cubital vein, 89, 89f
medical assistants, 2, 7
medical office risk management, 32, 48
medical technicians, 4
medical technologists, 4
Medicare, 184
medication treatment, monitoring effects of, 3
megakaryocyte, 129, 134
memory B cells
   in active immunity, 213, 214f
   defined, 210
   in humoral immunity, 213f
memory T cells, 210, 213
meningitis, 265t
menstrual period, urine specimen collection and, 56

INDEX

mercury poisoning, toxicology tests for, 285
metabolic panels, basic and comprehensive
   cardiac panel, 201, 201f
   electrolyte panel, 173–174
   hepatic panel, 200–201
   individual analytes and their disease associations, 201, 202t–204t
   overview of, 199–201, 200f
   renal panel, 199
   thyroid panel, 201
metabolism stage, pharmacokinetics, 275, 284–285
metabolites
   defined, 274
   of drugs of abuse, 275, 276t–278t
methadone, screening for, 276t–278t
methamphetamines, screening for, 276t–278t
methicillin-resistant Staphylococcus aureus (MRSA), 270t
metric units, in laboratory reports, 9–11
mg/dL (milligrams per deciliter)
   lab metric for analytes, 14t
   lab report metric, 9–11, 13t
   measuring glucose in urine, 64
MIC (minimum inhibitory concentration) sensitivity test, 262, 262f
microaerophilic, 237
microaerophilic organisms, 258
microalbuminuria, screening for, 66–67
microbiology
   acid-fast stains, 245, 245f
   biochemical testing, 261, 261f
   bioterrorism and. *see* bioterrorism
   classification of microorganisms, 237–238
   collecting blood culture specimen, 241, 242f
   collecting Chlamydia specimen, 241, 242f
   collecting fecal specimen (for ova and parasites), 241, 243f
   collecting Gonorrhea specimen, 241, 243f
   collecting pinworm specimen, 246–251, 246f
   collecting specimens, 240f
   collecting throat specimen, 241, 247b
   collecting urine culture specimen, 241, 242f
   culturing methods, 259–260, 260f–261f
   defined, 237
   emerging infectious diseases, 264, 270t
   equipment for, 259, 260f
   Gram stain. *see* Gram stain reaction
   growth requirements of bacteria, 257–258, 258f
   history of infection control, 237, 238t
   media for growing bacteria, 258–259
   nomenclature of microorganisms, 238
   overview of, 237–243, 240f
   parasites and protozoa, common diseases of, 268t
   parasites and protozoa seen in POLs, 264, 269f
   pathogenic bacteria, common diseases of, 263t–264t
   pathogenic bacteria seen in POLs, 262, 269f
   pathogenic fungi seen in POLs, 262–264
   potassium hydroxide preparation, 246, 251b
   review question answers, 273
   review questions, 272

microbiology (*Continued*)
   sensitivity testing, 261–262, 261f–262f
   structural characteristics of bacteria, 239, 239f
   transporting specimens, 240, 240f, 243, 243f
   urine cultures, 260–261, 273b
   websites, 273b
   wet mounts, 245–246, 246f, 251b
microbiology, CLIA-waived tests
   in ambulatory care setting, 7
   influenza, 252–257, 255b–257b
   Streptococcus Group A, 251–252, 252f, 253b–255b
   types of, 34t–35t
microcollection
   capillary tubes and, 92
   defined, 86
microcollection tubes, 92f, 93
microhematocrit procedures, general spun, 147, 148f
microorganisms
   defined, 237
   history of infection control, 238t
   overview of, 237–251
microorganisms, classification of
   bacteria, 237
   fungi, 237–238
   nomenclature of, 238
   overview of, 237–238
   parasites, 238
   viruses, 237
MicroScan identification kit, 261, 261f
microscopic procedure
   identifying foundational structures, 36
   identifying illuminating structures, 37–38
   identifying magnifying structures, 38–41
   identifying parts and functions, 36–41, 37f
   overview of, 36–41
   review question answers, 50
   review questions, 50
   working with, 38, 38b–40b
microscopic urinalysis
   artifacts in, 75, 80f
   bacteria in, 75, 79f
   calculating, 75, 81t
   casts, granular, 74, 77f
   casts, hyaline, 73–74, 77f
   casts, overview of, 73–74
   casts, red blood cell, 74, 77f
   casts, renal epithelial cell, 74, 77f
   casts, waxy, 74, 77f
   casts, white blood cell, 74, 77f
   cells, epithelial, 73, 76f
   cells, overview of, 73
   cells, red blood, 73, 76f
   cells, white blood, 73, 76f
   crystals, abnormal, 74–75, 79f
   crystals, acid urine, 74, 78f
   crystals, alkaline urine, 74, 78f
   crystals, overview of, 74–75
   mucous in, 75, 80f
   overview of, 72–75
   parasites in, 75, 80f
   procedure for preparation of, 82b–84b
   sperm in, 75
   yeast in, 75, 79f
microvascular problems, type 1 diabetes, 177
micturition (voiding or urination), 52, 54
milligrams per deciliter. *see* mg/dL (milligrams per deciliter)
minerals panel, possible disease associations, 202t–204t

minimum inhibitory concentration (MIC) sensitivity test, 262, 262f
mL or ml (milliliter), metrics for liquids, 11
mm (millimeters), metrics for test tube/capillary tube, 11
molds, growing fungi on, 237–238
monitoring tests
   in hospital laboratories, 6
   reasons for ordering, 3
   in reference laboratories, 4–6
monocytes, 129, 134
monocytes, WBCs identifying, 138
monocytic leukemia, 163
mononucleosis (kissing disease)
   overview of, 163, 165f, 217
   test procedure, 217, 221b–223b
monounsaturated fats, lowering cholesterol, 180
morbidity
   of bioterrorism agents, 264
   defined, 237
mortality
   of bioterrorism agents, 264
   defined, 237
motivation, of laboratory professional, 8
MRSA (methicillin-resistant Staphylococcus aureus), 270t
MSDS (material safety data sheets)
   chemical hazard training, 5f, 22–23
   labeling hazardous chemicals, 23–24
mucous membranes, 210–212
mucus, in microscopic urinalysis, 75, 80f
Multistix Pro10LS urinalysis strip, 66
musty odor of urine, 62
myalgia
   bubonic plague symptom, 267
   defined, 237
mycelium, 237–238
mycelium, in molds, 237–238
mycobacterial diseases, acid-fast staining for, 62
mycoplasma, diseases caused by, 266t
myeloblasts, 129, 131–132, 131f
myelocytes, 131–132, 131f, 133f
myocardial infarction (heart attack)
   hepatic panel tests for, 201
   lipid panel determining risk for, 181
   monitoring patient risk for, 3
myoglobin, 172, 201

N

Na (sodium), i-STAT testing of, 198–199
Na+ (sodium), renal panel testing of, 199
National Fire Protective Association (NFPA), labeling hazardous chemicals, 24, 25f
National Paint and Coatings Association (NPCA), 23
natural immunity, 213, 214f
natural killer cells, 210–212
needle sticks, federal laws for, 89–90
neonatal capillary puncture
   appropriate site for, 94, 94f
   avoiding bandages, 94
   depth of heel stick, 91
   filter paper and screening forms for, 96f
   lancets used for, 91, 91f
   neonatal screening blood collection, 94–95
   placing blood on screening form, 95f
   procedure for, 109b–111b
neonatal diseases, hemolytic disease of newborn, 226, 232b–233b

nephron
   defined, 52
   formation and flow of urine in. see urine formation and flow
   in urinary system, 52–54, 53f
neurological problems, from phlebotomy, 125
neutro- prefix, 129
neutrophils
   defined, 129
   indications of bacterial infection, 163
   overview of, 132
   as WBC found in urine, 73
   WBCs identifying, 138
NFPA (National Fire Protective Association), labeling hazardous chemicals, 24, 25f
NIDDM (non-insulin-dependent diabetes mellitus), type2, 177, 178t
nitrites, measuring in urine, 67
nocturia, 52
nomenclature, of microorganisms, 238
nongonococcal urethritis/vaginitis, Chlamydia causing, 266t
nongranulocytes (agranulocytes), 129, 132
non-insulin-dependent diabetes mellitus (NIDDM), type2, 177, 178t
noninvasive infrared absorption technology, glucose monitoring with, 183
nonspecific immunity
   defined, 210–211, 211f
   first line of defense, 211
   second line of defense, 211–212
normal biota, 237
normal flora, 210–212, 237
normoblasts, red cell production, 132f
normocytes, 129–131
nosepiece, microscope, 37f, 38
nosocomial infections
   chain of infection causing, 15
   defined, 2
   hand hygiene preventing, 16
   history of, 238t
NPCA (National Paint and Coatings Association), 23
nucleus, 129, 131–132
nutrients
   bacterial growth and, 258
   bacterial growth requirements, 258
   blood plasma, 172

O
O (universal donor) blood type, 225–226, 226t
obese patients, venipuncture precautions in, 125
objective lens settings, microscopes, 37f, 38, 38b–40b
occult. see also fecal occult blood testing
occupational exposure, 2, 18
Occupational Safety and Health Administration. see OSHA (Occupational Safety and Health Administration)
ocular lenses, microscopes, 37f, 38
odor of urine, urinalysis, 62
OGTT (oral glucose tolerance test), 2-hour PP blood sugar test, 178
oil immersion
   objective, 38
   setting up microscope for, 38b–40b
oliguria, 52, 55
opiates
   CLIA-waived tests screening for, 281
   defined, 274
   drug urine screening tests for, 276t–278t
   time intervals for detecting drugs in urine, 278t

OPIM (other potentially infections material)
   laboratory housekeeping guidelines, 21
   OSHA biohazard training in, 18–22
opportunistic infections, 2, 19
optical tests
   principle of photometers and spectrophotometers, 181–183, 182f
   quality assurance when using, 182
   Westgard's rules for monitoring QC results, 182–183
optics check, 32, 45
ORA Quick test, for HIV, 218
oral glucose tolerance test (OGTT), 2-hour PP blood sugar test, 178
order of draw
   for capillary puncture, 93, 93t
   for venipuncture, 102–104
organizational skills, of laboratory professional, 8
OSHA (Occupational Safety and Health Administration)
   biohazard training in BBPS. see BBPS (Bloodborne Pathogens Standard)
   Blood Borne Pathogen Quiz, 26
   compliance after exposure to blood, 22
   needle stick safety, 89
   regulations for disease prevention, 15
   work practice controls, 19
OSOM influenza A & B Test, 253–257, 255b–257b
osteomyelitis, 87, 93–94
OTC (over-the-counter) drugs of abuse, 275–281
other potentially infections material (OPIM)
   laboratory housekeeping guidelines, 21
   OSHA biohazard training in, 18–22
ova collection kits, 241
ovarian cancer (CA 125) antigen test, 228t–229t
OXY (oxycodone), screening for, 276t–278t
oxygen
   hemoglobin's affinity for, 131
   requirements for bacterial growth, 257–258

P
palpating, 87
panels
   defined, 2, 172
   laboratory requisitions listing, 9
   on reference laboratory blood chemistry requisition, 174, 175f
panic value, as test result, 4
parasites
   collection kit for, 241
   common diseases of, 268t
   commonly seen in POLs, 264, 269f
   lines of defense against harmful. see immune process
   microscopic urinalysis detecting, 75, 80f
   overview of, 238
   wet mounts detecting, 62–64, 76f
parenteral contact
   Bloodborne Pathogens Standard for, 18
   defined, 2
passive immunity
   defined, 210
   overview of, 215
passive immunity, acquiring, 213–215, 214f

pathogens
   analyzing specimens for presence of, 4, 6f
   cross-contamination of, 17
   defined, 2
   fewer than 1% of microorganisms as, 237
   OSHA biohazard training in BBPS, 18–22
pathologists, reference laboratory, 4
patient compliance, 2
patient identification
   blood collection, 90
   laboratory requisitions, 9
patient positioning, blood collection, 90
PCA (Portable Clinical Analyzer), I-STAT, 6
PCP (phencyclidine), detecting, 276t–278t
penicillin, discovery of, 238t
PEP (postexposure prophylaxis), 2, 22
peptic ulcers, caused by H. pylori, 217
peptidoglycan, 237, 244
percutaneous injury, 2, 21–22
permanent immunity, 214f
pernicious anemia, CBC tests indicating, 162
personal protective equipment. see PPE (personal protective equipment)
personnel, types of laboratory, 8t
petechiae, 87
Petri dish, 237
pH
   defined, 52
   i-STAT testing of, 198, 198t
   measuring in urine, 64, 65f
phagocytes, 210–211
phagocytosis, 210–211
pharmacokinetics, 274, 283–285
phencyclidine (PCP), detecting, 276t–278t
phenylketonuria (PKU), neonatal screening for, 94–95
PHI (protected health information), 32, 48
-phil suffix, 129, 132
phlebotomy, 87
photometers
   monitoring QC results, 182–183
   principle of, 181–183, 182f
   QA for optical instruments, 182
physical hazards
   defined, 2
   in medical laboratories, 15
   safety training in laboratory, 24–25
physical routine urinalysis
   appearance, 62, 62f
   becoming proficient at, 52, 67f
   color, 61–62, 61f
   odor, 62
   overview of, 61–62
physician identification, on requisitions, 9
Piccolo Xpress Chemistry Analyzer, 199
pinworms
   overview of, 268t
   parasites commonly seen in POL, 264
   specimen collection and microscopic results, 246–251, 246f
PKU (phenylketonuria), neonatal screening for, 94–95
plagues, caused by bacilli, 263t–264t
plasma
   activated in humoral immunity, 213f
   in blood, 172–173, 173f
   defined, 87, 210
   formed elements suspended in, 130
   vacuum collection tubes indicating, 95–96
plastic supplies, preventing exposure incidents with, 19

INDEX

platelets (thrombocytes)
  in complete blood count, 162
  defined, 129
  identification and description, 130f, 139
  overview of, 134–135, 134f–135f
  QBC STAR providing information on, 166
PMN (polymorphonuclear), 129, 131–132
Pneumocystis pneumonia, 267t
pneumonia
  cocci causing, 265t
  fungi causing Pneumocystis, 267t
  most commonly seen in POL, 262
  mycoplasma causing walking, 266t
POCT (point-of-care testing) collection devices
  in ambulatory care settings, 6
  capillary puncture devices, 91–92, 92f
  in hospitals, 6, 7f
  i-STAT. *see* i-STAT blood analyzer
poikilocytosis, 129, 139
POL (physician's office laboratory)
  benefits of medical testing methods in, 2
  specimens for CLIA-waived chemistry tests, 174
POL (physician's office laboratory), pathogenic organisms seen in
  diseases caused by bacilli, 263t–264t
  diseases caused by cocci, 265t
  diseases caused by fungi, 267t
  diseases caused by parasites and protozoa, 268t
  diseases caused by rickettsia, chlamydia and mycoplasma, 266t
  diseases caused by spirilla, 266t
  overview of, 262–264
  parasites and protozoa, 264, 269f
  pathogenic bacteria, 262, 269f
  pathogenic fungi, 262–264
  tularemia, 268
polychromia, 129, 139
polycythemia, 129, 159–162
polydipsia, 2, 4
polymorphonuclear (PMN), 129, 131–132
polyphagia, 2, 4
polyunsaturated fats, lowering cholesterol, 180
polyuria
  defined, 2, 52
  in diabetes mellitus diagnosis, 4
porphyrin, 52, 62
Portable Clinical Analyzer (PCA), I-STAT, 6
portal of entry, 2
portal of exit, 2
postexposure prophylaxis (PEP), 2, 22
potassium (K), i-STAT testing of, 198–199
potassium (K+), testing, 199
potassium hydroxide (KOH) preparation, 246, 251b
PPE (personal protective equipment)
  proper use of, 26, 27b–30b
  safety training in laboratory, 18
  as Standard Precaution, 15–16
PPMP (PPM Procedures) Certificate, 35–36, 36t
precision (reproducibility)
  analyzing control results, 47, 47f
  defined, 32
prediabetes. *see also* glucose screening/monitoring tests
preeclampsia, 66
pregnancy, gestational diabetes occurring in, 178

pregnancy testing
  HCG hormone test, 228t–229t
  overview of, 216–217, 216f, 219b–220b
  in vitro, 215, 216f
preservatives, in routine urinalysis, 60
preventive measures, minimizing exposure, 19–21
problem-solving, of laboratory professional, 8
procedure preparation, blood collection, 90, 90f
procedure sheets, reagent strip quality control, 64
professionals, laboratory
  attributes of, 8–9
  extensive training of, 5
  laboratory testing personnel, 7, 8t
  physician's office, 7
  preventing spread of disease, 15
profiles. *see* panels
prokaryotic
  bacteria classified as, 237
  defined, 237
Proper Use of Personal Protective Equipment, 26
protected health information (PHI), 32, 48
proteins
  Bence Jones, 67
  in blood plasma, 172–173
  defined, 66t
  measuring in urine, 66–67
  venous vs. capillary blood, 87
proteinuria, 52, 66
prothrombin
  in blood plasma, 173
  defined, 129
  theory of hemostasis, 139
prothrombin time. *see* PT (prothrombin time)
protime test, 129, 139
protozoa
  common diseases of, 268t
  overview of, 238
  seen in POLs, 264, 269f
provider-performed microscopy, complexity testing, 35–36, 36t
PT (prothrombin time)
  becoming proficient at, 149–159, 157b–159b
  monitoring patient with thrombosis, 139
  overview of, 144f, 149
pulmonary anthrax, 267
pyloric ulcers, caused by spirilla, 266t
pyuria, 52, 73

Q

QA (quality assurance)
  chemical urinalysis and, 62–64
  defined, 32
  monitoring testing procedures for, 35
  for optical instruments, 182
  overview of, 41–44, 43t
  for QBC STAR, 167
QBC STAR Centrifugal Hematology System, 166–167, 166f
QC (quality control)
  for accurate test results. *see* Piccolo Express Chemistry Analyzer
  defined, 32
  electronic medical records and bar coding, 48–49, 49f
  external controls, 45–48, 45f–47f
  good laboratory practices, 41, 42f
  HIPAA Privacy Rule, 48
  implementing for each test, 44–48

QC (quality control) *(Continued)*
  monitoring testing procedures for, 35
  optics check, 45
  qualitative waived tests, 44, 44f
  quality assurance in. *see* QA (quality assurance)
  quantitative waived tests, 45–48
  reagent strips and, 63–64, 63f, 68b–71b
  review question answers, 50
  review questions, 50
  risk management and, 48
  semiquantitative waived tests and, 44–45
quadrant (isolation) technique, inoculation of media, 259–260, 260f
qualitative drug screening, 274–275
qualitative waived tests
  defined, 32, 62
  fecal occult blood test as, 181
  monitoring QC in, 44, 44f
  semiquantitative tests vs., 44–45
quality assurance. *see* QA (quality assurance)
quality control. *see* QC (quality control)
quantitative drug screening, 274–275
quantitative waived tests
  defined, 33, 62
  monitoring QC in, 45–48
  most CLIA-waved blood chemistry tests as, 181
quarantine practices, history of, 238t
QuickVue iFOB test, 218–225, 218f
QuickVue+ Helicobacter pylori gII Test procedure, 218, 224b–225b
QuickVue+ Mononucleosis Test Procedure, 217, 221b–223b

R

random glucose test, 178
random urine specimen, 56
rapid strep testing, 252, 253b–255b
RBC (red blood cell) casts, microscopic urinalysis, 74, 77f
RBC indices, 129, 159–162
RBCs (red blood cells)
  in complete blood count, 159, 163t
  identification and description, 139, 139f, 142f, 144f
  indicating anemia in CBC test results, 162
  measuring bilirubin in urine, 65
  in microscopic urinalysis, 73, 76f
  overview of, 130–131, 132f
reabsorption, formation of urine and, 54
reagent strips
  defined, 62
  quality control and, 63–64, 63f, 68b–71b
  as time dependent, 62
  in urinalysis chemistry strips, 62, 63f
reagents
  defined, 2, 33
  monitoring QC in qualitative tests with, 44
red blood cells. *see* RBCs (red blood cells)
red bone marrow. *see* bone marrow
reducing substances, 52, 65
reference (or referral) laboratories
  certification regulations for, 33–35
  comprehensive reports for blood tests, 4, 5f
  organizational chart for, 4, 7f
  overview of, 4–6
  specimens for blood chemistry tests, 173–174, 174f–175f
  trained professionals staffing, 4, 4–5

reference range
	analyzing specimens by measuring, 3–4, 6f
	for complete blood count, 159, 163t
	defined, 2
	monitoring patients with diabetes, 3
	when test result is far from, 4
referral laboratories. see reference (or referral) laboratories
reflectance photometry, 172, 182
refrigeration
	quality assurance for optical tests and, 182
	for routine urinalysis, 60
	temperature for laboratory tests, 11, 14f
regulations. see CLIA government regulations
reliability
	analyzing control results, 47, 47f
	defined, 33
renal corpuscle, 52, 53f, 54
renal epithelial cell casts, 74, 77f
renal panel, 199, 202t–204t
renal threshold level, 52, 54
renal tubular epithelial (RTE) cells, 73, 76f
renal tubules, 52, 54
reports. see laboratory reports
requisitions
	blood collection, 90
	CBC, 159, 160f
	defined, 2
	example forms, 10f–11f
	laboratory process stage, 9, 13f
	overview of, 9, 10f
	reference laboratory blood chemistry, 174, 175f
	sending with specimen to reference lab, 5–6
	urinalysis, 60, 61f
reservoir host, 2
respiratory syncytial virus (RSV) test, 228t–229t
reticulocytes
	defined, 129
	red cell production and, 130–131, 132f
retractable nonreusable lancets, capillary puncture, 91, 91f
retroperitoneal space, 52
Rh blood types
	antibody titer tests and, 227
	antigenic responses of, 225–226
	hemolytic disease of newborn and, 226, 232b–233b
	overview of, 226
	procedure for testing, 232b–233b
rheumatoid factor (arthritis) test, 228t–229t
rheumatoid fever, 251–252
RhoGAM (Rh gamma globulin), hemolytic disease of newborn, 226
rickettsia, diseases caused by, 266t
ringworm, fungi causing, 267t
risk management
	blood collection and, 126
	overview of, 48
RNA (ribonucleic acid), in viruses, 237
Rocky Mountain spotted fever, 266t
rouleaux formation, 129, 148
RSV (respiratory syncytial virus) test, 228t–229t
RTEs (renal tubular epithelial) cells, 73, 76f
Rubella (German measles) test, 228t–229t

S

S. pyogenes (strep throat)
	commonly seen in POL, 262
	Streptococcus Group A tests, 251–252

safety training in laboratory
	CDC standard precautions for infection control, 15–18
	centrifuge, 104f, 105–123
	chemical hazard training, 22–24
	hand hygiene, 15–18
	hazards, 14–26
	laboratory safety evaluation, 26
	OSHA biohazard training in BBPS. see BBPS (Bloodborne Pathogens Standard)
	personal protective equipment, 18
	physical hazard training, 24–25
	review question answers, 31
	review questions, 30
	transmission and chain of infection, 15, 15f
	websites, 31b
safety transfer device, syringes, 116b–118b
salts, in blood plasma, 172
SARS (severe acute respiratory syndrome), 270t
scabies, 268t
scarlet fever, 251–252
screening tests
	detecting presence of common pathogens, 4, 6f
	reasons for ordering, 3
SD (standard deviation), 33, 45–46, 45f
sealants, capillary tube, 92
second line of defense, immune process, 211–212
secretion, formation of urine and, 54
sediment, microscopic urinalysis and, 52, 72
selective media, growing bacteria, 258
self-antigens, 210
semiquantitative tests, 33, 62
sensitivity testing, 261–262, 261f–262f
serology department, 210
serology tests
	defined, 210
	performing in vitro, 215
	waived status of, 34t–35t
serum
	defined, 87, 173
	reference laboratory blood chemistry testing, 173–174, 174f
	vacuum collection tubes obtaining, 95–97
serum separator tube (SST), blood chemistry testing, 173–174, 174f
severe acute respiratory syndrome (SARS), 270t
sexually transmitted diseases
	collecting Chlamydia specimens, 241
	collecting Gonorrhea specimens, 241
	detecting Trichomonas vaginalis, 62–64, 76f
	HIV. see HIV (human immunodeficiency virus)
sharps container
	for butterfly method, 118b–123b
	for syringes, 116b–118b
	for Vacutainer needle, 112b–115b
sharps injury log, after exposure to blood, 22
shifts, analyzing, 46–47, 47f
shingles test, 228t–229t
sickle cell disease, CBC test results indicating, 162
site preparation
	capillary puncture, 94
	venipuncture, 99–100
site selection, capillary puncture, 93–94, 94f

skin puncture. see capillary puncture
slides
	microscope procedures, 38b–40b
	urine microscopic, 72–73
smallpox, in bioterrorism, 268–271
smears
	Gram stain, 244–245, 245f, 248b–250b
	preparing blood, 135–139, 136f–138f, 145b–146b, 246
	WBC identification and differential, 136–139, 138f
sodium (Na), i-STAT testing of, 198–199
sodium (Na+), renal panel testing of, 199
Spanish flu, 252
specific gravity, 52, 64–67
specific immunity, 210–211, 211f, 213–215, 214f
specimen analysis
	general methods of, 3–4
	in hospital laboratories, 6
	in reference laboratories, 4–6
	requisition procedures, 9
	stages in laboratory process, 9, 13f
specimens
	CLIA-waived chemistry tests, 174
	preparing blood for laboratory pickup, 104–123, 104f
	reference laboratory blood chemistry tests, 173–174
	requisition procedures, 9
spectrophotometers
	principle of, 181–183, 182f
	QA for optical instruments, 182
	Westgard's rules for monitoring QC results, 182–183
sperm, in microscopic urinalysis, 75
spirillum (spirilla)
	characteristics of, 239
	diseases caused by, 266t
spores, bacterial structure of, 239
sporotrichosis, fungi causing, 267t
squamous epithelial cells, in microscopic urinalysis, 73, 76f
SST (serum separator tube), blood chemistry testing, 173–174, 174f
stage, microscope, 36, 37f
stains
	acid-fast, 62
	Gram. see Gram stain reaction
standard deviation. see SD (standard deviation)
Standard Precautions for infection control, CDC, 2, 15–18, 16f, 238t
Staphylococci, cocci bacterial structure of, 239
Staphylococcus infections, 238t
sterile disposable loop, inoculation, 260f
steroid therapy, causing transient diabetes, 178
strep throat. see also Streptococcus Group A tests
	caused by cocci, 265t
	most commonly seen in POL, 262
Streptococci, cocci bacterial structure of, 239
Streptococcus Group A tests
	bacitracin method, 252
	overview of, 251–252, 252f
	procedure for, 253b–255b
	rapid strep testing, 252, 253b–255b
	screening tests, 4, 6f
sulfonamide crystals, 75, 79f
supernatant, in microscopic urinalysis, 52, 72
suppressor T cells (TS), in cell-mediated immunity, 210, 213

INDEX

SureStep Pregnancy Test, 217
susceptible host, 2
sweet odor of urine, 62
swine flu, 252, 270t
syncope, and phlebotomy, 87, 124
synovial fluid, 172
syphilis
　caused by spirilla, 266t
　immunology test for, 228t–229t
syringe method, venipuncture
　equipment for, 101f, 103f
　I-STAT using, 174
　order of draw for, 102–104
　overview of, 100
　procedure for, 116b–118b

T

T cells
　cell-mediated immunity activating, 212–213, 212f
　helper. see helper T cells (TH4 or CD4)
　as third line of defense, 212–215
T lymphocytes, 134, 134f
T_3 (triiodothyronine) uptake, thyroid panel testing, 201
T_4 (thyroxine), thyroid panel testing, 201
tapeworms, 268t
TC/HDL (total cholesterol/high-density lipoprotein) ratio, 181
TDM (therapeutic drug monitoring)
　drug half-life and specimen collection, 285
　overview of, 283–285
　therapeutic ranges/toxic levels in, 283t
temperature for laboratory tests
　quality assurance for optical tests, 182
　routine urinalysis, 60
　sensitivity of specimens, 11, 14f
　warming site for capillary punctures, 94
temporary immunity, 214f
test kits, detecting pathogens, 4
test tubes, metrics for length of, 11
tests, laboratory
　general ways to analyze specimens, 3–4
　in hospital laboratories, 6
　in reference laboratories, 4–6
　reports giving results of, 9
　requisitions listing, 9
　why they are ordered, 3
tetanus (lockjaw), 239, 263t–264t
tetrads, cocci bacterial structure, 239
TH4 (helper T cells)
　in cell-mediated immunity, 212
　defined, 209
　HIV destroying, 218
thalassemia, CBC test results indicating, 162
therapeutic drug monitoring. see TDM (therapeutic drug monitoring)
third line of defense, immune process, 212–215
throat specimen, collecting, 241, 247b
thrombocytes. see platelets (thrombocytes)
thromboplastin, 91
thrombosis (internal clots)
　defined, 129
　drugs for, 139
　monitoring patient treatment for, 3
thrombus
　defined, 129
　theory of hemostasis, 139
thrush, fungi causing, 267t
thyroid panel
　overview of, 201
　possible disease associations, 202t–204t

thyroid-stimulating hormone (TSH), thyroid panel testing, 201
thyroxine (T_4), thyroid panel testing, 201
timed urine specimen
　24-hour urine specimen, 56–60, 57f, 60b
　overview of, 56–60
tissue fluid, defined, 91
titers, 210, 227
total cholesterol/high-density lipoprotein (TC/HDL) ratio, 181
tourniquet, Vacutainer collection and, 99–100, 103f
toxic shock, caused by cocci, 265t
toxicity, 274
toxicology
　blood collection for alcohol testing, 279b
　CLIA-waived drug screening tests, 281–283
　drug half-life and specimen collection, 285, 285f
　drugs of abuse, 275–281, 276t–278t
　ethanol content in alcoholic beverages, 278t
　overview of, 275
　pharmacokinetics, 283–285
　review questions, 286
　review questions answers, 286
　summary, 285
　therapeutic drug monitoring, 283, 284t
　typical time intervals for detecting drugs in urine, 278t
　urine collection for drug screening, 279b
　urine drug panel testing procedure, 282b–283b
　websites, 287b
toxoplasmosis, 268t
training, of laboratory professionals, 5
trans fats, 172, 180
transient microorganisms
　cross-contamination of, 17
　defined, 2
transitional epithelial cells, 73, 76f
transmission, chain of infection and, 2, 15, 15f
transmittance photometry, 172, 182
transporting microbiological specimens
　by mail, 243, 243f
　overview of, 239–243, 240f
trends, analyzing, 46
Trichinosis, 268t
Trichomonas vaginalis
　parasites commonly seen in POL, 264
　wet mounts detecting, 62–64, 76f
tricyclic antidepressants, detecting, 276t–278t
triglycerides
　lipid panel testing, 180–181
　overview of, 181
triiodothyronine (T_3) uptake, thyroid panel testing, 201
triple phosphate crystals, 74, 78f
Troponin I and T
　defined, 172
　hepatic panel testing, 201
TSH (thyroid-stimulating hormone), thyroid panel testing, 201
tuberculosis
　acid-fast staining for, 62
　history of infection control, 238t
tuberculosis, caused by bacilli, 263t–264t
tularemia, 268
turbid appearance of urine, 62, 62f

24-hour urine specimen
　container, 57f
　overview of, 57–60
　procedure for, 60b
　as timed urine specimen, 56–57
2 hr PP (2-hour postprandial) blood sugar test, 178
Typhus, 266t
tyrosine crystals, 75

U

universal donor (O) blood type, 225–226, 226t
Universal Precautions, 2, 18, 238t
ureters, 52, 54
urethra, 52, 54
urethral meatus, 52, 54
uric acid, 199
uric acid crystals, 74, 78f
urinalysis
　microscopic. see microscopic urinalysis
　review question answers, 85
　review questions, 84–85
　urinary system function, 52
　urinary system structures. see urinary system structures
　urine formation and flow. see urine formation and flow
　urine specimen collection. see urine specimen collection
　websites, 85b
urinalysis, CLIA-waived tests
　in ambulatory care setting, 6
　becoming proficient at, 67–72
　chemical urinalysis, 62–64, 63f
　chemical urinalysis- automated click method, 64, 64f
　chemical urinalysis- reagent strip quality control, 63–64, 63f, 68b–69b
　chemical urinalysis-quality assurance, 62–64
　overview of, 60–72, 61f
　physical routine urinalysis, 61–62, 61f–62f
　urine test strips, 64–67, 65f, 66t
　waived status of, 34t–35t
urinary bladder, 52, 54
urinary system structures
　defined, 52–54, 52f
　kidneys, 52–54, 53f
　ureters, 54
　urethra, 54
　urinary bladder, 54
urinary tract infection. see UTI (urinary tract infection)
urinary tract infections, 262, 263t–264t
urination, 52, 54
urine culture
　collecting specimen, 241, 242f
　culturing method for, 260–261, 273b
urine drug screening tests
　CLIA-waived, 281
　common drugs of abuse detected on multiple, 276t–278t
　detecting drugs of abuse in pregnant mothers, 285
　drug half-life and, 285
　overview of, 275
　procedure for, 282b–283b
　ruling out impaired employees with, 285
　time intervals for detecting drugs in, 278t
　urine collection for, 279b

urine formation and flow
  composition of urine, 54–55
  filtration, 54
  flow of blood and urine through kidney, 54
  overview of, 54
  reabsorption, 54
  secretion, 54
urine specimen collection
  24-hour procedure, 57–60, 57f, 60b
  clean-catch midstream, 56, 56f, 57b–59b
  first morning, 56
  overview of, 55–60, 55f
  random, 56
  timed, 56–60
urine test strips
  becoming proficient at urinalysis, 52
  Bence Jones protein, 67
  for bilirubin, 65–66
  for blood, 66
  for glucose, 65
  for ketones, 65
  for leukocytes, 67
  measuring specific gravity, 64–67
  for nitrites, 67
  overview of, 64–67
  for pH, 64, 65f
  for proteins, 66, 66t
  for urobilinogen, 66
urobilinogen, 65–66
UTI (urinary tract infection)
  clean-catch midstream urine specimen for, 56, 56f, 57b–59b
  foul odor of urine indicating, 62
  presence of WBCs in urine indicating, 67

V

vaccination
  defined, 210
  development of, 210
Vacutainer collection system
  of blood culture specimen, 241
  order of draw for, 102–104
  overview of, 98
  preparing blood smear from, 135–136, 136f
  procedure for, 112b–115b
  tourniquet for, 99–100, 103f
  Vacutainer holder for, 98–99, 99f, 101f, 103f
  Vacutainer needle for, 98–99, 99f–100f, 103f
vacuum collection tubes, venipuncture
  additives/color-coded hemoguard tubes, 97–98, 98t
  CLIA-waived tests from physician's office laboratory using, 174
  overview of, 95–97, 97f
  table for, 105t
  using Vacutainer tubes. see Vacutainer collection system

varicella zoster (chickenpox and shingles) test, 228t–229t
vascular site, capillary punctures, 93–94
vein finder, 123–124, 125f
veins
  in closed circuit system, 88f
  composition of, 87
  defined, 87
  layers within, 89f
  most commonly used, 89, 89f
  overview of, 87
venipuncture
  additives/color-coded hemoguard tubes for, 97–98, 98t
  becoming proficient at, 87
  butterfly method, 100–104, 102f–103f, 118b–123b
  CLIA-waived tests from physician's office laboratory using, 174
  defined, 2
  order of draw for, 102–104
  OSHA biohazard training in, 18
  overview of, 95–104
  syringe method, 100, 101f, 102–104, 103f, 116b–118b
  Vacutainer method. see Vacutainer collection system
  vacuum collection tube method, 95–97, 97f, 105t
very-low-density lipoproteins (VLDLs), 180–181
viral hemorrhagic fever, in bioterrorism, 271
viral infections
  immunology test for, 228t–229t
  indications of, 163
  QBC STAR giving WBC information on, 166
viruses
  in bioterrorism, 268–271
  lines of defense against. see immune process
  mutation of influenza, 252
  overview of, 237
vision, laboratory professional attributes, 9
vitamin B12, pernicious anemia and, 162
vitamin D, cholesterol helping absorption of, 180
vitamin K
  defined, 129
  PT test for patients deficient in, 149
VLDLs (very-low-density lipoproteins), 180–181
voiding, 52, 54

W

walking (atypical) pneumonia, 266t
waste products, blood plasma, 172
waste receptacles, laboratory housekeeping, 21, 22f–23f
waxy casts, in microscopic urinalysis, 74, 77f

WBC (white blood cell) casts, in microscopic urinalysis, 74, 77f
WBCs (white blood cells)
  in complete blood count, 138f, 162
  Diff staining procedure for, 145b–146b
  disorders, 163, 165f
  granulocytes, 131–134, 131f, 133f
  identification and differential, 136–139, 138f, 141t
  in microscopic urinalysis, 73, 76f
  nongranulocytes, 132, 134f
  overview, 131–134
  QBC STAR providing information on, 166
  screening leukocytes in urine, 67
websites
  blood collection, 127b
  chemistry, 208b
  CLIA government regulations, 50b
  CLIA-waived tests, 50b
  clinical laboratory introduction, 31b
  hematology, 170b
  immunology, 235b
  microbiology, 273b
  safety training in laboratory, 31b
  toxicology, 287b
  urinalysis, 85b
Western immunoblot method, for HIV, 218
Westgard's rules, monitoring QC results with, 182–183
wet mounts, 245–246, 246f, 251b
wheal, allergy testing, 210, 215, 215f
white blood cells. see WBCs (white blood cells)
whole blood specimen, CLIA-waived tests using, 174
whole numbers, for laboratory measurements, 11
whooping cough, caused by bacilli, 263t–264t
work practice controls, 19, 33
wound infections, 262, 265t

Y

yeast
  fungi causing, 267t
  growing fungi on, 237–238
  infections most commonly seen in POL, 262–264
  in microscopic urinalysis, 75, 79f
Yersinia pestis (plague), 267–268